Oxorn-Foote

HUMAN LABOR & BIRTH

Sixth Edition

Oxorn-Foote

HUMAN LABOR & BIRTH

Sixth Edition

GLENN D. POSNER, MDCM, MEd, FRCSC
Associate Professor, The University of Ottawa
Department of Obstetrics and Gynecology
The Ottawa Hospital
Ottawa, Ontario, Canada

JESSICA DY, MD, MPH, FRCSC
Assistant Professor, The University of Ottawa
Department of Obstetrics and Gynecology
The Ottawa Hospital
Ottawa, Ontario, Canada

AMANDA BLACK, MD, MPH, FRCSC
Associate Professor, The University of Ottawa
Department of Obstetrics and Gynecology
The Ottawa Hospital
Division of Pediatric Gynecology, Children's Hospital of Eastern Ontario
Ottawa, Ontario, Canada

GRIFFITH D. JONES, MBBS, MRCOG, FRCSC
Assistant Professor, The University of Ottawa
Medical Director, Obstetrics & Gynecology Ultrasound
Division of Maternal–Fetal Medicine
Department of Obstetrics and Gynecology
The Ottawa Hospital
Ottawa, Ontario, Canada

McGraw Hill Education (India) Private Limited
NEW DELHI

McGraw Hill Education Offices
New Delhi New York   St Louis   San Francisco   Auckland   Bogotá   Caracas
Kuala Lumpur   Lisbon   London   Madrid   Mexico City   Milan   Montreal
San Juan   Santiago   Singapore   Sydney   Tokyo   Toronto

McGraw Hill Education (India) Private Limited

Human Labor & Birth, Sixth Edition

Copyright © 2013 by The McGraw Hill Companies, Inc. All rights reserved. No part of this publication may be reproduced or distributed in any form or by any means, or stored in a database or retrieval system, without the prior written permission of the publisher.

International Edition ISBN 978-0-07-180124-9; MHID 0-07-180124-3
Copyright © 2013 Exclusive rights by The McGraw Hill Companies, Inc., for manufacture and export. This book cannot be re-exported from the country to which it is consigned by McGraw Hill. The International Edition is not available in North America.

McGraw Hill Education (India) Edition 2013

RQALCRYOLLRRR

Reprinted in India by arrangement with The McGraw-Hill Companies, Inc., New York

Sales territories: India, Pakistan, Nepal, Bangladesh, Sri Lanka and Bhutan

Library of Congress Cataloging-in-Publication Data

Oxorn-Foote human labor & birth.—6th ed. / [edited by] Glenn D. Posner...[et al.]
    p. ; cm
Oxorn-Foote human labor and birth
Human labor & birth
Includes bibliographical references and index.
ISBN 978-0-07-174028-9 (pbk. : alk. paper)—ISBN 0-07-174028-7 (pbk. : alk. paper)
1.   Posner, Glenn D. II. Foote, William R. (William Rodgers), 1908- III. Oxorn, Harry, 1920- IV. Title : Oxorn-Foote human labor and birth. V. Title: Human labor & birth.
[DNLM: 1. Labor, Obstetric. 2. Delivery, Obstetric. 3. Parturition. WQ 300]
                                                                    2012018751

ISBN-13: 978-93-5134-287-8
ISBN-10: 93-5134-287-5

Published by McGraw Hill Education (India) Private Limited,
P-24, Green Park Extension, New Delhi 110 016, and printed at
Gopsons Papers Limited, A-2 & 3, Sector 64, NOIDA 201301

To Dr. Harry Oxorn. We hope you'd be proud.

DEDICATION

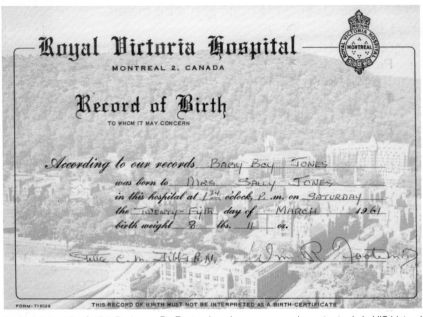

Birth record of Dr. Griffith D. Jones. Dr. Foote played an even more important role in HIS history!

Contributors   xi
Preface   xv
Acknowledgments   xvii

Part I: Clinical Anatomy   1

1   Pelvis: Bones, Joints, and Ligaments   3

2   The Pelvic Floor   9

3   Perineum   15

4   Uterus and Vagina   21

5   Obstetric Pelvis   37

6   The Passenger: Fetus   53

7   Fetopelvic Relationships   65

8   Engagement, Synclitism, Asynclitism   77

Part II: First Stage of Labor   87

9   Examination of the Patient   89

10   Normal Mechanisms of Labor   101

11   Clinical Course of Normal Labor   119

12   Fetal Health Surveillance in Labor   143

13   Induction of Labor   173

14   Labor Dystocia   193

15   Abnormal Cephalic Presentations   211

Part III: Second Stage of Labor   263

16 The Second Stage of Labor   265

17 Operative Vaginal Delivery   283

18 Shoulder Dystocia   333

Part IV: Third Stage of Labor   351

19 Delivery of the Placenta, Retained
Placenta, and Placenta Accreta   353

20 Postpartum Hemorrhage   367

21 Episiotomy, Lacerations, Uterine Rupture, and
Inversion   389

Part V: Complicated Labor   431

22 Cesarean Section   433

23 Trial of Labor After Previous
Cesarean Section   457

24 Obesity in Pregnancy   463

25 Breech Presentation   471

26 Transverse Lie   515

27 Compound Presentations   523

28 The Umbilical Cord   529

29 Multiple Pregnancy   537

Part VI: Other Issues   567

30 Preterm Labor   569

31 Antepartum Hemorrhage   587

32 Maternal Complications in Labor   601

33 Labor in the Presence of Fetal Complications   635

34 Intrapartum Infections   647

35 Postterm Pregnancy   663

36 Obstetric Anesthesia and Analgesia   671

37 Intrapartum Imaging   695

38 The Puerperium   707

39 The Newborn Infant   725

Index   747

Numbers in brackets refer to the chapter(s) written or co-written by the contributor.

Yaa Amankwah, MBCHB, FRCSC
Assistant Professor, The University of Ottawa
Department of Obstetrics and Gynecology
The Ottawa Hospital
Ottawa, Ontario, Canada [18]

Nadya Ben Fadel, MD, FAAP, FRCPC
Assistant Professor, The University of Ottawa
Division of Neonatology
Department of Pediatrics
Children's Hospital of Eastern Ontario
Ottawa, Ontario, Canada [39]

Dan Boucher, MD, MSc
Clinical Fellow, The University of Ottawa
Department of Medicine
The Ottawa Hospital
Ottawa, Ontario, Canada [32]

Yvonne Cargill, MD, FRCSC
Assistant Professor, The University of Ottawa
Division of Maternal–Fetal Medicine
Department of Obstetrics and Gynecology
The Ottawa Hospital
Ottawa, Ontario, Canada [28]

Darine El-Chaar, MD, FRCSC
Clinical Fellow, The University of Toronto
Division of Maternal–Fetal Medicine
Department of Obstetrics and Gynecology
The Toronto University Health Network
Toronto, Ontario, Canada [12, 15, 22, 23, 24, 25]

Ramadan El Sugy, MD, FRCSC
Department of Obstetrics and Gynecology
William Osler Health System
Brampton, Ontario, Canada [21]

Karen Fung Kee Fung, MD, FRCSC, MHPE
Associate Professor, The University of Ottawa
Division of Maternal–Fetal Medicine
Department of Obstetrics and Gynecology
The Ottawa Hospital
Ottawa, Ontario, Canada [29]

Laura M. Gaudet, MD, MSc, FRCSC
Assistant Professor, Dalhousie University
Division of Maternal–Fetal Medicine
Department of Obstetrics & Gynecology
The Moncton Hospital, Horizon Health Network
Moncton, New Brunswick, Canada [33, 35]

Catherine Gallant, MD, FRCPC
Assistant Professor, The University of Ottawa
Department of Anesthesiology
The Ottawa Hospital
Ottawa, Ontario, Canada [36]

Andrée Gruslin, MD, FRCSC
Professor, The University of Ottawa
Division of Maternal–Fetal Medicine
Departments of Obstetrics and Gynecology & Cellular and Molecular Medicine
The Ottawa Hospital
Ottawa, Ontario, Canada [34]

Samantha Halman, MD
Clinical Fellow, The University of Ottawa
Department of Medicine
The Ottawa Hospital
Ottawa, Ontario, Canada [32]

Alan Karovitch, MD, MEd, FRCPC
Associate Professor, The University of Ottawa
Division of General Internal Medicine
Departments of Medicine & Obstetrics and Gynecology
The Ottawa Hospital
Ottawa, Ontario, Canada [32]

Erin Keely, MD, FRCPC
Professor, The University of Ottawa
Division of Endocrinology and Metabolism
Departments of Medicine & Obstetrics and Gynecology
The Ottawa Hospital
Ottawa, Ontario, Canada [32]

Felipe Moretti, MD
Assistant Professor, The University of Ottawa
Division of Maternal–Fetal Medicine
Department of Obstetrics and Gynecology
The Ottawa Hospital
Ottawa, Ontario, Canada [38]

Lawrence Oppenheimer, MD, MA, FRCSC, FRCOG
Professor, The University of Ottawa
Division of Maternal–Fetal Medicine
Department of Obstetrics and Gynecology
The Ottawa Hospital
Ottawa, Ontario, Canada [16, 19]

Dante Pascali, MD, FRCSC
Assistant Professor, The University of Ottawa
Division of Urogynecology and Pelvic Reconstructive Surgery
Department of Obstetrics and Gynecology
The Ottawa Hospital
Ottawa, Ontario, Canada [1, 2, 3, 4]

Samira Samiee, MD, FRCPC
Clinical Fellow, The University of Ottawa
Division of Neonatology
Department of Pediatrics
Children's Hospital of Eastern Ontario
Ottawa, Ontario, Canada [39]

Gihad Shabib MD, MRCOG, FRCSC
Assistant Professor, The University of Ottawa
Department of Obstetrics and Gynecology
The Ottawa Hospital
Ottawa, Ontario, Canada [17]

George Tawagi, MD, FRCSC
Assistant Professor, The University of Ottawa
Division of Maternal–Fetal Medicine
Department of Obstetrics and Gynecology
The Ottawa Hospital
Ottawa, Ontario, Canada [26, 27]

This latest edition of Dr. Harry Oxorn's text is the result of collaboration between numerous physicians in the Department of Obstetrics and Gynecology at the Ottawa Hospital. Although modern medicine relies heavily on science and technology, the most astute accoucheurs still practice the art of obstetrics embraced in this book. Much has changed, but much has remained the same. Although every chapter has been revised and refreshed, we've endeavored to stay true to the utilitarian spirit of the book that Dr. Oxorn intended. This textbook is not a treatise on theoretical evidence-based obstetrics that can only be practiced at tertiary centers; rather, it is a handbook of useful information for practitioners in the trenches who need real advice on how to manage real problems. New additions, such as a chapter on the challenges of obesity in pregnancy, descriptions of modern techniques for the management of postpartum hemorrhage, and an expanded treatment of multiples, reflect the modernization of Dr. Oxorn's work.

It has always been our intention to bring this text into the twenty-first century while respecting its heritage. As such, we owe a great debt to the previous contributors for giving us such a solid foundation; their legacy resides both within these pages as well as in the halls of the labor wards in Ottawa.

We would like to thank our project manager, Erica Phillips-Posner, for keeping us on schedule and making this textbook happen.

ACKNOWLEDGMENTS

PART I

Clinical
Anatomy

CHAPTER 1

Pelvis: Bones, Joints, and Ligaments

Dante Pascali

PELVIC BONES

The pelvis is the bony basin in which the trunk terminates and through which the body weight is transmitted to the lower extremities. In females, it is adapted for childbearing. The pelvis consists of four bones: the two innominates, the sacrum, and the coccyx. These are united by four joints.

Innominate Bones

The innominate bones are placed laterally and anteriorly. Each is formed by the fusion of three bones—the ilium, ischium, and pubis—around the acetabulum.

Ilium

The ilium is the superior bone: It has a body (which is fused with the ischial body) and an ala. Points of note concerning the ilium include:

1. The anterior superior iliac spine gives attachment to the inguinal ligament
2. The posterior superior iliac spine marks the level of the second sacral vertebra. Its presence is indicated by a dimple in the overlying skin
3. The iliac crest extends from the anterior superior iliac spine to the posterior superior iliac spine

Ischium

The ischium consists of a body in which the superior and inferior rami merge.

1. The body forms part of the acetabulum
2. The superior ramus is posterior and inferior to the body
3. The inferior ramus fuses with the inferior ramus of the pubis
4. The ischial spine separates the greater sciatic from the lesser sciatic notch. It is an important landmark. Part of the levator ani muscle is attached to it
5. The ischial tuberosity is the inferior part of the ischium and is the bone on which humans sit

Pubis

The pubis consists of the body and two rami.

1. The body has a rough surface on its medial aspect. This is joined to the corresponding area on the opposite pubis to form the symphysis pubis. The levator ani muscles are attached to the pelvic aspect of the pubis

2. The pubic crest is the superior border of the body
3. The pubic tubercle, or spine, is the lateral end of the pubic crest. The inguinal ligament and conjoined tendon are attached here
4. The superior ramus meets the body of the pubis at the pubic spine and the body of the ilium at the iliopectineal line, where it forms a part of the acetabulum
5. The inferior ramus merges with the inferior ramus of the ischium

Landmarks can be identified:

1. The iliopectineal line extends from the pubic tubercle back to the sacroiliac joint. It forms the greater part of the boundary of the pelvic inlet
2. The greater sacrosciatic notch is between the posterior inferior iliac spine superiorly and the ischial spine inferiorly
3. The lesser sacrosciatic notch is bounded by the ischial spine superiorly and the ischial tuberosity inferiorly
4. The obturator foramen is delimited by the acetabulum, the ischial rami, and the pubic rami

Sacrum

The sacrum is a triangular bone with the base superiorly and the apex inferiorly. It consists of five vertebrae fused together; rarely, there are four or six. The sacrum lies between the innominate bones and is attached to them by the sacroiliac joints.

The upper surface of the first sacral vertebra articulates with the lower surface of the fifth lumbar vertebra. The anterior (pelvic) surface of the sacrum is concave, and the posterior surface is convex.

The sacral promontory is the anterior superior edge of the first sacral vertebra. It protrudes slightly into the cavity of the pelvis, reducing the anteroposterior diameter of the inlet.

Coccyx

The coccyx (tail bone) is composed of four rudimentary vertebrae. The superior surface of the first coccygeal vertebra articulates with the inferior surface of the fifth sacral vertebra to form the sacrococcygeal joint. Rarely, there is fusion between the sacrum and coccyx, with resultant limitation of movement.

The coccygeus muscle, levator ani muscles, and sphincter ani externus are attached to the anterior aspect of the coccyx. They are important to pelvic floor function.

CLINICAL ANATOMY

PELVIC JOINTS AND LIGAMENTS

The sacrum, coccyx, and two innominate bones are linked by four joints: the symphysis pubis, the sacrococcygeal, and the two sacroiliac synchondroses (Fig. 1-1).

Sacroiliac Joint

The sacroiliac joint lies between the articular surfaces of the sacrum and the ilium. The weight of the body is transmitted through it to the pelvis and then to the lower limbs. It is a synovial joint and permits a small degree of movement. The capsule is weak, and stability is maintained by the muscles around it as well as by four primary and two accessory ligaments.

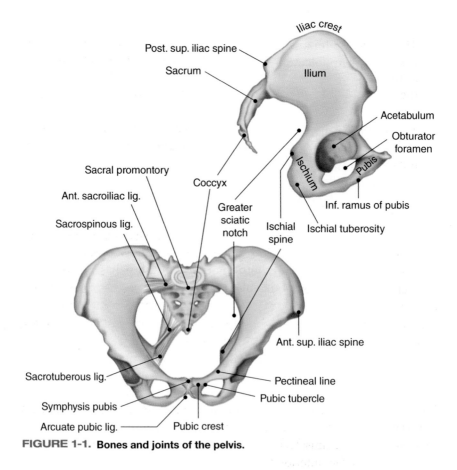

FIGURE 1-1. **Bones and joints of the pelvis.**

Primary Ligaments

1. The anterior sacroiliac ligaments are short and transverse, running from the preauricular sulcus on the ilium to the anterior aspect of the ala of the sacrum
2. The interosseus sacroiliac ligaments are short, strong transverse bands that extend from the rough part behind the auricular surface on the ilium to the adjoining area on the sacrum
3. The short posterior sacroiliac ligaments are strong transverse bands that lie behind the interosseus ligaments
4. The long posterior sacroiliac ligaments are each attached to the posterosuperior spine on the ilium and to the tubercles on the third and fourth sacral vertebrae

Accessory Ligaments

1. The sacrotuberous ligaments are attached on one side to the posterior superior iliac spine; posterior inferior iliac spine; tubercles on the third, fourth, and fifth sacral vertebrae; and lateral border of the coccyx. On the other side, the sacrotuberous ligaments are attached to the pelvic aspect of the ischial tuberosity
2. The sacrospinous ligament is triangular. The base is attached to the lateral parts of the fifth sacral and first coccygeal vertebrae, and the apex is attached to the ischial spine

Sacrococcygeal Joint

The sacrococcygeal joint is a synovial hinge joint between the fifth sacral and the first coccygeal vertebrae. It allows both flexion and extension. Extension, by increasing the anteroposterior diameter of the outlet of the pelvis, plays an important role in parturition. Overextension during delivery may break the small cornua by which the coccyx is attached to the sacrum. This joint has a weak capsule, which is reinforced by anterior, posterior, and lateral sacrococcygeal ligaments.

Symphysis Pubis

The symphysis pubis is a cartilaginous joint with no capsule and no synovial membrane. Normally, there is little movement. The posterior and superior ligaments are weak. The strong anterior ligaments are reinforced

CLINICAL ANATOMY

by the tendons of the rectus abdominis and the external oblique muscles. The strong inferior ligament in the pubic arch is known as the arcuate pubic ligament. It extends between the rami and leaves a small space in the subpubic angle.

MOBILITY OF PELVIS

During normal pregnancy, under the influence of progesterone and relaxin, there is increased flexibility of the sacroiliac joints and the symphysis pubis. Hyperemia and softening of the ligaments around the joints also take place. The pubic bones may separate by 1 to 12 mm. Excessive mobility of the symphysis pubis leads to pain and difficulty in walking. It has been shown that, besides the local changes that may take place in the pelvic ligaments, a generalized change in the laxity of joints occurs in pregnancy.

MALE AND FEMALE PELVISES

At birth, there is no difference between male and female pelvises. Sexual dimorphism does not take place until puberty. A female pelvis develops in offspring born with no gonads. Thus, ovaries and estrogen are not necessary for the formation of the female-type pelvis, but the presence of a testis that is producing androgen is essential for development of the male-type pelvis.

ADOLESCENCE

Adolescent girls' pelvises are smaller than those of mature women. The pattern of growth of the pelvic basin is different from that of bodily stature. Among girls, the growth in stature decelerates rapidly in the first year after menarche and ceases within 1 or 2 years. The pelvic basin, on the other hand, grows more slowly and more steadily during late adolescence. At the same time, it changes from an anthropoid to a gynecoid configuration. Thus, maturation of the reproductive system and attainment of adult size do not indicate that the growth and development of the pelvis are complete. The smaller pelvic capacity in adolescent girls may contribute to the higher incidence of cephalopelvic disproportion and other dystocias in primigravidous girls younger than the age of 15 years.

CHAPTER 2

The Pelvic Floor

Dante Pascali

THE PELVIC FLOOR

The pelvic floor (Fig. 2-1) is a muscular diaphragm that separates the pelvic cavity above from the perineal space below. It is formed by the levator ani and coccygeus muscles and is covered completely by parietal fascia.

The urogenital hiatus is an anterior gap through which the urethra and vagina pass. The rectal hiatus is posterior, and the rectum and anal canal pass through it.

PELVIC FLOOR FUNCTIONS

1. The pelvic floor supports the pelvic viscera in humans
2. To build up effective intraabdominal pressure, the muscles of the diaphragm, abdominal wall, and pelvic floor must contract together
3. During parturition, the pelvic floor helps the anterior rotation of the presenting part and directs it downward and forward along the birth passage

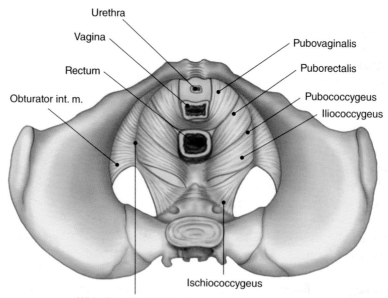

FIGURE 2-1. Pelvic floor.

PELVIC FLOOR MUSCLES

1. Levators ani, each composed of two muscles:

   a. Pubococcygeus, which has three divisions: pubovaginalis, puborectalis, and pubococcygeus proper
   b. Iliococcygeus

2. Coccygeus (ischiococcygeus)

Levator Ani Muscle

The levator ani muscle has a lateral origin and a central insertion, where it joins with the corresponding muscle from the other side. The direction of the muscle from origin to insertion is inferior and medial. The origin of each levator ani is from the:

1. Posterior side of the pubis
2. Arcuate tendon of the pelvic fascia (the white line of the pelvic fascia)
3. Pelvic aspect of the ischial spine

   The insertion, from anterior to posterior, is into:

1. Vaginal walls
2. Central point of the perineum
3. Anal canal
4. Anococcygeal body
5. Lateral border of the coccyx

Pubococcygeus Muscle

The pubococcygeus is the most important, most dynamic, and most specialized part of the pelvic floor. It lies in the midline; is perforated by the urethra, vagina, and rectum; and is often damaged during delivery. It originates from the posterior side of the pubis and from the white line of the pelvic fascia anterior to the obturator canal. The muscle passes posterior and medially in three sections: (1) pubovaginalis, (2) puborectalis and (3) pubococcygeus proper.

Pubovaginalis Muscle. The most medial section of the pubococcygeus, this muscle is shaped like a horseshoe, open anteriorly. The fibers make contact and blend with the muscles of the urethral wall, after which they form a loop around the vagina. They insert into the sides and back of the vagina and into the central point of the perineum.

The principal function of the pubovaginalis is to act as a sling for the vagina. Since the vagina helps to support the uterus and appendages, bladder and urethra, and rectum, this muscle is the main support of the female pelvic organs. Tearing or overstretching predisposes to uterovaginal prolapse. The muscle also functions as the vaginal sphincter, and when it goes into spasm, the condition is called *vaginismus*.

Puborectalis Muscle. The intermediate part of the pubococcygeus, this muscle forms a loop around the anal canal and rectum. The insertion is into the lateral and posterior walls of the anal canal between the sphincter ani internus and externus, with whose fibers the puborectalis joins. It inserts also in the anococcygeal body.

The puborectalis suspends the rectum, but since this organ does not support the other pelvic viscera, the puborectalis plays a small role in holding up the pelvic structures. The main work of this muscle is in controlling the descent of feces and in so doing it acts as an auxiliary sphincter for the anal canal. When the anococcygeal junction is pulled forward, the puborectalis increases the anorectal flexure and slows the descent of feces.

Pubococcygeus Proper. This muscle is composed of the most lateral fibers of the pubococcygeus muscle. It has a Y-shaped insertion into the lateral margins of the coccyx. When it contracts, it pulls the coccyx anteriorly, increasing the anorectal juncture. Thus, in combination with the external sphincter ani, it helps control the passage of feces.

Iliococcygeus Muscle

The iliococcygeus muscles arise from the white line of the pelvic fascia posterior to the obturator canal. They join with the pubococcygeus muscle proper and insert into the lateral margins of the coccyx. These are less dynamic than the pubovaginalis and act more like a musculofascial layer.

Ischiococcygeus Muscle

The ischiococcygeus or coccygeus muscles originate from the ischial spines and insert into the lateral borders of the coccyx and the fifth sacral vertebra. These muscles supplement the levators ani and occupy most of the posterior portion of the pelvic floor.

PELVIC FLOOR DURING PARTURITION

When the presenting part has reached the proper level during the second stage of labor, the central point of the perineum becomes thin. The levator ani muscles and the anal sphincter relax, and the muscles of the pelvic floor are drawn over the advancing head. Tearing and overstretching these muscles weaken the pelvic floor and may cause extensive damage.

CLINICAL ANATOMY

CHAPTER 3

Perineum

Dante Pascali

The perineum is a diamond-shaped space that lies below the pelvic floor (Fig. 3-1). Its boundaries are as follows:

1. Superiorly: the pelvic floor made up of the levator ani muscles and the coccygei
2. Laterally: the bones and ligaments that make up the pelvic outlet; from front to back, these are the subpubic angle, ischiopubic rami, ischial tuberosities, sacrotuberous ligaments, and coccyx
3. Inferiorly: the skin and fascia

This area is divided into two triangles: anteriorly, the urogenital triangle; posteriorly, the anal triangle. These are separated by a transverse band composed of the transverse perineal muscles and the base of the urogenital diaphragm.

UROGENITAL TRIANGLE

The urogenital triangle is bounded:

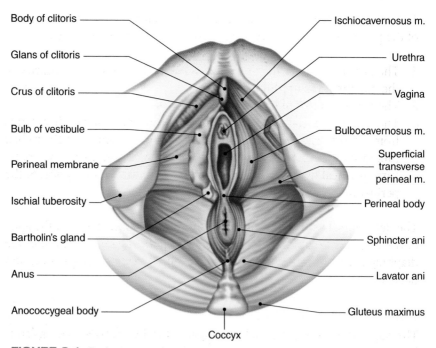

Body of clitoris — Ischiocavernosus m.
Glans of clitoris — Urethra
Crus of clitoris — Vagina
Bulb of vestibule — Bulbocavernosus m.
Perineal membrane — Superficial transverse perineal m.
Ischial tuberosity — Perineal body
Bartholin's gland — Sphincter ani
Anus — Lavator ani
Anococcygeal body — Gluteus maximus
Coccyx

FIGURE 3-1. Perineum.

1. Anteriorly: by the subpubic angle
2. Laterally: by the ischiopubic rami and the ischial tuberosities
3. Posteriorly: by the transverse perineal muscles and the base of the urogenital diaphragm

The urogenital triangle contains:

1. Opening of the vagina
2. Terminal part of the urethra
3. Crura of the clitoris with the ischiocavernosus muscles
4. Vestibular bulbs (erectile tissue) covered by the bulbocavernosus muscles
5. Bartholin's glands and their ducts
6. Urogenital diaphragm
7. Muscles that constitute the central point of the perineum (perineal body)
8. Perineal pouches, superficial and deep
9. Blood vessels, nerves, and lymphatics

Urogenital Diaphragm

The urogenital diaphragm (triangular ligament) lies in the anterior triangle of the perineum. It is composed of muscle tissue covered by fascia.

1. The two muscles are the deep transverse perineal and the sphincter of the membranous urethra
2. The superior layer of fascia is thin and weak
3. The inferior fascial layer is a strong fibrous membrane. It extends from a short distance beneath the arcuate pubic ligament to the ischial tuberosities. The fascial layers fuse superiorly and form the transverse perineal ligament. Inferiorly, they join in the central point of the perineum

The deep dorsal vein of the clitoris lies in a small space between the apex of the urogenital diaphragm and the arcuate pubic ligament. Through the diaphragm pass the urethra, the vagina, blood vessels, lymphatics, and nerves.

Superficial Perineal Pouch

The superficial perineal pouch is a space that lies between the inferior layer of the urogenital diaphragm and Colles fascia.

Superficial Transverse Perineal Muscles

The superficial transverse perineal muscles are the superficial parts of the deep muscles and have the same origin and insertion. These are outside the urogenital diaphragm. Sometimes they are entirely lacking.

Ischiocavernosus Muscles

The ischiocavernosus muscles cover the clitoral crura. The origin of each is the inferior ramus of the pubis, and they insert at the lateral aspect of the crus. These muscles compress the crura and by blocking the venous return cause the clitoris to become erect.

Bulbocavernosus Muscle

The bulbocavernosus muscle surrounds the vagina. With the external anal sphincter, it makes a figure eight around the vagina and rectum. It is also called the *bulbospongiosus*. It originates from the central point of the perineum and inserts into the dorsal aspect of the clitoral body. The muscle passes around the orifice of the vagina and surrounds the bulb of the vestibule.

The bulbocavernosus muscle compresses the erectile tissue around the vaginal orifice (bulb of the vestibule) and helps in clitoral erection by closing its dorsal vein. It acts as a weak vaginal sphincter. The real sphincter of the vagina is the pubovaginalis section of the levator ani.

Deep Perineal Pouch

The deep perineal pouch lies between the two fascial layers of the urogenital diaphragm.

Sphincter of the Membranous Urethra

The sphincter of the membranous urethra lies between the fascial layers of the urogenital diaphragm. It is also called the *compressor of the urethra*.

The voluntary fibers have their origin from the inferior rami of the ischium and pubis. They join with the deep transverse perineal muscles. Their action is to expel the last drops of urine.

The involuntary fibers surround the urethra and act as its sphincter.

Deep Transverse Perineal Muscles

The deep transverse perineal muscles lie between the layers of fascia of the urogenital diaphragm. They blend with the sphincter of the membranous urethra. The origin is the ischiopubic ramus on each side, and they insert at the central point of the perineum (perineal body).

ANAL TRIANGLE

The anal triangle is bounded:

1. Anteriorly: by the transverse perineal muscles and the base of the urogenital diaphragm
2. Laterally: by the ischial tuberosities and the sacrotuberous ligaments
3. Posteriorly: by the coccyx

The anal triangle contains the following:

1. Lower end of the anal canal and its sphincters
2. Anococcygeal body
3. Ischiorectal fossa
4. Blood vessels, lymphatics, and nerves

Sphincter Ani Externus

The sphincter ani externus has two parts.

1. The superficial portion surrounds the anal orifice. Its fibers are voluntary and act during defecation or in an emergency. The origin is the tip of the coccyx and the anococcygeal body. Insertion is in the central point of the perineum
2. The deep part is an involuntary muscle that surrounds the lower part of the anal canal and acts as a sphincter for the anus. It blends with the levators ani and the internal anal sphincter. When inactive, the deep circular fibers are in a state of tonus, occluding the anal orifice

Anococcygeal Body

The anococcygeal body is composed of muscle tissue (levators ani and external sphincter ani) and fibrous tissue. It is located between the tip of the coccyx and the anus.

PERINEAL BODY

The central point of the perineum or perineal body lies between the posterior angle of the vagina in front and the anus behind. In obstetrics, it is referred to as the *perineum*. It is often torn during delivery. The following muscles meet to form this structure:

1. Sphincter ani externus
2. Two levator ani muscles
3. Superficial and deep transverse perineal muscles
4. Bulbocavernosus muscle

CHAPTER 4

Uterus and Vagina

Dante Pascali

UTERUS

The normal uterus is a small muscular organ in the female pelvis. It is composed of three layers:

1. An outer, covering, serous peritoneal layer—the perimetrium
2. A thick middle layer made up of muscle fibers—the myometrium
3. An inner mucous layer of glands and supporting stroma—the endometrium—which is attached directly to the myometrium

The *myometrium* is made up of three layers of muscle:

1. An outer layer of mainly longitudinal fibers
2. An inner layer whose fibers run, for the most part, in a circular direction
3. A thick middle layer whose fibers are arranged in an interlacing pattern and through which the blood vessels course. When these fibers contract and retract after the products of conception have been expelled, the blood vessels are kinked and constricted. In this way, postpartum bleeding is controlled

Uterine Shape

In the nonpregnant condition and at the time of implantation, the uterus is pear shaped. By the third month of gestation, the uterus is globular. From the seventh month to term, the contour is again pyriform.

Uterine Size

The uterus grows from the nonpregnant dimensions of about 7.5 × 5.0 × 2.5 cm to 28 × 24 × 21 cm. The weight rises from 30 to 60 g to 1000 g at the end of pregnancy. The uterus changes from a solid organ in the nullipara to a large sac, the capacity increasing from almost nil to 4000 mL.

Uterine Location

Normally, the uterus is entirely in the pelvis. As it enlarges, it gradually rises, and by the fourth month of gestation, it extends into the abdominal region.

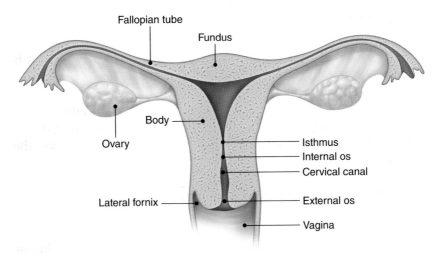

FIGURE 4-1. Uterus, cervix, and vagina.

Uterine Divisions

1. The fundus (Fig. 4-1) is the part superior to the openings of the fallopian tubes
2. The body (corpus) is the main part; it has thick walls, lies between the tubal openings and the isthmus, and is the main contractile portion. During labor, the contractions force the baby downward, distend the lower segment of the uterus, and dilate the cervix
3. The isthmus is a small constricted region of the uterus. It is about 5 to 7 mm in length and lies superior to the internal os of the cervix
4. The cervix (Fig. 4-2) is composed of a canal with an internal os superiorly, separating the cervix from the uterine cavity, and an external os inferiorly which closes off the cervix from the vagina. The cervix is about 2.5 cm in length. The lower part pierces the anterior wall of the vagina, and its tissue blends with that of the vagina

MYOMETRIUM

Most of the uterine growth takes place in the myometrium of the body and fundus. During the first half of pregnancy, the main factor in uterine growth is hyperplasia (formation of new muscle fibers). In the second half, hypertrophy predominates (enlargement of existing myometrial cells). Individual myometrial fibers increase 10-fold during pregnancy from a

24

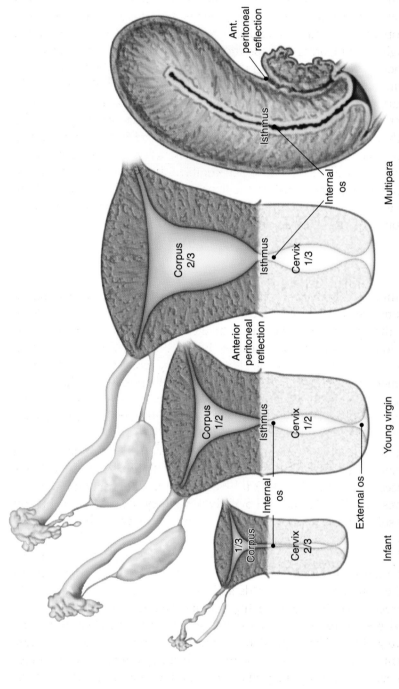

FIGURE 4-2. Isthmus of a pregnant uterus.

nonpregnant length of 50 to 100 μ to 500 to 800 μ during pregnancy. At term, the estimated number of cells is 200 billion. The myometrial fibers are composed of four major proteins: myosin, actin, tropomyosin, and troponin. The main stimulus to growth is provided by 17 β-estradiol, although some myometrial hypertrophy occurs in response to stretch.

There is also an increase in the number and size of the blood vessels and lymphatics, as well as a marked overgrowth of connective tissue.

During early pregnancy, the uterine walls are thicker than in the non-pregnant state. As gestation continues, the lumen becomes larger and the walls thinner. At the end of the fifth month, they are 3 to 5 mm thick and remain so until term. Thus, during late pregnancy, the uterus is a large muscular sac with thin, soft, easily compressible walls. This makes the corpus indentable and enables the fetus to be palpated. The walls of the uterus are so malleable that the uterus changes shape easily and markedly to accommodate to changes in fetal size and position.

Isthmus

The isthmus lies between the body of the uterus and the cervix. In humans, its boundaries are not well defined, and it is important as a physiologic rather than as an anatomic entity. In the nonpregnant uterus it is 5 to 7 mm long. It differs from the corpus in that it is free of mucus-secreting glands. The upper limit of the isthmus corresponds to a constriction in the lumen of the uterus, which marks the lower boundary of the body of the uterus (the anatomic internal os of Aschoff). The lower limit is the site of transition from the mucosa of the isthmus to the endocervical mucous membrane (histologic internal os).

Although the isthmus is of little importance in the normal state, in pregnancy, it plays an important role. As the uterus grows, the isthmus increases in length (Fig. 4-3) to about 25 mm and becomes soft and compressible. The Hegar sign of early pregnancy depends on palpation of the soft isthmus between the body of the uterus above and the cervix below.

The ovum implants, in the great majority of cases, in the upper part of the uterus. At about the third month, the enlarging embryo grows into the isthmus, which unfolds and expands to make room for it. As this process continues, the isthmus is incorporated gradually into the general uterine cavity, and the shape of the uterus changes from pyriform to globular. The expanded isthmus forms part of the lower uterine segment of the uterus during labor. The histologic internal os becomes the internal os of pregnancy, and the anatomic internal os becomes the physiologic retraction ring of normal labor (and pathologic retraction ring of obstructed labor).

The unfolding of the isthmus continues until it has reached the firm cervix, where it stops. After the seventh month, most of the enlargement takes place in the body and fundus, and the uterus becomes pear shaped again. At the onset of labor, the lower uterine segment comprises about one-third of the whole uterus. Although this area is not the passive part it was once thought to be, its contractions during normal labor are extremely weak when compared with those of the body.

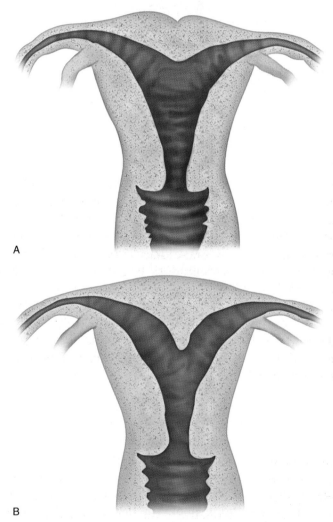

A

B

FIGURE 4-3. A. Arcuate uterus. **B.** Septate uterus, partial. **C.** Septate uterus, complete.

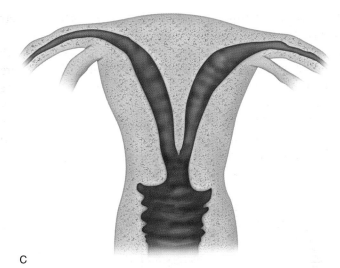

C

FIGURE 4-3. *(Continued)*

CLINICAL ANATOMY

Cervix

The cervix is composed mostly of connective tissue interspersed with muscle fibers. It feels hard and fibrous in the nonpregnant state. During pregnancy, the cervix becomes progressively softer. This is caused by increased vascularity, general edema, and hyperplasia of the glands. The compound tubular glands become overactive and produce large quantities of mucus. The secretion accumulates in the cervical canal and thickens to form the so-called mucous plug. This inspissated mucus effectively seals off the canal from the vagina and prevents the ascent of bacteria and other substances into the uterine cavity. The plug is expelled early in labor.

At the end of gestation and during labor, the internal os gradually disappears, and the cervical canal also becomes part of the lower uterine segment, leaving only the external os.

VAGINA

The vagina is a fibromuscular membranous tube surrounded by the vulva inferiorly, the uterus superiorly, the bladder anteriorly, and the rectum posteriorly. Its direction is obliquely superior and posterior. The cervix uteri enters the vagina through the anterior wall, and for this reason, the anterior wall of the vagina (6-8 cm) is shorter than the posterior wall

(7-10 cm). The protrusion of the cervix into the vagina divides the vaginal vault into four fornices: an anterior, a posterior, and two lateral fornices. The posterior fornix is much deeper than the others.

The wall of the vagina is made up of four layers:

1. The mucosa is the epithelial layer
2. The submucosa is rich in blood vessels
3. The muscularis is the third layer
4. The outer connective tissue layer connects the vagina to the surrounding structures

Even in the normal condition, the vagina is capable of great distention, but in pregnancy, this ability is increased many times. In the pregnant state, there is greater vascularity, thickening and lengthening of the walls, and increased secretion, so that most women have varying quantities of vaginal discharge during the period of gestation.

UTERINE ABNORMALITIES

Prolapse of the Uterus

Prolapse of the uterus during pregnancy is rare but troublesome. As a rule, the uterus rises out of the pelvis by the end of the fourth month. Occasionally, it fails to do so. In most cases, it is only the cervix, with or without an associated hypertrophic elongation, that protrudes through the vagina. Occasionally, the whole uterus is involved. Pregnancy cannot carry to term with the uterus completely out of the vagina.

Complications

Antepartum

1. Abortion and premature labor
2. Cervical edema, ulceration, and sepsis
3. Urinary retention and infection
4. Possible consideration of prolonged bed rest

Intrapartum

1. Cervical dilatation may begin outside the vagina, offering resistance to progress
2. The edema and fibrosis may cause cervical dystocia

3. Lacerations of the cervix are common
4. Obstructive labor may lead to uterine rupture

Postpartum
Puerperal infection is increased.

Treatment

Antepartum

1. Bed rest in the Trendelenburg position to reduce edema and permit repositioning of the uterus
2. Pessary to maintain the position of the uterus

Intrapartum

1. Most patients have a normal vaginal delivery, but arrest of progress may ensue

2. If cervical dystocia develops, several procedures may be considered:

    a. Dührssen incisions of the cervix
    b. Pitocin augmentation of labor
    c. Cesarean section

Postpartum
A pessary should be inserted to elevate the uterus and support the ligaments.

ANOMALIES OF THE UTERUS

Abnormal fusion of the Müllerian ducts or failure of absorption of the septum leads to a variety of congenital malformations of the uterus. The reported incidence is between one in 1200 and one in 600 fertile women. Most Müllerian anomalies are never detected because of the absence of clinical symptoms. Only about 25 percent of women with uterine anomalies have serious reproductive problems. Concurrent renal abnormalities are common.

Fetal wastage occurs in all trimesters, including abortion, early or late, and preterm labor and delivery. Malpresentation, especially breech, is common. Women with uterine anomalies are in a high-risk group and have to be controlled carefully during pregnancy, labor, and delivery.

The theoretical reasons for reproductive failure include:

1. Poor vascularization of the endometrium
2. Distortion of the uterine cavity
3. Incompetent cervix

Diagnosis

During pregnancy, a uterine anomaly may be suspected when the following conditions are present:

1. Notching and broadening of the uterine fundus
2. Abnormal lie
3. Recurring breech
4. Trapped or retained placenta
5. Prolonged third stage of labor
6. Recurrent spontaneous abortion
7. Axial deviation of the uterus
8. Flanking of the fetal limbs
9. Cervix located in the lateral fornix of the vagina
10. Presence of a vaginal septum

In any suspicious case, hysterography should be performed postpartum.

Complications

1. Breech presentation
2. Transverse lie; the fetus often assumes the hammock position with the head in one horn and the feet in the other
3. Incoordinate uterine action may result in failure of progress necessitating cesarean section
4. Premature rupture of membranes
5. Placenta previa
6. Obstruction of descent of the fetus by the nonpregnant horn
7. Obstruction by a thick vaginal septum

Labor and Delivery

In many cases, labor progresses without incident and terminates in a normal delivery. Therefore, a trial of labor is indicated. Failure to progress is treated by cesarean section. The incidence of the latter is higher than in normal patients.

Postpartum Complications

1. Retained placenta
2. Subinvolution of the placental site
3. Postpartum hemorrhage

Arcuate Uterus

The uterine fundus has a midline curved indentation that projects into the cavity of the uterus (Fig. 4-3A). The external contours of the uterus are not affected and, seen at laparoscopy, the uterus appears normal. Hysteroscopy and hysterosalpingography help in establishing the diagnosis. It is rare for this abnormality to lead to fetal loss from either abortion or preterm delivery. Most pregnancies are normal, and the diagnosis is not made.

Septate Uterus

The longitudinal septum may be complete (Fig. 4-3B), extending down to the internal or external os of the cervix, or incomplete or partial (Fig. 4-3C), when it extends part way from the uterine fundus. Fetal loss in the first half of pregnancy is common. In such cases, the septum should be excised hysteroscopically.

Unicornuate Uterus

This is a uterus with a single horn (Fig. 4-4). A normal vagina and a single normal tube are present in most cases. The other half of the uterus is absent or rudimentary. In many patients, the kidney is absent on the same side as the uterine abnormality.

In this condition, there is an increased incidence of difficulty or inability to conceive, spontaneous abortion, preterm labor, abnormal presentation of the fetus, and intrauterine growth restriction. A possible explanation of the latter is that, with one uterine artery being absent, there are inadequate perfusion of the uterus and reduced fetal nutrition. On the other hand, there may be insufficient room in the uterus for normal growth. An incompetent cervix is often present.

If there is a rudimentary horn, transmigration of sperm or ova can occur with a resultant pregnancy. In such cases, the rudimentary horn should be

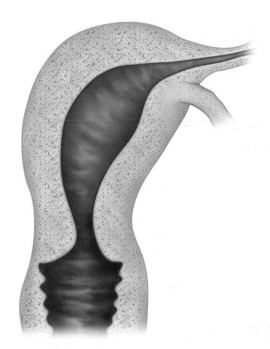

FIGURE 4-4. Unicornuate uterus.

excised. If the patient is unable to conceive, removal of the contralateral ovary and rudimentary horn may be followed by a successful pregnancy.

Bicornuate Uterus

The division down the middle of the uterus is complete to the internal os (Fig. 4-5). Diagnosis is made by palpation, postpartum exploration of the uterine cavity, during curettage, by hysteroscopy, by hysterosalpingography, and by laparoscopy. Abortion, incompetent cervix, premature rupture of membranes, preterm labor, abnormal presentation (especially breech and transverse lie), and cesarean section are all more common than when the uterus is normal. Fetal salvage is good in many cases. When fetal loss recurs, a unification operation should be performed.

Labor proceeds to vaginal delivery in many cases. Cesarean section is indicated only for obstetric reasons and not because of the anomaly per se. Dystocia may be caused by uterine inertia, obstruction by the nongravid horn, and hypertrophy of a septum. Occasionally, the nonpregnant horn may rupture during labor.

Retained placenta occurs in some 20 percent of cases and may lead to postpartum hemorrhage.

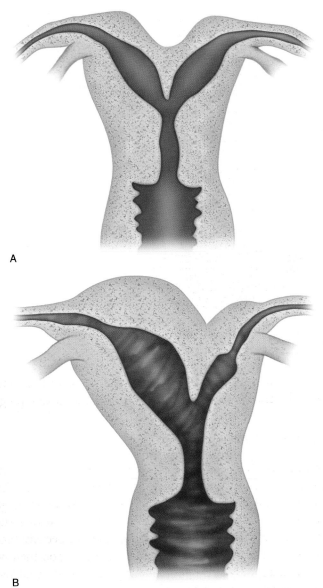

A

B

FIGURE 4-5. A. Bicornuate uterus. **B.** Bicornuate uterus with a rudimentary horn.

Double Uterus: Uterus Didelphys

The reported incidence of complete duplication of the female reproductive tract is between one in 1500 and one in 15,000 pregnant women (Fig. 4-6). The cervices are externally united, and the uterine fundi are

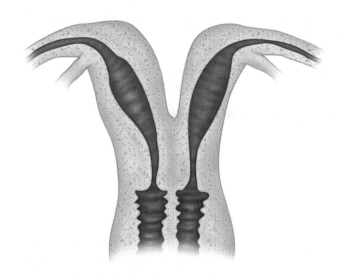

FIGURE 4-6. Double uterus: uterus didelphys.

externally separate. In most cases, there are two vaginas. The halves of the uterus are often of different sizes.

Ineffectual contractions and slowly dilating cervices are common during the first stages of labor. Postpartum atony leading to hemorrhage is observed often. Sloughing of a decidual cast from the nonpregnant uterus can cause excessive bleeding. The cervix of the nongravid uterus may interfere with the descent and rotation of the fetal presenting part and may so obstruct progress that cesarean section is necessary. Many women have normal vaginal deliveries, however. Preterm labor is common. Unification is indicated only when fetal wastage occurs repeatedly.

TORSION OF PREGNANT UTERUS

Uterine torsion is defined as rotation of the uterus on its long axis of more than 45°. Torsion of the pregnant uterus is rare; the condition was first reported in animals in 1662 and in the human 200 years later. The exact cause is not known, but some uterine malformation or tumor is present in many instances.

Most pregnant uteri show a slight degree of rotation, to the right in 80 percent and toward the left in 20 percent. In most abnormal situations, the rotation has been 180°, although a case was reported of a 540° torsion associated with uterine necrosis.

In 20 percent of cases, no causative factor is apparent. Predisposing conditions include:

1. Malpresentation, especially transverse lie
2. Uterine myomas
3. Anomalies of the uterus
4. Pelvic adhesions
5. Ovarian cyst
6. Uterine suspension
7. Abnormal pelvis
8. Placenta previa

Preoperative diagnosis is rare. The picture is one of an acute abdominal crisis, including pain, shock, bleeding, obstructed labor, and symptoms referable to the intestinal and urinary tracts. The most serious complication is uterine rupture. Acute torsion results in compromise of the uterine circulation. Treatment at or near term is by cesarean section. Before viability of the fetus has been reached, laparotomy is performed, the uterus is rotated to its normal position, and the pregnancy is allowed to continue to term.

SELECTED READING

Andrews MC, Jones HW Jr: Impaired reproductive performance of the unicornuate uterus: Intrauterine growth retardation, infertility, and recurrent abortion in five cases. Am J Obstet Gynecol 144:173, 1982
Ansbacher R: Uterine anomalies and future pregnancies. Clin Perinatol 10:295, 1983
Heinonen PK, Saarikoski S, Pystynen P: Reproductive performance of women with uterine anomalies. Acta Obstet Gynecol Scand 61:157, 1982
Nielsen TF: Torsion of the pregnant uterus without symptoms. Am J Obstet Gynecol 141:838, 1981
Visser AA, Giesteira MUK, Heyns A, Marais C: Torsion of the pregnant uterus. Case reports. Br J Obstet Gynaecol 90:87, 1983

CHAPTER 5

Obstetric Pelvis

Glenn D. Posner

THE PELVIS

The pelvis is made up of the two innominate bones (which occupy the front and sides) and the sacrum and coccyx (which are behind). The bones articulate through four joints. The sacroiliac joint is the most important, linking the sacrum to the iliac part of the innominate bones. The symphysis of the pubis joins the two pubic bones. The sacrococcygeal joint attaches the sacrum to the coccyx.

The *false pelvis* lies above the true pelvis, superior to the linea terminalis. Its only obstetric function is to support the enlarged uterus during pregnancy. Its boundaries are:

1. Posteriorly: lumbar vertebrae
2. Laterally: iliac fossae
3. Anteriorly: anterior abdominal wall

The *true pelvis* (Fig. 5-1A) lies below the pelvic brim, or linea terminalis, and is the bony canal through which the fetus must pass. It is divided into three parts: (1) the inlet, (2) the pelvic cavity, and (3) the pelvic outlet. The *inlet* (pelvic brim) is bounded:

1. Anteriorly by the pubic crest and spine
2. Laterally by the iliopectineal lines on the innominate bones
3. Posteriorly by the anterior borders of the ala and promontory of the sacrum

The *pelvic cavity* (Fig. 5-1B) is a curved canal.

1. The anterior wall is straight and shallow. The pubis is approximately 5 cm long
2. The posterior wall is deep and concave. The sacrum is approximately 10 to 15 cm long
3. The ischium and part of the body of the ilium are found laterally

The *pelvic outlet* is diamond shaped. It is bounded:

1. Anteriorly by the arcuate pubic ligament and the pubic arch
2. Laterally by the ischial tuberosity and the sacrotuberous ligament
3. Posteriorly by the tip of the sacrum

The *pelvic inclination* (Fig. 5-1C) is assessed when the woman is in the upright position. The plane of the pelvic brim makes an angle of about 60°

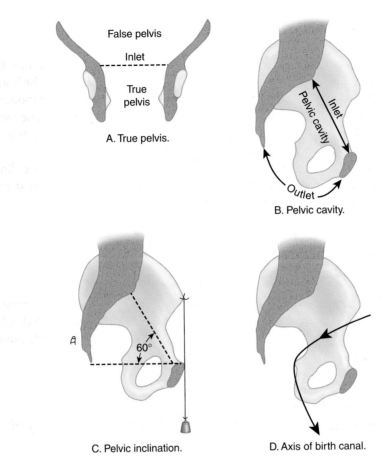

A. True pelvis.

B. Pelvic cavity.

C. Pelvic inclination.

D. Axis of birth canal.

FIGURE 5-1. Pelvic cavity.

CLINICAL ANATOMY

with the horizontal. The anterior superior iliac spine is in the same vertical plane as the pubic spine.

The *axis of the birth canal* (Fig. 5-1D) is the course taken by the presenting part as it passes through the pelvis. At first it moves downward and backward to the level of the ischial spines, which is the area of the bony attachment of the pelvic floor muscles. Here the direction changes and the presenting part proceeds downward and forward.

The *pelvic planes* (Fig. 5-2) are imaginary flat surfaces passing across the pelvis at different levels. They are used for the purposes of description. The important ones are as follows:

1. The plane of the inlet is also called the superior strait
2. The pelvic cavity has many planes, two of which are the plane of greatest dimensions and the plane of least dimensions

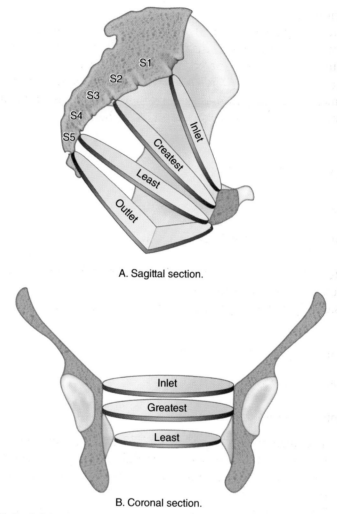

A. Sagittal section.

B. Coronal section.

FIGURE 5-2. **Pelvic planes.**

3. The plane of the outlet is also called the inferior strait

The *diameters* are distances between given points. Important ones are the following:

1. Anteroposterior diameters
2. Transverse diameters
3. Left oblique: Oblique diameters are designated left or right according to their posterior terminal

4. Right oblique
5. Posterior sagittal diameter: This is the back part of the anteroposterior diameter, extending from the intersection of the transverse and antero-posterior diameters to the posterior limit of the latter
6. Anterior sagittal diameter: This is the front part of the anteroposterior diameter, extending from the intersection of the transverse and antero-posterior diameter to the anterior limit of the latter

PELVIC INLET

Plane of Obstetric Inlet

The plane of the obstetric inlet is bounded:

1. Anteriorly by the posterior superior margin of the pubic symphysis
2. Laterally by the iliopectineal lines
3. Posteriorly by the promontory and ala of the sacrum

Diameters of Inlet

The diameters of the inlet are as follows:

1. Anteroposterior diameters:

   a. The anatomic conjugate (Fig. 5-3) extends from the middle of the sacral promontory to the middle of the pubic crest (superior surface of the pubis). It measures approximately 11.5 cm. It has no obstetric significance
   b. The obstetric conjugate extends from the middle of the sacral promontory to the posterior superior margin of the pubic symphysis. This point on the pubis, which protrudes back into the cavity of the pelvis, is about 1.0 cm below the pubic crest. The obstetric conjugate is approximately 11.0 cm in length. This is the important anteroposterior diameter because it is the one through which the fetus must pass
   c. The diagonal conjugate extends from the subpubic angle to the middle of the sacral promontory. It is approximately 12.5 cm in length. This diameter can be measured manually in the patient. It is of clinical significance because by subtracting 1.5 cm, an approximate length of the obstetric conjugate can be obtained

CLINICAL ANATOMY

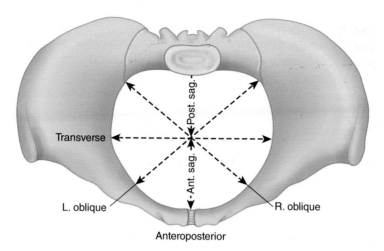

A. Anteroposterior view.

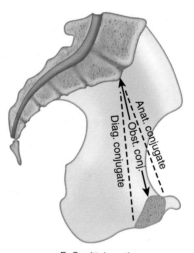

B. Sagittal section.

FIGURE 5-3. **Pelvic inlet.**

2. Transverse diameter is the widest distance between the iliopectineal lines and is approximately 13.5 cm

3. Left oblique diameter extends from the left sacroiliac joint to the right iliopectineal eminence and is approximately 12.5 cm

4. Right oblique diameter extends from the right sacroiliac joint to the left iliopectineal eminence and is approximately 12.5 cm

5. Posterior sagittal diameter extends from the intersection of the anteroposterior and transverse diameters to the middle of the sacral promontory and is approximately 4.5 cm long

PELVIC CAVITY

The pelvic cavity extends from the inlet to the outlet.

Plane of Greatest Dimensions

This is the roomiest part of the pelvis and is almost circular. Its obstetric significance is small. Its boundaries are:

1. Anteriorly: midpoint of the posterior surface of the pubis
2. Laterally: upper and middle thirds of the obturator foramina
3. Posteriorly: the junction of the second and third sacral vertebrae

The diameters of importance are:

1. The anteroposterior diameter extends from the midpoint of the posterior surface of the pubis to the junction of the second and third sacral vertebrae and measures approximately 12.75 cm
2. The transverse diameter is the widest distance between the lateral aspects of the plane and is approximately 12.5 cm

Plane of Least Dimensions

This is the most important plane of the pelvis (Fig. 5-4). It has the least room, and it is here that most instances of arrest of progress take place. This plane extends from the apex of the subpubic arch, through the ischial spines, to the sacrum, usually at or near the junction of the fourth and fifth sacral vertebrae. The boundaries are, from front to back:

1. Lower border of the pubic symphysis
2. White line on the fascia covering the obturator foramina
3. Ischial spines
4. Sacrospinous ligaments
5. Sacrum

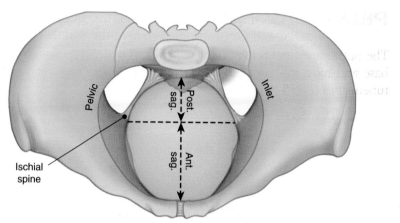

A. Anteroposterior view showing the anteroposterior and transverse diameters.

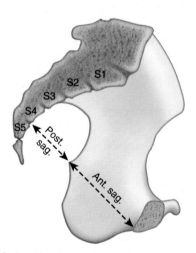

B. Sagittal section showing the anteroposterior diameter.

FIGURE 5-4. Pelvic cavity: the plane of least dimensions.

The diameters of importance are:

1. Anteroposterior diameter, extending from the lower border of the pubic symphysis to the junction of the fourth and fifth sacral vertebrae and measuring approximately 12.0 cm
2. Transverse diameter, lying between the ischial spines and measuring approximately 10.5 cm
3. Posterior sagittal diameter, extending from the bispinous diameter to the junction of the fourth and fifth sacral vertebrae and measuring approximately 4.5 to 5.0 cm

PELVIC OUTLET

The outlet is made up of two triangular planes, having as their common base and most inferior part the transverse diameter between the ischial tuberosities (Fig. 5-5).

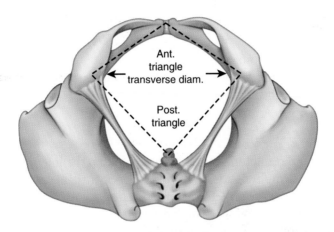

A. Inferior view.

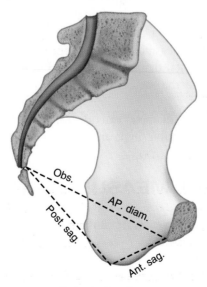

B. Sagittal section.

FIGURE 5-5. **Pelvic outlet.**

Anterior Triangle

The anterior triangle has the following boundaries:

1. The base is the bituberous diameter (transverse diameter)
2. The apex is the subpubic angle
3. The sides are the pubic rami and ischial tuberosities

Posterior Triangle

The posterior triangle has the following boundaries:

1. The base is the bituberous diameter
2. The obstetric apex is the sacrococcygeal joint
3. The sides are the sacrotuberous ligaments

Diameters of the Outlet

1. The anatomic anteroposterior diameter is from the inferior margin of the pubic symphysis to the tip of the coccyx. It measures approximately 9.5 cm. The obstetric anteroposterior diameter is from the inferior margin of the pubic symphysis to the sacrococcygeal joint. This measures approximately 11.5 cm. Because of the mobility at the sacrococcygeal joint, the coccyx is pushed out of the way by the advancing presenting part, increasing the available space
2. The transverse diameter is the distance between the inner surfaces of the ischial tuberosities and measures approximately 11.0 cm
3. The posterior sagittal diameter extends from the middle of the transverse diameter to the sacrococcygeal junction and is approximately 9.0 cm
4. The anterior sagittal diameter extends from the middle of the transverse diameter to the subpubic angle and measures approximately 6.0 cm

IMPORTANT MEASUREMENTS

In assessing the obstetric capacity of the pelvis, the most important measurements are the following:

1. Obstetric conjugate of the inlet
2. Distance between the ischial spines
3. Subpubic angle and bituberous diameter

4. Posterior sagittal diameters of the three planes
5. Curve and length of the sacrum

CLASSIFICATION OF THE PELVIS

Variations in the female pelvis and in the planes of any single pelvis are so great that a rigid classification is not possible. A pelvis of the female type in one plane may be predominantly male in another. Many pelves are mixed in that the various planes do not conform to a single parent type.

For the purpose of classification, the pelvis is named on the basis of the inlet, and mention is made of nonconforming characteristics. For example, a pelvis may be described as a female type with male features at the outlet.

The classification of Caldwell and Moloy is used commonly (Table 5-1 and Figs. 5-6 through 5-8).

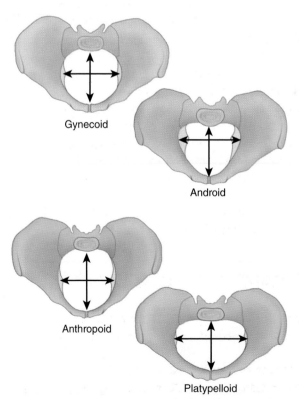

FIGURE 5-6. Pelvic outlet (Caldwell-Moloy classification).

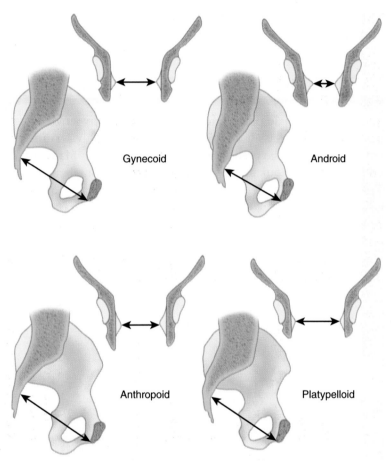

Gynecoid

Android

Anthropoid

Platypelloid

FIGURE 5-7. Midpelvis (Caldwell-Moloy classification).

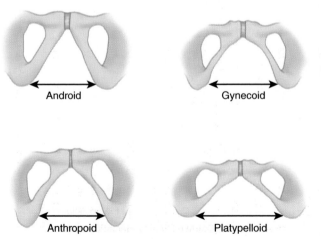

Android

Gynecoid

Anthropoid

Platypelloid

FIGURE 5-8. Pelvic outlet (Caldwell-Moloy classification).

TABLE 5-1: CLASSIFICATION OF PELVIS (CALDWELL AND MOLOY)

	Gynecoid	Android	Anthropoid	Platypelloid
INLET				
Sex type	Normal female	Male	Apelike	Flat female
Incidence	50%	20%	25%	5%
Shape	Round or transverse oval; transverse diameter is a little longer than the anteroposterior	Heart or wedge shaped	Long anteroposterior oval	Transverse oval
Anteroposterior diameter	Adequate	Adequate	Long	Short
Transverse diameter	Adequate	Adequate	Adequate but relatively short	Long
Posterior sagittal diameter	Adequate	Very short and inadequate	Very long	Very short
Anterior sagittal diameter	Adequate	Long	Long	Short
Posterior segment	Broad, deep, roomy	Shallow; sacral promontory indents the inlet and reduces its capacity	Deep	Shallow
Anterior segment	Well rounded forepelvis	Narrow, sharply angulated forepelvis	Deep	Shallow

(Continued)

TABLE 5-1: CLASSIFICATION OF PELVIS (CALDWELL AND MOLOY) (Continued)

	Gynecoid	Android	Anthropoid	Platypelloid
PELVIC CAVITY: MIDPELVIS				
Anteroposterior diameter	Adequate	Reduced	Long	Shortened
Transverse diameter	Adequate	Reduced	Adequate	Wide
Posterior sagittal diameter	Adequate	Reduced	Adequate	Shortened
Anterior sagittal diameter	Adequate	Reduced	Adequate	Short
Sacrum	Wide, deep curve; short; slopes backward; light bone	Flat; inclined forward; long; narrow; heavy	Inclined backward; narrow; long	Wide, deep curve; often sharply angulated with enlarged sacral fossa
Sidewalls	Parallel, straight	Convergent; funnel pelvis	Straight	Parallel
Ischial spines	Not prominent	Prominent	Variable	Variable
Sacrosciatic notch	Wide; short	Narrow; long; high arch	Wide	Short
Depth: iliopectineal eminence	Average	Long	Long	Short
capacity	Adequate	Reduced in all diameters	Adequate	Reduced

50

TABLE 5-1: CLASSIFICATION OF PELVIS (CALDWELL AND MOLOY) (Continued)

	Gynecoid	Android	Anthropoid	Platypelloid
OUTLET				
Anteroposterior diameter	Long	Short	Long	Short
Transverse diameter (bituberous)	Adequate	Narrow	Adequate	Wide
Pubic arch	Wide and round; 90°	Narrow; deep; 70°	Normal or relatively narrow	Very wide
Inferior pubic rami	Short; concave inward	Straight; long	Long; relatively narrow	Straight; short
Capacity	Adequate	Reduced	Adequate	Inadequate
EFFECT ON LABOR				
Fetal head	Engages in transverse or oblique diameter in slight asynclitism; good flexion; occiput anterior (OA) position is common	Engages in transverse or posterior diameter in asynclitism; extreme molding	Engages in anteroposterior or oblique; often occiput posterior position	Engages in transverse diameter with marked asynclitism

(Continued)

TABLE 5-1: CLASSIFICATION OF PELVIS (CALDWELL AND MOLOY) *(Continued)*

	Gynecoid	Android	Anthropoid	Platypelloid
Labor	Good uterine function; early and complete internal rotation; spontaneous delivery; wide pubic arch reduces perineal tears	Deep transverse arrest is common; arrest as occiput posterior (OP) position with failure of rotation; delivery is often by difficult forceps application, rotation, and extraction; the narrow pubic arch may lead to major perineal tears	Delivery and labor usually easy; birth face to pubis is common	Delay at inlet
Prognosis	Good	Poor	Good	Poor; disproportion; delay at inlet; labor often terminated by cesarean section

CHAPTER 6

The Passenger: Fetus

Glenn D. Posner

GENERAL CONSIDERATIONS

1. Resemblance to the adult human form may be perceptible at the end of 8 weeks and is obvious at the end of 12 weeks
2. By the end of 12 weeks and sometimes sooner, the sexual differences in the external genitalia may be recognized in abortuses
3. Growth is greatest during the sixth and seventh months of intrauterine life
4. Quickening (the perception by the pregnant woman of fetal movements in utero) occurs between the 16th and 20th weeks of pregnancy. The time of quickening is too variable to be of value in determining the expected date of confinement or when term has been reached. Active intestinal peristalsis is the most common phenomenon mistaken for quickening
5. Depending on maternal body habitus, the fetal heart is audible using a fetal Doppler by the 12th to 13th weeks of gestation
6. The fetal heart is audible using a stethoscope by the 18th or 20th week
7. The average length of the fetus at term is 50 cm
8. Within wide variations, the average boy in Canada (7 pounds, 15 oz or ~3600 g) is a little heavier at birth (based on 40 weeks gestational age) than the average girl (7 pounds, 10 oz or ~3500 g)
9. In premature babies, the circumference of the head is relatively large compared with the shoulders. This fact is of clinical relevance when contemplating preterm breech delivery. As the fetus matures, the body grows faster than the head, so that at term, the circumferences of the head and the shoulders are nearly the same

FETAL OVOIDS

In its passage through the pelvis, the fetus presents two oval parts, movable on each other at the neck. The oval of the head is longer in its anteroposterior diameter, while that of the shoulders and body is longer transversely. Thus, the two ovoids are perpendicular to each other.

FETAL HEAD

From the obstetric standpoint, the fetal head (Fig. 6-1) is the most important part of the fetus. It is the largest, the least compressible, and the most frequently presenting part of the baby. Once the head has been born, rarely is there delay or difficulty with the remainder of the body.

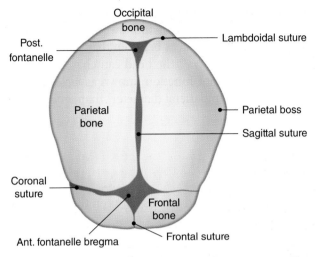

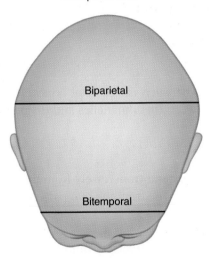

A. Superior view.

B. Transverse diameters.

FIGURE 6-1. Fetal skull.

Base of Skull

The bones of the base of the skull are large, ossified, firmly united, and not compressible. Their function is to protect the vital centers in the brain stem.

Vault of Skull: Cranium

The cranium is made up of several bones. Important ones are the occipital bone posteriorly, the two parietal bones on the sides, and the two temporal and the two frontal bones anteriorly. The bones of the cranial vault are laid down in membrane. At birth they are thin, poorly ossified, easily compressible, and joined only by membrane. This looseness of union of the bones (actually, there are spaces between them) permits their overlapping under pressure. In this way, the head can change its shape to fit the maternal pelvis, an important function known as *molding*. The top of the skull is wider posteriorly (biparietal diameter) than anteriorly (bitemporal diameter).

Sutures of Skull

Sutures are membrane-occupied spaces between the bones. They are useful in two ways (Fig. 6-1A):

1. Their presence makes molding possible
2. By identifying the sutures on vaginal examination, the position of the baby's head can be diagnosed. The important sutures include the following

Sagittal Suture
The sagittal suture lies between the parietal bones. It runs in an anteroposterior direction between the fontanelles and divides the head into left and right halves.

Lambdoidal Sutures
The lambdoidal sutures extend transversely from the posterior fontanelle and separate the occipital bone from the two parietals.

Coronal Sutures
The coronal sutures extend transversely from the anterior fontanelle and lie between the parietal and frontal bones (Fig. 6-1).

Frontal Suture
The frontal suture is between the two frontal bones and is an anterior continuation of the sagittal suture. It extends from the glabella to the bregma.

Fontanelles

Where the sutures intersect are the membrane-filled spaces known as fontanelles. Two are important, the anterior and the posterior. These areas are useful clinically in two ways (Fig. 6-1A):

1. Their identification helps in diagnosing the position of the fetal head in the pelvis
2. The large fontanelle is examined in assessing the condition of the child after birth. In dehydrated infants, the fontanelle is depressed below the surface of the bony skull. When the intracranial pressure is elevated, the fontanelle is bulging, tense, and raised above the level of the skull

Anterior Fontanelle
The anterior fontanelle (bregma) is at the junction of the sagittal, frontal, and coronal sutures. It is by far the larger of the two, measuring about 3 × 2 cm, and is diamond shaped. It becomes ossified by 18 months of age. The anterior fontanelle facilitates molding. By remaining patent long after birth, it plays a part in accommodating the remarkable growth of the brain.

Posterior Fontanelle
The posterior fontanelle (lambda) is located where the sagittal suture meets the two lambdoidals. The skull is not truly deficient at this point, and the area is a meeting point of the sutures rather than a true fontanelle. It is much smaller than the anterior one. The intersection of the sutures makes a Y with the sagittal suture as the base and the lambdoidals as the arms. This fontanelle closes at 6 to 8 weeks of age.

Landmarks of Skull

From posterior to anterior, certain areas are identified (Fig. 6-2A).

1. Occiput: the area of the back of the head occupied by the occipital bone. It is behind and inferior to the posterior fontanelle and the lambdoidal sutures
2. Posterior fontanelle
3. Vertex: the area between the two fontanelles. It is the top of the skull and is bounded laterally by the parietal bosses
4. Bregma or large anterior fontanelle
5. Sinciput (or brow): the region bounded superiorly by the bregma and the coronal sutures, inferiorly by the glabella and the orbital ridges
6. Glabella: the elevated area between the orbital ridges
7. Nasion: the root of the nose
8. Parietal bosses: two eminences, one on the side of each parietal bone. The distance between them is the widest transverse diameter of the fetal head

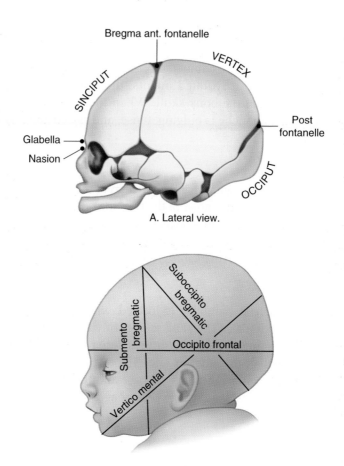

A. Lateral view.

B. Anteroposterior diameters.

FIGURE 6-2. **Landmarks and diameters of fetal skull.**

Diameters of Fetal Skull

The diameters are distances between given points on the fetal skull (Fig. 6-2B). Their size varies, and the particular anteroposterior diameter that presents to the maternal pelvis depends on the degree of flexion or extension of the fetal head.

1. The biparietal diameter (Fig. 6-1B) is between the parietal bosses. It is the largest transverse diameter and measures approximately 9.5 cm
2. The bitemporal diameter lies between the lateral sides of the temporal bones. It is approximately 8.0 cm in length and is the shortest transverse diameter of the skull

3. The suboccipitobregmatic diameter extends from the undersurface of the occipital bone, where it meets the neck, to the center of the bregma. It is approximately 9.5 cm long. It is the anteroposterior diameter that presents when the head is flexed well
4. The occipitofrontal diameter presents in the military attitude, neither flexion nor extension. It extends from the external occipital protuberance to the glabella and is approximately 11.0 cm long
5. The verticomental diameter is involved in brow presentations (halfway extension of the head). It runs from the vertex to the chin, measures approximately 13.5 cm, and is the longest anteroposterior diameter of the head
6. The submentobregmatic is the diameter in face presentations (complete extension of the head). Reaching from the junction of the neck and lower jaw to the center of the bregma, it is approximately 9.5 cm long

Circumferences of Fetal Skull and Shoulders

1. In the occipitofrontal plane, the circumference of the head is approximately 34.5 cm
2. In the suboccipitobregmatic plane, it is approximately 32 to 34 cm
3. At term, the bisacromial diameter of the shoulders is approximately 33 to 34 cm

Molding

Molding is the ability of the fetal head to change its shape and so adapt itself to the unyielding maternal pelvis (Fig. 6-3). This property is of the greatest value in the progress of labor and descent of the head through the birth canal.

The fetal bones are joined loosely by membranes so that actual spaces exist between the edges of the bones. This permits the bones to alter their relationships to each other as pressure is exerted on the head by the bony pelvis; the bones can come closer to each other or move apart. The side-to-side relationships of the bones are changeable, and one bone is able to override the other. When such overlapping takes place, the frontal and occipital bones pass under the parietal bones. The posterior parietal bone is subjected to greater pressure by the sacral promontory; therefore, it passes beneath the anterior parietal bone. A contributing factor to molding is the softness of the bones.

Compression in one direction is accompanied by expansion in another, and hence the actual volume of the skull is not reduced. Provided that

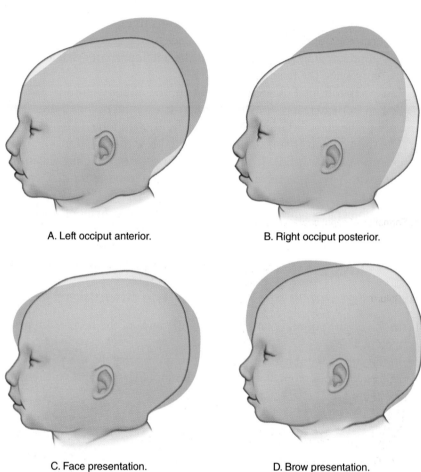

A. Left occiput anterior.   B. Right occiput posterior.

C. Face presentation.   D. Brow presentation.

FIGURE 6-3. **Molding.**

molding is not excessive and that it takes place slowly, no damage is done to the brain.

Alteration of the shape of the head is produced by compression of the presenting diameter, with resultant bulging of the diameter that is at right angles. For example, in the occipitoanterior position, the suboccipitobregmatic is the presenting diameter. The head therefore is elongated in the verticomental diameter, with bulging behind and above.

Caput Succedaneum

The caput succedaneum is a localized swelling of the scalp formed by the effusion of serum (Fig. 6-4). Pressure by the cervical ring causes obstruction of the venous return, so that the part of the scalp that lies within the

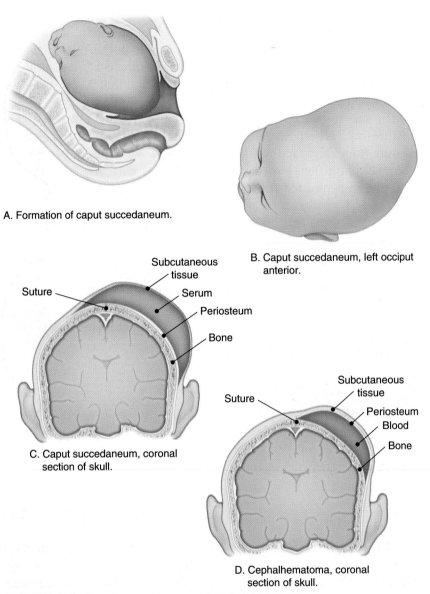

A. Formation of caput succedaneum.

B. Caput succedaneum, left occiput anterior.

C. Caput succedaneum, coronal section of skull.

D. Cephalhematoma, coronal section of skull.

FIGURE 6-4. **Caput succedaneum and cephalohematoma.**

cervix becomes edematous. The caput forms during labor and after the membranes have been ruptured. It is absent if the fetus is dead, the contractions are poor, or the cervix is not applied closely to the head.

The location of the caput varies with the position of the head. In occipitoanterior (OA) positions, the caput forms on the vertex, to the right of the sagittal suture in left (LOA), and to the left in right (ROA). As flexion becomes more pronounced during labor, the posterior part of the vertex becomes the presenting part and the caput is found in that region, a little to the right or left as before. Thus, when the position is LOA, the caput is on the posterior part of the right parietal bone, and in ROA on the posterior part of the left parietal bone.

The size of the caput succedaneum is an indication of the amount of pressure that has been exerted against the head. A large one suggests strong pressure from above and resistance from below. A small caput is present when the contractions have been weak or the resistance feeble. The largest are found in contracted pelves after long, hard labor. In the presence of prolonged labor, a large caput suggests disproportion or occipitoposterior position, and a small one indicates uterine inertia.

In performing vaginal examinations during labor, one must take care to distinguish between the station of the caput and that of the skull. The enlarging caput may make the accoucheur believe that the head is descending, when in reality it means that advancement of the head is delayed or arrested. A growing caput is an indication for reassessing the situation.

The caput is present at birth, begins to disappear immediately afterward, and is usually gone after 24 to 36 hours.

Cephalohematoma

Cephalohematoma (also spelled cephalhematoma) is a hemorrhage under the periosteum of one or more of the bones of the skull (Fig. 6-4D). It is situated on one or, rarely, both parietal bones and is similar in appearance to a caput succedaneum. A cephalohematoma is caused by trauma to the skull, including:

1. Prolonged pressure of the head against the cervix, perineum, or pubic bones
2. Damage from forceps blades or ventouse
3. Difficult manual rotation of the head
4. Rapid compression and relaxation of the forces that act on the fetal head, as in precipitous births

This injury may occur also during normal spontaneous delivery.

Because the hemorrhage is under the periosteum, the swelling is limited to the affected bone and does not cross the suture lines; this is one way of distinguishing it from a caput succedaneum. The swelling appears within a few hours of birth, and since absorption is slow, it takes 6 to 12 weeks to disappear. The blood clots early at the edges and remains fluid to the center. Rarely, ossification takes place in the clot and may cause a permanent deformity of the skull. The health of the child is not affected, and the brain is not damaged.

The prognosis is good. No local treatment is indicated, but observation of the fetus and measurement of the head circumference to ensure that the hematoma is not expanding are appropriate (to differentiate from subgaleal hematoma). Vitamin K may be given to reduce further bleeding. The area should be protected from injury, but no attempt is made to evacuate the blood. Rarely, infection ensues with formation of an abscess that must be drained. The differential diagnosis of caput succedaneum and cephalohematoma includes these criteria:

Caput Succedaneum	Cephalohematoma
Present at birth	May not appear for several hours
Soft; pits on pressure	Soft; does not pit
Diffuse swelling	Sharply circumscribed
Lies over and crosses the sutures	Limited to individual bones; does not cross suture lines
Movable on skull; seeks dependent portions	Fixed to original site
Is largest at birth and immediately begins to grow smaller, disappearing in a few hours	Appears after a few hours, grows larger for a time, and disappears only after weeks or months

Subgaleal Hematoma

A subgaleal hemorrhage or hematoma refers to bleeding in the potential space between the periosteum of the skull and the galea aponeurosis of the scalp. These injuries are more commonly seen as a result of the traction related to vacuum-assisted vaginal delivery. This traction can rupture the connections between dural sinus and scalp veins, leading to an accumulation of blood under the aponeurosis of the scalp muscle superficial to the periosteum. The presence of the rare subgaleal hematoma should alert the clinician to seek other associated complications of head trauma such as intracranial hemorrhage or skull fracture.

Subgaleal hematoma is diagnosed based on a fluctuant boggy mass developing over the scalp and superficial skin bruising. The swelling develops gradually 12 to 72 hours after delivery, although in severe cases, it can be seen more quickly after delivery. The hematoma can slowly spread across the whole head and conceal a large quantity of blood. As such, neonates with subgaleal hemorrhage could descend into hemorrhagic shock.

As opposed to the cephalohematoma, the subgaleal hematoma can cross suture lines, and if enough blood accumulates, a visible fluid wave may be seen. The long-term prognosis is good; management consists of close observation to rule out progression and fluid resuscitation. Transfusion may be required if blood loss is significant, and the fetus should also be monitored for hyperbilirubinemia.

Meningocele

A meningocele is a hernial protrusion of the meninges. It is a serious congenital deformity and must be distinguished from caput succedaneum and cephalohematoma. The meningocele always lies over a suture or a fontanelle and becomes tense when the baby cries.

CHAPTER 7

Fetopelvic Relationships

Glenn D. Posner

Definitions

LIE Relationship of the long axis of the fetus to the long axis of the mother.

PRESENTATION The part of the fetus that lies over the inlet. The three main presentations are cephalic (head first), breech (pelvis first), and shoulder.

PRESENTING PART The most dependent part of the fetus, lying nearest the cervix. During vaginal examination, it is the area with which the finger makes contact first.

ATTITUDE Relationship of fetal parts to each other. The basic attitudes are flexion and extension. The fetal head is in flexion when the chin approaches the chest and in extension when the occiput nears the back. The typical fetal attitude in the uterus is flexion, with the head bent in front of the chest, the arms and legs folded in front of the body, and the back curved forward slightly.

DENOMINATOR An arbitrarily chosen point on the presenting part of the fetus used in describing position. Each presentation has its own denominator (i.e. occiput, sacrum, mentum, frontum).

POSITION Relationship of the denominator to the front, back, or sides of the maternal pelvis.

LIE

The two lies are (1) longitudinal, when the long axes of the fetus and mother are parallel, and (2) transverse, or oblique, when the long axis of the fetus is perpendicular or oblique to the long axis of the mother.

All terms of direction refer to the mother in the standing position. Upper means toward the maternal head, and lower toward the feet. Anterior, posterior, right, and left refer to the mother's front, back, right, and left, respectively.

Longitudinal Lies

Longitudinal lies are grouped into (1) cephalic, when the head comes first, and (2) breech, when the buttocks or lower limbs lead the way (Table 7-1).

TABLE 7-1: FETOPELVIC RELATIONSHIPS ACCORDING TO FETAL POSITION

Presentation	Attitude	Presenting Part	Denominator
Longitudinal lie (99.5%)			
Cephalic (96%-97%)	Flexion	Vertex (posterior part)	Occiput (O)
	Military	Vertex (median part)	Occiput (O)
	Partial extension	Brow	Forehead (frontum) (Fr)
	Complete extension	Face	Chin (mentum) (M)
Breech (3%-4%)			
Complete	Flexed hips and knees	Buttocks	Sacrum (S)
Frank	Flexed hips, extended knees	Buttocks	Sacrum (S)
Footling: single, double	Extended hips and knees	Feet	Sacrum (S)
Kneeling: single, double	Extended hips; flexed knees	Knees	Sacrum (S)
Transverse or oblique lie (0.5%)			
Shoulder	Variable	Shoulder, arm, trunk	Scapula (Sc)

Cephalic Presentations

Cephalic presentations are classified into four main groups, according to the attitude of the fetal head:

1. Flexion is present when the baby's chin is near his or her chest (Fig. 7-1A). The posterior part of the vertex is the presenting part, and the occiput is the denominator

2. The position with neither flexion nor extension is called the military attitude or the median vertex presentation (Fig. 7-1B). The vertex (area between the two fontanelles) presents, and the occiput is the denominator

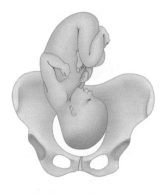

A. Flexion of head.

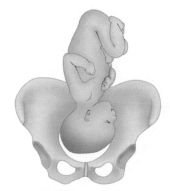

B. Military attitude.

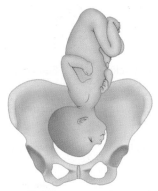

C. Brow presentation, partial extension.

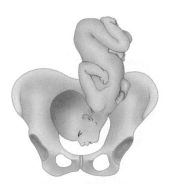

D. Face presentation, complete extension.

FIGURE 7-1. Attitude.

3. In brow presentation (Fig. 7-1C), there is halfway extension. The frontum (forehead) leads the way and is also the denominator
4. When extension is complete, the presenting part is the face (Fig. 7-1D), and the denominator is the mentum (chin)

Breech Presentations

Breech or pelvic presentations are classified according to the attitudes at the hips and knees (Fig. 7-2).

1. The breech is complete when there is flexion at both hips and knees. The buttocks are the presenting part
2. Flexion at the hips and extension at the knees change it to a frank breech. The lower limbs lie anterior to the baby's abdomen. The buttocks lead the way

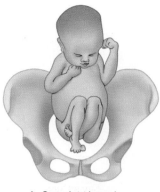

A. Complete breech.

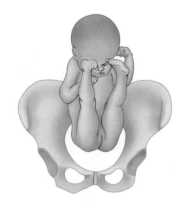

B. Frank breech.

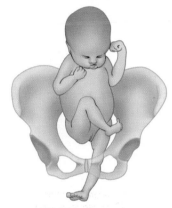

C. Footling breech.

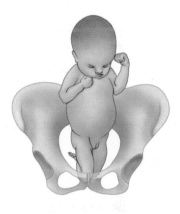

D. Kneeling breech.

FIGURE 7-2. Breech.

3. When there is extension both at the hips and at the knees, it is a footling breech—single if one foot is presenting and double if both feet are down
4. Extension at the hips and flexion at the knees make it a kneeling breech, single or double. Here the knees present

In all variations of breech presentation, the sacrum is the denominator.

Transverse or Oblique Lie

Transverse or oblique lie (Fig. 7-3) exists when the long axis of the fetus is perpendicular or oblique to the long axis of the mother. Most often the shoulder is the presenting part, but it may be an arm or some part of the trunk, such as the back, abdomen, or side. The scapula is the denominator.

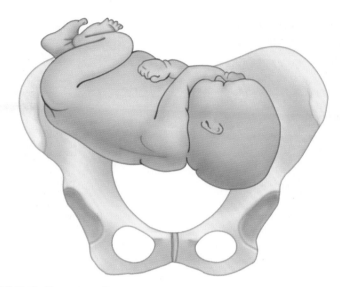

FIGURE 7-3. Transverse lie.

The position is anterior or posterior depending on the situation of the scapulas and right or left according to the location of the head.

POSITION

Position is the relationship of the denominator to the front, back, or sides of the mother's pelvis. The pelvic girdle has a circumference of 360°. The denominator can occupy any part of the circumference. In practice, eight points, 45° from each other, are demarcated, and the position of the fetus is described as the relationship between the denominator and one of these landmarks.

Three sets of terms are used to describe position: (1) the *denominator;* (2) *right* or *left,* depending on which side of the maternal pelvis the denominator is in; and (3) *anterior, posterior,* or *transverse,* according to whether the denominator is in the front, in the back, or at the side of the pelvis.

With the patient lying in the lithotomy position, the pubic symphysis is anterior and the sacrum posterior. Starting at the symphysis and moving in a clockwise direction, eight positions are described in succession, each 45° from the preceding one (Fig. 7-4A).

1. Denominator anterior (DA): The denominator is situated directly under the pubic symphysis
2. Left denominator anterior (LDA): The denominator is in the anterior part of the pelvis, 45° to the left of the midline

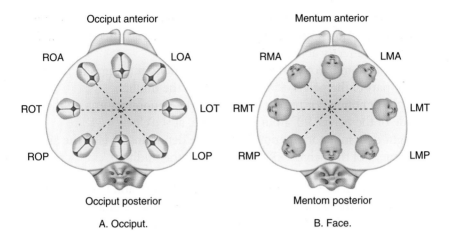

A. Occiput.

B. Face.

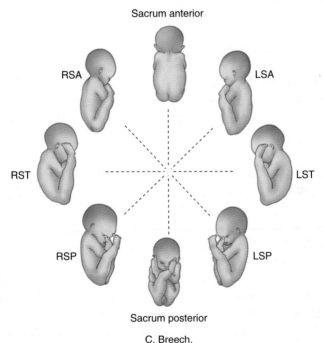

C. Breech.

FIGURE 7-4. Position.

3. Left denominator transverse (LDT): The denominator is on the left side of the pelvis, 90° from the midline, at 3 o'clock

4. Left denominator posterior (LDP): The denominator is now in the posterior segment of the pelvis and is 45° to the left of the midline

5. Denominator posterior (DP): The denominator has rotated a total of 180 and is now in the posterior part of the pelvis, directly in the midline and directly above the sacrum
6. Right denominator posterior (RDP): The denominator is in the posterior part of the pelvis, 45° to the right of the midline
7. Right denominator transverse (RDT): The denominator is on the right side of the pelvis, 90° from the midline, at 9 o'clock
8. Right denominator anterior (RDA): The denominator is in the anterior segment of the pelvis, 45° to the right of the midline

Further rotation of 45° completes the circle of 360°, and the denominator is back under the symphysis pubis in the denominator anterior position.

This method of describing position is used for every presentation. Each presentation has its own denominator, but the basic descriptive terminology is the same.

Figure 7-4A demonstrates the various positions in which the vertex is the presenting part. The occiput (back of the head) is the denominator, and the eight positions (moving clockwise) are OA—LOA—LOT—LOP—OP—ROP—ROT—ROA—OA.

In face presentations (Fig. 7-4B), the chin (mentum) is the denominator, and the sequence of positions is MA—LMA—LMT—LMP—MP—RMP—RMT—RMA—MA.

A further example is in breech presentations in which the sacrum is the denominator (Fig. 7-4C). Here the eight positions are SA—LSA—LST—LSP—SP—RSP—RST—RSA—SA.

CEPHALIC PROMINENCE

The cephalic prominence is produced by flexion or extension (Fig. 7-5). When the head is well flexed, the occiput is lower than the sinciput, and the forehead is the cephalic prominence. When there is extension, the occiput is higher than the sinciput, and the occiput or back of the head is the cephalic prominence. The cephalic prominence can be palpated through the abdomen by placing both hands on the sides of the lower part of the uterus and moving them gently toward the pelvis. When there is a cephalic prominence, the fingers abut against it on that side and on the other side meet little or no resistance. The location of the cephalic prominence aids in diagnosing attitude. When the cephalic prominence and the back are on opposite sides, the attitude is flexion. When the cephalic prominence and the back are on the same side, there is extension. When

CLINICAL ANATOMY

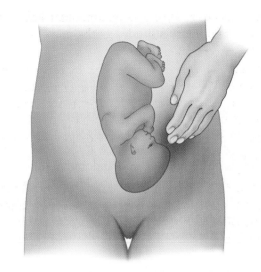

A. Flexion.

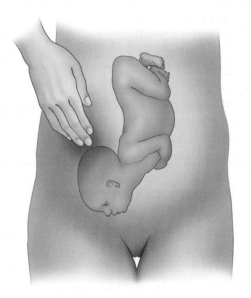

B. Extension.

FIGURE 7-5. **Cephalic prominence.**

no cephalic prominence is palpable, there is neither flexion nor extension, and the head is in the military attitude.

LIGHTENING

Lightening is the subjective sensation felt by the patient as the presenting part descends during the latter weeks of pregnancy. It is not synonymous with engagement, although both may take place at the same time. Lightening is caused by the tonus of the uterine and abdominal muscles and is part of the adaptation of the presenting part to the lower uterine segment and to the pelvis. In the latter weeks of pregnancy, the cervix is taken up and the isthmus becomes part of the lower uterine segment. As this area expands, there is more room in the lower part of the uterus, and the fetus drops into it. Symptoms include:

1. Less dyspnea
2. Decreased epigastric pressure
3. A feeling that the child is lower
4. Increased pressure in the pelvis
5. Low backache
6. Urinary frequency
7. Constipation
8. Initial appearance or aggravation of already present hemorrhoids and varicose veins of the lower limbs
9. Edema of the legs and feet
10. More difficulty in walking

GRAVIDITY AND PARITY

Gravidity

1. A *gravida* is a pregnant woman
2. The word *gravida* refers to a pregnancy regardless of its duration
3. A woman's *gravidity* relates to the total number of her pregnancies regardless of their duration
4. A *primigravida* is a woman pregnant for the first time
5. A *secundagravida* is a woman pregnant for the second time, although this term is rarely used in modern practice
6. A *multigravida* is a woman who has been pregnant several times, although common usage of this term is for a woman who has delivered at least once before

Parity

1. The word *para* alludes to past pregnancies that have reached viability
2. *Parity* refers to the number of past pregnancies that have gone to viability and have been delivered regardless of the number of children involved. (For example, the birth of triplets increases the parity by only one)
3. A *nullipara* is a woman who has never delivered a child who reached viability
4. A *primipara* is a woman who has delivered one pregnancy in which the child has reached viability, without regard to the child's being alive or dead at the time of birth. Alas, the common use of this term is to describe a woman who is pregnant with her first child
5. A *multipara* is a woman who has had two or more pregnancies that terminated at the stage when the children were viable, although this term is often used to describe a parturient who is delivering her second child
6. A *parturient* is a woman in labor

Nomenclature: Gravida and Para

1. A woman pregnant for the first time is a primigravida and is described as gravida 1, para 0
2. If she aborts before viability, she remains gravida 1, para 0. Specifically, she would be gravida 1, para 0, aborta 1
3. If she delivers a fetus who has reached viability, she becomes a primipara, regardless of whether the child is alive or dead. She is now gravida 1, para 1
4. During a second pregnancy, she is gravida 2, para 1
5. After she delivers the second child, she is gravida 2, para 2
6. A patient with two abortions and no viable children is gravida 2, para 0, aborta 2. When she becomes pregnant again, she is gravida 3, para 0, aborta 2. When she delivers a viable child, she is gravida 3, para 1, aborta 2
7. Multiple births do not affect the parity by more than one. A woman who has viable triplets in her first pregnancy is gravida 1, para 1

Nomenclature: The GTPAL System

A different way of describing the patient's obstetrical situation is as follows:

1. G: Gravidity
2. T: Term deliveries
3. P: Preterm deliveries
4. A: Abortions
5. L: Living children

CHAPTER 8

Engagement, Synclitism, Asynclitism

Glenn D. Posner

ENGAGEMENT

When the presenting part of the fetus is entirely out of the pelvis and is freely movable above the inlet, it is said to be floating (Fig. 8-1A).

When the presenting part has passed through the plane of the inlet but engagement has not occurred, it is said to be dipping (Fig. 8-1B).

By definition, engagement (Fig. 8-1C) has taken place when the widest diameter of the presenting part has passed through the inlet. In cephalic presentations, this diameter is the biparietal, between the parietal bosses. In breech presentation, it is the intertrochanteric.

In most women, once the head is engaged, the bony presenting part (not the caput succedaneum) is at or nearly at the level of the ischial spines. Radiologic studies have shown that this relationship is not constant and that in women with deep pelves, the presenting part may be as much as 1 cm above the spines even though engagement has occurred.

The presence or absence of engagement is determined by abdominal or vaginal examination. In primigravidas, engagement usually takes place 2 to 3 weeks before term. In multiparas engagement, engagement may occur any time before or after the onset of labor. Engagement tells us that the pelvic inlet is adequate. It gives no information as to the midpelvis or the outlet. Although failure of engagement in a primigravida is an indication for careful examination to rule out disproportion, abnormal presentation, or some condition blocking the birth canal, it is no cause for alarm. The occurrence of engagement in normal cases is influenced by the tonus of the uterine and abdominal muscles.

STATION

Station is the relationship of the presenting part to an imaginary line drawn between the ischial spines (Fig. 8-2). The location of the buttocks in breech presentations or the bony skull (not the caput succedaneum) in cephalic presentations at the level of the spines indicates that the station is zero. Above the spines, the station is −1, −2, and so forth, depending on how many centimeters above the spines the presenting part is. At spines −5, it is at the inlet. Below the spines, it is +1, +2, and so forth. There are various relationships between station and the progress of labor.

CLINICAL ANATOMY

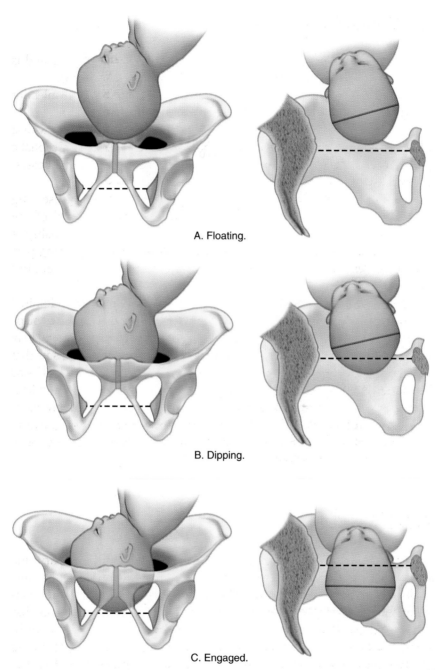

A. Floating.

B. Dipping.

C. Engaged.

FIGURE 8-1. **The process of engagement.**

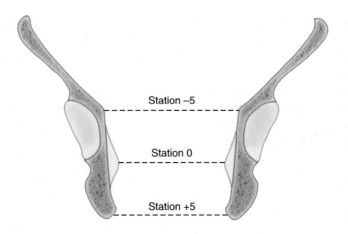

Station –5

Station 0

Station +5

A. Anteroposterior view.

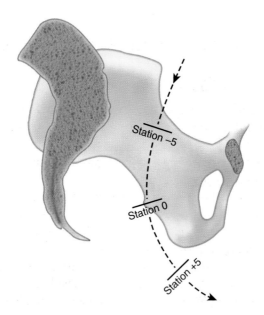

Station –5

Station 0

Station +5

B. Lateral view.

FIGURE 8-2. Station of the presenting part.

1. In nulliparas entering labor with the fetal head well below the spines, further descent is often delayed until the cervix is fully dilated

2. In nulliparas beginning labor with the head deep in the pelvis, descent beyond the spines often takes place during the first stage of labor

3. An unengaged head in a nullipara at the onset of labor may indicate disproportion and warrants investigation. This condition is not rare, however, and in many cases, descent and vaginal delivery take place
4. The incidence of disproportion is more common when the head is high at the onset of labor
5. Patients who start labor with high fetal heads usually have lesser degrees of cervical dilatation. There is a tendency for lower stations to be associated with cervices that are more effaced and dilated, both at the onset of labor and at the beginning of the active phase
6. Other factors being equal, the higher the station, the longer the labor
7. Dysfunctional labor is more frequent when the station is high
8. A high head that descends rapidly is usually not associated with abnormal labor

SYNCLITISM AND ASYNCLITISM

Engagement in Synclitism

In cephalic presentations, engagement has occurred when the biparietal diameter has passed through the inlet of the pelvis. The fetal head engages most frequently with its sagittal suture (the anteroposterior diameter) in the transverse diameter of the pelvis. Left occiput transverse is the most common position at engagement.

When the biparietal diameter of the fetal head is parallel to the planes of the pelvis, the head is in *synclitism*. The sagittal suture is midway between the front and the back of the pelvis. When this relationship does not occur, the head is said to be in *asynclitism*.

Engagement in synclitism takes place when the uterus is perpendicular to the inlet and the pelvis is roomy (Fig. 8-3). The head enters the pelvis with the plane of the biparietal diameter parallel to the plane of the inlet, the sagittal suture lies midway between the pubic symphysis and the sacral promontory, and the parietal bosses enter the pelvis at the same time.

Posterior Asynclitism

In most women, the abdominal wall maintains the pregnant uterus in an upright position and prevents it from lying perpendicular to the plane of the pelvic inlet. As the head approaches the pelvis, the posterior parietal

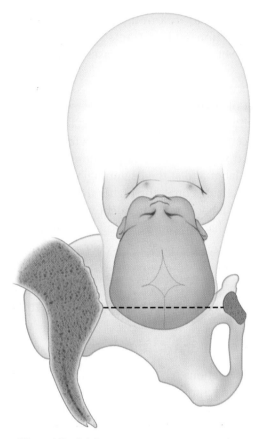

FIGURE 8-3. Synclitism at the inlet.

bone is lower than the anterior parietal bone, the sagittal suture is closer to the symphysis pubis than to the promontory of the sacrum, and the biparietal diameter of the head is in an oblique relationship to the plane of the inlet. This is posterior asynclitism (Fig. 8-4). It is the usual mechanism in normal women and is more common than engagement in synclitism or anterior asynclitism.

As the head enters the pelvis, the posterior parietal bone leads the way, and the posterior parietal boss (eminence) descends past the sacral promontory. At this point, the anterior parietal boss is still above the pubic symphysis and has not entered the pelvis. Uterine contractions force the head downward and into a movement of lateral flexion. The posterior parietal bone pivots against the promontory, the sagittal suture moves posteriorly toward the sacrum, and the anterior parietal boss descends

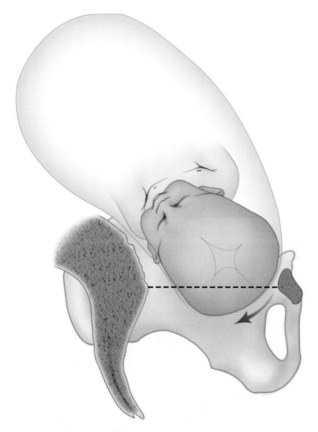

FIGURE 8-4. Posterior asynclitism.

past the symphysis and into the pelvis. This brings the sagittal suture midway between the front and back of the pelvis, and the head is now in synclitism.

Anterior Asynclitism

When the woman's abdominal muscles are lax and the abdomen is pendulous so that the uterus and baby fall forward, or when the pelvis is abnormal and prevents the more common posterior asynclitism, the head enters the pelvis by anterior asynclitism (Fig. 8-5). In this mechanism, the anterior parietal bone descends first, the anterior parietal boss passes by the pubic symphysis into the pelvis, and the sagittal suture lies closer to the sacral promontory than to the pubic symphysis. When the anterior parietal bone becomes relatively fixed behind the symphysis, a movement of lateral

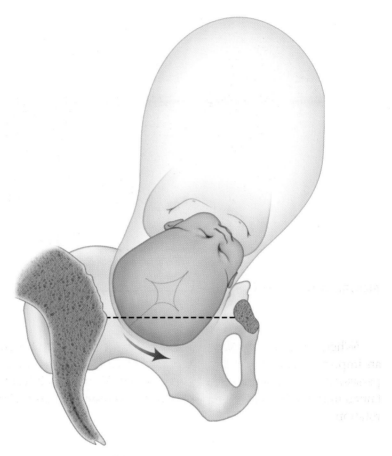

FIGURE 8-5. Anterior asynclitism.

flexion takes place so that the sagittal suture moves anteriorly toward the symphysis and the posterior parietal boss squeezes by the sacral promontory and into the pelvis. The mechanism of engagement in anterior asynclitism is the reverse of that with posterior asynclitism.

There is a mechanical advantage to the head's entering the pelvis in asynclitism. When the two parietal bosses enter the pelvic inlet at the same time (synclitism), the presenting diameter is the biparietal of about 9.5 cm. In asynclitism, the bosses come into the pelvis one at a time, and the diameter is the subsuperparietal of approximately 8.75 cm. Thus, engagement in asynclitism enables a larger head to pass through the inlet than would be possible if the head entered with its biparietal diameter parallel to the plane of the inlet (Fig. 8-6).

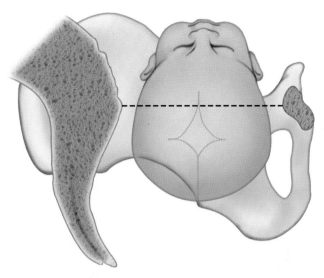

FIGURE 8-6. Synclitism in the pelvis.

Whenever there is a small pelvis or a large head, asynclitism plays an important part in enabling engagement to take place. Marked and persistent asynclitism, however, is abnormal. When asynclitism is maintained until the head is deep in the pelvis, it may prevent normal internal rotation.

PART II

First Stage of Labor

CHAPTER 9

Examination of the Patient

Jessica Dy

Examination of the patient is important before the onset of labor to assess the fetal position with respect to the pelvis. This can be done clinically by abdominal palpation, vaginal examination, or fetal heart auscultation. Sonography can also be used to confirm fetal position in certain cases.

ABDOMINAL INSPECTION AND PALPATION (LEOPOLD'S MANEUVERS)

The position of the baby in utero is determined by inspecting and palpating the mother's abdomen, with these questions in mind:

1. Is the lie longitudinal, transverse, or oblique?
2. What presents at or in the pelvic inlet?
3. Where is the back?
4. Where are the small parts?
5. What is in the uterine fundus?
6. On which side is the cephalic prominence?
7. Has engagement taken place?
8. How high in the abdomen is the uterine fundus?
9. How big is the baby?

The patient lies on her back with the abdomen uncovered (Fig. 9-1). To help relax the abdominal wall muscles, the shoulders are raised a little and the knees are drawn up slightly. If the patient is in labor, the examination is carried out between contractions.

First Maneuver: What Is the Presenting Part?

The examiner stands at the patient's side and grasps the lower uterine segment between the thumb and fingers of one hand to feel the presenting part (Fig. 9-2A). The other hand may be placed on the fundus to steady

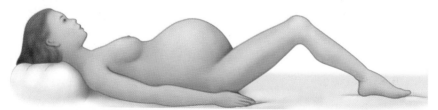

FIGURE 9-1. Position of patient for abdominal palpation.

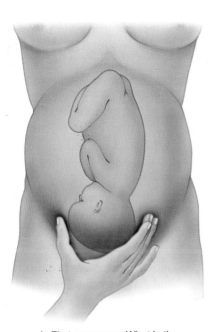

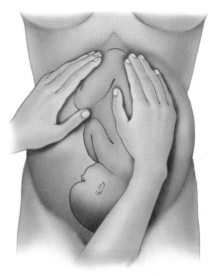

C. Third maneuver: What is in
the fundus?

A. First maneuver: What is the
presenting part?

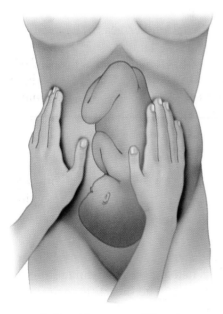

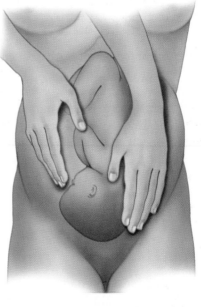

D. Fourth maneuver: What is
the cephalic prominence?

B. Second maneuver: Where is
the back?

FIGURE 9-2. **Abdominal palpation.**

the uterus. This maneuver should be performed first. Since the head is the part of the fetus that can be identified with the most certainty and since it is at or in the pelvis in 90 percent of cases, the logical thing to do first is to look for the head in its most frequent location. Once it has been established that the head is at the inlet, two important facts are known: (1) that the lie is longitudinal and (2) that the presentation is cephalic. An attempt is made to move the head from side to side to see whether it is outside the pelvis and free (floating) or in the pelvis and fixed (engaged). In contrast to the breech position, the head is harder, smoother, more globular, and easier to move. A groove representing the neck may be felt between the head and the shoulders. The head can be moved laterally without an accompanying movement of the body. When the head is in the fundus and when there is sufficient amniotic fluid, the head can be ballotted.

When a floating rubber ball is forced under water, it returns to the surface as soon as it is released; so the fetal head can be pushed posteriorly in the amniotic fluid, but as soon as the pressure on it is relaxed, it rises back and abuts against the examining fingers.

Second Maneuver: Where Is the Back?

The examiner stands at the patient's side facing her head. The hands are placed on the sides of the abdomen using one hand to steady the uterus while the other palpates the fetus (Fig. 9-2B). The location of the back and of the small parts is determined.

The side on which the back is located feels firmer and smoother and forms a gradual convex arch. Resistance to the palpating fingers (as pressure is exerted toward the umbilicus) is even in all regions. On the other side, the resistance to pressure is uneven, the fingers sinking deeper in some areas than they do in others. The discovery of moving limbs is diagnostic.

Third Maneuver: What Is in the Fundus?

The hands are moved up the sides of the uterus and the fundus is palpated (Fig. 9-2C). In most cases, the breech is here. It is a less definite structure than the head and is not identified as easily. The breech is softer, more irregular, less globular, and not as mobile as the head. It is continuous with the back, there being no intervening groove. When the breech is moved laterally, the body moves as well. Finding moving small parts in the vicinity of the breech strengthens the diagnosis.

Fourth Maneuver: Where Is the Cephalic Prominence?

The examiner turns and faces the patient's feet. Gently the fingers are moved down the sides of the uterus toward the pubis (Fig. 9-2D). The cephalic prominence is felt on the side where there is greater resistance to the descent of the fingers into the pelvis. In attitudes of flexion, the forehead is the cephalic prominence. It is on the opposite side from the back. In extension attitudes, the occiput is the cephalic prominence and is on the same side as the back. In addition, it is noted whether the head is free and floating or fixed and engaged.

Relationship of the Head to the Pelvis

1. The floating head lies entirely above the symphysis pubis, so that the examining fingers can be placed between the head and the pubis. The head is freely movable from side to side
2. When the head is engaged, the biparietal diameter has passed the inlet, and only a small part of the head may be palpable above the symphysis. The head is fixed and cannot be moved laterally. Sometimes it is so low in the pelvis that it can barely be felt through the abdomen
3. The head may be midway between the previous two locations. Part of it is felt easily above the symphysis. It is not freely movable but is not fixed; nor is it engaged. The head is described as lying in the brim of the pelvis, or dipping

AUSCULTATION OF FETAL HEART

In most cases, there is a constant relationship between the location of the baby's heart and the fetal position in the uterus. In attitudes of flexion, the fetal heart sound is transmitted through the scapula and the back of the shoulder. It is, therefore, heard loudest in that area of the mother's abdomen to which the fetal back is closest. In attitudes of extension, the fetal heart beat is transmitted through the anterior chest wall of the baby.

In cephalic presentations, the fetal heart beat is loudest below the umbilicus; in anterior positions, it is clearest in one or the other lower quadrant of the mother's abdomen. The relationship of the fetal back and the fetal heart to the midline of the maternal abdomen is similar. As the one comes nearer to or moves away from the midline, so does the other. In posterior positions, the fetal heart is loudest in the maternal flank on the

FIRST STAGE OF LABOR

side to which the back is related. Having the patient lie in a lateral position may bring the fetal heart closer to the midline and can be heard more easily in some women. In breech presentation, the point of maximum intensity of the baby's heart sound is above the umbilicus.

The position of the fetal heart changes with descent and rotation. As the baby descends, so does the fetal heart. The anterior rotation of an occipitoposterior position can be followed by listening to the fetal heart as it moves gradually from the maternal flank toward the midline of the abdomen.

The location of the fetal heart (Fig. 9-3) may be used to check, but should not be relied upon to make, the diagnosis of presentation and position. Occasionally, the point of maximum intensity of the fetal heart beat is not in the expected location for a given position. For example, it is not unusual in breech presentations for the fetal heart to be heard loudest below the umbilicus instead of above it. The diagnosis made by careful abdominal palpation is the more reliable finding. Locating the fetal

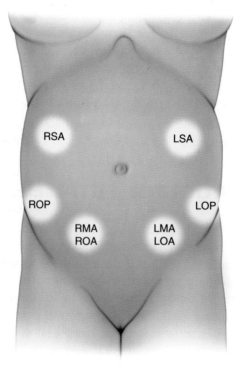

FIGURE 9-3. Location of the fetal heart beat in relation to the various positions. LMA, left mentum anterior; LOA, left occiput anterior; LOP, left occiput posterior; LSA, left sacrum anterior; RMA, right mentum anterior; ROA, right occiput anterior; ROP, right occiput posterior; RSA, right sacrum anterior.

heart sound in an unexpected place is an indication for reexamination by palpation of the position of the infant. If the findings on palpation are confirmed, the locale of the fetal heart tones should be disregarded.

VAGINAL EXAMINATION

Several recent studies demonstrated that there is no greater danger of infection with vaginal than with rectal examination. Points in favor of the vaginal examination in the management of labor are as follows:

1. Vaginal examination is more accurate than rectal examination in determining the condition and dilatation of the cervix. With a dilated cervix, important, accurate information on the station and position of the presenting part and relationship of the fetus to the pelvis can be obtained
2. Vaginal examination takes less time, requires less manipulation, and gives more information than the rectal approach
3. Vaginal examination causes less pain
4. Prolapse of the umbilical cord can be diagnosed early, as can compound presentations
5. Cultures taken during the puerperium from women whose vaginas were sterile on admittance to hospital showed no higher incidence of positive results in those who had vaginal examinations during labor than those who had only rectal evaluations
6. Clinical studies have shown that maternal morbidity is no higher after vaginal than after rectal examinations
7. It is important to remember that a clean or sterile glove is different from the contaminated finger of Semmelweis's time, when doctors went from infected surgical cases to the maternity ward without using aseptic precautions

The examination must be done gently, carefully, thoroughly, and under aseptic conditions. Sterile gloves should be used. We prefer the lithotomy or dorsal position, finding the examination and orientation easier. This is the best position for determining proportion between the presenting part and the pelvis.

Palpation of Cervix

1. Is the cervix soft or hard?
2. Is it thin and effaced or thick and long?

FIRST STAGE OF LABOR

3. Is it anterior or posterior to the fetal head?
4. Is it closed or open/dilated? If it is open, estimate the length of the diameter of the cervical ring (cervical dilatation)

Presentation

1. What is the presentation—breech, cephalic, shoulder, or compound?
2. Is there a caput succedaneum, and is it small or extensive? Is there significant moulding?
3. What is the station? What is the relationship of the presenting part (not the caput succedaneum) to a line between the ischial spines? If it is above the spines, it is −1, −2 or −3 cm. If it is below the spines, it is +1, + 2, or + 3 cm

Position

1. If it is a breech, where is the sacrum? Are the legs flexed or extended?
2. With a cephalic presentation, identify the sagittal suture (Fig. 9-4A). What is its direction? Is it in the anteroposterior, oblique, or transverse diameter of the pelvis?
3. Is the sagittal suture midway between the pubis and the sacrum (synclitism), is it near the sacral promontory (anterior asynclitism), or is it near the pubic symphysis (posterior asynclitism)?
4. Where is the posterior fontanelle (Fig. 9-4B)? (It is Y shaped and has three sutures)
5. Is the bregma right or left, anterior or posterior? (It is diamond shaped and is the meeting point of four sutures [Fig. 9-4C])
6. Is the head in flexion (occiput lower than sinciput) or is there extension (sinciput lower than occiput)?
7. When there is difficulty in identifying the sutures, palpation of an ear (Fig. 9-4D) helps establish the direction of the sagittal suture and thus the anteroposterior diameter of the long axis of the head. The tragus points to the face

Membranes

Feeling the bag of waters is evidence that the membranes are intact. The drainage of fluid, passage of meconium, and palpation of fetal hair indicate that the membranes have ruptured. If membrane rupture is uncertain, a sterile speculum examination should be performed and vaginal fluid examined for the presence of ferning.

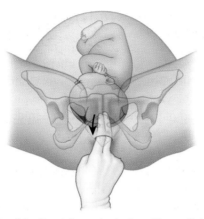

A. Determining the station and palpation of the sagittal suture.

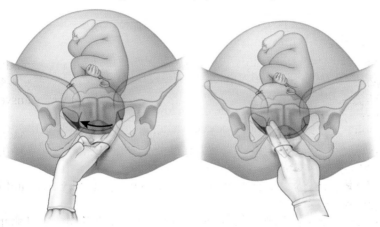

B. Identification of the posterior fontanelle.   C. Identification of the anterior fontanelle.

FIRST STAGE OF LABOR

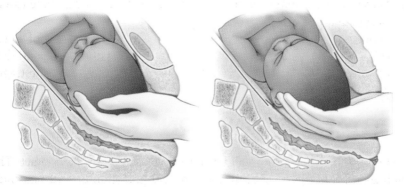

D. Palpation of the posterior ear.

FIGURE 9-4. A–D. Diagnosis of station and position. *(From Douglas and Stromme. Operative Obstetrics, 4th ed., 1982. Courtesy of Appleton-Century-Crofts.)*

General Assessment of Pelvis

1. Can the sacral promontory be reached? The diagonal conjugate can be measured clinically. It extends from the inferior margin of the pubic symphysis to the middle of the sacral promontory, and its average length is 12.5 cm. During the vaginal examination, the promontory is palpated. When the distal end of the finger reaches the middle of the promontory, the point where the proximal part of the finger makes contact with the subpubic angle is marked (Figs. 9-5A, B, and C). The fingers are withdrawn from the vagina, and the distance between these two points is measured. By deducting 1.5 cm from the diagonal conjugate (Fig. 9-5C), the approximate length of the obstetric conjugate can be obtained. In many women, the promontory cannot be reached, and this is accepted as evidence that the anteroposterior diameter of the inlet is adequate. If the promontory can be felt, the obstetric conjugate may be short

2. Is the pelvic brim symmetrical?

3. Are the ischial spines prominent and posterior?

4. Is the sacrum long and straight or short and concave?

5. Are the side walls parallel or convergent?

6. Is the sacrosciatic notch wide or narrow?

7. Is there any bony or soft tissue encroachment into the cavity of the pelvis?

8. How wide is the subpubic angle? The distance between the ischial tuberosities (average, 10.5 cm) can be measured roughly by placing a fist between them (Fig. 9-5D). If this can be done, the transverse diameter of the outlet is considered adequate

9. Are the soft tissues and the perineum relaxed and elastic or hard and rigid?

Fetopelvic Relationship

1. How does the presenting part fit the pelvis?

2. If engagement has not taken place, can the presenting part be pushed into the pelvis by fundal and suprapubic pressure?

3. Does the presenting part ride over the pubic symphysis?

RECTAL EXAMINATION

The course of labor in normally progressing cases was followed by rectal examinations in the past because of fear of an increased risk of ascending infections from multiple vaginal examinations. However, rectal examination is rarely performed today to assess labor progress for the following reasons:

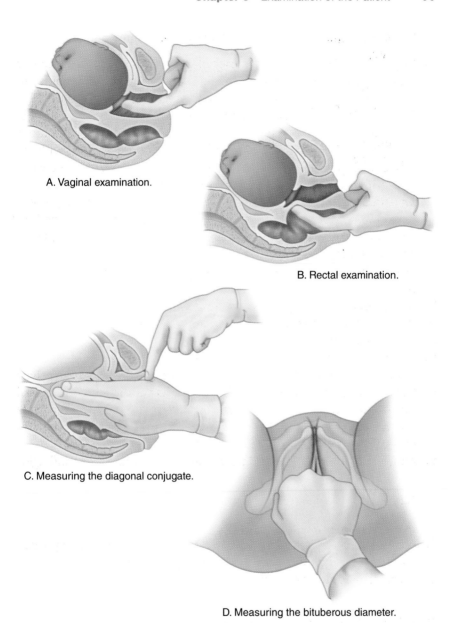

A. Vaginal examination.

B. Rectal examination.

C. Measuring the diagonal conjugate.

D. Measuring the bituberous diameter.

FIGURE 9-5. A–D. Pelvic assessment.

FIRST STAGE OF LABOR

1. It is less accurate than vaginal examination and must not be relied on in problem cases
2. The condition and dilatation of the cervix is often difficult to determine, especially when a bag of waters is present
3. The caput succedaneum may be mistaken for the skull, resulting in erroneous diagnoses of station
4. It is unreliable in breech presentation
5. Rectal examination is painful

CHAPTER 10

Normal Mechanisms of Labor

Jessica Dy

LEFT OCCIPUT ANTERIOR: LOA

LOA is a common longitudinal cephalic presentation (Fig. 10-1). Two-thirds of occiput anterior positions are in the LOA position. The attitude is flexion, the presenting part is the posterior part of the vertex and the posterior fontanelle, and the denominator is the occiput (O).

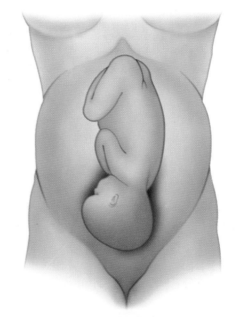

A. Abdominal view.

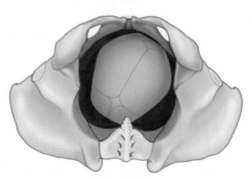

B. Vaginal view.

FIGURE 10-1. Left occiput anterior.

Diagnosis of Position: LOA

Abdominal Examination

1. The lie is longitudinal. The long axis of the fetus is parallel to the long axis of the mother
2. The head is at or in the pelvis
3. The back is on the left and anterior and is palpated easily except in obese women
4. The small parts are on the right and are not felt clearly
5. The breech is in the fundus of the uterus
6. The cephalic prominence (in this case the forehead) is on the right. When the attitude is flexion, the cephalic prominence and the back are on opposite sides. The reverse is true in attitudes of extension

Fetal Heart
The fetal heart is heard loudest in the left lower quadrant of the mother's abdomen. In attitudes of flexion, the fetal heart rate is transmitted through the baby's back. The point of maximum intensity varies with the degree of rotation. As the child's back approaches the midline of the maternal abdomen, so does the point where the fetal heart is heard most strongly. Therefore, in a left anterior position, it is heard below the umbilicus and somewhere to the left of the midline, depending on the exact situation of the back.

Vaginal Examination

1. The station of the head is noted—whether it is above, at, or below the ischial spines
2. If the cervix is dilated, the suture lines and the fontanelles of the baby's head can be felt. In the LOA position, the sagittal suture is in the right oblique diameter of the pelvis
3. The small posterior fontanelle is anterior and to the mother's left
4. The bregma is posterior and to the right
5. Since the head is probably flexed, the occiput is a littler lower than the brow

Normal Mechanism of Labor: LOA

The mechanism of labor as we know it today was described first by William Smellie during the 18th century. It is the way the baby adapts itself to and passes through the maternal pelvis. There are six movements, with considerable overlapping:

FIRST STAGE OF LABOR

1. Descent
2. Flexion
3. Internal rotation
4. Extension
5. Restitution
6. External rotation

The following description is for left anterior positions of the occiput.

Descent

Descent, which includes engagement in the right oblique diameter of the pelvis, continues throughout normal labor as the baby passes through the birth canal. The other movements are superimposed on it. In primigravidas, considerable descent should have taken place before the onset of labor (Figs. 10-2A and B) in the process of engagement, provided there is no disproportion and the lower uterine segment is well formed. In multiparas, engagement may not take place until good labor has set in. Descent is brought about by the downward pressure of the uterine contractions, aided in the second stage by the bearing-down efforts of the patient and to a minimal extent by gravity.

Flexion

Partial flexion exists before the onset of labor since this is the natural attitude of the fetus in utero. Resistance to descent leads to increased flexion. The occiput descends in advance of the sinciput, the posterior fontanelle

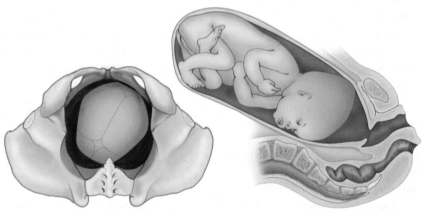

A. Vaginal view.   B. Lateral view.

FIGURE 10-2. Mechanism of labor: left occiput anterior.

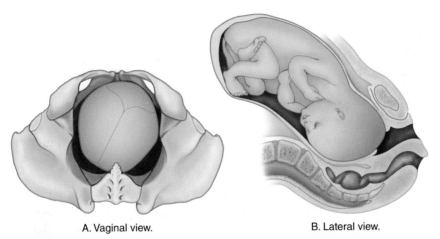

A. Vaginal view.   B. Lateral view.

FIGURE 10-3. **Descent and flexion of the head.**

is lower than the bregma, and the baby's chin approaches his or her chest (Figs. 10-3A and B). This usually takes place at the inlet, but it may not be complete until the presenting part reaches the pelvic floor. The effect of flexion is to change the presenting diameter from the occipitofrontal of 11.0 cm to the smaller and rounder suboccipitobregmatic of 9.5 cm. Since the fit between fetal head and maternal pelvis may be snug, the reduction of 1.5 cm in the presenting diameter is important.

Internal Rotation

In the majority of pelves, the inlet is a transverse oval. The anteroposterior diameter of the midpelvis is a little longer than the transverse diameter. The outlet is an anteroposterior oval, as is the fetal head. The long axis of the fetal head must fit into the long axis of the maternal pelvis. Hence, the head, which entered the pelvis in the transverse or oblique diameter, must rotate internally to the anteroposterior diameter in order to be born. This is the purpose of internal rotation (Fig. 10-4).

The occiput now leads the way to the midpelvis, where it makes contact with the pelvic floor (the levator ani muscles and fascia). Here the occiput rotates 45° to the right (toward the midline). The sagittal suture turns from the right oblique diameter to the anteroposterior diameter of the pelvis: LOA to occiput anterior (OA). The occiput comes to lie near the pubic symphysis and the sinciput near the sacrum.

The head rotates from the right oblique diameter to the anteroposterior diameter of the pelvis. The shoulders, however, remain in the left oblique diameter. Thus, the normal relationship of the long axis of the

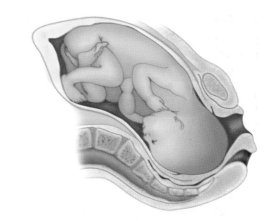

A. Lateral view.

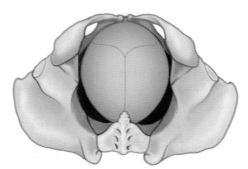

B. Vaginal view.

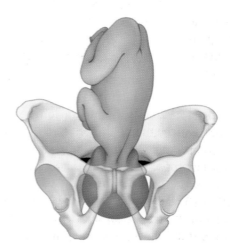

C. Anteroposterior view.

FIGURE 10-4. Internal rotation: left occiput anterior to occiput anterior.

head to the long axis of the shoulders is changed, and the neck undergoes a twist of 45°. This situation is maintained as long as the head is in the pelvis.

We do not know accurately why the fetal head, which entered the pelvis in the transverse or oblique diameter, rotates so that the occiput turns anteriorly in the great majority of cases and posteriorly in so few. One explanation is based on pelvic architecture. Both the bones and the soft tissues play a part. The ischial spines extend into the pelvic cavity. The sidewalls of the pelvis anterior to the spines curve forward, downward, and medially. The pelvic floor, made up of the levator ani muscles and fascia, slopes downward, forward, and medially. The part of the head that reaches the pelvic floor and ischial spines first is rotated anteriorly by these structures. In most cases, the head is well flexed when it reaches the pelvic floor, and the occiput is lower than the sinciput. Hence the occiput strikes the pelvic floor first and is rotated anteriorly under the pubic symphysis.

This does not explain why some well-flexed heads in the left occiput transverse (LOT) and right occiput transverse (ROT) positions (proved by radiography) do not rotate posteriorly. Nor do the theories based on pelvic architecture explain the situation in which, in the same patient, the head rotates anteriorly during one labor and posteriorly in another. In truth, we do not know the exact reasons internal rotation takes place in the way it does. In most labors, internal rotation is complete when the head reaches the pelvic floor or soon after. Early internal rotation is frequent in multiparas and in patients having efficient uterine contractions. Internal rotation takes place mainly during the second stage of labor.

Extension

Extension (Fig. 10-5) is basically the result of two forces: (1) uterine contractions exerting downward pressure and (2) the pelvic floor offering resistance. It must be pointed out that the anterior wall of the pelvis (the pubis) is only 4 to 5 cm long, but the posterior wall (the sacrum) is 10 to 15 cm. Hence, the sinciput has a greater distance to travel than the occiput. As the flexed head continues its descent, there is bulging of the perineum followed by crowning. The occiput passes through the outlet slowly, and the nape of the neck pivots in the subpubic angle. Then by a rapid process of extension, the sinciput sweeps along the sacrum, and the bregma, forehead, nose, mouth, and chin are born in succession over the perineum.

FIRST STAGE OF LABOR

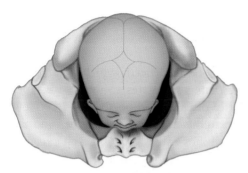

A. Vaginal view.

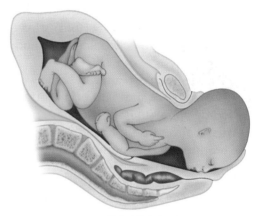

B. Lateral view.

FIGURE 10-5. Extension.

Restitution

When the head reaches the pelvic floor, the shoulders enter the pelvis (Fig. 10-6). Since the shoulders remain in the oblique diameter while the head rotates anteriorly, the neck becomes twisted. Once the head is born and is free of the pelvis, the neck untwists, and the head restitutes back 45° (OA to LOA) to resume the normal relationship with the shoulders and its original position in the pelvis.

External Rotation

External rotation of the head is really the outward manifestation of internal rotation of the shoulders. As the shoulders reach the pelvic floor, the lower anterior shoulder is rotated forward under the symphysis, and the bisacromial diameter turns from the left oblique to the anteroposterior diameter

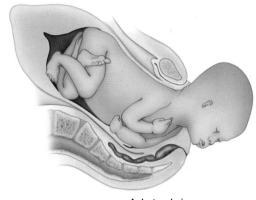

A. Lateral view.

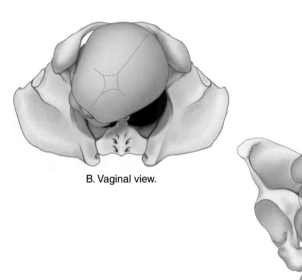

B. Vaginal view.

C. Anteroposterior view.

FIGURE 10-6. Restitution: occiput anterior to left occiput anterior.

of the pelvis. In this way, the long diameter of the shoulders can fit the long diameter of the outlet. The head, which had already restituted 45° to resume its normal relationship to the shoulders, now rotates another 45° to maintain it: LOA to LOT (Fig. 10-7). A summary of the mechanism of labor to this point is seen in Figure 10-8.

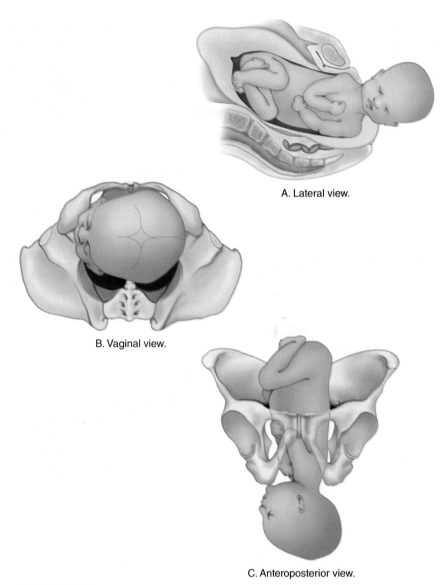

A. Lateral view.

B. Vaginal view.

C. Anteroposterior view.

FIGURE 10-7. **External rotation: left occiput anterior to left occiput transverse.**

Mechanism of the Shoulders

When the head appears at the outlet, the shoulders enter the inlet. They engage in the oblique diameter opposite that of the head. For example, in LOA, when the head engages in the right oblique diameter of the inlet, the shoulders engage in the left oblique.

The uterine contractions and the bearing-down efforts of the mother force the baby downward. The anterior shoulder reaches the pelvic floor first and rotates anteriorly under the symphysis. Anterior rotation of the shoulders takes place in a direction opposite to that of anterior rotation of the head. The anterior shoulder is born under the pubic symphysis

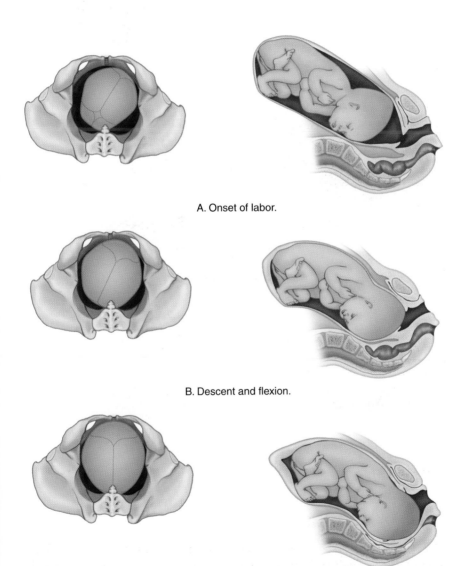

A. Onset of labor.

B. Descent and flexion.

C. Internal rotation: LOA to OA.

FIGURE 10-8. Summary of mechanism of labor: left occiput anterior.

FIRST STAGE OF LABOR

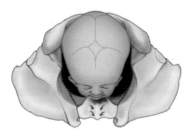 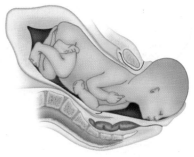

D. Extension.

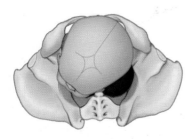 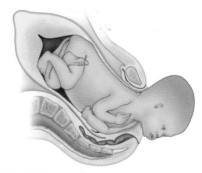

E. Restitution: OA to LOA.

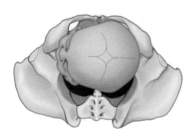 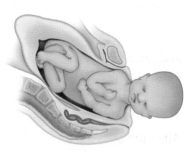

F. External rotation: LOA to LOT.

FIGURE 10-8. (Continued)

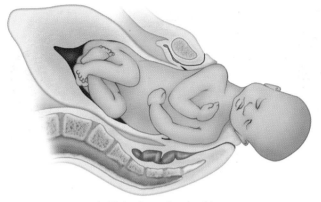

A. Birth of anterior shoulder.

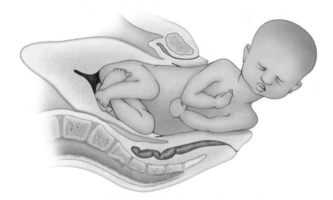

B. Birth of posterior shoulder.

FIGURE 10-9. Delivery of the shoulders.

FIRST STAGE OF LABOR

and pivots there (Fig. 10-9A). Then the posterior shoulder slides over the perineum by a movement of lateral flexion (Fig. 10-9B).

Birth of the Trunk and Extremities

After the shoulders have been born, the rest of the child is delivered by the mother's forcing down, with no special mechanism and with no difficulty.

Moulding

In LOA, the presenting suboccipitobregmatic diameter is diminished, and the head is elongated in the verticomental diameter (Fig. 10-10).

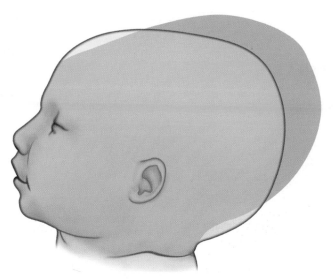

FIGURE 10-10. Moulding.

BIRTH OF THE PLACENTA

Separation of the Placenta

Within a few minutes of delivery of the child, the uterine contractions begin again. Because the fetus is no longer in the uterus, the extent of the retraction of the upper segment is larger than during the first and second stages. This retraction greatly decreases the area where the placenta is attached (Fig. 10-11A). The size of the placenta itself, however, is not reducible. The resultant disparity between the size of the placenta and its area of attachment leads to a cleavage in the spongy layer of the decidua, and in this way, the placenta is separated from the wall of the uterus (Fig. 10-11B). During the process of separation, blood accumulates between the placenta and uterus. When the detachment is complete, the blood is released and gushes from the vagina; some lengthening of the umbilical cord is noted.

Expulsion of the Placenta

Soon after the placenta has separated, it is expelled into the vagina by the uterine contractions. From there, it is delivered by the bearing-down efforts of the patient. Two methods of expulsion have been described. In the Duncan method, the lower edge of the placenta comes out first, with the maternal and fetal surfaces appearing together, and the rest of the

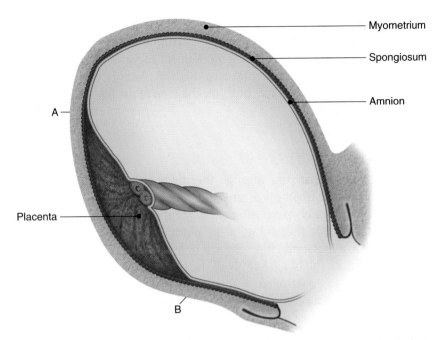

A. Placenta attached to uterine wall.

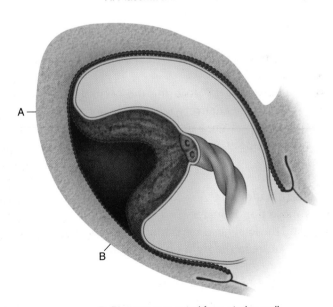

B. Placenta separated from uterine wall.

FIGURE 10-11. Birth of the placenta.

FIRST STAGE OF LABOR

organ slides down. In the Schultze method, the placenta comes out like an inverted umbrella, the shiny fetal side appearing first and the membranes trailing after. Although the Schultze mechanism suggests fundal implantation and the Duncan method intimates that the placenta was attached to the wall of the uterus, the exact birth mechanism of the placenta is of little practical significance.

Control of Hemorrhage

The blood vessels that pass through the myometrium are tortuous and angular. The muscle fibers are arranged in an interlacing network through which the blood vessels pass. After the placenta has separated, retraction leads to a permanent shortening of the uterine muscle fibers. This compresses, kinks, twists, and closes the arterioles and venules in the manner of living ligatures. The blood supply to the placental site is effectively shut off, and bleeding is controlled. If the uterus is atonic and fails to retract properly after separation of the placenta, the vessels are not closed off, and postpartum hemorrhage may take place. It is therefore important to wait for the uterus to retract and the cleavage plane to occur before attempting to deliver the placenta.

CLINICAL COURSE OF LABOR: LOA

Almost always, an LOA turns 45° to bring the occiput under the pubic arch, from where spontaneous delivery takes place. Occasionally, because of minor degrees of disproportion, a rigid perineum, or generalized fatigue, the patient may not be able to complete the second stage. Arrests may take place in two positions:

1. It can occur after rotation to OA is complete, so that the sagittal suture is in the anteroposterior diameter
2. Rotation may fail, the fetal head remaining in the original LOA position with the sagittal suture in the right oblique diameter of the pelvis

Management of arrested occipitoanterior positions consists of the following steps:

1. If rotation to OA has occurred, forceps are applied to the sides of the baby's head, which is then extracted. (See Chapter 25 for details of technique)

2. If rotation has failed, the forceps are applied to the sides of the baby's head. First the head is rotated with the forceps from LOA to OA and then it is extracted. (See Chapter 25 for details of technique)

RIGHT OCCIPUT ANTERIOR: ROA

ROA is less common than LOA. The physical findings and the mechanism of labor are similar but opposite of LOA. The difference lies in the fact that in ROA the occiput and back of the fetus are on the mother's right side, and the small parts are on the left.

FIRST STAGE OF LABOR

CHAPTER 11

Clinical Course
of Normal Labor

Jessica Dy

Definitions

LABOR The physiologic process by which the products of conception (fetus, amniotic fluid, placenta, and membranes) are separated and expelled from the uterus through the vagina into the outside world. It is defined by the presence of regular uterine contractions accompanied by cervical effacement and dilatation and fetal descent.

PRETERM LABOR The onset of labor in a gravid woman whose period of gestation is less than 37 completed weeks (less than 259 days) from the first day of the last menstrual period.

DYSTOCIA Abnormally slow and protracted labor.

EXPECTED DATE OF CONFINEMENT On an average, this is 280 days from the first day of the last menstrual period or 267 days from conception. It is calculated by going back 3 months from the first day of the last menses and adding 7 days (Naegle's rule)

ONSET OF LABOR

Causes of Onset of Labor

Hippocrates' concept that a fetus determines the time of his or her birth has been proven correct in some animals. In humans, however, it appears that the placenta and fetal membranes play the major role in the initiation of labor, while the fetus may modulate the timing of labor. Although the exact cause of and mechanism for labor are not known, evidence is mounting in support of a hormonal basis.

In sheep, it is clear that maturation of the fetal hypothalamo–hypophyseal–adrenal axis during late pregnancy is responsible for initiating labor by inducing changes in the pattern of placental steroid genesis and, ultimately, by increasing the production of intrauterine prostaglandin. Birth can be induced by infusing adrenocorticotropic hormone (ACTH) or glucocorticoids to the fetal lamb in utero before term has been reached. These preterm fetuses are viable and are able to expand their lungs, indicating that the fetal glucocorticoids play a role in pulmonary maturation as well as in parturition. In sheep as in humans, the nature of the stimulus that leads to increased pituitary–adrenal activity in late pregnancy is not known.

At the present time, there is no evidence that human fetuses play the same pivotal role in determining the time they are born as do sheep. The belief that anencephaly and adrenal hypoplasia predispose to prolongation of pregnancy has been challenged. In both humans and monkeys, the administration of glucocorticoids does not bring on labor, nor is there evidence to show that fetal cortisol sets off parturition in humans.

Estrogen

Although some evidence shows that estrogen is involved in human parturition, its mode of action has not been well defined. The placenta is the main source of estrogen biosynthesis in pregnancy. Estrogens upregulate myometrial gap junctions and receptors responsible for myometrial contractions (e.g., calcium channels and oxytocin receptors).

Progesterone

In some animals, progesterone plays a part in maintaining uterine quiescence. In primates, the role of progesterone is unclear. Recent evidence suggests that supplemental progesterone may reduce the risk of preterm birth in select women at risk of preterm labor. On the other hand, administration of progesterone receptor antagonists does not seem to induce labor at term, and progesterone withdrawal does not occur in all women before the spontaneous onset of labor. There is, to the contrary, some evidence that the levels of free progesterone may rise as parturition approaches.

Oxytocin

Maternal serum oxytocin levels do not increase before the onset of spontaneous labor; therefore, it is unlikely that oxytocin provides the trigger for the initiation of human parturition. However, the sensitivity of the uterus to oxytocin increases in late pregnancy mainly because of the 100- to 200-fold increase in the concentration of oxytocin receptors in the myometrium. And with an increase in the pulsatile release of oxytocin as labor progresses, oxytocin during labor results in stronger uterine contractions.

Prostaglandin

Three lines of evidence support the part played by prostaglandin in human parturition: (1) There is an increase in the production of prostaglandin at term. (2) Myometrial contractility and preterm labor can be suppressed by the use of inhibitors of the synthesis of prostaglandin (including cyclooxygenase inhibitors such as indomethacin). (3) Exogenous prostaglandins stimulate the primate uterus to contract. Whether the primary effect of prostaglandin at term is exerted by increased biosynthesis, by increased myometrial sensitivity, or both is not yet known.

FIRST STAGE OF LABOR

Phenomena Preliminary to the Onset of Labor

1. Lightening occurs 2 to 3 weeks before term and is the subjective sensation felt by the mother as the baby settles into the lower uterine segment
2. Engagement takes place 2 to 3 weeks before term in primigravidas
3. Vaginal secretions increase in amount
4. Loss of weight is caused by the excretion of body water
5. The mucous plug is discharged from the cervix
6. Bloody show is noted
7. The cervix becomes soft and effaced
8. Persistent backache is present
9. False labor pains occur with variable frequency

NORMAL UTERINE CONTRACTIONS

Definitions

CONTRACTION The shortening of a muscle in response to stimulus with return to its original length after the contraction has worn off.

RETRACTION The muscle shortens in response to a stimulus but does not return to its original length when the contraction has passed. The muscle becomes fixed at a relatively shorter length, but the tension remains the same. In this way, the slack is taken up, and the walls of the uterus maintain contact with the contents. Retraction is responsible for descent. Without this property, the fetus would move down with the contraction, only to return to the original level once the contraction had ceased. With retraction, on the other hand, the fetus remains at a slightly lower level each time. During contraction, it is as though three steps are taken forward and then three backward. With retraction, three steps are taken forward and then two backward. In this way, a little ground is gained each time. In the control of postpartum bleeding, retraction is essential. Without it, many patients might bleed to death.

PHYSIOLOGIC RETRACTION RING As labor and retraction proceed, the upper part of the uterus becomes progressively shorter and thicker, and the lower portion gets longer and thinner. The boundary between the two segments is the physiologic retraction ring (Fig. 11-1).

PATHOLOGIC RETRACTION RING In cases of obstructed labor, the physiologic ring becomes extreme and is known as the pathologic retraction (Bandl) ring.

CONSTRICTION RING A localized segment of myometrial spasm that grips the fetus tightly and prevents descent.

TONUS The lowest intrauterine (intraamniotic) pressure between contractions. It is expressed in millimeters of mercury (mm Hg). The normal resting tension is 8 to 12 mm Hg.

INTENSITY Also known as amplitude, it is the rise in intrauterine pressure brought about by each contraction. It is measured from the baseline, resting pressure (tonus) rather than from zero. The normal is 30 to 50 mm Hg.

FREQUENCY Caldeyro-Barcia defined this as the number of contractions per 10 minutes. For the patient to be in good labor, the frequency must be at least two contractions per 10 minutes.

UTERINE ACTIVITY The Montevideo unit (MU) was introduced by Caldeyro-Barcia and represents the average intensity of the uterine contractions multiplied by the number of contractions observed during a 10-minute period of monitoring (intensity × frequency). To incorporate the third variation, duration of the contraction, the Alexandria unit (AU) was evolved. It represents the product of the average intensity of the contractions in millimeters of mercury, the frequency of contractions per 10 minutes, and the average duration of the contractions in minutes (intensity × frequency × duration).

FIRST STAGE OF LABOR

Uterine contractions occur spontaneously in patterns that are characteristic of individuals and of various stages of gestation. The frequency, duration, and strength of the myometrial contractions can be estimated by feeling them with a hand placed on the mother's abdomen or by electronic techniques. The latter use either a noninvasive external tocodynamometer that consists of a pressure sensor held in place on the abdomen over a prominent part of the uterus or by an internal method using an open-ended, fluid-filled catheter placed through the cervix into the uterine cavity. The last is the most accurate technique of monitoring uterine contractions.

The recorded curve of a normal uterine contraction is bell shaped. The steep crescentic slope leading to the apex of the curve represents the actual power of the contraction and comprises only one-third of the total contraction. The period of relaxation makes up two-thirds of the process and is shown by a curve that is, initially, a steep decrescentic slope that becomes more horizontal in the last third, reflecting the gradualness of the final stage of relaxation.

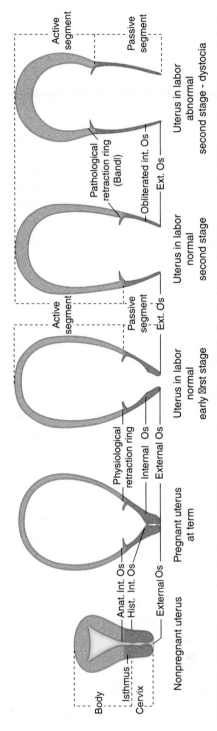

FIGURE 11-1. Progressive development of the segments and rings of the uterus at term. Note the comparison between the nonpregnant uterus, uterus at term, and uterus in labor. The passive segment is derived from the lower uterine segment (isthmus) and cervix; the physiologic retraction ring forms the anatomic internal os. The pathologic ring that forms under abnormal conditions develops from the physiologic ring. *(From Pritchard, MacDonald and Gant Williams Obstetrics, 17th ed., 1985. Courtesy of Appleton-Century-Crofts.)*

Caldeyro-Barcia has published a logical and understandable description of the normal uterine contraction wave.

Triple Descending Gradient of Caldeyro-Barcia

Each contraction wave has three components:

1. *The propagation* of the wave is from above downward. It starts at the pacemaker and works its way to the lower part of the uterus
2. *The duration* of the contraction diminishes progressively as the wave moves away from the pacemaker. During any contraction, the upper portion of the uterus is in action for a longer period of time than the lower
3. *The intensity* of the contraction diminishes from the top to the bottom of the uterus. The upper segment of the uterus contracts more strongly than the lower

For normal labor to take place, all parts of the triple descending gradient must perform properly. The activity of the upper part dominates and is greater than that of the lower part. All parts of the uterus contract, but the upper segment does so more strongly than the lower segment; in turn, the latter's contractions are stronger than those of the cervix. Were this not so, there would be no progress.

The normal contractions are regular and intermittent. There is contraction (systole) and relaxation (diastole). The most efficient uterus is one showing moderately low tonus and strong contractions.

Pacemakers

Normally, there are two, one situated at each uterine end of the fallopian tube. Since one pacemaker is responsible for initiation of a contraction, their activities must be coordinated. In the abnormal uterus, new pacemakers may spring up anywhere in the organ, resulting in incoordinate uterine action.

Propagation

The wave begins at the pacemaker and proceeds downward to the rest of the uterus. A small wave goes up to the fundal portion of the uterus above the level of the pacemaker.

Coordination

Coordination is such that, while the wave begins earlier in some areas than in others, the contraction attains its maximum in the different parts

FIRST STAGE OF LABOR

of the uterus at the same time. The places where the contraction starts later achieve their acme more rapidly. Thus, at the peak of the contraction, the entire uterus is acting as a unit. Relaxation, on the other hand, starts simultaneously in all parts of the uterus. For normal uterine action, there must be good coordination between the two halves of the uterus as well as between the upper and lower segments.

Dilatation of the Cervix

Dilatation of the cervix is caused by two mechanisms:

1. The pressure on the cervix by the presenting part: When this part of the fetus is regular and well fitting (e.g., the flexed head), it favors effective uterine action and smooth cervical dilatation. The bag of waters does not play an important role in helping promote good contractions and rapid cervical opening
2. The longitudinal traction on the cervix by the upper part of the uterus as it contracts and retracts: After each contraction, the upper segment becomes shorter and thicker; the lower uterine segment becomes longer, thinner, and more distended; and the cervix becomes more and more dilated

Cervical dilatation is the result of a gradient of diminishing activity from the fundus through the lower uterine segment.

Round Ligament Contraction

These ligaments contain muscle, and they contract at the same time as the upper segment of the uterus. This anchors the uterus, prevents its ascending in the abdomen, and so helps force down the presenting part.

Uterine Contractions During Pregnancy

Some uterine activity goes on throughout pregnancy. During the first 30 weeks, the frequency and strength of the contractions are low, less than 20 Montevideo units.

After 30 weeks and especially after 35 weeks, the contractions become more frequent and may be noticed by the patient. Sometimes they are painful and are called false labor pains. Prelabor, as evidenced in the increasing activity of the uterus during the later weeks of pregnancy, is an integral part of the process of evacuating the human uterus. The contractions of this period are associated with steadily increasing uterine activity, cervical ripening, and general readiness for true labor (Braxton Hicks contractions). Prelabor merges into clinically recognizable labor by such small degrees that the exact point at which so-called true labor begins is difficult to determine.

PAIN OF LABOR

Pain during labor is related to contractions of the uterus. In normal labor, the pain is intermittent. It starts as the uterus contracts, becomes more severe as the contraction reaches its peak, and disappears when the uterus relaxes. The degree of pain varies in different patients, in the same patient during succeeding labors, and at different stages in the same labor. In some cases, the contractions are painless.

Causes

1. Distention of the lower pole of the uterus
2. Stretching of the ligaments adjacent to the uterus
3. Pressure on or stretching of the nerve ganglia around the uterus
4. Contractions of the muscle while it is in a relatively ischemic state (similar to angina pectoris). This occurs especially when the uterine tonus is too high or when the contractions are too frequent and last too long. Adequate amounts of blood do not get to the muscles, and they become hypoxic

Pain in the Lower Abdomen
Pain in the lower abdomen seems to be related to activity in the upper uterine segment and is present during efficient labor.

Pain in the Back
Pain in the back is related to tension in the lower uterus segment and the cervix. In normal labor, back pain is prominent only at the start of a contraction and in the early stages of cervical dilatation. When the cervix is abnormally resistant, the backache is severe. Backache is prominent also in posterior positions. In general, the less the backache, the more efficient the uterus.

FIRST STAGE OF LABOR

Pain in the Incoordinate Uterus

1. An excessive amount of pain is felt in the back
2. Because of persistent high tonus or spasm in some parts of the uterus, the pain seems to be present even in the intervals between contractions
3. The patient complains of pain before the uterus is felt to harden, and the pain persists even after the uterus relaxes

TRUE AND FALSE LABOR

Signs of True Labor

1. Uterine contractions occur at regular intervals. Coming every 20 or 30 minutes at the beginning, the contractions get closer together and occur every 3 to 5 minutes in the active phase. As labor proceeds, the contractions increase in duration and severity
2. The uterine systoles are painful
3. Hardening of the uterus is palpable
4. Pain is felt both in the back and in the front of the abdomen
5. True labor is effective in shortening and dilating the cervix
6. The presenting part descends
7. Bulging of the membranes is a frequent result

False Labor Pains

False labor pains are inefficient contractions of the uterus that usually last only a few seconds. They appear a few days to 1 month before term. Usually they start on their own. They are irregular and short and are felt more in the front than in the back. The uterus does not become stony hard and can be indented with the finger. These contractions are inefficient in pushing down the presenting part and do not bring about progressive effacement and dilatation of the cervix.

False labor pains can have the harmful effect of tiring the patient, so that when true labor does begin, she is in poor condition, both mentally and physically. The treatment is directed to the cause if there is one, or the physician can prescribe efficient analgesia that stops the false labor pains but does not interfere with true labor. It is also important to ensure that the patient has adequate hydration and rest. Appropriate sedatives may be given judiciously to allow the patient to have some rest before the onset of true labor.

TRUE LABOR	FALSE LABOR
Pains at regular intervals	Irregular
Intervals gradually shorten	No change and inconsistent
Duration and severity increase	No change and inconsistent
Pain starts in back and moves to front	Pain mainly in front
Walking increases the intensity	No change
Association between the degree of uterine hardening and intensity of pain	No relationship
Bloody show often present	No show
Cervix effaced and dilated	No change in cervix
Descent of presenting part	No descent
Head is fixed between pains	Head remains free
Sedation does not stop true labor	Efficient sedative stops false labor pains

The strength of the uterine contractions can be estimated clinically by using the criteria shown in Table 11-1.

TABLE 11-1: STRENGTH OF UTERINE CONTRACTIONS

	Frequency	Duration	Indentibility of Uterus
Good	Every 2-3 min	45-60 sec	None
Fair	Every 4-5 min	30-45 sec	Slight
Poor	Every 6+ min	<30 sec	Easy

STAGES OF LABOR

First Stage. From the onset of true labor to complete dilatation of the cervix. It lasts 6 to 18 hours in a nulliparous woman and 2 to 10 hours in parous women.

FIRST STAGE OF LABOR

Second Stage. From complete dilatation of the cervix to the birth of the baby. It takes 30 minutes to 3 hours in a nulliparous woman and 5 to 30 minutes in a parous woman. The median duration is slightly under 20 minutes in multiparas and just under 50 minutes for nulliparous women.

Third Stage. From the birth of the baby to delivery of the placenta. It takes 5 to 30 minutes.

Fourth Stage. From the birth of the placenta to 1 hour postpartum.

First Stage of Labor

The first stage of labor lasts from the onset of true labor to full dilatation of the cervix. The contractions are intermittent and painful, and the uterine hardening is felt easily by a hand on the abdomen. The pains become more frequent and more severe as labor proceeds. As a rule, they begin in the back and pass to the front of the abdomen and the upper thighs.

Effacement and Dilatation of the Cervix

During most of pregnancy, the cervix uteri is about 3.0 to 4.0 cm in length and closed. Toward the end of the period of gestation, progressive changes occur in the cervix, including softening, effacement (shortening), dilatation, and movement from a posterior to an anterior position in the vagina. The internal os starts to disappear as the cervical canal becomes part of the lower segment of the uterus. The extent to which these changes have taken place correlates with the proximity of the onset of labor and with the success of attempts to induce labor.

Ideally, the cervix should be ripe at the onset of labor. A ripe cervix (1) is soft, (2) is less than 1.3 cm in length or 80% effaced, (3) admits a finger easily, and (4) is dilatable. The presence of a ripe cervix is one indication that the uterus is ready to begin labor. During labor, the cervix shortens further, and the external os dilates. When the cervix has opened enough (average, 10 cm) to permit passage of the fetal head, it is described as being fully dilated (Fig. 11-2).

Ripening of the cervix is a gradual process that merges into labor. The rigid collagen bundles rearrange themselves in a more flexible pattern so that the fibers are able to slide over each other more freely. During pregnancy, this process takes place gradually, resulting in softening, shortening, and partial dilatation of the cervix. These changes may begin as

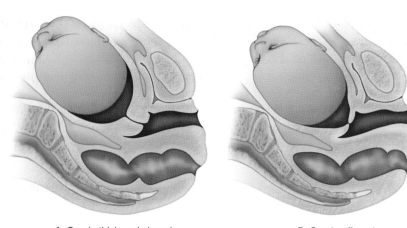

A. Cervix thick and closed.   B. Cervix effaced.

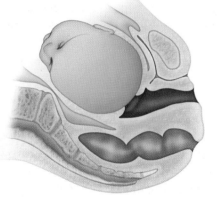

C. Cervix effaced and dilated 2 to 3 cm.

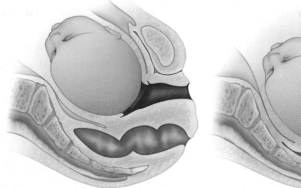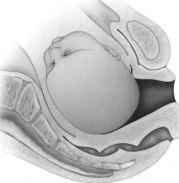

D. Cervix half open.   E. Cervix fully dilated and retracted.

FIGURE 11-2. Dilatation of the cervix.

FIRST STAGE OF LABOR

early as the 24th to 28th week of pregnancy. The mechanisms that control cervical ripening are not well understood, but they are linked with those that control parturition. Factors that play a part include Braxton Hicks contractions (usually painless) of the uterus pulling on the cervix and hormones such as estrogen, progesterone, relaxin, oxytocin, and prostaglandin.

The changes in the cervix during pregnancy can be correlated to the time of onset of labor. Women whose cervices ripen early are likely to begin labor before 40 weeks. When the cervix remains unripe until late in pregnancy, prolongation of the gestation past 40 weeks is common.

Phases of the First Stage of Labor

The Latent Phase. The onset of the latent phase of the first stage of labor is difficult to accurately define because it begins when the patient first perceives strong, regular uterine contractions. The rate of cervical change is slow and gradual during this phase (Fig. 11-3). However, the contractions are becoming coordinated, stronger, polarized, and more efficient. At the same time, the cervix is becoming softer, pliable, and more elastic. The average latent phase lasts 8.6 hours in nulliparas and 5.3 hours in multiparas (Table 11-2). The normal latent phase does not exceed 20 hours in the former and 14 hours in the latter. Patients who enter labor with a ripe cervix have a shorter latent phase than those whose cervix is unripe.

The Active Phase. The diagnosis of the onset of the active phase requires an assessment of both uterine contractions and cervical changes. The dilatation of the cervix usually has reached 3 to 4 cm for nulliparas and 4 to 5 cm for multiparas. Although there may be no great change in the uterine contractions, the cervix has undergone important alterations that make

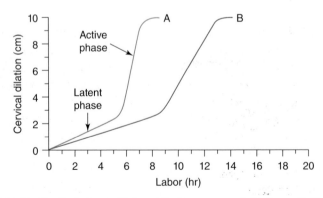

FIGURE 11-3. The first stage of labor: Friedman curve. A, Multipara. **B,** Nullipara.

TABLE 11-2: LENGTHS OF THE PHASES OF LABOR

	Nulliparas		Multiparas	
	Average	Upper Normal	Average	Upper Normal
Latent phase	8.6 hr	20 hr	5.3 hr	14 hr
Active phase	5.8 hr	12 hr	2.5 hr	6 hr
First stage of labor	13.3 hr	28.5 hr	7.5 hr	20 hr
Second stage labor	57 min	2.5 hr	18 min	50 min
Rate of cervical dilatation during active phase	1.2 cm/hr	0.5 cm/hr	1.5 cm/hr	0.8 cm/hr

it more responsive, and cervical dilatation proceeds more rapidly at this time. The average length of the active phase is 5.8 hours in nulliparas and 2.5 hours in multiparas, with the upper limits of normal being 12 and 6 hours, respectively (Table 11-2).

The mean and upper limits of the duration of the different stages of labor were established by Friedman in the early 1950s. More recent data suggest that the upper limit of a normal active phase may be longer and rate of cervical dilatation slower than those set by Friedman. In these studies, only half of nulliparous women in the active phase of the first stage of labor dilated at a rate greater than 1.2 cm/hr. These studies suggest that labor progress in low-risk nulliparous women who enter labor spontaneously at a rate greater than 0.5 cm/hr should be considered normal. *With the more frequent use of regional anesthesia and an older obstetric population with higher maternal body mass index, these time parameters should only be used as a guideline.*

Descent of the Presenting Part. During the latent and early active phase of cervical dilatation, fetal descent may be minimal. When the phase of rapid cervical dilatation has begun, steady fetal descent usually begins. The greatest degree of descent takes place when the cervix nears full dilatation and in the second stage of labor. When descent begins, it should be progressive. Descent of less than 1 cm/hr in nulliparas and 2 cm/hr in multiparas is abnormal, and investigation is indicated (see Chapter 16).

Bag of Waters: Amniotic Membranes

The fetus lies in a sac with an inner layer of amnion and an outer covering of chorion. The sac is filled with the amniotic fluid. As labor proceeds and

FIRST STAGE OF LABOR

the internal os becomes effaced and opens, the membranes separate from the lower uterine segment. The lower pole of the membranes bulges a little with each contraction and may adopt various shapes:

1. The protruding part may have the shape of a watch glass (Fig. 11-4A) containing a small amount of amniotic fluid. This is called the forewaters
2. In other cases, the membranes point into the cervix like a cone (Fig. 11-4B)

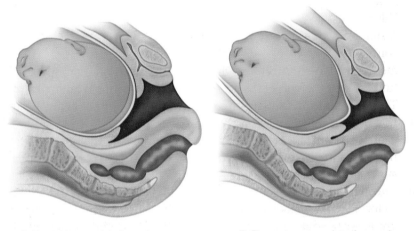

A. Forewaters: watchglass shape.   B. Forewaters: cone into the cervix.

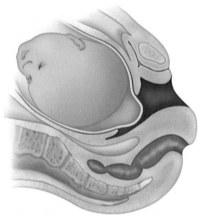

C. Bag of waters in the vagina.   D. No forewaters.

FIGURE 11-4. **The membranes.**

3. Still again, the bag may hang into the vagina (Fig. 11-4C)
4. In some cases, the membranes are applied so tightly to the fetal head that no bag forms (Fig. 11-4D)

Frequently, the membranes rupture near the end of the second stage, but this event can take place at any time during or before labor. When the membranes rupture, the fluid may come away with a gush or may dribble away. On occasion, it is difficult to know whether the membranes are ruptured or intact. Methods of determining whether the bag of waters has ruptured include:

1. Observation of the escape of fluid from the vagina spontaneously or as a result of manual pressure on the fundus of the uterus or simple Valsalva maneuvers
2. A sterile speculum in the vagina and directly observing amniotic fluid coming out from the cervical canal is the best method for confirming membrane rupture. The amount may be increased by pressure on the fundus of the uterus or by Valsalva maneuvers
3. The passage of meconium
4. Use of Nitrazine paper to determine the pH of the vaginal fluid. The vagina, normally acidic, becomes neutral or alkaline when contaminated with alkaline amniotic fluid. Hence, an alkaline pH in the vagina suggests that the membranes are ruptured
5. The arborization test depends on the property of dried amniotic fluid to form crystals in an arborization pattern. A few drops of vaginal fluid are aspirated from the vagina by a bulb syringe and are placed on a clean, dry glass slide. After waiting 5 to 7 minutes for drying to take place, the slide is examined under a low-power microscope for identification of the arborization (or ferning) pattern
6. The AmniSure test is a commercially available kit that detects trace amounts of placental alpha macroglobulin-1 protein in vaginal fluid with high sensitivity and specificity for membrane rupture. It is a relatively expensive test but may aid in diagnosing membrane rupture in difficult cases

A bag of waters that hangs into the vagina is of little or no help in dilating the cervix; it may impede labor by filling the vagina and preventing descent of the fetal head. The intact bag of amniotic fluid does little to help labor progress. In normal cases after the membranes have ruptured (spontaneously or artificially), the uterine contractions are more efficient, and labor progresses faster. Routine amniotomy, however, does not accelerate spontaneous labor. Amniotomy should be avoided in women with known vasa previa, active genital Herpes Simplex or untreated HIV infection.

FIRST STAGE OF LABOR

Indications for amniotomy include:

1. Atypical or abnormal fetal heart rate
2. To detect the presence of meconium
3. To facilitate the use of an internal scalp electrode or an internal intrauterine pressure catheter
4. To induce or augment labor

Several conditions should be present before amniotomy is performed to improve likelihood of a normal vaginal birth:

1. Labor is in progress, as indicated by presence of regular uterine contractions and observed changes in the cervix
2. The cervix is at least 3 cm dilated and effaced
3. The head is fixed in the pelvis and applied to the cervix
4. The patient does not have active genital herpes simplex virus infection or have a high HIV viral load

Passage of Meconium in Cephalic Presentations

The passage per vagina of meconium or meconium-stained amniotic fluid when the fetal presentation is cephalic may be a sign of fetal distress. It is believed to result from relaxation of the rectal sphincter and increased peristalsis as a consequence of fetal hypoxia. However, the passage of meconium may represent nothing more than fetal maturity. In most cases, no cause is found.

The incidence of meconium staining is around 5 percent. The occurrence of stillbirth when this is the only sign is low, but the number of newborns requiring resuscitation is higher than the overall incidence.

When meconium is passed, the fetal heart must be observed closely, preferably by continuous external fetal monitoring. Should there be a significant alteration in the rate and rhythm of the fetal heart, immediate delivery may be needed to save the child. Operative delivery is not indicated on the basis of meconium staining alone, however.

In breech presentations the passage of meconium is caused by pressure of the uterine contractions on the fetal intestines and is not accepted as a sign of anoxia or fetal distress.

Management of the First Stage of Labor

1. As long as the patient is healthy, the presentation normal, the presenting part engaged, and the fetus in good condition, the parturient may walk about, sit in a chair, shower or bathe in a tub, or may be in bed,

as she wishes. Women who are ambulatory, have frequent positional changes, and adopt a more upright position (e.g., sitting, standing, kneeling, squatting) have a shorter first stage of labor. There is also less need for analgesia and for augmentation of labor with oxytocin in women who are ambulatory during labor compared with those who remain in bed. Women should be encouraged to ambulate and to adopt whatever position they find most comfortable throughout labor

2. Continuous close supportive care should be given to the laboring patient. Appropriate support during labor may reduce the need for analgesia and decrease the rate of operative delivery. The patient should receive continual reassurance, frequent encouragement, and judicious use of analgesia

3. Breathing and relaxation techniques to help the patient cope with pain in labor should be encouraged. Such relaxation helps the patient rest, assists her in keeping control, and accelerates the progress of labor. Laboring in water is recommended for pain relief. When the pains are severe, inhalational, intramuscular, intravenous, or regional analgesia may be given, depending on the progress of labor and maternal and fetal well-being. Since there is a limit to the amount of opioids that can be administered without harming the baby or interfering with labor, these must be given in logical dosage and sequence (see Chapter 36)

4. During the first stage, the patient is impressed continually with the importance of relaxing with the contractions. Bearing down must be avoided because it does nothing to improve progress. Bearing down comes into its own use when the cervix is fully dilated and not before. During the first stage, it has only bad effects:

   a. It delays cervical dilatation and can make the cervix edematous
   b. It tires the patient needlessly
   c. It forces down the uterus and stretches the supporting ligaments, predisposing to later prolapse

5. Adequate amounts of fluid and nourishment are essential. In most normal labors, isotonic drinks or clear soups can be taken by mouth. A light diet may be given in established labor. However, since solid foods remain in the stomach during labor, tend to be vomited, and increase the danger of aspiration pneumonitis, they should be avoided if the risk of a general anesthetic is high. If the patient is unable to take enough fluids orally, an intravenous infusion of crystalloid solution is given

FIRST STAGE OF LABOR

6. Although an intravenous crystalloid infusion should not be used routinely in normal labor, it should be considered in certain situations for the following reasons:

   a. Fluids and nourishment can be given without provoking emesis. A woman who cannot take adequate fluids by mouth or who is nauseated or vomiting can be maintained in a state of good hydration

   b. Analgesics in small amounts can be administered for rapid effect. Fluid preloading is also recommended if regional anesthesia is to be used to avoid hypotension

   c. When uterine action is inefficient, oxytocin added to the intravenous solution improves labor

   d. When there is excessive bleeding in the third or fourth stages, oxytocic agents can be given quickly

   e. Blood and plasma expanders may be infused without delay

   f. When hypotension has occurred, the veins often collapse, and it is difficult to insert a needle. Having an infusion already underway obviates this problem

7. The patient's condition and progress is checked periodically. The pulse, temperature, and blood pressure are measured every 4 hours or more often if necessary

8. The fetal heart should be auscultated for a minimum of 1 minute every 15 minutes in the active phase of the first stage of labor and every 5 minutes in the active second stage of labor. These should be done immediately after a contraction. If the fetal heart is abnormal by auscultation, continuous electronic fetal monitoring should be considered (see Chapter 12)

9. The progress of labor is followed by abdominal and vaginal examination to note the position of the baby, station of the presenting part, and dilatation of the cervix. A partogram should be started when a patient enters the active phase of labor. Vaginal examinations should be done at one to four hourly intervals and should be done only often enough to ensure safe conduct of labor. Routine hourly examinations should be discouraged in the first stage of labor when labor is progressing normally

10. Artificial rupture of membranes (amniotomy). Many physicians perform amniotomy as soon as patients are admitted to the hospital in well-established labor. However, evidence shows that routine

amniotomy does not accelerate spontaneous labor and may cause more harm when performed in certain conditions

a. Advantages of amniotomy:
  i. It enables the condition of the amniotic fluid to be observed, especially the presence or absence of meconium
  ii. When continuous fetal heart rate monitoring is indicated, the electrode can be placed directly on the fetal scalp, providing a better tracing than is obtained by an electrode on the mother's abdomen
  iii. A recording catheter can be placed inside the uterus and can measure intrauterine pressure directly and accurately
  iv. It may shorten the duration of labor when performed in the setting of dysfunctional labor. It is believed that the better application of the fetal head to the cervix improves the pattern of dilatation and that direct pressure on the cervix leads to improved uterine contractions by reflex action
b. Disadvantages of amniotomy:
  i. The reduction in the amount of amniotic fluid may increase compression of the umbilical cord and result in transient reduced blood flow to the fetus and abnormal fetal heart rate patterns
  ii. There may be a slight increase in the risk of cesarean section
  iii. There may be a risk of umbilical cord prolapse if performed when the presenting part is not well applied against the cervix or in cases of unstable lie of the fetus

11. Proper hygiene measures should be implemented when caring for women in labor. Standard hand hygiene practices and single use non-sterile gloves are appropriate to reduce cross-contamination among women, babies, and health care professionals

12. Enemas should not be routinely given to the patient when she is admitted to the labor ward. Studies have shown that giving an enema made no difference in labor progress or in the incidence of fecal contamination. Many women object to having an enema

13. Overdistention of the bladder is obviated by urging the patient to pass urine every few hours. Occasionally, catheterization may be necessary if epidural analgesia is in place. The distensible part of the bladder is largely abdominal during the active phase of labor, and it is rare for a full bladder to interfere with progress in a normal case.

FIRST STAGE OF LABOR

Since catheterization does not improve the progress of labor and does increase the risk of infection, it should be carried out only when absolutely necessary

Second Stage of Labor

The second stage of labor lasts from the end of the first stage, when the cervix has reached full dilatation, to the birth of the baby. As the patient passes through the end of the first stage and into the second stage, the contractions become more frequent and are accompanied by some of the worst pain of the whole labor. After the second stage has been achieved, the discomfort is less (see Chapter 16).

Third Stage of Labor

Delivery of the placenta occurs in two stages: (1) separation of the placenta from the wall of the uterus and into the lower uterine segment and/or the vagina and (2) actual expulsion of the placenta out of the birth canal (see Chapter 19).

Fourth Stage of Labor

The patient is kept in the delivery suite for 1 hour postpartum under close observation. She is checked for bleeding, the blood pressure is measured, and the pulse is counted. The third stage and the hour after delivery are more dangerous to the mother than any other time.

Before the doctor leaves the patient, he or she must do the following:

1. Feel the uterus through the abdomen to be sure it is firm and not filling with blood
2. Look at the perineum and vagina to see that any lacerations have been repaired adequately and that there is no hemorrhage
3. See that the mother's vital signs are normal and that she is in good condition
4. Examine the baby to be certain that he or she is breathing well and that the color and tone are normal

SELECTED READING

Atwood RJ: Parturitional posture and related birth behaviour. Acta Obstet Gynecol Scand (Suppl) 57, 1976

Challis JRG, Mitchell BF: Hormonal control of preterm and term parturition. Semin Perinatal 5:192, 1981

Drover JW, Casper RF: Initiation of parturition in humans. Can Med Assoc J 128:387, 1983

Kenepp NB, Kumar S, Shelley WC, et al: Fetal and neonatal hazards of maternal hydration with 5% dextrose before cesarean section. Lancet 1:1150, 1982

Kerr-Wilson RH, Parham GP, Orr JW Jr: The effect of a full bladder on labor. Obstet Gynecol 62:319, 1983

Mendiola J, Grylack LJ, Scanlon JW: Effects of intrapartum maternal glucose infusion on the normal fetus and newborn. Anesth Analg 6:32, 1982

Neal JL, Lowe NK, et al: "Active labor" duration and dilation rates among low risk, nulliparous women with spontaneous labor onset: A systematic review. J Midwifery Womens Health 55: 308-318, 2010.

Shepherd JH, Knuppel RA: The role of prostaglandins in ripening the cervix and inducing labor. Clin Perinatol 8:49, 1981

Stewart P, Kennedy JH, Calder AA: Spontaneous labour: When should the membranes be ruptured? Br J Obstet Gynaecol 89:39, 1982

Tita AT, Rouse DJ: Progesterone for preterm birth prevention: an evolving intervention. Am J Obstet Gynecol 200:219, 2009

Smyth RM, Alldred SK, Markham C: Amniotomy for shortening spontaneous labour. Cochrane Database Syst Rev(4):CD006167, 2007

Zhang J, Landy HJ, Branch DW, et al. Contemporary patterns of spontaneous labor with normal neonatal outcomes. Obstet Gynecol 116:1281, 2010

FIRST STAGE OF LABOR

CHAPTER 12

Fetal Health Surveillance in Labor

Darine El-Chaar

INDICATIONS FOR FETAL ASSESSMENT

There are numerous situations in which it is important to ascertain both the maturity and the health of the fetus while it is still in utero. Among these are the following:

During Pregnancy

Patients at Risk for Uteroplacental Insufficiency

1. Diabetes mellitus
2. Hypertension and preeclampsia
3. Renal disease
4. Previous stillbirth
5. Intrauterine growth restriction, suspected
6. Postterm pregnancy (over 42 weeks)
7. Isoimmunization
8. Preterm premature rupture of membranes
9. Multiple gestation
10. History of placental abruption
11. Chronic abruption
12. Maternal obesity
13. Abnormal maternal serum screening in the absence of fetal anomaly
14. Oligohydramnios or polyhydramnios

Obstetric Reasons

1. Previous cesarean section

2. When induction of labor is necessary
   a. In the interests of the mother
   b. In the interests of the fetus

During Labor

Obstetric Reasons

1. Clinically detected abnormalities of the fetal heart rate (FHR)
2. Passage of meconium

3. Oxytocin stimulation of labor
4. Preterm labor
5. Slow progress in labor
6. Abnormal presentation

DETERMINATION OF FETAL HEALTH: ANTEPARTUM

In North America, antenatal and intrapartum deaths are rare. The reduction in the perinatal mortality rate has been achieved largely by the decrease in the rate of neonatal death. The prevention of fetal death represents a major therapeutic goal, and is the reason for antepartum fetal surveillance.

Biochemical assessment of the fetus has largely been replaced by biophysical and biometric evaluation. Fetal biophysical activities are initiated, modulated, and regulated by mechanisms of the central nervous system (CNS). A fetus compromised by hypoxia demonstrates one or both of the following changes:

1. A decrease or cessation of biophysical activity
2. A significant reduction in the volume of amniotic fluid that becomes evident as oligohydramnios on sonography

The fetal CNS is exquisitely sensitive to changes in PO_2. Hypoxia and its resultant metabolic acidosis produce pathologic CNS depression with changes in biophysical activity. Any biophysical response, however, has its own inherent periodicity and circadian (diurnal) rhythm. Hence, the absence of a given biophysical event may reflect physiologic periodicity, and a normal "sleep state" in a fetus must be differentiated from the comatose state of hypoxic CNS depression.

The important principle in antepartum testing, regardless of the method used, is that a normal test result is reliable in indicating present fetal well-being and is an accurate predictor of a good outcome. However, the diagnosis of fetal jeopardy, based on a single absent or abnormal biophysical event, is frequently inaccurate. Hence, in any scheme of antepartum testing, the goal must be to reduce and, if possible, eliminate the incidence of falsely positive results. This is achieved by increasing the period of observation for any single biophysical event and/or using multiple observations. The demonstration of several biophysical activities showing a normal pattern collectively negates a single abnormal result.

FIRST STAGE OF LABOR

Fetal Movement

Fetal movement, first perceived by the mother at 16 to 20 weeks' gestation, may be recorded subjectively or objectively using active or passive techniques. Fetal movements are not random phenomena. Rather, they are regulated and modulated by complex CNS mechanisms and reflexes. They occur in cyclic periods or in epochs associated and integrated with respiratory, cardiac, behavioral, and "sleep" cycles. The acceleration of the FHR, which occurs after certain fetal movements, provides the basis of the nonstress test (NST). Movements lasting more than 3 seconds elicit FHR accelerations 99.8 percent of the time. Movements of lesser duration rarely do so.

It is well established that reduced fetal activity may be a good predictor of fetal compromise. The significance of fetal movement counting should be discussed with all healthy pregnant women to be aware of in the third trimester. It is the only antenatal surveillance technique recommended for all pregnant women regardless of the presence or absence of risk factors. There is no evidence that fetal movement counting increases maternal stress or anxiety.

In pregnancies at high risk for adverse perinatal outcome, daily fetal movement monitoring should be initiated from 26 to 32 weeks. In healthy pregnancies with no risk factors, fetal movement counting becomes more important in the third trimester. In these low-risk pregnancies, fetal movement count should be initiated when the woman perceives decreased movements.

Counting Methods

1. The "count to 10" method: In this simple method the patient counts fetal movements starting at 9 AM. After 10 movements are perceived, the counting comes to an end. This routine is carried on daily, and the patient is asked to alert her physician if:

   a. Fewer than 10 movements occur after 12 hours on 2 successive days or

   b. No movements are perceived after 12 hours in a single day. In such a situation, an NST should be performed

   In most pregnancies, 10 movements are perceived within 1 hour of counting

2. Ideally, counting fetal movements should be over a shorter period of time. This is more convenient for women to do on a daily basis. Recent

recommendations propose counting fetal movements until six. If the six movements are not reached in a period of 2 hours, the woman should seek medical attention for further antenatal testing

Fetal activity may be decreased in late pregnancy but only slightly in a normal fetus. The possible reasons for the reduction in fetal movement at this time include decreasing amounts of amniotic fluid and the larger fetus having less room to move in the uterus. It could also be related to sleep states, which are thought to occur for longer periods in mature fetuses. Finally, sedatives and drugs that produce autonomic blockade reduce fetal activity.

Nonstress Test

This test is performed in patients who are not in labor. It uses the observation that the occurrence of accelerations of the FHR in response to fetal movement or a uterine contraction is a reliable indicator of current healthy fetal well-being.

Advantages

1. There are no contraindications and no complications
2. The test is simple, inexpensive, and takes less time than a contraction stress test or a biophysical profile
3. It can be used in an office setting and provides an immediate answer
4. Performance of the test requires no special expertise

Indications

1. Patients at risk for uteroplacental insufficiency (see previous section of this chapter)
2. The absence of normal fetal movements

Instrumentation and Technique

1. An FHR tracing is obtained using external ultrasonography for at least 20 minutes
2. The recording is obtained with the patient in the lateral recumbent position or with a lateral tilt so as to avoid supine hypotension. The uterus should be relaxed, and it is recommended that the woman have an empty bladder before testing

Frequency of Testing

1. Weekly testing is indicated and adequate in most conditions

2. The test must be repeated immediately if any change in the clinical condition of the mother or fetus occurs

3. Certain conditions may require twice-weekly testing:

    a. Maternal diabetes
    b. Postterm pregnancy
    c. Fetal growth retardation with oligohydramnios
    d. Maternal hypertension requiring medications

Timing of Testing

In most patients, testing is instituted at 32 to 34 weeks of gestation. In selected cases, such as poor past obstetric performance or specific high-risk condition in the current pregnancy, testing may begin at 26 to 28 weeks. At this time, many fetuses may show atypical or abnormal (previously called *nonreactive*) patterns because of immaturity, and the significance of the test is questionable. However, the finding of a normal (previously called *reactive*) pattern in early gestation has a reassuring value.

Classification

1. Normal NST result

    a. The presence of two or more accelerations of the FHR in a 20-minute period of observation (Fig. 12-1)
        i. Each acceleration with fetal movement must be of amplitude >15 beats per minute (bpm) and of duration >15 seconds
    b. The baseline FHR
        i. Is within the normal range of 110 to 160 bpm
    c. There is moderate FHR variability of 6 to 26 bpm
    d. There are no periodic decelerations. An occasional variable below 30 sec is acceptable

2. Atypical NST result

    a. Fewer than two accelerations meeting criteria have occurred in 40 to 80 minutes
    b. The occurrence of variable decelerations lasting 30 to 60 seconds in duration

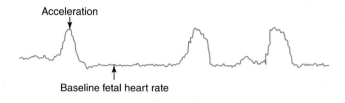

Acceleration

Baseline fetal heart rate

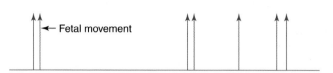

Fetal movement

FIGURE 12-1. Normal nonstress test. Showing accelerations of fetal heart rate with fetal movement. Amplitude more than 15 bpm, duration longer than 15 seconds.

  c. The baseline FHR:
    i. Is within 100 to 110 bpm
    ii. Is over 160 bpm for <30 minutes
    iii. Has a rising baseline
  d. There is absent or minimal FHR variability of 5 bpm or less for 40 to 80 minutes

3. Abnormal NST result

  a. Fewer than two accelerations meeting criteria have occurred in >80 minutes
  b. The occurrence of variable decelerations lasting >60 seconds in duration or the occurrence of late deceleration(s)
  c. The baseline FHR
    i. Bradycardia <100 bpm
    ii. Tachycardia >160 bpm for >30 minutes
    iii. Erratic baseline
  d. There is absent or minimal FHR variability ≤5 bpm for >80 minutes. There is high fetal heart variability (>25 bpm) >10 minutes or a sinusoidal FHR pattern

Significance of the Nonstress Test

1. Normal nonstress test result: The normal (reactive) NST result is a reliable indicator of present fetal health. The risk of fetal death within 1 week of a reactive pattern is only 3.2 per 1000. Hence, the test is highly sensitive, with a falsely negative rate (normal test, abnormal fetus) of less than 0.5 percent

2. Atypical nonstress test result: An atypical pattern may be caused by the following:

   a. Hypoxia
   b. Effects of drugs
      i. Sedative or tranquilizing agents
      ii. Parasympatholytic drugs (e.g., atropine)
      iii. Sympatholytic drugs (beta-blockers)
   c. Fetal immaturity
   d. Fetal sleep cycle

   In contrast to the reliability of the normal NST, the false-positive (abnormal test, normal fetus) rate of an atypical NST is high. This is, almost certainly, a reflection of the normal periodicity of the function of the fetal CNS. Hence, an atypical NST result, defined as above, requires either prolonged observation or repeated testing. The primary care provider should be made aware of this to initiate further assessment as needed

3. Abnormal nonstress test result: This can be caused by the same reasons described above in atypical NST. This tracing requires urgent action, with an assessment of the situation, and further investigation by ultrasound or biophysical profile is warranted. This may also be an indication for immediate delivery

Other Methods of Antenatal Fetal Assessment

In certain pregnancies with risk factors for adverse perinatal outcomes, further antenatal assessment of fetal well-being may be indicated. Where facilities and expertise exist, this may include measurement of the biophysical profile, uterine artery Doppler, and umbilical artery Doppler through ultrasonography (see Chapter 37).

DETERMINATION OF FETAL HEALTH: INTRAPARTUM

Intermittent Auscultation of Fetal Heart

Intermittent auscultation using handheld devices such as fetoscope or Doppler of the fetal heart beat is the recommended method of fetal surveillance in labor in healthy women, without obstetric risk factors.

In the first stage of labor, the fetal heart is auscultated every 15 minutes to 30 minutes for at least 30 seconds, immediately after a uterine contraction. Ideally, listening for a 60-second period for auscultation improves accuracy, but 30-second periods are more feasible. In the second stage of labor, auscultation is performed every 5 minutes.

Intermittent FHR auscultation is an acceptable method of assessing the fetal condition in women at low risk for intrapartum fetal distress. Interpretation of auscultated FHR data must be done on the basis of an understanding of the relationship between changes in the FHR and the uterine contractions. To achieve excellence with this method, an almost one-to-one relationship is necessary between the patient and an experienced nurse. Auscultation of the FHR every 1 to 2 hours, seen frequently on a busy obstetric service, is inadequate observation of the laboring patient.

Advantages of Intermittent Auscultation

This technique is not expensive, is less invasive, and has increased freedom of movement for the patient.

Disadvantages of Intermittent Auscultation

1. It is not continuous, and variable or prolonged decelerations may be missed
2. The proper categorization of a deceleration in relationship to uterine contractions cannot often be made
3. Studies show that intermittent auscultation is of no value in diagnosing early fetal distress
4. Fetal heart rate variability, which is the most important component of the FHR record in the assessment of fetal status, cannot be evaluated
5. There is no permanent record to allow for the progressive analysis or retrospective evaluation. This may be of medicolegal importance
6. It may be difficult to auscultate FHR in more obese patients

Uterine Activity Recording

Technique

1. External: An external tocodynamometer or pressure transducer is placed on the abdominal wall. Semiquantitative recordings are obtained, which do not actually reflect intrauterine pressure. However, they do indicate when the contractions begin, peak, and end. The advantage of this method is that it is noninvasive

FIRST STAGE OF LABOR

2. Internal: A transcervical intrauterine catheter, connected to a strain gauge transducer, is used to obtain direct pressure measurements, which are recorded on the second channel of the apparatus. Insertion of the intrauterine pressure catheter has been attended by rare, occasional complications. The reported incidence of uterine perforation ranges from one per 1400 to one per 376 monitored cases

Indications for Internal Uterine Pressure Catheter

1. Patients with a previous cesarean section undergoing a trial of labor. Sudden loss of uterine pressure will be the first sign of uterine rupture in these cases
2. In obstructed labor, the assessment of the strength of uterine contractions may be helpful in ruling out uterine inertia. It is useful to monitor the strength of uterine contractions more accurately when augmentation of labor with oxytocin is used
3. Useful to monitor contractions in obese patients, given the difficulty to palpate or pick up contractions externally in this setting

Terminology

1. Normal: ≤5 contractions in 10 minutes, averaged over 30 minutes
2. Tachysystole: >5 contractions in 10 minutes, averaged over 30 minutes

Continuous Electronic FHR Recording

The FHR is modulated by reflex neurogenic mechanisms. A normal rate and variability of the FHR indicates an intact fetal CNS with normal cardiac responsiveness. Changes in the fetal PO_2 produce alterations in the CNS. Biochemical changes (metabolic acidosis), through their effect on the CNS, ultimately produce hemodynamic alterations. The clinical use of continuous electronic FHR monitoring is based on the assumption that there is metabolic evidence of asphyxia and hemodynamic change before permanent neurologic damage occurs.

All conventional FHR monitors provide a continuous record of the rate derived from serial calculations of instantaneous or beat-to-beat heart rate. A counter processes each consecutive pair of cardiac signals and measures the elapsed time between each beat. The reciprocal of this beat-to-beat interval is used to calculate the instantaneous heart rate required to produce that time interval. This is then printed out on the FHR record in beats per minute. As the interval of each cardiac cycle changes with varying neurogenic input, the instantaneous heart rate, as recorded by the monitor, changes constantly. This allows evaluation of intrinsic variability within the heart rate signal as well as the baseline rate.

The Role of Continuous FHR Monitoring

Continuous bioelectronic FHR monitoring was developed to improve the predictive accuracy of intermittent auscultation. At present, bioelectronic fetal monitoring during labor is a widely used and clinically accepted technique. As with most fetal assessment methods, the incidence of false-negative results is extremely low. Great care in the interpretation of abnormal tracings must be exercised, however, in order to reduce the incidence of false-positive results. Failure to do this will lead to an increased incidence of interference and unnecessary cesarean sections. A proper understanding of the physiologic and pathologic basis of FHR changes allows knowledgeable physicians to make effective use of electronic monitoring. Some institutions use adjunctive fetal scalp pH estimations in an attempt to reduce the errors of the fetal monitoring. As better understanding of the significance of changes in the FHR develops, the need for fetal scalp blood sampling is reduced. Careful attention to the entire FHR record and the assessment of the degree of FHR variability allows for accurate and reliable assessment of immediate fetal status.

Indications for Continuous FHR Monitoring

1. Clinically detected abnormalities of the FHR
2. Meconium in the amniotic fluid
3. Oxytocin stimulation of labor
4. Premature labor
5. Slow progress in labor
6. Abnormal presentation
7. Patients at risk for uteroplacental insufficiency

Methods of Recording

1. Internal or direct: With this technique, an electrode is applied to the fetal scalp or buttocks by means of which a fetal electrocardiogram signal is obtained

   a. Advantages:
      i. Accurate
      ii. Helpful in monitoring obese patients
   b. Disadvantages:
      i. Invasive
      ii. Abscess of the scalp is a rare and usually benign complication. The lesions are single and localized in most cases. They are more

common after prolonged labor and an extended period of monitoring of the fetal heart. In most instances, spontaneous evacuation takes place after local treatment. Occasionally, incision and drainage is needed. Rarely, parenteral antibiotics are given

2. External or indirect: A fetal heart tracing is obtained by using a Doppler ultrasonic technique. The transducer is applied to the mother's abdomen. In Doppler ultrasound detection of fetal cardiac motion, a transducer of ultrasound crystals directs a broad ultrasound beam toward the fetal heart. Continuous or repetitive bursts of ultrasound energy are emitted from the crystal, which serves both as a transmitter and a receiver for ultrasound energy. Moving cardiac structures produce a Doppler shift in reflected frequencies. The fastest moving objects, usually the cardiac valves, produce the greatest Doppler shift and the greatest increase in frequency. These changes in frequency are detected by the ultrasound crystal and converted to an electronic signal. This signal is measured by the cardiotachometer, which calculates an instantaneous heart rate from measuring the time interval between two heart beats

   a. Advantages:
      i. Noninvasive
      ii. Suitable in patient with intact membranes or closed cervix
      iii. Allows for antepartum monitoring
   b. Disadvantages:
      i. High level of artifact
      ii. May artificially increase the variation in instantaneous heart rate and give an erroneous interpretation of FHR variability
      iii. Need for readjustment with maternal or fetal movement
      iv. Difficult to obtain clear tracing in obese women and in polyhydramnios

Components of the FHR Tracing

1. Baseline fetal heart rate

2. Baseline variability

3. Periodic changes:
   a. Accelerations
   b. Decelerations

Baseline FHR

The baseline FHR is the average rate observed when the patient is not in labor or between uterine contractions.

Definitions

1. Normal range: 110 to 160 bpm

2. Tachycardia

   a. Atypical: >160 bpm for >30 minutes to <80 minutes
   b. Abnormal: >160 bpm for >80 minutes

3. Baseline bradycardia

   a. Atypical: 100 to 110 bpm
   b. Abnormal: <100 bpm

The baseline FHR decreases with advancing gestational age, reflecting increased parasympathetic control. The baseline FHR is the least sensitive indicator of the degree of fetal oxygenation, and a compromised fetus could have a normal baseline rate. On the other hand, changes in the baseline rate should be considered as indicating asphyxia until it has been ruled out by other evidence. In cases of asphyxia, changes in the baseline rate are usually accompanied by late or variable decelerations and decreased beat-to-beat variability. By definition, to be accepted as a baseline change, the alteration in the FHR must be sustained for longer than 10 minutes.

Tachycardia. *Tachycardia* is defined as a rate over 160 bpm. It reflects increased adrenergic tone with decreased vagal input. Tachycardia is usually accompanied by some decrease in heart rate variability.

1. Causes of tachycardia

   a. Fetal hypoxia
   b. Fetal anemia
   c. Fetal cardiac failure
   d. Fetal tachyarrhythmia
   e. Prematurity
   f. Maternal fever (and therefore elevated fetal temperature)
   g. Maternal anxiety
   h. Maternal or fetal hyperthyroidism

FIRST STAGE OF LABOR

   i. Chorioamnionitis

   j. Parasympatholytic drugs (atropine, Atarax, phenothiazines)

   k. Betamimetic drugs (ritodrine, salbutamol, isoxsuprine)

2. Outcome

   a. The outcome is good if decelerations are absent and FHR variability is normal

   b. The outcome is poor if decelerations, with or without a decrease in FHR variability, are present

     Tachycardia alone is not a good indicator of fetal infection or asphyxia. It may, however, be an early sign of hypoxia and indicates fetal distress when accompanied by periodic changes and absent variability. There is some evidence that, in postterm fetuses, fetal distress is manifest as a tachycardia with loss of variability. These changes may precede fetal death without the appearance of late or variable decelerations.

Bradycardia. An FHR less than 110 bpm is defined as bradycardia. Any bradycardia in the presence of good heart rate variability is usually benign. Bradycardias must be distinguished from prolonged decelerations (periodic bradycardia) because the significance and subsequent management are different in the two situations.

1. Causes of bradycardia:

   a. Asphyxia (usually a late sign)

   b. Physiologic

   c. Arrhythmia

   d. Drug effect

   e. Maternal hypotension

   f. Maternal position

   g. Congenital heart block (maternal systemic lupus erythematous)

   h. Umbilical cord compression

   i. Fetal vagal response in cephalic presentations

2. Outcome: Fetal bradycardia is a late sign of fetal distress when:

   a. Variability and accelerations are absent

   b. There are periodic decelerations. However, in a severely compromised fetus, late decelerations may be absent because the fetus is so acidotic that it can neither accelerate nor decelerate its heart rate

Baseline Variability of the FHR

In the normal FHR, there is a beat-to-beat variation of 6 to 25 bpm. A minor baseline irregularity is normal and indicates that the CNS is functioning normally and is capable of controlling the FHR (Fig. 12-2A).

In predicting the immediate status of the fetus, variability of the baseline FHR is a most significant parameter. Moderate variability is good indicator of normal fetal acid–base balance. Loss of variability indicates that the fetus may have hypoxia and acidosis and correlates well with the measurement of the pH of blood obtained from the fetal scalp antepartum and the cord blood postpartum.

Fetal heart variability may be divided into four types:

Absent: undetectable change in amplitude
Minimal: ≤5 bpm in range
Moderate: range of 6 to 25 bpm
High: >25 bpm in range

1. Changes in variability

   a. Marked or high variability: If the high variability (>25 bpm) is over 10 minutes, then the FHR tracing is abnormal. There are several possible explanations:
      i. Mild fetal hypoxia. High variability is one of the early FHR signs of a decrease in fetal oxygenation
      ii. Fetal hemorrhage. In this case, there is usually an accompanying tachycardia. A Kleihauer test on maternal blood will reveal fetal red blood cells. Assessment of the hematocrit from a scalp sample will show anemia
      iii. Vulnerable cord syndrome. This results from the compression of an umbilical cord made vulnerable by shortening or oligohydramnios
   b. Absent or minimal variability: A tracing is atypical if variability is ≤5 bpm for 40 to 80 minutes. A tracing becomes abnormal when the variability is <5 bpm for >80 minutes. Decreased variability is caused by several factors:
      i. Fetal hypoxia. This is the most serious situation
      ii. Physiologic sleep cycle. In labor, this lasts 20 to 40 minutes
      iii. Central nervous system–depressing drugs
      iv. Parasympatholytic drugs cause decreased variability and tachycardia
      v. Sympatholytic drugs lead to decreased variability and bradycardia

FIRST STAGE OF LABOR

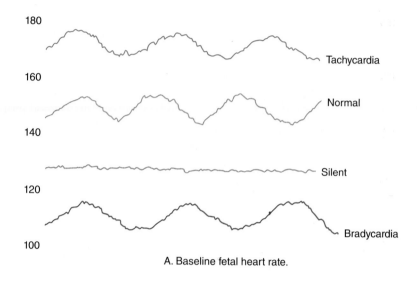

180

160

140

120

100

Tachycardia

Normal

Silent

Bradycardia

A. Baseline fetal heart rate.

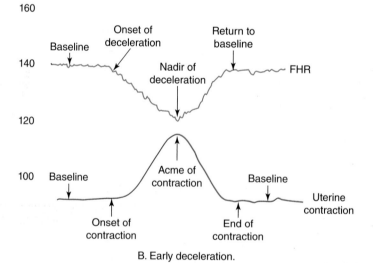

180

160

140

120

100

Baseline

Onset of
deceleration

Return to
baseline

Nadir of
deceleration

FHR

Baseline

Acme of
contraction

Onset of
contraction

Baseline

End of
contraction

Uterine
contraction

B. Early deceleration.

FIGURE 12-2. **Fetal heart rate (FHR) patterns.**

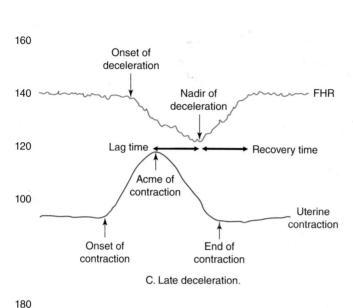

C. Late deceleration.

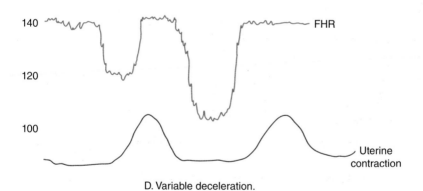

D. Variable deceleration.

FIGURE 12-2. (*Continued*)

2. Interpretation: When absent or minimal variability is the result of hypoxia, there are, in most cases, periodic changes (decelerations) in the FHR with or without a change in the baseline rate. Decreased variability occurs during fetal sleep, and if the tracing is normal in other respects, no action need be taken. Normal variability will return either spontaneously or after stimulation of the fetus

A difficult pattern to evaluate is one in which the baseline rate is persistently flat but the FHR is within the normal range and there are no abnormal periodic changes. Possible causes include:

a. Congenital anomalies of the heart or CNS
b. Prematurity
c. Previous hypoxia
d. Some cases are idiopathic, and no etiologic factor is identifiable. Estimation of fetal pH from a sample of scalp blood should be performed before active treatment is instituted

Poor or absent variability may not show up on tracings from an external monitor. Therefore, in problem cases, a scalp electrode should be applied so a more accurate assessment can be made. However, absence of variability, demonstrated by the external monitor, is significant because the true variability is never more than that displayed on the external monitor.

Periodic Changes in the FHR

Accelerations. These occur most commonly in the antepartum period, in early labor, and along with variable decelerations. The acceleration is a change of 15 bpm or greater above the baseline lasting over 15 seconds but less than 2 minutes. Atypical FHR tracing have an absence of acceleration despite fetal scalp stimulation. Abnormal FHR tracings usually have absent accelerations.

There are two possible physiologic mechanisms for accelerations:

1. They represent an intact CNS in a state of arousal, indicating a healthy fetus
2. Partial cord occlusion results in compression of the umbilical vein while the umbilical artery remains patent. This causes decreased fetal cardiac output and fetal hypotension. Hypotension elicits a baroreceptor response, resulting in an FHR acceleration. Hence, these accelerations are often seen just at the start of a uterine contraction and often precede a variable deceleration

Decelerations. Four types are identified according to their shape and temporal relationship to uterine contractions.

SIGNIFICANT FEATURES

In interpreting the FHR patterns (Fig. 12-2), the following features are significant:

1. The baseline FHR
2. The increase or decrease of the FHR in response to a uterine contraction
3. Whether the curve of the FHR is uniform or variable
4. The time relationship between the onset of the contraction and the start of the deceleration of the FHR
5. The lag time, that is, the interval between the peak of the intrauterine pressure curve and the lowest level of the FHR
6. The recovery time, that is, the interval from the nadir of the FHR until its return to the baseline

CLASSIFICATION

1. Uniform: When the pattern of the FHR relates to the curve of the uterine contraction

   a. Early deceleration (Fig. 12-2B)
   b. Late deceleration (Fig. 12-2C)

2. Variable: When there is no relationship between the uterine contraction and the FHR (Fig. 12-2D). They can be divided into two groups, defined later in this section

   a. Uncomplicated
   b. Complicated

EARLY DECELERATION OF FHR

1. Characteristics: All the following must apply (Fig. 12-2B):

   a. The shape of the curve is uniform and appears the same from one contraction to the next
   b. The pattern of the FHR mirrors that of the contraction
   c. Onset of the deceleration is early in the contraction cycle. Onset of deceleration to nadir is ≥30 seconds
   d. Nadir of the deceleration occurs at the peak of the contraction

    e. The FHR returns to the baseline before the contraction is over

    f. The lowest amplitude is proportional to the strength of the contraction

    g. Baseline FHR rarely falls below 100 bpm

    h. The amplitude of deceleration is usually <30 bpm

    i. The pattern is repetitive in most cases

    j. Baseline beat-to-beat variation is maintained

2. Proposed mechanism: Early deceleration is believed to be the result of fetal head compression, resulting in altered cerebral blood flow, which initiates a vagal reflex and cardiac slowing. This deceleration may be abolished by atropine

3. Interpretation: This is a benign FHR pattern. It is not usually associated with baseline changes or loss of beat-to-beat variability. It is not associated with fetal hypoxia, acidosis, or low APGAR scores. It may represent a physiologic mechanism by which the fetus conserves energy in labor. During a uterine contraction, the fall in placental perfusion results in decreased transfer of oxygen. Slowing of the fetal heart at this time would conserve cardiac glycogen at a time when the energy yield is lowest

4. Management: No treatment is indicated

LATE DECELERATION OF FHR

1. Characteristics: All the following must apply (Fig. 12-2C):

    a. The shape of the curve is uniform; one is similar to the next

    b. The onset of the deceleration occurs late in the uterine contraction cycle, 20 to 30 seconds after the start of the contraction

    c. The FHR does not return to baseline until after the end of the uterine contraction. The deceleration may persist for 30 to 60 seconds after the contraction

    d. The lag time (interval between the peak of the uterine contraction and the lowest level of the FHR) is >20 seconds

    e. The duration of the deceleration of the FHR is proportional to the uterine contraction

    f. The amplitude of the deceleration is proportional to the strength of the contraction

    g. The deceleration is usually 20 to 30 bpm. Rarely does it exceed 40 bpm

    h. The pattern is usually repetitive

2. Proposed mechanism:

   a. Decreased uterine blood flow (uteroplacental insufficiency)
   b. Reduction of Po_2 below a critical level during the peak of contraction
   c. Initially mediated by hypoxic depression of CNS
   d. Severe hypoxia also leads to direct depression of fetal myocardium

3. Interpretation: Late decelerations are potentially ominous, and a repetitive pattern may lead to fetal acidosis. Management of this pattern is often based on whether the cause of the uteroplacental insufficiency is considered to be potentially reversible or is known to be irreversible

   a. Potentially reversible causes:
      i. Hyperstimulation with oxytocic agents
      ii. Maternal hypotension
         i. Supine position
         ii. Associated with epidural anesthesia
         iii. Maternal hypovolemia
   b. Usually irreversible causes:
      i. Fetal growth restriction
      ii. Diabetes
      iii. Hypertension
      iv. Postmaturity
      v. Placental abruption

4. Management:

   a. Corrective measures:
      i. Relief of maternal hypotension by turning the patient on her side
      ii. Reduction of uterine tachysystole by discontinuing oxytocin
      iii. Administration of oxygen to the mother by tight-fitting face mask
   b. If the pattern persists for more than 15 minutes, preparation should be made for early delivery
   c. The presence of good FHR variability would indicate the absence of fetal acidosis. In this situation, if delivery is anticipated within 1 hour, a fetal scalp pH should be performed. If the pH is normal, then vaginal delivery may be awaited
   d. Persistent late decelerations, accompanied by baseline changes (bradycardia or tachycardia) and decreased FHR variability, indicate significant fetal distress and acidosis. Delivery should be carried out immediately, by cesarean section, if necessary

FIRST STAGE OF LABOR

e. In certain situations, persistent late decelerations in the face of normal heart rate variability or normal scalp pH, delivery by cesarean section may still be carried out. An example is late decelerations appearing in a patient known to have an irreversible cause for placental insufficiency in early labor. In this situation, although the presence of normal variability or the demonstration of a normal scalp pH would indicate absence of fetal acidosis at that time, it is obvious that the fetus would eventually become compromised during the course of many hours of labor

Variable Deceleration of FHR

1. Characteristics:

   a. Variable shape and wave form. It may be U, V, or W shaped, and so on. It differs from one deceleration to the next (Fig. 12-2D)
   b. Variable onset
   c. Variable lag time
   d. Variable amplitude and duration
   e. Need not be repetitive. For any single contraction, a variable deceleration can mimic an early or late deceleration
   f. It is frequently preceded or followed by accelerations ("shoulders")

2. Proposed mechanism:

   a. Cord compression initially produces obstruction of umbilical vein blood flow while the umbilical artery remains patent. This produces a fall in fetal cardiac output, hypotension, and a baroreceptor response. The baroreceptor response initiates a period of FHR acceleration
   b. As umbilical cord compression proceeds, the flow through the umbilical artery is finally impaired. This isolates the fetal cardiovascular system from the low-pressure placental unit. The increased peripheral vascular resistance in the fetus increases fetal blood pressure. This always provokes a vagal reflex response as seen by a slowing of the FHR. If cord compression is sustained and persistent, it may eventually lead to hypoxia and metabolic acidosis. Hence, a variable deceleration has two components:

      i. A neurogenic or reflex vagal deceleration, usually accompanied by a reversible respiratory acidosis caused by the accumulation of carbon dioxide and increased P_{CO_2} in the fetus

ii. A late component caused by hypoxic depression of the CNS after sustained or persistent cord compression. When this occurs, metabolic acidosis will supervene

3. Interpretation: Variable decelerations are the most common periodic change observed in labor. There is a higher incidence in association with a nuchal, short, or prolapsed cord and when oligohydramnios is present. The potential for cord compression exists each time there is fetal movement or a uterine contraction.

Variable decelerations are also noted with occipitoposterior positions. In this situation, the deceleration does not result from compression of the umbilical cord but from other mechanisms. The distinguishing feature is the absence of the "shoulders" (accelerations of the FHR) that usually accompany variable decelerations caused by compression of the cord.

Variable decelerations can be divided into two categories:

a. Uncomplicated: Decelerations present as initial acceleration, rapid deceleration of FHR to the nadir, and a rapid return to baseline FHR pattern. Variable decelerations in this circumstance are not associated with low APGAR scores or fetal acidosis

b. Complicated: Decelerations will have the following features and may be a predictor of fetal hypoxia
   i. Deceleration to <70 bpm for >60 seconds
   ii. Minimal variability in the baseline FHR and in the trough of the deceleration
   iii. Biphasic deceleration
   iv. Overshoot acceleration after deceleration lasting >20 bpm for >20 seconds
   v. Slower return to baseline FHR
   vi. Establishing lower baseline rate than before deceleration
   vii. Evidence of fetal bradycardia or tachycardia

4. Management: When any of these criteria are exceeded, it may mean that the fetus is becoming hypoxic and acidotic. Treatment varies and is based on the clinical situation.

Characteristics of a normal FHR tracing will have no, or only occasional, uncomplicated variables or early decelerations. A tracing becomes atypical when there are three or more uncomplicated variable decelerations in a 20-minute tracing. Atypical tracing may also have occasional late decelerations or a single prolonged deceleration over 2 minutes but less than 3 minutes.

An abnormal tracing, requiring intervention as clinically indicated, involves the presence of three or more complicated variables as described above. It can also be an abnormal tracing because of the presence of late decelerations with more than half of the contractions or if there is a single prolonged deceleration over 3 minutes but less than 10 minutes.

a. A patient in early labor having variable decelerations of a severity exceeding the above criteria is treated best by delivery by cesarean section. It is unreasonable to expect any improvement as labor progresses since variable deceleration tends to worsen as descent of the fetus increases traction on the umbilical cord

b. On the other hand, a patient in the second stage of labor, having variable decelerations that exceed the stated criteria, may be managed expectantly. As long as FHR variability is present and there is no progressive rise in the FHR, it is unlikely that fetal acidosis is present. Variable decelerations that occur repetitively during the second stage and last more than 1 minute are seen frequently. Difficult operative vaginal deliveries are best avoided as long as heart rate variability is maintained. Fetal scalp sampling is of limited use and may be misleading in patients with variable deceleration. Any interpretation of a scalp sample performed in association with variable decelerations must take account of the profound but reversible respiratory acidosis that may occur during and just after the deceleration

The presence of beat-to-beat variability in this situation is a good guide to the absence of significant acidosis. Careful correlation of persistent severe variable decelerations with variability and other baseline changes will obviate unnecessary intervention. It may be stated that variable decelerations are responsible for most unnecessary cesarean sections when inexperienced personnel overreact to their significance

Summary

1. A normal FHR tracing with normal heart rate variability indicates a healthy fetus and is associated with normal APGAR scores virtually 100 percent of the time

2. FHR changes represent a hemodynamic response to a fetal *stress* and should not be interpreted to mean the presence of fetal *distress*. According to the new nomenclature from the 2008 National Institute of Child Health and Human Development workshop, fetal heart tracing should be assessed as normal (category I), atypical (category II), or abnormal (category III) tracings:

a. Normal or category I: FHR patterns that are "normal": Associated with fetal well-being. No interventions are required in this setting
   i. Baseline rate: 110 to 160 bpm
   ii. Baseline FHR variability: moderate
   iii. Late or variable decelerations: absent
   iv. Early decelerations: present or absent
   v. Accelerations: present or absent

b. Atypical or category II: FHR patterns that are "indeterminate": Inconsistently associated with fetal acidemia. Requires evaluation and continued surveillance, depending on clinical scenario
   i. Baseline rate <110 bpm without absent variability
   ii. Baseline >160 bpm
   iii. Marked variability
   iv. Absent variability without decelerations
   v. Absence of accelerations after fetal stimulation
   vi. Prolonged decelerations (>2 minutes but <10 minutes)
   vii. Recurrent late decelerations with moderate variability
   viii. Recurrent variable decelerations with minimal or moderate variability

c. Abnormal or category III: FHR patterns that are "abnormal": Consistently associated with fetal acidemia. This requires prompt evaluation and management, including maternal reposition, oxygen, discontinue labor stimulus, or emergency delivery
   i. Absent variability and any of the following:
   ii. Recurrent late decelerations
   iii. Recurrent variable decelerations
   iv. Baseline rate <110 bpm
   v. Sinusoidal pattern

PSYCHOLOGICAL RESPONSE TO FETAL MONITORING

Proper use of both intermittent auscultation and continuous electronic fetal monitoring, in both high- and low-risk patients, should include an explanation to the patient of the purpose of these examinations and a

FIRST STAGE OF LABOR

discussion with her about her concerns and wishes. Ideally, this should take place during the prenatal visits and again upon her admittance to the labor suite. As valuable as the fetal monitor is, it transforms the labor room into an intensive care environment, and some patients manifest strong reactions.

Positive Response

Many women find that their state of anxiety is relieved, the machine providing valuable information that is otherwise unavailable. The clicking of the monitor confirms that the baby is alive. Both the patient and husband can tell when the next contraction is coming and are able to prepare for it. Women who have had a fetal loss in a previous pregnancy are strongly in favor of fetal monitoring.

Negative Response

Patients complain about the discomfort from the abdominal transducers and from the wires of the intravaginal electrode, which hangs between their thighs. They are unhappy with their enforced immobility, the loss of privacy, and their loss of control of the labor. Some are concerned that the electrode may damage the baby or that fetal monitoring is carried on only in dangerous situations and become anxious by variations in the FHR. A few resent the doctor and the husband paying more attention to the equipment than to the patient and believe that they are being used as guinea pigs.

The solution to these problems lies in educating the patient in the antepartum period. A description and demonstration of the apparatus, correction of erroneous impressions as to the purposes of and indications for fetal monitoring, reference to the scalp electrode as a small clip attached to the skin, and reassurance that the procedure is not part of a research project will make electronic monitoring more acceptable.

During labor, the working and purposes of the monitor should be explained, the patient should be allowed as much mobility as possible, her comfort must be a paramount consideration, and her privacy maintained.

BIOCHEMICAL ANALYSIS OF FETAL CAPILLARY BLOOD

When significant fetal hypoxia occurs, metabolic acidosis develops. As anaerobic metabolism proceeds, increasing amounts of lactic acid progressively lower the pH of fetal blood. Saling developed a method of testing fetal blood for acidosis before birth. A blood sample is obtained from the presenting part. Microanalysis is performed mainly to measure the pH, P_{CO_2}, and bicarbonate levels, but glucose, electrolytes, blood type, and antibodies can be determined.

It must be emphasized that a proper interpretation of fetal scalp pH requires a complete analysis of fetal blood gases.

Indications

1. When an atypical or abnormal FHR pattern is present with some elements that suggest fetal hypoxia
2. When there is a sustained baseline heart rate without variability but showing no ominous periodic changes
3. When uncorrectable late decelerations, in the presence of good variability, occur in a patient where vaginal delivery may be anticipated within 60 minutes
4. In gestational age greater than 34 weeks

Technique

To be successful, fetal capillary blood sampling requires an organized routine, availability of equipment for immediate analysis, and operators with expertise. The membranes must be ruptured, the presenting part fixed in the pelvis, the position known, the cervix dilated more than 3 cm, and good lighting available. Under aseptic conditions and with the patient lying preferably in the left lateral position, an amnioscope is introduced into the posterior fornix of the vagina. Slow withdrawal of the scope at an angle allows the end to slip through the cervix and, with light pressure, to come against the fetal scalp (or rarely, the buttocks). The site for sampling is wiped clean of maternal blood and amniotic fluid, and a thin layer of silicone gel is applied to induce beading of blood to aid in its collection. The commercially available scalpels are preset so that the depth of incision is 3 mm. A cruciate incision is made, and a brief, moderate flow of blood follows. The volume collected is depending on the commercial kit used. The samples must be analyzed immediately. Excessive or prolonged bleeding is rare; it is easily controlled by pressure. In fewer than 1 percent of cases, a mild localized infection occurs.

Correlation Between FHR Patterns, Fetal pH, and Outcome

A normal fetus has a pH of 7.25 to 7.35 before the start of labor. During labor, there is a gradual shift in pH toward 7.25. If fetal hypoxia produces metabolic acidosis, fetal pH falls through preacidosis (7.20-7.24) to frank acidosis (<7.20).

FIRST STAGE OF LABOR

Certain correlations between fetal pH and neonatal condition have been observed:

1. pH over 7.25: More than 90 percent of these neonates will be healthy and nondepressed with high APGAR scores and would have shown normal FHR patterns during labor
2. pH between 7.20 and 7.24: This level indicates mild preacidosis. It is often associated with a prolonged second stage of labor and mild hypoxemia. FHR patterns often demonstrate late or variable decelerations, but beat-to-beat variability is normal. Most of these neonates have high APGAR scores. Operative intervention is not indicated, but the sampling should be repeated in 30 minutes
3. pH less than 7.20: This is usually indicative of significant fetal acidosis. In 80 percent of neonates, the APGAR score is under 6. FHR patterns often show persistent late or persistent severe variable decelerations with loss of heart variability
4. pH less than 7.10: This indicates profound asphyxia. Significant neonatal depression is present in 90 percent of cases

The correlation between fetal scalp pH measurements and neonatal APGAR score increases as the sample is taken closer to the time of birth. If taken within 5 minutes of delivery, Hon and associates have shown a high correlation between low pH and low APGAR scores. However, there appears to be a poor correlation between fetal pH and APGAR scores between 7 and 10. This could be accounted for partially by local factors that may make the fetal pH low at the scalp when the central fetal circulation is normal, especially at the time of delivery when caput formation is greatest.

A low fetal pH should not be interpreted in isolation. A full review of the entire blood gas picture must be carried out. An assessment of the P_{CO_2}, bicarbonate, and base deficit values are required to substantiate a diagnosis of metabolic acidosis. Respiratory acidosis, unassociated with hypoxia, may follow cord compression. Hence, if a scalp sample is obtained during or just after a variable deceleration, an extremely low fetal pH caused by respiratory acidosis may be obtained. Interpreted in isolation of other acid–base parameters, this would lead to erroneous diagnosis of severe fetal distress and result in unnecessary intervention.

False Results

1. False normal results (pH >7.20, low APGAR score) occur in association with sedative drugs, anesthesia, obstruction of the airway, congenital

anomalies, prematurity, hypoxia subsequent to the sampling, trauma of delivery, or a previous episode of asphyxia (the acid–base balance returns to normal, but the CNS does not)

2. False abnormal results (pH <7.20, good APGAR score) may occur in the presence of maternal acidosis. Hence, it is important to measure the maternal pH when low values are obtained in the fetus before definitive action is taken

Management During Labor

1. An abnormal FHR is an indication for analysis of the fetal blood
2. If the pH is over 7.25, labor is allowed to go on, and the analysis is repeated only if the FHR remains abnormal
3. When the pH is 7.20 to 7.24, another sampling is performed in 30 minutes
4. With the pH under 7.20, another sample is collected, and preparations are made for operative delivery. If the second analysis confirms the first one, delivery is carried out immediately

SELECTED READING

Cordero L, Anderson CW, Zuspan FP: Scalp abscess: A benign and infrequent complication of fetal monitoring. Am J Obstet Gynecol 146:126, 1983

Elias S: Fetoscopy in prenatal diagnosis. Clin Perinatol 10:357, 1983

Electronic fetal heart rate monitoring: research guidelines for interpretation. National Institute of Child Health and Human Development Research Planning Workshop. Am J Obstet Gynecol 177:1385, 1997

Freeman RK, Garite TJ: Fetal Heart Rate Monitoring. Baltimore/London: Williams and Wilkins, 1981, pp 84-112

Leveno KJ, William ML, DePalma RT, Whalley PJ: Perinatal outcome in the absence of antepartum fetal heart acceleration. Obstet Gynecol 61:347, 1983

Liston R, Sawchuck D, Young D: Fetal health surveillance: antepartum and intrapartum consensus guideline. J Obstet Gynaecol Can 29 (9 Suppl 4) S3, 2007

Macones GA, Hankins GD, Spong CY, et al: The 2008 National Institute of Child Health and Human Development Workshop Report on Electronic Fetal Monitoring: Update on definitions, interpretation, and research guidelines. Obstet Gynecol 112:661, 2008

Madanes AE, David D, Cetrulo C: Major complications associated with intrauterine pressure monitoring. Obstet Gynecol 59:389, 1982

Manning FA, Lange IR, Morrison I, Harman CR: Determination of fetal health: Methods for antepartum and intrapartum fetal assessment. Curr Prob Obstet Gynecol 7(4), 1983

FIRST STAGE OF LABOR

Miller RC: Meconium staining of the amniotic fluid. Clin Obstet Gynecol 6:359, 1979

Molfese V, Sunshine P, Bennett A: Reactions of women to intrapartum fetal monitoring. Obstet Gynecol 59:705, 1982

Pearson JF, Weaver JB: Fetal activity and fetal wellbeing: an evaluation. Br Med J, 1:1305, 1976

Young DC, Gray JH, Luther ER, et al: Fetal scalp blood pH sampling: Its value in an active obstetric unit. Am J Obstet Gynecol 136:276, 1980

CHAPTER 13

Induction of Labor

Jessica Dy

Induction of labor is the artificial initiation of labor before its spontaneous onset. It should be considered when the benefits of earlier delivery outweigh the potential risks to the mother and baby associated with induction of labor and prolongation of pregnancy. A careful and well-documented discussion should be made between the health care provider and the patient and should include the reason for induction, method of induction, and risks associated with induction of labor. Some of the common indications for induction of labor are discussed below.

MATERNAL INDICATIONS

PRELABOR SPONTANEOUS RUPTURE OF MEMBRANES
If membrane rupture occurs beyond 37 weeks and labor does not begin after 24 hours, induction of labor is appropriate and recommended to reduce the risk of infection to both the mother and the baby. If preterm (<37 weeks) spontaneous rupture of membranes occur, induction of labor should be considered after 34 weeks.

PREECLAMPSIA Induction of labor should be considered in women with gestational hypertension. In the presence of preeclampsia, toxemia, or other adverse conditions (to the mother or baby), induction of labor is recommended.

POLYHYDRAMNIOS There is no evidence to support routine labor induction in otherwise uncomplicated pregnancies with polyhydramnios. Induction of labor is sometimes carried out if an unstable lie places the woman at high risk for an umbilical cord prolapse if the membranes rupture spontaneously.

ANTEPARTUM BLEEDING Induction of labor may be indicated in cases of stable low-lying placenta and placental abruption in which bleeding is persistent.

INTRAUTERINE FETAL DEATH (IUFD) In cases of IUFD where there is evidence of ruptured membranes, infection, bleeding, or coagulopathy, immediate induction of labor is recommended. If the woman is otherwise well, labor induction may be delayed. Induction of labor may also be considered in women with a history of IUFD near term in past pregnancies. The timing of induction should be individualized but is usually carried out 1 week prior to the gestation of a previous stillbirth.

ELECTIVE When induction of labor is being carried out for the convenience of the patient and/or the doctor, it is called an *elective induction*. Elective inductions should be avoided as much as possible. In exceptional circumstances (e.g., a history of rapid labors or the patient lives far from a hospital), induction may be considered at or after 40 weeks.

FETAL INDICATIONS

POSTTERM PREGNANCY There is strong evidence to support a recommendation of induction of labor between 41^{+0} and 42^{+0} weeks of gestation. Beyond 42^{+0} weeks, there is an increased risk of perinatal death and meconium aspiration to the baby. For the mother, the risk of cesarean section is reduced when induction of labor is carried out between 41^{+0} and 42^{+0} weeks gestation.

MATERNAL DIABETES There is a risk of fetal death in utero associated with insulin-dependent diabetes during the later weeks of pregnancy. In cases of preexisting diabetes or insulin-dependent diabetes or in the presence of complications associated with diabetes, labor induction is indicated. The timing of induction should be individualized.

INTRAUTERINE GROWTH RESTRICTION (IUGR) Some experts advocate induction of labor in cases of suspected IUGR to reduce the risk of stillbirth.

MACROSOMIA There is a higher risk of shoulder dystocia and brachial plexus injury when the baby has a birthweight above 4500 g. This risk is increased if the mother has diabetes or if a previous delivery had shoulder dystocia. Because an accurate estimate of fetal weight is difficult, induction of labor when there is suspected macrosomia should not be carried out routinely.

CHORIOAMNIONITIS Induction of labor is indicated in cases of suspected chorioamnionitis.

ISOIMMUNIZATION When the fetus is being sensitized or when there has been isoimmunization or fetal death in utero during previous pregnancies, induction of labor is indicated. The timing of induction should be individualized.

FIRST STAGE OF LABOR

OLIGOHYDRAMNIOS There is no evidence to support routine labor induction in otherwise uncomplicated pregnancies with isolated oligohydramnios. However, some experts advocate induction of labor to reduce perinatal mortality and morbidity.

CONTRAINDICATIONS FOR LABOR INDUCTION

PLACENTA PREVIA OR VASA PREVIA

NONCEPHALIC PRESENTATION Induction of labor is contraindicated if the baby is in a transverse lie or is a footling breech. It is generally not recommended if the baby is in a breech presentation.

PRIOR CLASSICAL CESAREAN SECTION OR INVERTED T UTERINE INCISION

PRIOR SIGNIFICANT UTERINE SURGERY (e.g., full-thickness myomectomy)

PRIOR UTERINE RUPTURE

ACTIVE GENITAL HERPES

INVASIVE CERVICAL CARCINOMA

RISKS ASSOCIATED WITH LABOR INDUCTION

IATROGENIC PRETERM OR LATE PRETERM BIRTH

INCREASED OPERATIVE VAGINAL DELIVERY

PROLONGED LABOR

INCREASED CESAREAN DELIVERY

UMBILICAL CORD PROLAPSE

TACHYSYSTOLE (excessive uterine activity)

ABNORMAL FETAL HEART RATE PATTERNS

UTERINE RUPTURE

EREQUISITES AND CONDITIONS R SUCCESSFUL LABOR DUCTION

ESENTATION The presentation should be cephalic. Labor is never ced in the presence of attitudes of extension, transverse lies, or compound ntations and almost never when the breech presents.

TION The head must be engaged to avoid umbilical cord prolapse when otomy is performed. The lower the head, the easier and safer the procedure.

RVICAL RIPENESS One of the most important predictors for induc-success is the prelabor status of the cervix. The cervix must be effaced, less 1.3 cm (0.5 inch) in length, soft, dilatable, and open to admit at least one r and preferably two. The firm ring of the internal os should not be present. dvantageous for the cervix to be in the center of the birth canal or anterior. n the cervix is posterior, conditions for induction are less favorable.

RITY The success rate for vaginal delivery within 24 hours is better for parous women than nulliparous women.

TERNAL HEIGHT AND WEIGHT Successful induction is associ-with women who are taller and have a lower body mass index.

STATIONAL AGE The closer the gestation is to term, the more ssful is the induction, likely because of a more favorable cervix. When rm termination of pregnancy is necessary, tests for fetal lung maturity can rformed.

FIRST STAGE OF LABOR

PRE-INDUCTION CERVICAL RIPENING

The changes in the uterine cervix that take place before the onset of labor include physically detectable softening, shortening, and dilatation of the os. This process is known as *ripening*. The collagen fibrils become disaggregated and no longer tightly bound by the glycosaminoglycans so that they will slide apart more readily and allow the cervix to dilate.

In most normal pregnancies, the cervix is ripe at the onset of labor. A ripe cervix is soft, less than 1.3 cm in length, admits a finger easily, and is dilatable. The length of labor and the success of induction in both nulliparous and multiparous women depend on the degree of cervical ripeness. There are many situations, however, in which labor and vaginal delivery are indicated when the cervix is not ripe. In such cases, the cervix is unlikely to respond favorably to uterine activity.

Evaluation of the Cervix

Before inducing labor or using a modality to prime or ripen a cervix, one must differentiate between a cervix that is unprepared and one that is already ripe. The most readily used methods to make the assessment depend on the physical characteristics of the cervix.

Bishop was the first to attempt to quantify the physical examination of the cervix by the use of a numeric scoring system (Fig. 13-1). This is based on a number of criteria, including dilatation, effacement, consistency, and position of the cervix in the vagina. Each of the criteria is evaluated and assigned a number of points. Of all these parameters, dilatation

		Points			
		0	1	2	3
	Dilatation of cervix (cm)	0	1–2	3–4	5–6
	Effacement of cervix (%)	0–30	40–50	60–70	80
Factor	Consistency of cervix	Firm	Medium	Soft	
	Position of cervix in the vagina	Posterior	Mid	Anterior	
	Station	−3	−2	−1, 0	+1, +2

FIGURE 13-1. Bishop score.

is the most significant and position of the cervix the least important. The higher the score, the shorter will the length of labor be and the more likely will induction be successful.

When a high score is present, it can be assumed that cervical ripening has taken place, and no further attempts to prime the cervix are needed. According to Bishop's system, the maximal total score is 13. When the score is 9 or more, there is a high likelihood that induction of labor will be successful. When the score is 4 or less, failure of induction is common, and preinduction cervical priming should be performed.

Lange and associates suggested that the factor of crucial significance to inducibility of labor is the condition of the cervix and that cervical dilatation should be weighted by at least twice the value given it by Bishop. The results of their modified score are the same as those achieved by other methods, but theirs is simpler in that only three parameters are used: station of the presenting part, dilatation of the cervix, and length of the cervix. When the score is 5 to 7, the rate of successful induction is over 75 percent. When it is under 4, the rate of failure is considerable (Fig. 13-2).

Mechanical Methods of Cervical Priming

Mechanical methods to ripen the cervix have the advantage of low cost, stability at room temperature, low risk of tachysystole, and few systemic side effects. However, there is generally a small increased risk of infection (depending on the type of mechanical method used) to both the mother and the baby.

Station	−3	−2	−1, 0	+1, +2
Points	0	1	2	3
Dilatation of cervix (cm)	0	1–2	3–4	>4
Points	0	2	4	6
Length of cervix (cm)	3	2	1	0
Points	0	1	2	3

FIGURE 13-2. Lange score.

FIRST STAGE OF LABOR

Hygroscopic Dilators

Hygroscopic dilators are safe and effective for dilating the cervix but are inadequate for induction of labor. Hygroscopic dilators may be a synthetic product or made from dried natural seaweed (laminaria tents). They are primarily used for pregnancy termination rather than for preinduction cervical ripening of term pregnancies.

Hygroscopic dilators expand when coming in contact with moisture. It gradually swells within the cervical canal to three to five times its original diameter. In so doing, it brings about gradual softening and dilatation of the cervix. The most rapid swelling occurs in the first 4 to 6 hours, and the maximal effect is achieved in 24 hours. The effect is entirely local. Uterine hyperactivity is rare. There is some evidence that the insertion of the hygroscopic dilators leads to the production of endogenous prostaglandin (PG), and this may play a part in the ripening process.

Technique

1. In the evening before the day of induction, two to five laminaria are placed in the cervix. The number depends on the capacity of the cervix. As many as possible are inserted. Insertion of multiple small-diameter hygroscopic dilators (2 or 3 mm) is better than using a few large ones. The number of dilators inserted should be documented
2. Care is taken not to rupture the membranes
3. One or two 4 × 4 sterile gauze is placed against the cervix to hold the laminaria in place. The number of gauze inserted should be documented
4. The next morning, the dilators are removed
5. Amniotomy is performed when the presenting part is well applied against the cervix
6. An infusion of oxytocin may be started immediately. However, some obstetricians prefer to use oxytocin only if labor does not begin after a few hours

Complications

1. Mild pelvic cramps occur occasionally
2. Cervical bleeding has been reported
3. There is a small risk of infection, especially if the interval between the insertion of the tents and the emptying of the uterus is prolonged

Intracervical Balloon Catheters

Commercially available balloons for cervical ripening or a regular Foley catheter (#16 with a 30-80 cc balloon) can be used. Use of a balloon catheter results in a mean change of 3.3 to 5.3 in the Bishop score. They are generally as effective as PGs for cervical ripening. Compared with those receiving PGs, women who had balloon catheters for cervical ripening required more use of oxytocin for labor induction and augmentation. Balloon catheters are also associated with less uterine hyperstimulation or tachysystole compared with PGs.

Balloon catheters for cervical ripening are generally reserved for use in women with intact membranes. There is a small but non-significant increased risk in maternal infection.

Technique

1. With a speculum in the vagina and the cervical os well visualized, a deflated balloon catheter is passed through the internal cervical os and into the extra-amniotic space
2. Ring forceps can be used to aid in passing the catheter through the cervical os
3. When in the extra-amniotic space, the balloon is filled with 30 to 60 cc of saline or water. This dilates the balloon to about 2-3 cm
4. The clinician ensures that the balloon is not just resting in the vagina
5. The catheter is retracted so the balloon rests against the internal os. Some clinicians believe in pulling on the balloon so there is some weight or traction against the internal os
6. The catheter is left in place until it spontaneously falls out (usually when the cervix is more favorable and about 2-3 cm dilated). This usually occurs within 12 to 24 hours of catheter placement
7. If the catheter does not fall out spontaneously, it should be removed in 24 hours to avoid increased risk of infection
8. An amniotomy is performed or oxytocin induction is usually started after the balloon catheter has been removed

Pharmacologic Methods of Cervical Priming

Prostaglandin

PGs have been shown to be effective in ripening the cervix and sometimes as an initiator of active labor. It is likely that the effect is twofold: (1) PG brings about biochemical changes in the collagenous matrix of the cervix that result in softening, and (2) PG stimulates the uterus to contract gently, leading to retraction and partial dilatation of the cervix.

Prostaglandin E2 and E1 are the PGs currently used for cervical ripening. The optimal route, dose, and frequency of PG administration have not been determined. Locally administered PG preparations (intravaginal or

FIRST STAGE OF LABOR

endocervical) appear to have good clinical response while minimizing systemic side effects and are therefore the preferred routes. Side effects from PG include fever, chills, vomiting, and diarrhea. PGs are also associated with excessive uterine activity. Fetal heart rate (FHR) monitoring should be done after administration of PG.

Prostaglandin E2 (dinoprostone) preparations are widely used for cervical ripening. It is available for intracervical or vaginal administration. Depending on the preparation of PGE2 used, it remains in the posterior vaginal fornix for 6 to 12 hours or until active labor begins.

Misoprostol (Cytotec) is a PGE1 analog that is approved for use for treatment and prevention of peptic ulcers. It has been used "off label" for cervical ripening and labor induction. The dose required for cervical ripening and labor induction in the third trimester is much lower than in the first or second trimester because the myometrium has increased sensitivity to PGs with advancing gestational age. It is usually available as 100- or 200-mcg tablets, so the misoprostol tablets need to be broken down. The recommended dose is 25 mcg vaginally or 50 mcg orally every 4 to 6 hours. If necessary, oxytocin may be initiated no earlier than 4 hours after the last misoprostol dose was given.

In all PGE1 and PGE2 preparations, contractions of low amplitude can begin within a couple of hours. These are similar to the contractions of early spontaneous labor. Not infrequently, active labor begins during the period of cervical ripening, so that use of oxytocin is less when PGs are used. It is recommended that PGs be administered in settings where uterine activity and FHR patterns can be monitored. It is prudent to monitor the FHR pattern for up to 2 hours post-administration, or longer if there is increased uterine activity noted. *There is an increased incidence of tachysystole with PG use.*

Prostaglandins (PGE1 and PGE2) are not recommended as induction agents in women who have had a previous uterine scar because of the increased incidence of uterine tachysystole and uterine rupture.

If labor has not started within 24 hours and the cervix has become favorable, amniotomy is performed and, if necessary, an oxytocin infusion is set up. When the cervix does not respond, the case must be reevaluated.

Oxytocin

Oxytocin does induce contractions of the pregnant myometrium, but it has not been proven to be an efficient priming agent of the cervix. Given as an intravenous infusion, oxytocin does improve the Bishop score but to a much smaller extent than that achieved by PGs or mechanical balloon catheters. Oxytocin is an inefficient ripening agent.

METHODS OF INDUCING LABOR

Castor oil and soapsuds enemas have not been proven to be effective in inducing labor in any randomized studies and therefore should not be used.

Membrane Stripping

Membrane stripping or sweeping is a common practice. It involves examining the cervix, reaching beyond the internal cervical os with the examining finger, and rotating the finger circumferentially to detach the fetal membranes from the lower uterine segment. When performed at 40 weeks of gestation, membrane stripping may reduce the need for labor induction for postterm pregnancy because a majority of women enter spontaneous labor within 72 hours. There does not appear to be an increase in the risk of bleeding, infection, or membrane rupture with membrane stripping.

Artificial Rupture of Membranes

Artificial rupture of membranes, or amniotomy, can be a simple and effective means of inducing labor when the cervix is favorable and the presenting part is well applied against the cervix. However, in some cases, amniotomy alone will not be enough to initiate labor, and oxytocin infusion is usually required to establish labor.

Technique

1. The fetal heart is checked carefully

2. Sterile vaginal examination is made to determine that the necessary conditions and prerequisites are present

3. With a finger placed between the cervix and the bag of waters, the cervix is rimmed, stripping the membranes away from the lower uterine segment

4. If necessary, pressure is maintained on the uterine fundus through the abdomen to keep the head well down

5. Using a uterine dressing forceps, an Allis forceps, a Kelly clamp, or a membrane hook, the bag of waters is torn or punctured

6. A gush of fluid from the vagina is proof of success

FIRST STAGE OF LABOR

7. The fetal heart is checked carefully after successful amniotomy

8. Although the head may be pushed upward slightly to allow escape of the amniotic fluid, this must be done with caution because there is danger of umbilical cord prolapse

9. Artificial rupture of the membranes can be performed through a vaginal amnioscope. Advantages include:

   a. The procedure is carried out under direct vision, which adds to safety
   b. The color of the fluid and the presence of meconium can be ascertained before the membranes are ruptured
   c. The presence of a low-lying umbilical cord or vasa previa can be ruled out
   d. Amniotic fluid, uncontaminated by vaginal contents, can be collected for biochemical analysis
   e. The amnioscope provides a sterile pathway to the cervix and reduces the danger of amnionitis

Contraindications to Artificial Rupture of the Membranes

1. High presenting part
2. Presentation other than vertex
3. Unripe cervix
4. Active genital herpes and HIV infection with high viral load

Oxytocin

Oxytocin, an octapeptide, is produced in the supraoptic and paraventricular nuclei of the hypothalamus. The hormone migrates down the supraoptic–neurohypophyseal nerve pathways and is stored in the posterior pituitary gland. Oxytocin-releasing stimuli include (1) cervical dilatation; (2) coitus; (3) emotional reactions; (4) suckling; and (5) drugs such as acetylcholine, nicotine, and certain anesthetics.

Maternal levels of oxytocin increase throughout gestation; secretion seems to occur in a pulsatile fashion. Fetal blood contains much more oxytocin at the end of the second stage of labor than does maternal blood. The blood in the umbilical cord of anencephalic infants, however, has no oxytocin. It is possible that the fetus may be an important source of oxytocin during parturition. In experimental animals, the establishment of neurohypophyseal deficiency leads to difficulty in parturition. The same is not true in humans. Pregnant patients who have had an hypophysectomy or have idiopathic diabetes insipidus experience no difficulty in labor.

The exact role of oxytocin in human labor is not known. It may be that oxytocin has only a facilitating role in the physiology of uterine activity during pregnancy and not a primary role in the initiation and maintenance of labor.

Pituitrin, Pitocin, and Pitressin

Posterior pituitary extract has been used for many years to stimulate uterine contractions. In the beginning, whole posterior pituitary extract (Pituitrin) was used. It contains mainly an oxytocic agent and an antidiuretic-hypertensive factor. To eliminate the undesirable side effects of the latter, the extract has been divided into its two main components—an almost pure oxytocic factor (Pitocin) and a hypertensive agent (Pitressin).

During the early 1950s, DuVigneaud and his colleagues succeeded in the purification, chemical identification, and synthesis of oxytocin and vasopressin. The natural and synthetic products are equally efficient in regard to their action on the myometrium. Synthetic oxytocin is a chemically pure substance and is free from the danger of reaction to animal protein.

At the present time, all commercial preparations of oxytocin used in obstetrics are synthetic. It is the most commonly used method of induction for women with a viable pregnancy.

Artificial rupture of the membranes increases the efficiency of inducing labor with oxytocin.

Effects of Oxytocin

Uterus
In causing the uterus to contract, oxytocin is believed to act on the myometrial cell membrane. It increases the normal excitability of the muscle but adds no new properties. The myometrial sensitivity to oxytocin rises as pregnancy progresses because of increasing oxytocin receptors on the myometrium.

Cardiovascular System
Oxytocin has numerous effects on the cardiovascular system.

1. Heart rate: a small to moderate increase
2. Systemic arterial blood pressure: a decrease results mainly from a lowering of peripheral resistance
3. Cardiac output: given as a single dose, oxytocin causes a rise in cardiac output followed by a fall; continuous infusion results in an increased cardiac output

FIRST STAGE OF LABOR

4. Renal blood flow: no significant change
5. Skin: the blood vessels are sensitive to the vasodilatory action of oxytocin, and flushing of the face, neck, and hands may occur
6. Uterine flow: the decrease is caused mainly by the extravascular resistance around the uterine blood vessels as the result of the increased uterine contractions

Kidneys

Oxytocin can induce antidiuresis. The human kidney is not damaged, the excretion of electrolytes is not changed, and renal blood flow is not reduced. The antidiuretic action probably occurs by resorption of water from the distal convoluted tubules and the collecting ducts.

Breast

Oxytocin stimulates the myoepithelial cells of the breasts and causes the passage of milk from the alveoli to the mammary ducts.

Administration

Routes of administration include intramuscular or repeated subcutaneous injections of small or large doses and the placing of a cotton pledget soaked in 5 or 10 units of oxytocin in the nostril, whence the drug is absorbed. However, the intravenous infusion of a dilute solution of oxytocin is so superior to other methods that it is the procedure of choice for labor induction to the virtual exclusion of the others.

Advantages of the Intravenous Route

1. The amount of oxytocin entering the bloodstream can be regulated. With other techniques, the amount given to the patient is known, but there is no control over the rate of absorption. It can be fast or slow, regular or intermittent, and it may accumulate in the tissues to be released later in a large amount and high concentration
2. Minute amounts are effective
3. The blood level and the activity of oxytocin are constant as long as the rate of the drip is maintained. It can be speeded up or slowed down with instant changes in effect
4. The plasma of pregnant women near term contains an enzyme, pitocinase, in such high concentration that half of an intravenously given dosage of Pitocin is destroyed in 2 to 3 minutes. Thus, within 3 to

4 minutes of shutting off an intravenous infusion, the oxytocic activity
has ceased

5. The contractions brought on by this technique seem to be mainly of
   the normal triple-descending gradient type

Technique of Intravenous Administration

The two methods of intravenous infusion are by the use of a constant infusion pump or by a Murphy drip. For safety reasons, the constant rate infusion pump should be used. Changes in the patient's position or movement
will not affect the speed at which the solution is being infused.

Whichever system is used, it is advisable to start the drip at a rate of
1.0 mU/min to test for untoward reactions. If none occurs, the oxytocin
infusion should be gradually increased by 1 to 2 mU/min or 4 to 6 mU/min
at 20- to 30-minute intervals until adequate uterine contractions are
achieved. The physiologic dose of oxytocin that will produce regular uterine
contractions is 8 to 12 mU/min. The maximum safe dose is 20 mU/min. In
most cases, doses of less than 10 mU/min are adequate. The aim is to bring
about strong uterine contractions lasting 40 to 50 seconds and recurring
every 2 to 3 minutes. Care must be exercised to avoid tumultuous contractions so frequent and prolonged that there is no interval between them.
This carries the danger of uterine rupture, placental separation, and fetal
asphyxia.

The popular strengths of the solutions are 5, 10, or 20 units of oxytocin
in 1 L of crystalloid solution (e.g., normal saline or Ringer's lactate). The
advantages of a dilute solution are that the dose is physiologic rather than
pharmacologic, the control is easier, and the danger of excessive uterine contraction is reduced. The disadvantage is that too much fluid may be given.
When used for induction or augmentation of labor, it is advisable to maintain the infusion for 1 hour postpartum to obviate uterine atony. To avoid
water intoxication, the amount of oxytocin and fluid must be controlled: less
than 45 mU/min of the former and 1 L per 24 hours of the latter.

When the drip method is used, the two-bottle system is advised. One
bottle contains 1 L of crystalloid solution. The other contains 1 L of crystalloid to which the oxytocin has been added; this must be labeled clearly.
The two tubes leading from the bottles are connected by a Y adapter, which
connects to the needle in the vein. The Y adapter should be close to the
needle so that a change from one solution to the other will be immediate.

The drip is started with the crystalloid solution. When it is running at
10 to 15 drops a minute, the switch is made to the oxytocin solution. Careful observation is made as to the type, strength, and duration of the contractions and to their effect on the fetal heart. If no untoward reactions are noted,

FIRST STAGE OF LABOR

the drip is continued. If excessive uterine contractions occur, or if there is fetal bradycardia (<100 bpm), tachycardia (>160 bpm), or irregularity of the heart, the oxytocin is stopped and plain crystalloid is infused. Oxytocin is a potent drug. It may vary a hundredfold in its actions on different people. The dosage is regulated by the effect on the individual receiving it. The speed of the drip is determined by and correlated to the frequency, intensity, and duration of the resulting contractions rather than by any arbitrary number of drops per minute.

Prerequisites for the Use of Oxytocin

1. The presenting part should be well engaged
2. The cervix must be ripe, effaced, soft, and partially dilated
3. There must be no fetopelvic disproportion
4. The fetus should be in normal position
5. The fetus should be in good condition with normal fetal heart
6. Adequate personnel must be available to watch the patient
7. The patient must be examined carefully before the oxytocin is started
8. The doctor in charge of the case should be in the hospital and available while the drip is running

Contraindications to the Use of Oxytocin

1. Absence of proper indication
2. Absence of the prerequisites
3. Disproportion, generally contracted pelvis, and obstruction by tumors
4. Grand multiparity: There is too great a chance of uterine rupture
5. Previous classical cesarean section or extensive myomectomy
6. Hypertonic or incoordinate uterus: The hypertonic or incoordinate uterus is made worse by oxytocin and may lead to a constriction ring
7. Maternal exhaustion: This condition should be treated by rest and fluids, not by oxytocin stimulation
8. Abnormal FHR pattern: Not only should oxytocin not be given, but the appearance of an irregular or slow heart while the drip is running demands that the drip be stopped
9. Abnormal presentation and position of all types
10. Unengaged head
11. Congenital anomalies of the uterus
12. Placenta previa

Dangers of Oxytocin

Maternal Dangers

1. Tachysystole is defined as having more than five contractions in 10 minutes over a 30-minute period. This can be associated with a normal or abnormal FHR pattern. Prolonged or excessive uterine contractions can occur with the use of PGs and oxytocin
2. Uterine rupture. If the patient is oversensitive to the drug, she may get hard and even tetanic contractions, enough to rupture the uterus, but normal contractions would do no harm. The risk of uterine rupture is doubled when she has had a previous cesarean section
3. Cervical and vaginal lacerations can be caused by too rapid passage of the baby through the pelvis
4. Uterine atony and postpartum hemorrhage may develop when the oxytocin is discontinued. This is more likely to occur in situations of prolonged labor
5. Abruptio placentae has been reported
6. Water intoxication is induced by retention in the body of large amounts of water in excess of electrolytes

Water Intoxication

Oxytocin has an antidiuretic effect that begins when the rate of infusion is 15 mU/min and is maximal at 45 mU/min. Single doses have no effect; the antidiuretic activity seems to depend on the maintenance of a constant and critical level. The action is on the distal convoluted tubules and collecting ducts of the kidneys, causing increased resorption of water from the glomerular filtrate. The combination of oxytocin and large amounts of electrolyte-free glucose in water leads to retention of fluid, low serum levels of sodium chloride, and often progressive oliguria.

The symptoms range from headache, nausea, vomiting, mental confusion, and seizures to coma and death. These have been attributed to edema and swelling of the brain.

Management of Water Intoxication

1. Prevention: A more concentrated solution of oxytocin can be used (20-40 units of oxytocin in 1 L of crystalloid solution). Patients receiving an infusion of oxytocin should not receive more than 1 L of electrolyte-free fluid in 24 hours
2. Mild cases: Discontinue the oxytocin and withhold all fluids

FIRST STAGE OF LABOR

3. Severe cases require, in addition, the infusion of hypertonic (3.0%) sodium chloride intravenously. This will withdraw fluid from the tissues and bring about a diuresis. The rate of infusion must be slow and should be discontinued when the diuretic phase ends to avoid overcorrection, lest the cerebral effects of hypernatremia be imposed upon those of water intoxication

Fetal Dangers From Oxytocin

1. Anoxia caused by contractions that are too hard, too frequent, and last too long. The uterus never relaxes enough to maintain adequate circulation. In some cases, separation of the placenta (placental abruption) has taken place
2. Forcing the fetus through a pelvis too small for it
3. Abnormal FHR patterns. In a large series, it was shown that the signs of abnormal FHR patterns are more common in patients receiving an oxytocin drip than in those without stimulation of labor. In almost all instances, slowing or stopping the oxytocin infusion resulted in the rapid return to normal of the fetal heart. The incidence of emergency obstetric intervention was no higher, and the final fetal results were comparable

SELECTED READING

Binkin NJ, Schulz KF, Grimes DA, Cates W: Urea-prostaglandin versus hypertonic saline for instillation abortion. Am J Obstet Gynecol 146:947, 1983

Crane JM: Factors predicting labour induction success: A critical analysis. Clin Obst Gynecol 49:3, 2006

Gower RH, Toraya J, Miller JM: Laminaria for preinduction cervical ripening. Obstet Gynecol 60:617, 1982

Kazzi GM, Bottoms SF, Rosen MG: Efficacy and safety of *Laminaria digitata* for preinduction ripening of the cervix. Obstet Gynecol 60:440, 1982

Kennedy JH, Stewart P, Barlow DH, et al: Induction of labour: A comparison of a single prostaglandin E$_2$ vaginal tablet with amniotomy and intravenous oxytocin. Br J Obstet Gynaecol 89:704, 1982

Lange AP, Secher NJ, Westergaard JG, et al: Prelabour evaluation of inducibility. Obstet Gynecol 60:137, 1982

Mozurkewich E, Chilimigras J, Koepke E, King V: Indications for induction of labour: a best-evidence review. BJOG 2009; 116:626-636

Sawyer MM, Lipshitz J, Anderson GD, et al: Third-trimester uterine rupture associated with vaginal prostaglandin E$_2$. Am J Obstet Gynecol 140:710, 1981

Shepherd JH, Bennett MJ, Laurence D, et al: Prostaglandin vaginal suppositories: A simple and safe approach to the induction of labour. Obstet Gynecol 58:596, 1981

Shepherd JH, Knuppel RA: The role of prostaglandins in ripening the cervix and inducing labour. Clin Perinatol 8:49, 1981

Steiner AL, Creasy RK: Methods of cervical priming. Clin Obstet Gynecol 26:37, 1983

Vaknin Z, Kurzweil Y, Sherman D: Foley catheter balloon vs locally applied prostaglandins for cervical ripening and labour induction: A systematic review and metaanalysis. Am J Obstet Gynecol 203:418, 2010

FIRST STAGE OF LABOR

Labor Dystocia

Jessica Dy

Labor dystocia refers to a slow and abnormal progression of labor. It is the most common problem associated with labor and primarily affects nulliparous women. A Danish study reported a 37% incidence of dystocia among uncomplicated pregnancies in nulliparous women. Labor dystocia is the leading indication for primary cesarean sections.

DEFINITION

The definition of *dystocia* is based on the deviations from the normal labor curve established by Friedman. Because it is difficult in many cases to be certain exactly when labor began, dystocia is rarely diagnosed with absolute certainty. A commonly accepted definition of dystocia is a rate of cervical dilatation less than 0.5 cm/hr over 4 hours in the active phase of the first stage of labor or fetal descent of less than 1 cm/hr in the second stage. These definitions are based on the 95th percentile for duration of labor in low-risk women with spontaneous labor. The term *failure to progress* has also been commonly used and refers to either a lack of progressive cervical dilatation or a lack of fetal descent or both.

ETIOLOGY AND RISK FACTORS

The principal causes of dystocia are related to the 4 Ps: power, passenger, passage, and psyche.

Power

Uterine contractions may be infrequent, hypotonic, or incoordinate such that they are unable to dilate the cervix. This is commonly seen in primary dysfunctional labor. Normal uterine contractions in the active phase have been defined as uterine contraction pressures greater than 200 Montevideo units. Maternal exhaustion or dense motor blockage from regional anesthesia can result in ineffective maternal expulsive efforts in the second stage.

Passenger

Fetal malposition and malpresentation (e.g., asynclitism, persistent occiput posterior, brow presentation) are associated with dystocia. If the fetus is disproportionately large relative to the maternal pelvis or if there is a congenital anomaly (hydrocephalus), prolonged labor can also ensue.

Passage

Examination of the pelvis may reveal an inadequate pelvis. Any prominent ischial spines, a narrow pubic arch, or other soft tissue mass (e.g., tumors, septums) may impede progressive descent of the fetus. True *cephalopelvic disproportion* refers to a disparity between the pelvic architecture or size and the fetal head that precludes vaginal delivery.

Inlet Contraction

Inlet contraction is present when the anteroposterior diameter (obstetric conjugate) is less than 10 cm or the transverse diameter is less than 12 cm. Inlet contraction may result from rickets or from generally poor development.
Effects on the fetus are:

1. Failure of engagement
2. Increase in malpositions
3. Deflexion attitudes
4. Exaggerated asynclitism
5. Extreme molding
6. Formation of a large caput succedaneum
7. Prolapse of the umbilical cord. This becomes a complication because the presenting part does not fit the inlet well

Effects on labor include:

1. Dilatation of the cervix is slow and often incomplete
2. Premature rupture of the membranes is common
3. Inefficient uterine action is a frequent accompaniment

Midpelvic Contraction

Midpelvic contraction is basically a reduction in the plane of least dimensions, the one that passes from the apex of the pubic arch through the ischial spines to meet the sacrum usually at the junction of the fourth and fifth segments.

When the distance between the ischial spines is less than 9.0 cm or when the sum of the interspinous (normal, 10.5 cm) and the posterior sagittal (normal, 4.5-5.0 cm) distances is less than 13.5 cm (normal is 15.0-15.5 cm), contraction of the midpelvis is probably present. To obtain accurate measurement of these diameters, x-ray pelvimetry is essential. Clinical suspicion of a small midpelvis is aroused by the finding on manual examination of a small pelvis, the palpation of large spines that jut into the cavity, and the observation that the distance between the ischial tuberosities is less than 8.0 cm.

Midpelvic contraction is a common cause of dystocia and operative delivery. It is more difficult to manage than inlet contraction because if the fetal head cannot even enter the inlet, there is no doubt that abdominal delivery is necessary. However, when the head has descended into the pelvis, one is loath to perform cesarean section, hoping that the head will come down to a point where it can be extracted with forceps. A danger here is that with molding and caput formation, the head may appear lower than it actually is. Instead of the projected midforceps delivery, one is engaged in a high forceps operation, often with disastrous results for both the mother and infant.

Midpelvic contractions may prevent anterior rotation of the occiput and may direct it into the hollow of the sacrum. Failure of rotation and deflexion attitudes are associated frequently with a small pelvic cavity.

Outlet Contraction

Outlet contraction is present when the distance between the ischial tuberosities is less than 8.0 cm. Dystocia may be expected when the sum of the inter-tuberous diameter and the posterior sagittal diameter is much less than 15.0 cm. Diminution of the intertuberous diameter and the subpubic angle forces the head backward, so the prognosis depends on the capacity of the posterior segment, the mobility at the sacrococcygeal joint, and the ability of the soft tissues to accommodate the passenger. The sides of the posterior triangle are not bony. Although outlet contraction causes an increase in perineal lacerations and a greater need for forceps deliveries, only rarely is it an indication for cesarean section. Because the bituberous diameter can be measured manually, however, and since it may warn us that there is contraction higher in the pelvis, it should always be assessed as part of the routine examination.

Psyche

Pain, anxiety, and stress can inhibit progressive cervical dilatation, especially in the latent phase.

Other Risk Factors for Labor Dystocia

Other risk factors associated with labor dystocia include:

1. Advanced maternal age
2. Obesity

3. Nulliparity
4. Short maternal stature (<150 cm)
5. Medical complications in pregnancy
6. Induction of labor
7. Prelabor rupture of membranes
8. Prolonged latent phase
9. Epidural anesthesia
10. Chorioamnionitis
11. Postterm pregnancy (>41 weeks)
12. Estimated fetal weight large for gestational age
13. Malpositioning or malpresentation (occiput posterior position, face presentation)

These factors may act alone or in concert. A marked abnormality of one or a minor deviation in several can prevent successful spontaneous vaginal birth. Whereas normal delivery is impossible in the presence of absolute cephalopelvic disproportion, a mild disparity between the size of the pelvis and that of the fetus can be overcome by strong and effective uterine contractions. The pelvis may be sufficiently large to accommodate an occipitoanterior presentation but too small for an occipitoposterior one. It is a matter of balance.

COMPLICATIONS OF LABOR DYSTOCIA

Although prolonged labor is worrisome, maternal and neonatal outcomes are generally good. However, if labor dystocia is not recognized and proper interventions are not carried out, it can be associated with serious maternal and neonatal morbidity.

Maternal Complications

1. Postpartum hemorrhage
2. Chorioamnionitis
3. Injuries to the pelvic floor (especially from a prolonged second stage)
4. Increased risk of operative deliveries

Neonatal Complications

Prolonged labor has been associated with a higher risk of meconium-stained fluid at the time of delivery and an increased risk of neonatal

FIRST STAGE OF LABOR

infection and bacteremia. There may also be an increased incidence of transient depression at birth requiring immediate resuscitation of the newborn. However, most studies looking at neonatal outcomes in labors with dystocia report overall good neonatal outcomes with no increased risk for fetal asphyxia, lower APGAR scores, or admission to neonatal intensive care unit.

GRAPHIC ANALYSIS OF LABOR

Friedman described a graphic analysis of labor, also called a *partogram* (Fig. 14-1), correlating the duration of labor with the rate of cervical dilatation. On graph paper, the cervical dilatation in centimeters is placed on the ordinate, and the time in hours is plotted on the abscissa. Joining the points of contact makes a sigmoid curve. The rate of cervical dilatation, as shown by the slope of the curve, is described in centimeters per hour.

Once the active phase of labor begins, changes in cervical dilatation usually proceed at a much faster rate, and labor is closely monitored to ensure adequate progress. The partogram is the documentation of serial assessments of the cervical dilatation and fetal descent as soon as the active phase of labor begins. It is an easy and simple way of visually summarizing the progress of labor, or the lack of progress, and allows early and objective identification of labor that has deviated from the normal labor curve.

The mean and longest acceptable duration of labor and rates of cervical dilatation were historically established by Friedman in the early 1950s based on a mixed population of women, including women who were in spontaneous and induced labor and fetuses in breech presentations. Friedman's data showed a nonlinear (sigmoid) curve of labor progress in the active phase that encompassed dilatation of the cervix from 2.5 cm

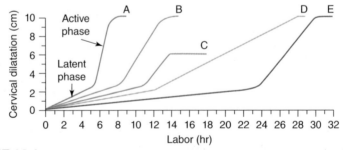

FIGURE 14-1. **Normal and abnormal labor during the first stage. A,** Average multipara. **B,** Average primigravida. **C,** Secondary arrest of dilatation. **D,** Primary dysfunctional labor. **E,** Prolonged latent phase.

to 10 cm. The average duration of the active phase of labor for nulliparous women was 4.6 hours, and the longest normal duration (mean + 2 standard deviation) was 11.7 hours. The average rate of cervical dilatation was 3 cm/hr, and the slowest acceptable rate was 1.2 cm/hr.

More recently, Zhang et al studied 1329 nulliparous women with a single-term vertex presentation in spontaneous labor and demonstrated a markedly different curve than Friedman. Almost half of the women included in Zhang's study received regional anaesthesia (48%) and oxytocin augmentation (50%). Although both labor curves depict a relatively slow rate of cervical dilatation in the latent phase, the transition from latent phase to active phase was less obvious in Zhang's labor curve. In Zhang's study, cervical dilatation from 4 to 10 cm took 5.5 hours instead of 2.5 hours in Friedman's curve, and the rate of cervical change was more gradual. Women in the fifth percentile rate of cervical dilatation were all below 1 cm/hr.

CLASSIFICATION OF PROLONGED LABOR

Prolonged Latent Phase

False labor and the latent phase of labor initially share similar characteristics, so determining the actual duration of the latent phase accurately is problematic. The latent phase begins with the onset of true labor and lasts until the beginning of the active phase of cervical dilatation, when the cervix has usually reached 3 to 4 cm dilatation in nulliparous women. In nulliparous women, the average length of the latent phase is 8.6 hours, with the upper limit of normal at 20 hours (Table 14-1). For multiparas, the figures are 5.3 and 14 hours. In general, a latent phase that exceeds 20 hours in a nullipara or 14 hours in a multipara is considered prolonged and abnormal.

Wide variations occur, and a prolonged latent period does not necessarily mean that the active phase will be abnormal. The unripe cervix prolongs only the latent phase, and most cervices open normally once effacement is achieved. Even when the latent phase lasts more than 20 hours, many patients advance to normal cervical dilatation when the active phase begins. A diagnosis of labor dystocia should not be made before the onset of the active phase when the cervix is less than 4 cm.

Risk factors for prolonged latent phase include (1) an unripe cervix at the onset of labor, (2) abnormal position of the fetus (occiput transverse

FIRST STAGE OF LABOR

TABLE 14-1: AVERAGE DURATION OF THE PHASES OF LABOR

	Primigravidas		Multiparas	
	Average	Upper Normal	Average	Upper Normal
Latent phase (hr)	8.6	20	5.3	14
Active phase (hr)	5.8	12	2.5	6
First stage of labor (hr)	13.3	28.5	7.5	20
Rate of cervical dilatation during active phase (cm/hr)	1.2	0.5	1.5	0.8

or posterior positions), (3) cephalopelvic disproportion, (4) dysfunctional labor, (5) induction of labor, (6) prelabor rupture of amniotic membranes, (7) early administration of regional anesthetic with heavy motor block. Maternal age, infant birth weight, pelvic capacity, and gestational age do not affect the duration of the latent phase.

Prolonged Active Phase

The active period lasts from the end of the latent phase to full dilatation of the cervix. The curve changes from the almost horizontal slope of the latent phase to a nearly vertical incline representing a period of steady and rapid cervical dilatation. Recent studies on contemporary labor patterns suggest that this phase is actually more gradual than that suggested by Friedman's curve and in some cases may not actually start until cervical dilatation has reached 5 to 6 cm in a nulliparous woman.

There is considerable variation in the duration of labor and rate of cervical dilatation in the active phase of labor. An active phase longer than 12 hours in a nullipara and longer than 6 hours in a multipara was considered abnormal based on Friedman's data on normal labor. More important than the length of this phase is the speed of cervical dilatation. According to Friedman's data, a rate less than 1.2 cm/hr in nulliparas and 1.5 cm/hr in multiparas is evidence of some abnormality and should alert the attendant.

A recent systematic review of labor duration in nulliparous women in spontaneous labor shows that the upper limit of a normal active phase appears to be longer and rate of cervical dilatation appears to be slower that those set by Friedman. Only half of nulliparous women in the active phase dilated at a rate greater than 1.2 cm/hr. For all of these labor curves, it is evident that the duration of labor varies from woman to woman, and the rate of cervical change is faster in the active first stage and in parous women. These studies suggest that in low-risk nulliparous women with a spontaneous onset of labor, labors progressing at a rate greater than 0.5 cm/hr should be considered normal.

A diagnosis of prolonged active phase is made when the cervix dilates less than 0.5 cm/hr over a 4-hour observation period (*primary dysfunctional labor*) or if there is complete cessation of cervical dilatation over a 2-hour period (*secondary arrest of dilatation*) in the active phase when the cervix has reached at least 4 cm.

In cases of primary dysfunctional labor, there is progress being made, albeit at a very slow rate of cervical dilatation. In cases of secondary arrest of dilatation, there are two subgroups: (1) the uterine contractions become insufficient to maintain progressive dilatation of the cervix and (2) cervical dilatation ceases despite strong and efficient uterine contractions. Although this is a different entity from the primary dysfunctional labor, both can occur in the same patient, and the etiology can be related. Thus, either a slowly dilating cervix or one that had been opening normally may stop advancing.

Accurate assessment of the situation and diagnosis of etiology is vital. Keeping in mind that inefficient uterine action is often associated with disproportion and abnormal position of the fetus, one must not blame the lack of progress on poor contractions until mechanical factors have been ruled out. When ineffective labor (often myometrial fatigue) is the sole cause, half the patients resume progress after no more than treatment with rest and adequate hydration. In this group, amniotomy and oxytocin stimulation work well. When there are complications such as disproportion or abnormal position, the treatment must be aimed in their direction.

FIRST STAGE OF LABOR

Descent of the Presenting Part

Once active descent begins late in the first stage of labor, it should advance progressively throughout the course of the second stage. Interruption of descent usually suggests malpositioning, cephalopelvic disproportion, or abnormalities of uterine action. Diagnosis is based on the demonstration of there being no change in the station of the fetal presenting part over the period of at least 2 hours. Cesarean section and assisted vaginal deliveries are frequently associated with this problem. With difficult or failed operative vaginal deliveries, maternal and fetal trauma are common.

Prolonged Second Stage

Prolonged labor in the second stage was formerly defined as labor exceeding 2 hours in a nullipara and 1 hour in a multipara. Because of the concept of passive and active second stage, these time limits are no longer appropriate definitions of dystocia in the second stage (see Chapter 16). In general, birth should be expected to occur within 3 hours of the start of the active second stage in a nullipara and within 2 hours in a multipara. Delay in the active second stage should therefore be recognized and diagnosed when it has lasted 2 hours in the nullipara and 1 hour in the multipara. Labor dystocia in the second stage has also been defined as a lack of descent or descent less than 1 cm/hr of the fetal presenting part in the active phase of the second stage of labor.

Etiology of Prolonged Second Stage

1. Cephalopelvic disproportion

   a. Small pelvis
   b. Large baby

2. Malpresentation and malposition

3. Ineffective labor

   a. Primary inefficient uterine contractions
   b. Myometrial fatigue: secondary inertia
   c. Constriction (Bandl's ring)
   d. Inability or refusal of the patient to bear down (maternal exhaustion)
   e. Excessive motor block from regional anesthesia

4. Soft tissue dystocia

   a. Narrow vaginal canal
   b. Rigid perineum

Under conditions of good fetal well-being, the second stage can be extended if there appears to be good progress being made and vaginal delivery is likely. Factors that affect the duration of second stage include:

1. Parity
2. Regional anesthesia

3. Duration of first stage of labor
4. Maternal height and weight
5. Fetal weight
6. Fetal position

A prolonged second stage is associated with increased maternal risks, including chorioamnionitis, postpartum hemorrhage, operative vaginal delivery, and third- and fourth-degree perineal lacerations.

MANAGEMENT OF LABOR DYSTOCIA

Management of labor includes several components, including a strict and disciplined approach to the diagnosis of labor, regular assessment of maternal and fetal well-being, and careful monitoring of labor progress. Once labor dystocia is recognized and confirmed, management depends on the etiology and stage or phase of labor. Appropriate and timely intervention with oxytocin augmentation may reduce maternal and neonatal morbidity.

Prevention Strategies

1. Good prenatal care and preparation for childbirth reduce the incidence of prolonged labor. Continuous close support during labor has also been shown to prevent the incidence of labor dystocia
2. Labor should not be induced in the absence of a medical indication for induction and/or when the cervix is not favorable
3. The patient's general physical and mental condition is assessed with respect to fatigue, morale, hydration, and nourishment
4. False labor is treated by adequate rest, hydration, and support. Judicious use of appropriate analgesia in the early phase of labor should also be given
5. Admission to the birthing unit should be delayed until the woman has entered the active phase of labor as long as maternal and fetal well-being are confirmed
6. Avoid routine amniotomy, especially in the latent phase of labor
7. Avoid a diagnosis of labor dystocia in the latent phase of labor
8. Assess adequacy of labor progress. By charting the progress of labor on a partogram (see Fig. 14-1), we can ascertain whether cervical dilatation is occurring at a normal rate, too slowly, or has ceased altogether. The type of abnormality can be diagnosed, and the point at which intervention is necessary is indicated

FIRST STAGE OF LABOR

Vaginal Examination

Once labor dystocia is diagnosed and confirmed, vaginal examination should be performed at 2-hour intervals in the first stage and 1-hour intervals in the second stage of labor to ensure adequate progress in labor. A careful assessment of the cervix and fetal station and position is performed.

Cervix

Has there been any progress or further dilatation since the last examination? Is the cervix swollen suggestive of obstructed labor? Is an anterior cervical lip caught between the head and the symphysis?

Station of Presenting Part

The station of the bony presenting part is determined. Is it at, above, or below the spines? Has engagement taken place? Is there a caput? Is molding excessive?

Position

The position must be diagnosed accurately. In all cases of prolonged labor, malpositions such as brow presentation and occiput posterior should be kept in mind.

Failure of Descent

What seems to be holding up the presenting part? Is the cause of arrest in the bony pelvis or the cervix? Is the head too big for the pelvis? Or is the problem not the pelvis, the cervix, or the fetus, but in the uterine contractions, and will a few hours of really good labor achieve progress to successful delivery?

Uterine Contractions

The uterine contractions are assessed in terms of strength and frequency. Is the basic problem in the type of labor, or is the main problem elsewhere and the poor uterine action a secondary complication? If the contractions are judged to be efficient, then the reason for the failure of progress must be in another field. Because inefficient uterine action is almost entirely a disorder of primigravidas, multiparas with prolonged labors must be investigated for other factors carefully before a diagnosis of poor labor is made. A woman who has delivered a 7-pound baby with no trouble may not be able to do the same with a 9-pound baby.

The strength of the contractions may be assessed manually or with the use of an electronic external or internal uterine pressure monitoring system.

Dystocia in the First Stage

Mechanical factors must be ruled out. In some cases, there is cephalopelvic disproportion, and cesarean section is indicated. For the rest, hypotonic uterine contractions account for the majority of slowly progressive labor, and medical management is carried out as long as the fetus and mother are in good condition. Nothing is done to complicate the situation further. Slow progress is accepted. Support, reassurance, rest, fluids, and analgesia are provided. Premature and traumatic vaginal operations are not recommended.

Therapeutic Rest

Therapeutic rest involves providing pain relief by effective support and analgesia. Some women who experience excessive pain or anxiety during labor produce high endogenous catecholamines, which has a direct inhibitory effect on uterine contractions. This leads to a vicious cycle of inefficient uterine contractions, poor labor progress, increased anxiety, and higher catecholamines. Nonpharmacologic and pharmacologic options for pain management should be provided.

Parenteral narcotics with a short half-life are effective in providing short-term pain relief. Epidural anesthesia has an advantage of providing effective pain relief for the duration of labor and allows women to rest (see Chapter 36). In particular, it allows the administration of oxytocin augmentation for women with labor dystocia without increasing the amount of labor pain significantly.

Epidural anesthesia is associated with prolonged labor in the first and second stages of labor, an increased incidence of fetal malposition, an increased use of oxytocin augmentation, and an increased risk of assisted vaginal deliveries. It has not been shown to increase the risk of cesarean section, although studies are conflicting.

Amniotomy

Amniotomy alone when used in the latent phase of labor is usually insufficient to result in significant augmentation of labor. Routine and early amniotomy has also not been shown to accelerate spontaneous labor or increase the chance of a successful vaginal delivery. However, in the setting of prolonged or delayed labor in the active phase, amniotomy is recommended in all women with intact membranes. Performing an amniotomy increases local prostaglandin levels and may increase the strength and frequency of uterine contractions. Amniotomy in this setting has also been shown to shorten the duration of the first stage of labor.

Oxytocin

When all other more conservative measures have been attempted to stimulate more effective contractions and in the setting of stable maternal and fetal conditions, it is recommended that labor augmentation be started with oxytocin before a caesarean delivery being performed for "failure to progress." Oxytocin should be initiated in cases of labor dystocia caused by inadequate of inefficient uterine contractions. Oxytocin, when administered intravenously as a constant infusion, increases the frequency, force and duration of uterine contractions. Several studies have shown that oxytocin augmentation decreases the duration of labor and increases the rate of successful spontaneous vaginal delivery.

It should be used with caution when cephalopelvic disproportion is suspected, in cases of hypersensitivity to oxytocin, uteroplacental insufficiency, abnormal fetal heart rate (FHR), and previous cesarean section.

When oxytocin is used, an initial dose of 1 to 2 mU/min of oxytocin is started. It should be titrated slowly to achieve a contraction pattern of four or five contractions in 10 minutes. This should be done gradually with a 30-minute interval between dose increases. While most patients achieve a response to stimulation at oxytocin concentrations between 4 and 10 mU/min, a proportion of nullipara require higher doses of oxytocin. When 20 mU/min of oxytocin is reached, a careful reevaluation of the labor progress and maternal and fetal well-being should be carried out before further increases in oxytocin titration. Continuous electronic fetal heart rate monitoring (EFM) should be implemented whenever oxytocin is used.

Tachysystole

Oxytocin use is associated with an increased incidence of tachysystole. *Tachysystole* is defined as a contraction frequency of more than five contractions in 10 minutes with less than 60 seconds of resting tone or uterine contractions lasting for more than 2 minutes. It can occur with or without FHR abnormalities. Persistent uterine tachysystole with FHR abnormalities can lead to fetal hypoxia if not corrected. Appropriate use and titration of the oxytocin dose to achieve minimally effective strength and frequency of uterine contractions, without causing too much, is usually sufficient to correct tachysystole.

Uterine tachysystole is associated with (1) high-dose oxytocin titration regimens (4-6 mU/min oxytocin increments) and (2) when incremental increases in oxytocin dose are increased at intervals of less than 30 minutes.

Fetal Heart Rate Monitoring

Continuous FHR monitoring should be offered when labor dystocia is diagnosed. Whenever oxytocin is used, continuous external or internal FHR monitoring should be used (see Chapter 12).

Cervical Dystocia

The cervix may be holding up progress. A thick anterior lip or a thin, soft rim of cervix may be caught between the head and the symphysis pubis. This can be pushed over the head during a contraction, especially in multiparous women.

Arrest of Labor in the Second Stage

Clinical reassessment of labor progress should be done at hourly intervals in the second stage. It is vital that mechanical factors be ruled out carefully. These include malpositions and malpresentations as well as cephalopelvic disproportion. Cesarean section is performed in most cases of cephalopelvic disproportion.

Maternal and fetal well-being should be monitored carefully. Continuous EFM is recommended when there is a delay in the second stage to ensure that the fetus is tolerating labor. In the setting of good fetal well-being, support, rest, and adequate pain relief for the exhausted mother may be beneficial in the second stage. A passive second stage (or delayed pushing) allows for fetal descent to occur mainly from the action of the uterine contractions without exhausting the mother. Where membranes are still intact in the second stage, they should be artificially ruptured.

Oxytocin should be started as soon as labor dystocia is recognized in the second stage. The same principles for oxytocin use in the first stage of labor are applied in the second stage. It should be used with caution when cephalopelvic disproportion is suspected and in cases of hypersensitivity to oxytocin, uteroplacental insufficiency, abnormal FHR, and previous cesarean section.

If progress is being made and vaginal delivery is expected, the duration of the second stage alone should not mandate intervention with operative delivery.

FIRST STAGE OF LABOR

Operative Delivery

Delivery by cesarean section or assisted vaginal delivery is indicated when there is no further progress despite oxytocin augmentation. In the first stage of labor, an adequate trial of oxytocin augmentation with a minimum of 4 hours of minimally effective uterine contractions should be given before operative delivery is considered. Minimally effective uterine contractions is defined either as uterine contractions achieving 200 or more Montevideo units or three or four strong contractions every 10 minutes. In spontaneously laboring women with slow progress of labor at term, oxytocin augmentation for 4 hours can result in vaginal deliveries in approximately 80% of nulliparous women and 95% of multiparous women with no adverse effect on the mother or baby. After an adequate trial of oxytocin augmentation and complete arrest of dilatation of the cervix occurs in the first stage of labor (dilatation arrests at less than 10 cm), vaginal delivery is impossible at this time, and cesarean section must be performed.

When arrest of labor in the second stage is established, operative delivery is indicated when there is no further descent of the presenting part after 1 hour of active pushing with adequate contractions. If the presenting part is low in the pelvis, there is no disproportion, and the baby may be delivered by forceps or vacuum if the presentation is cephalic and by cesarean section if he or she is a breech. The decision to proceed with an assisted vaginal delivery versus a cesarean section should be made on the basis of the clinical assessment of the mother and fetus and the skill of the obstetrician.

At any sign fetal or maternal distress, early intervention and operative delivery are indicated. Preparations should be at hand for the treatment of postpartum hemorrhage and fetal distress.

SELECTED READING

American College of Obstetricians and Gynecologists: Dystocia and Augmentation of Labor. ACOG Practice Bulletin No. 49. Obstet Gynecol 102:1445-1454, 2003

Drouin P, Nasah BT, Nkounawa F: The value of the Partogramme in the management of labor. Obstet Gynecol 53:741, 1979

Friedman EA: Disordered labor. Objective evaluation and management. J Family Pract 2:167, 1975

Friedman EA, Sachtleben MR: Station of the fetal presenting part. Arrest in nulliparas. Obstet Gynecol 47:129, 1976

Kjaergaard H, Olsen J, Ottesen B, Dykes AK: Incidence and outcomes of dystocia in the active phase of labor in term nulliparous women with spontaneous labor onset. Acta Obstet Gynecol Scand 88:402, 2009

Maltau JM, Anderson HT: Epidural anesthesia as an alternative to cesarean section in the treatment of prolonged, exhaustive labour. Acta Anesthesiol Scand 19:349, 1975

National Institute for Health and Clinical Excellence: Intrapartum Care, care of healthy women and their babies during childbirth. http://guidance.nice.org.uk/CG55/ Guidance, 2007

Neal JL, Lowe NK, Ahijevych KL et al: Active labor duration and dilation rates among low-risk, nulliparous women with spontaneous labor onset: A systematic review. J Midwifery Womens Health 55:308-318, 2010

Rouse DJ, Owen J, Savage KG, Hauth, JC: Active phase labor arrest: oxytocin augmentation for at least 4 hours. Obstet Gynecol 93:323, 1999

Zhang J, Landy HJ, Branch DW, et al: Contemporary patterns of spontaneous labor with normal neonatal outcomes. Obstet Gynecol 116:1281, 2010

FIRST STAGE OF LABOR

CHAPTER 15

Abnormal
Cephalic
Presentations

Jessica Dy
Darine El-Chaar

MALPRESENTATIONS

The fetus enters the pelvis in a cephalic presentation approximately 95 percent to 96 percent of the time. In these cephalic presentations, the occiput may be in the persistent transverse or posterior positions. In about 3 percent to 4 percent of pregnancies, there is a breech-presenting fetus (see Chapter 25). In the remaining 1 percent, the fetus may be either in a transverse or oblique lie (see Chapter 26), or the head may be extended with the face or brow presenting.

Predisposing Factors

Maternal and Uterine Factors

1. Contracted pelvis: This is the most common and important factor
2. Pendulous maternal abdomen: If the uterus and fetus are allowed to fall forward, there may be difficulty in engagement
3. Neoplasms: Uterine fibromyomas or ovarian cysts can block the entry to the pelvis
4. Uterine anomalies: In a bicornuate uterus, the nonpregnant horn may obstruct labor in the pregnant one
5. Abnormalities of placental size or location: Conditions such as placenta previa are associated with unfavorable positions of the fetus
6. High parity

Fetal Factors

1. Large baby
2. Errors in fetal polarity, such as breech presentation and transverse lie
3. Abnormal internal rotation: The occiput rotates posteriorly or fails to rotate at all
4. Fetal attitude: Extension in place of normal flexion
5. Multiple pregnancy
6. Fetal anomalies, including hydrocephaly and anencephaly
7. Polyhydramnios: An excessive amount of amniotic fluid allows the baby freedom of activity, and he or she may assume abnormal positions
8. Prematurity

Placenta and Membranes

1. Placenta previa
2. Cornual implantation
3. Premature rupture of membranes

Effects of Malpresentations

Effects on Labor

The less symmetrical adaptation of the presenting part to the cervix and to the pelvis plays a part in reducing the efficiency of labor.

1. The incidence of fetopelvic disproportion is higher
2. Inefficient uterine action is common. The contractions tend to be weak and irregular
3. Prolonged labor is seen frequently
4. Pathologic retraction rings can develop, and rupture of the lower uterine segment may be the end result
5. The cervix often dilates slowly and incompletely
6. The presenting part stays high
7. Premature rupture of the membranes occurs often
8. The need for operative delivery is increased

Effects on the Mother

1. Because greater uterine and intraabdominal muscular effort is required and because labor is often prolonged, maternal exhaustion is common

2. There is more stretching of the perineum and soft parts, and there are more lacerations

3. Bleeding is more profuse, originating from:

   a. Tears of the uterus, cervix, and vagina
   b. Uterine atony from prolonged labor

4. There is a greater incidence of infection. This is caused by:

   a. Early rupture of the membranes
   b. Excessive blood loss
   c. Tissue damage
   d. Frequent rectal and vaginal examinations
   e. Prolonged labor

5. The patient's discomfort seems out of proportion to the strength of the uterine contractions. She complains bitterly of pain before the uterus is felt to harden and continues to feel the pain after the uterus has relaxed

6. Paresis of the bowel and bladder add to the patient's suffering

FIRST STAGE OF LABOR

Effects on the Fetus

1. The fetus fits the pelvis less perfectly, making passage through the pelvis more difficult and leading to excessive molding
2. The long labor is harder on the baby, with a greater incidence of a low arterial cord pH at the time of delivery. Without appropriate and timely intervention, this can lead to anoxia, brain damage, asphyxia, and intrauterine death
3. There is a higher incidence of operative delivery, increasing the danger of trauma to the baby
4. Prolapse of the umbilical cord is more common than in normal positions

TRANSVERSE POSITIONS OF THE OCCIPUT

Left Occiput Transverse: LOT

Engagement is more frequent in the transverse diameter of the inlet than in the oblique. Left occiput transverse (LOT) is the most common position at the onset of labor (Fig. 15-1).

Diagnosis of Position: LOT

Abdominal Examination

1. The lie is longitudinal
2. The head is at or in the pelvis
3. The back is on the left and toward the mother's flank
4. The small parts are on the right and sometimes can be felt clearly
5. The breech is in the fundus of the uterus
6. The cephalic prominence (forehead) is on the right

Fetal Heart. The fetal heart is heard loudest in the left lower quadrant of the mother's abdomen.

Vaginal Examination

1. The sagittal suture is in the transverse diameter of the pelvis. If the head is in synclitism (Fig. 15-1B), the sagittal suture is midway between the symphysis pubis and the promontory of the sacrum. If there is posterior

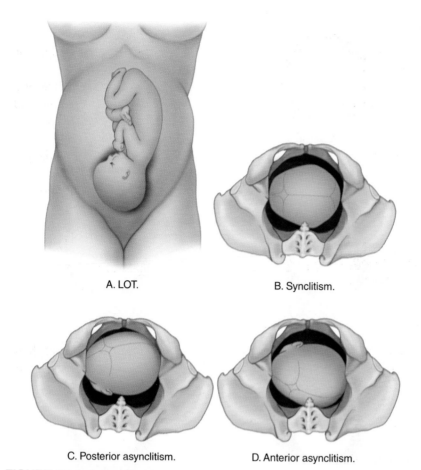

A. LOT. B. Synclitism.

C. Posterior asynclitism. D. Anterior asynclitism.

FIGURE 15-1. Left occiput transverse (LOT).

asynclitism (Fig. 15-1C), the sagittal suture is closer to the pubic symphysis. With anterior asynclitism (Fig. 15-1D), the sagittal suture is closer to the sacral promontory

2. The small posterior fontanel is toward the mother's left at 3 o'clock
3. The bregma is on the right at 9 o'clock
4. If there is flexion, the occiput is lower than the brow. If flexion is poor, the occiput and brow are almost at the same level in the pelvis

Mechanism of Labor: LOT

Descent. Descent includes engagement, which may have taken place before labor (Figs. 15-2A and B). Descent continues throughout labor.

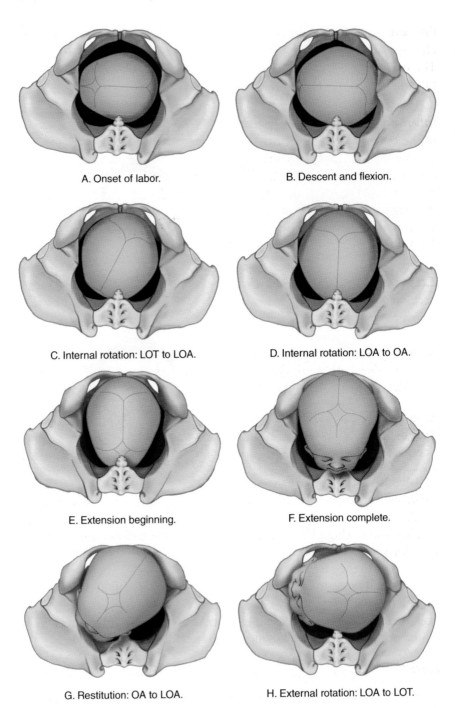

A. Onset of labor.

B. Descent and flexion.

C. Internal rotation: LOT to LOA.

D. Internal rotation: LOA to OA.

E. Extension beginning.

F. Extension complete.

G. Restitution: OA to LOA.

H. External rotation: LOA to LOT.

FIGURE 15-2. Mechanism of labor: left occiput transverse (LOT). LOA, left occiput anterior; OA, occiput anterior.

Flexion. Resistance to descent causes the head to flex (Fig. 15-2B) so that the chin approaches the chest. This reduces the presenting diameter by 1.5 cm. The occipitofrontal diameter of 11.0 cm is replaced by the suboccipito-bregmatic diameter of 9.5 cm.

Internal Rotation. The head enters the pelvis with the sagittal suture in the transverse diameter of the inlet and the occiput at 3 o'clock. The occiput then rotates 90° to arrive under the pubic symphysis. The sinciput comes to lie anterior to the sacrum. The sequence is LOT to left occiput anterior (LOA) to occiput anterior (OA) (Figs. 15-2A to 2D). The shoulders lag behind 45° so that when the sagittal suture of the head is in the anteroposterior diameter of the pelvis, the shoulders are in the left oblique. Thus, the neck is twisted.

Extension. Birth is by extension (Figs. 15-2E and F). The nape of the neck pivots under the pubis, while the vertex, bregma, forehead, face, and chin are born over the perineum.

Restitution. When the head has made its exit, the neck untwists, and the head turns back 45° to the left, resuming the normal relationship with the shoulders—OA to LOA (Fig. 15-2G).

External Rotation. The shoulders now rotate 45° to the left to bring their bisacromial diameter into the anteroposterior diameter of the pelvis. The head follows the shoulder and rotates externally another 45° to the left—LOA to LOT (Fig. 15-2H).

Birth of Shoulders, Trunk, and Placenta. Birth of the shoulders, trunk, and placenta is the same as described in Chapter 10, "Normal Mechanism of Labor." A summary of the mechanism of labor (LOT) is presented in Figure 15-3.

Clinical Course of Labor: LOT

Most fetuses who begin labor in the LOT position rotate the head 90° (LOT to LOA to OA) to bring the occiput under the pubic symphysis, from which position spontaneous delivery takes place.

Arrest of Progress. Arrest of progress can occur in any of these situations:

1. Anterior rotation of 90° to the OA position but spontaneous delivery does not take place
2. Anterior rotation of 45° with cessation of progress in the LOA position

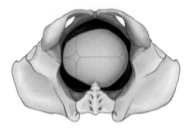

A. At onset of labor.

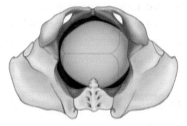

B. Descent and flexion.

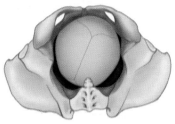

C. Internal rotation: LOT to LOA.

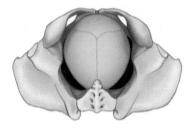

D. Internal rotation: LOA to OA.

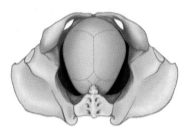

E. Extension beginning.

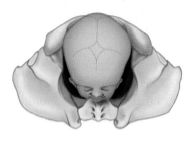

F. Extension complete.

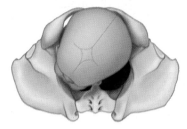

G. Restitution: OA to LOA.

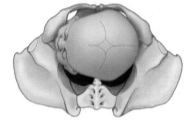

H. External rotation: LOA to LOT.

FIGURE 15-3. Summary of the mechanism of labor: left occiput transverse (LOT).
LOA, left occiput anterior; OA, occiput anterior.

3. No rotation. The head is arrested with the sagittal suture in the transverse diameter of the pelvis. This is known as transverse arrest
4. In the rare case posterior rotation takes place, LOT to left occiput posterior (LOP). The mechanism of labor then becomes that of occipito-posterior positions

Management of Arrested Cases. Providing the prerequisites for operative vaginal delivery are present (see Chapter 17), the following treatment is carried out:

1. Arrest in OA position: Forceps or vacuum are applied to the sides of the fetal head, which is then extracted

2. Arrest as LOA: Forceps or vacuum are applied to the fetal head, which is then rotated 45° to the OA position and extracted

3. Transverse arrest: LOT: Two operative techniques are available

   a. Manual rotation, 90°, LOT to LOA to OA, followed by forceps or vacuum extraction
   b. Application of the forceps to the sides of the baby's head, rotation by the forceps of 90°, LOT to LOA to OA, and then extraction by the forceps or vacuum

4. Arrest as an occiput posterior is treated like other occiput posterior deliveries

Right Occiput Transverse: ROT

Right occiput transverse (ROT) is similar to LOT. The difference is that the back and occiput are on the mother's right, and the limbs are on her left.

POSTERIOR POSITIONS OF THE OCCIPUT

General Considerations

Definition
The occiput and the small posterior fontanel are in the rear segment of the maternal pelvis, and the brow and bregma are in the anterior segment.

FIRST STAGE OF LABOR

Incidence

The incidence of this position is 15 to 30 percent of all cephalic presentations and is more common in nulliparous women. The exact incidence of posterior positions is difficult to ascertain since most of them rotate anteriorly and are considered erroneously as being originally occipitoanterior. The posterior positions that rotate anteriorly with no difficulty are often not diagnosed, and only the persistent posteriors are recognized regularly. Right occiput posterior (ROP) is five times as common as LOP.

Etiology

The etiology of posterior positions of the occiput is the same as the etiology of other abnormal positions. Cephalopelvic disproportion is a frequent and serious complicating factor that must be considered at all times. The shape of the pelvic inlet influences the position of the occiput. Where the forepelvis is narrow, there is a tendency for the back of the head with its long biparietal diameter to be pushed to the rear, so that the front of the head with its short bitemporal diameter can be accommodated by the small forepelvis. Hence, posterior positions of the occiput are found often in android and anthropoid pelvises.

Right Occiput Posterior: ROP

Diagnosis of Position: ROP

Abdominal Examination

1. The lie is vertical. The long axis of the fetus is parallel to the long axis of the mother (Fig. 15-4)
2. The head is at or in the pelvis
3. The fetal back is in the right maternal flank. In most cases, it cannot be outlined clearly
4. The small parts are easily felt anteriorly on the left side. The maternal abdomen has been described as being alive with little hands and feet
5. The breech is in the fundus of the uterus
6. The cephalic prominence is on the left. It is not felt as easily as in anterior positions because flexion is less marked

Fetal Heart. Fetal heart tones are transmitted through the scapula and hence are heard in the right maternal flank on the same side as the baby's back. Frequently, the fetal heart sounds are indistinct. They can be transmitted through the baby's chest and in some cases are loudest in the left

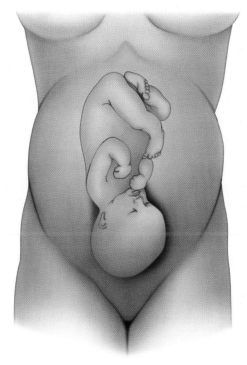

A. Abdominal view.

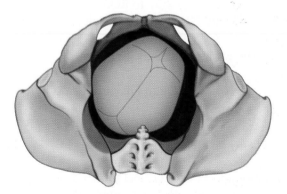

B. Vaginal view.

FIGURE 15-4. Right occiput posterior.

anterior lower quadrant of the abdomen. The location of the fetal heart sounds is not a reliable sign in determining how the baby is placed; hence, a carefully made diagnosis of posterior position should not be changed because of the situation of the fetal heart. As the back rotates anteriorly, the fetal heart tones approach the midline of the abdomen.

Vaginal Examination

1. The sagittal suture is in the right oblique diameter of the pelvis
2. The small posterior fontanel is in the right posterior segment of the pelvis
3. The bregma is anterior and to the left of the symphysis pubis
4. Since flexion is imperfect, the fontanels may be close to the same level in the pelvis
5. Where there is difficulty in diagnosis, the pinna (auricle) of the ear is found pointing to the occiput

Mechanism of Labor: ROP

Rotation of varying degree and direction can take place:

1. Anterior rotation:

    a. Long arc rotation of 135°, ROP to ROT to right occiput anterior (ROA) to OA. This occurs in 90 percent of occipitoposterior positions. The baby is born as an occipitoanterior
    b. Rotation of 90°, ROP to ROT to ROA
    c. Rotation of 45°, ROP to ROT. The result is deep transverse arrest

2. No rotation. The position remains ROP

3. Posterior rotation of 45°, ROP to OP with the occiput turning into the hollow of the sacrum

Spontaneous delivery can take place after:

1. Anterior rotation to OA with normal birth
2. Posterior rotation to OP with face to pubis delivery

Arrest of labor can occur:

1. High in the pelvis, with failure to engage. These are often problems of disproportion

2. In the midpelvis, with complete or partial failure of rotation
   a. Deep transverse arrest, ROT
   b. Arrest with the sagittal suture in the right oblique diameter of the pelvis, ROP
   c. Arrest with the occiput in the hollow of the sacrum, OP

3. Arrest at the outlet

Long Arc Rotation: 135° to the Anterior

DESCENT. The head enters the inlet with the sagittal suture in the right oblique diameter (Fig. 15-5A), and unless obstruction is encountered descent continues throughout labor. Engagement may be delayed, and the entire labor may take longer than in normal anterior positions.

FLEXION. Flexion (Fig. 15-5B) is imperfect and often is not complete until the head reaches the pelvic floor. The partial flexion and the resulting larger diameter of the presenting part contribute to the labor being longer and harder for both the mother and child.

INTERNAL ROTATION. The occiput rotates 135° anteriorly under the symphysis pubis—ROP to ROT to ROA to OA (Figs. 15-5C to E).

EXTENSION. The nape of the neck pivots in the subpubic angle, and the head is born by extension (Figs. 15-5F and G). The bregma, forehead, nose, mouth, and chin pass over the perineum in order.

RESTITUTION. Restitution (OA to ROA) takes place to the right (Fig. 15-5H). The extent of restitution depends on how far the shoulders have followed the head during internal rotation. In most cases, the shoulders turn with the head, lagging behind only 45°, and restitution is the usual 45°. Occasionally, the shoulders may lag behind more or may swing back. The head then restitutes 90° or even 135°.

EXTERNAL ROTATION. The anterior shoulder strikes the pelvic floor and rotates 45° toward the pubic symphysis so that the bisacromial diameter of the shoulders is in the anteroposterior diameter of the outlet. The head follows the shoulders, and the occiput rotates 45° to the right transverse position—ROA to ROT (Fig. 15-5I).

FIRST STAGE OF LABOR

Short Arc Rotation: 45° to the Posterior

DESCENT. The head enters the inlet with the sagittal suture in the right oblique (Fig. 15-6A). Descent continues throughout labor.

FLEXION. Flexion (Fig. 15-6B) is imperfect, resulting in a longer presenting diameter.

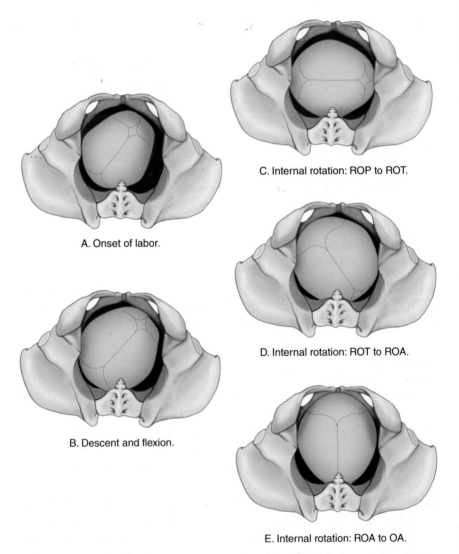

A. Onset of labor.

B. Descent and flexion.

C. Internal rotation: ROP to ROT.

D. Internal rotation: ROT to ROA.

E. Internal rotation: ROA to OA.

FIGURE 15-5. **Right occiput posterior (ROP): long arc rotation.** OA, occiput anterior; ROA, right occiput anterior.

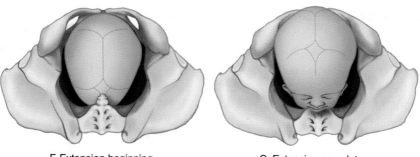

F. Extension beginning.   G. Extension complete.

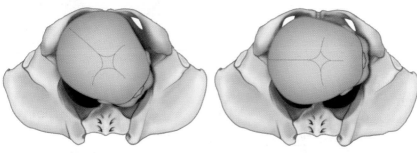

H. Restitution: OA to ROA.   I. External rotation: ROA to ROT.

FIGURE 15-5. (Continued)

FIRST STAGE OF LABOR

INTERNAL ROTATION. The occiput turns posteriorly 45° (ROP to OP) into the hollow of the sacrum (Fig. 15-6C). The sagittal suture is in the antero-posterior diameter of the pelvis. The bregma is behind the pubis.

BIRTH OF HEAD. Birth of the head is by a combination of flexion and extension (Fig. 15-6D-G).

There are two mechanisms of flexion:

1. Where there is good flexion, the area anterior to the bregma pivots under the symphysis pubis. The presenting diameter is the suboccipitofrontal of 10.5 cm. The bregma, vertex, small fontanel, and occiput are born by further flexion

2. Where flexion is incomplete, the root of the nose pivots under the symphysis. The presenting diameter is the larger occipitofrontal of 11.5 cm. This bigger diameter is more traumatic than the smaller one. By flexion, the forehead, bregma, vertex, and occiput are born over the perineum

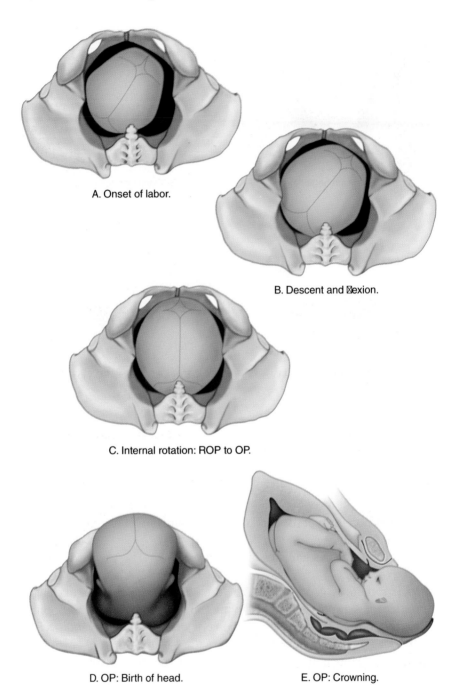

A. Onset of labor.

B. Descent and flexion.

C. Internal rotation: ROP to OP.

D. OP: Birth of head.

E. OP: Crowning.

FIGURE 15-6. Right occiput posterior (ROP): short arc rotation. OP, occiput posterior; ROT, right occiput transverse.

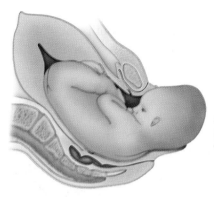

F. OP: Flexion beginning.

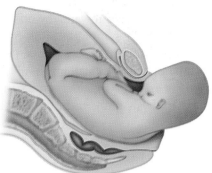

G. OP: Flexion complete.

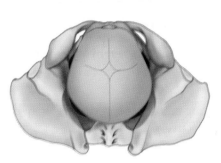

H. Extension: Vaginal view.

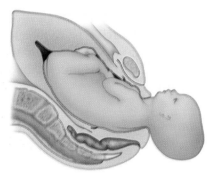

I. Extension: Lateral view.

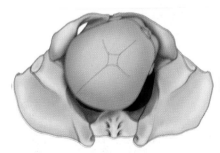

J. Restitution: OP to ROP.

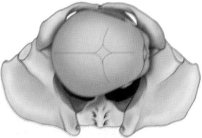

K. External rotation: ROP to ROT.

FIGURE 15-6. *(Continued)*

FIRST STAGE OF LABOR

After the top and back of the head have been born by flexion, the occiput falls back toward the anus, and the nose, mouth, and chin are born under the symphysis pubis by extension (Figs. 15-6H and I).

Restitution of the occiput is 45° to the right oblique (OP to ROP) to resume the normal relationship of the head to the shoulders (Fig. 15-6J).

The anterior shoulder strikes the pelvic floor and rotates 45° toward the symphysis pubis to bring the bisacromial diameter of the shoulders into the anteroposterior diameter of the pelvis (external rotation). The head follows, and the occiput rotates 45° to the right transverse position—ROP to ROT (Fig. 15-6K).

Molding. In persistent occipitoposterior positions, the head is shortened in the occipitofrontal and lengthened in the suboccipitobregmatic and mentobregmatic diameters. The head rises steeply in front and in back. The caput succedaneum is located over the bregma. Molding (Fig. 15-7) and extensive edema of the scalp make accurate identification of the sutures and fontanels difficult, thereby obscuring the diagnosis.

Summaries. Summaries of both long arc and short arc rotations may be reviewed in Figures 15-8 and 15-9, respectively.

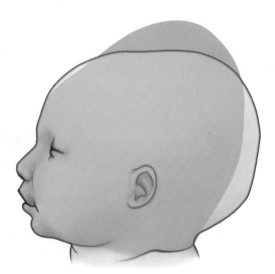

FIGURE 15-7. Molding: right occiput posterior.

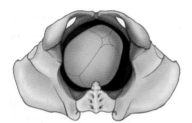

A. ROP: Onset of labor.

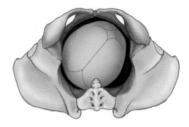

B. Descent and flexion.

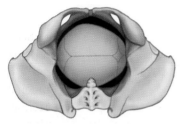

C. Internal rotation: ROP to ROT.

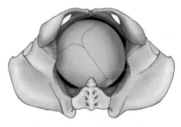

D. Internal rotation: ROT to ROA.

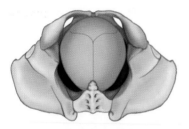

E. Internal rotation: ROA to OA.

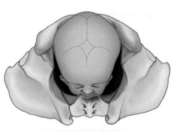

F. Extension.

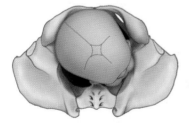

G. Restitution: OA to ROA.

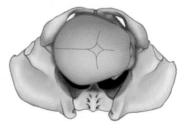

H. External rotation: ROA to ROT.

FIGURE 15-8. Summary of long arc rotation: right occiput posterior (ROP) to occiput posterior (OP). OA, occiput anterior; ROA, right occiput anterior; ROT, right occiput transverse.

FIRST STAGE OF LABOR

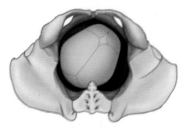

A. ROP: Onset of labor.

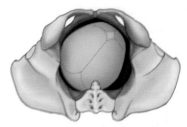

B. Descent and flexion.

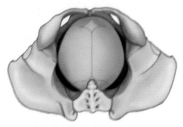

C. Internal rotation: ROP to OP.

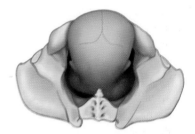

D. Birth by flexion.

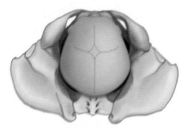

E. Head falls back in extension.

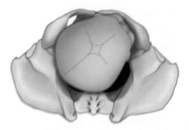

F. Restitution: OP to ROP.

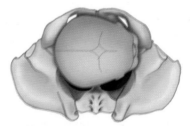

G. External rotation: ROP to ROT.

FIGURE 15-9. **Summary of short arc rotation: right occiput posterior (ROP) to occiput posterior (OP).** ROT, right occiput transverse.

Management of the Persistent Occiput Posterior Position

1. Expectant observation is the best policy. Given sufficient time, most posterior positions of the occiput rotate anteriorly, and the baby is delivered spontaneously or by low forceps or vacuum. Thus, as long as the fetus and mother are in good condition and labor is progressing, there is no justification for interference. The safe and wise rule is to leave occipitoposterior positions to nature, supplying only supportive measures until there is a definite indication for intervention

2. Placing the mother in forward-leaning or side-lying positions may help the rotation of the occiput. Forward-leaning positions such as kneeling, straddling, and hands and knees positions may enhance the rotation and reduce back pain. It is believed that anterior rotation is helped by the mother's lying on the same side toward which the occiput is already directed. So if the fetus is in the ROP position, the mother lies on her right side

3. Because the labor may be long and difficult for mother and child, care must be exercised to ensure adequate intake of fluids and nourishment. More judicious use of analgesia and sedation is required than in normal occipitoanterior positions

4. If effective labor does not begin, the uterus may be stimulated using an intravenous oxytocin infusion as per protocol developed in each institution. The drip is started slowly at a rate of about 1 to 2 milliunits/hr and then increased every half an hour by either 1 to 2 milliunits/hr. During this time, the effect on the contractions and the fetal heart is observed. The aim is to achieve good uterine contractions every 2 to 3 minutes, lasting 45 to 60 seconds (see Chapter 14)

5. Intact membranes do not always help labor and often even seem to delay it. Therefore, before the progress of labor can be considered halted, the membranes should be ruptured artificially and the patient given a further trial of labor. With these measures, the patient frequently makes good progress in rotation and descent, and spontaneous delivery takes place

6. When the head is delivered in the posterior position (face to pubis), the large back part of the head (biparietal diameter, 9.5 cm) causes greater stretching and more lacerations of the perineum than does the narrow anterior part of the head (bitemporal diameter, 8.0 cm). For this reason, an episiotomy may sometimes be helpful. Frequently, there is arrest at the perineum, and low forceps or vacuum is the management of choice

FIRST STAGE OF LABOR

7. With forceps or vacuum, the fetal head can be delivered in the posterior position or can be rotated to the anterior position before being extracted. The various maneuvers are described in Chapter 17. If an attempt at operative vaginal delivery fails, cesarean section is performed
8. If there has been no progress in the face of efficient uterine contractions and a diagnosis of fetopelvic disproportion has been made, cesarean section should be performed

Indications for Intervention
Although the basic strategy of nonintervention is, up to a point, a wise one, it is not safe to wait too long; fine judgment is needed to decide the point at which further delay is undesirable or even harmful. When the standard signs of fetal or maternal distress are present, the decision to interfere is based on clear-cut grounds.

Maternal Distress. Maternal distress is fatigue or exhaustion and is accompanied by the following signs:

1. Pulse >100 bpm
2. Temperature >100°F
3. Dehydration, dry tongue, dry skin, concentrated urine
4. Loss of emotional stability

Fetal Distress. Fetal distress is shown by:

1. Irregular fetal heart rate
2. Fetal heart rate <100 or >160 bpm between uterine contractions
3. Passage of meconium in a vertex presentation

Lack of Progress. The cessation of descent and/or rotation indicates that labor is arrested and that interference is mandatory. Reasons for failure of descent and rotation include:

1. Cephalopelvic disproportion
2. Android midpelvis
3. Ineffective uterine contractions
4. Deflexion of the head
5. Uterine contraction ring preventing the shoulders from rotating anteriorly
6. Multiparity, pendulous abdomen, poor abdominal and uterine tone
7. A weak pelvic floor, failing to guide the occiput anteriorly

BROW PRESENTATIONS

General Considerations

Definition

Brow presentation is an attitude of partial (halfway) extension in contrast to face presentation in which extension is complete. The presenting part is the area between the orbital ridges and the bregma. The denominator is the forehead (frontum: Fr). The presenting diameter is the verticomental, which, at 13.5 cm, is the longest anteroposterior diameter of the fetal head.

Incidence

The incidence is under 1 percent, ranging from 1 in 500 to 1 in 1400. Primary brow presentations—those that occur before labor has started—are rare. The majorities are secondary—that is, they occur after the onset of labor. Often the position is transitory, and the head either flexes to an occiput presentation or extends completely and becomes a face presentation.

Etiology

The causes are similar to those of face presentation and include anything that interferes with engagement in flexion.

1. Cephalopelvic disproportion is of great significance

2. Some fetal conditions prevent flexion

   a. Tumors of the neck (e.g., thyroid)
   b. Coils of umbilical cord around the neck
   c. Fetal anomalies

3. Increased fetal mobility

   a. Polyhydramnios
   b. Small or premature baby

4. Premature rupture of membranes when the head is not engaged. It is trapped in an attitude of extension

5. Uterine abnormalities

   a. Neoplasm of lower segment
   b. Bicornuate uterus

FIRST STAGE OF LABOR

6. Abnormal placental implantation: placenta previa

7. Iatrogenic: external version

Left Frontum Anterior: LFrA

Diagnosis of Position: LFrA

Abdominal Examination

1. The lie is longitudinal (Fig. 15-10A)
2. The head is at the pelvis but is not engaged
3. The back is on the mother's right and posterior; it may be difficult to palpate. The small parts are on the left and anterior
4. The breech is in the fundus of the uterus
5. The cephalic prominence (occiput) and the back are on the same side (the right)

Fetal Heart. Fetal heart sounds are heard best in the left lower quadrant of the maternal abdomen.

Vaginal Examination

1. The anteroposterior diameter of the head is in the right oblique diameter of the pelvis (Fig. 15-10B)
2. The brow, the area between the nasion and the bregma, presents and is felt in the left anterior quadrant of the pelvis
3. The vertex is in the right posterior quadrant
4. The bregma (anterior fontanel) is palpated easily
5. The frontal suture is felt, but the sagittal suture is usually out of reach
6. Identification of the supraorbital ridges is a key to diagnosis

Late and Failed Diagnosis. The difference, on vaginal examination, between the hard, smooth dome of the skull and the soft, irregular face is great enough to diagnose the abnormal position or at least to suspect it. On the other hand, the feel of the vertex and that of the forehead may be similar, and molding and edema add to the difficulty of differentiation. Hence, anything short of a most careful abdominal and vaginal examination with a high index of suspicion fails to identify the malposition. A good rule is that whenever there is failure of progress, one should examine the patient thoroughly, keeping brow presentation in mind.

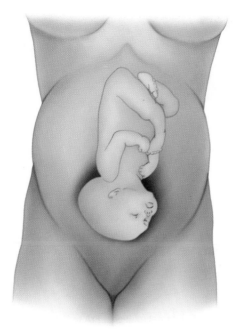

A. Abdominal view.

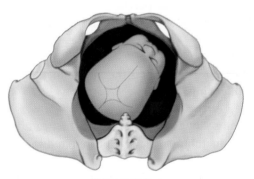

B. Vaginal view.

FIGURE 15-10. **Left frontum anterior.**

Mechanism of Labor: LFrA

The presenting diameter is the verticomental, measuring 13.5 cm. It is the longest anteroposterior diameter of the head. When engagement takes place, it is accompanied by extensive molding, and when progress occurs, it is slow.

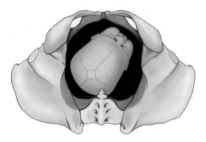

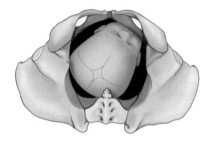

A. LFrA: Onset of labor.   B. Descent.

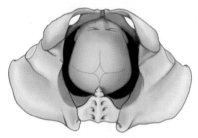

C. Internal rotation: LFrA to FrA.

FIGURE 15-11. Labor: left frontum anterior (LFrA). Descent, internal rotation. FrA, frontum anterior.

Spontaneous delivery is rare and can take place only when there is the combination of a large pelvis, strong uterine contractions, and a small baby. In these cases, the following mechanism of labor occurs (Fig. 15-11):

Extension. The head extends and the verticomental diameter presents, with the forehead leading the way.

Descent. Descent is slow and late. Usually the head does not settle into the pelvis until the membranes have ruptured and the cervix has reached full dilatation.

Internal Rotation. The forehead rotates anteriorly 45° so that the face comes to lie behind the pubic symphysis (LFrA to frontum anterior [FrA]). A considerable amount of internal rotation may take place between the ischial spines and the tuberosities.

Flexion. The face impinges under the pubis, and as the head pivots round this point, the bregma, vertex, and occiput are born over the perineum (Figs. 15-12A to C).

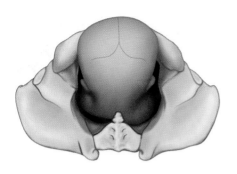

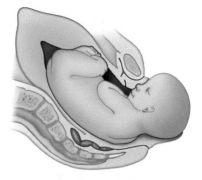

A. Birth by flexion.   B. Flexion beginning.

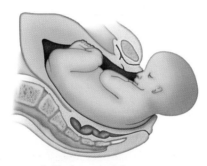

C. Flexion complete.

FIGURE 15-12.   Birth of brow and head by flexion.

Extension. The head then falls back in extension (Figs. 15-13A and B), and the nose, mouth, and chin slip under the symphysis.

Restitution. The neck untwists, and the head turns 45° back to the original side (Fig. 15-14A).

External Rotation. As the shoulder rotates anteriorly from the oblique to the anteroposterior diameter of the pelvis, the head turns back another 45° (Fig. 15-14B).

Molding. Molding is extreme (Fig. 15-15). The verticomental diameter is compressed. The occipitofrontal diameter is elongated markedly so that the forehead bulges greatly. The face is flattened, and the distance from the chin to the top of the head is long. This is exaggerated by the large caput succedaneum that forms on the forehead.

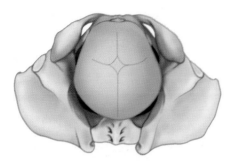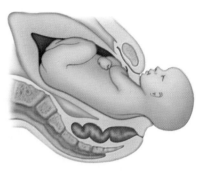

A. Vaginal view.   B. Lateral view.

FIGURE 15-13. Head falls back in extension.

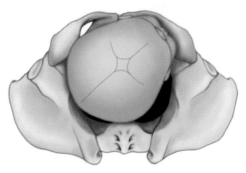

A. Restitution: FrA to LFrA.

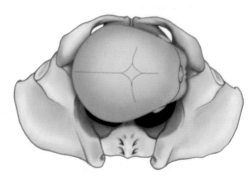

B. External rotation: LFrA to LFrT.

FIGURE 15-14. Restitution, external rotation. FrA, frontum anterior; LFra, left frontum anterior; LFrT, left frontum transverse.

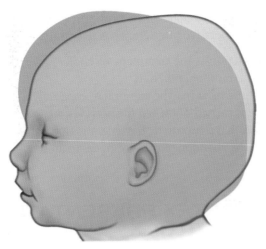

FIGURE 15-15. Molding: brow presentation.

Prognosis: Brow Presentations

Labor
In most cases, brow presentations do not deliver spontaneously. If the malposition is detected early in labor and if appropriate therapeutic measures are undertaken, the fetal and maternal results are good. Failure to recognize the problem leads to prolonged and traumatic labor.

Mother
Passage of a brow through the pelvis is slower, harder, and more traumatic to the mother than any other presentation. Perineal laceration is inevitable and may extend high into the vaginal fornices or into the rectum because of the large diameter offered to the outlet.

Fetus
The fetal mortality rate is high. The excessive molding may cause irreparable damage to the brain. Mistakes in diagnosis and treatment are the main causes of the poor fetal prognosis.

Management of Brow Presentations

1. *Trial of labor:* Since brow presentation may be transitory, a trial of labor is permissible in the hope that flexion to an occiput presentation or complete extension to a face presentation will take place

FIRST STAGE OF LABOR

2. *Persistent brow presentation:* Since brow presentations cannot deliver spontaneously, operative interference is necessary

   a. Cesarean section is the treatment of choice, giving the best results for both the mother and child
   b. Flexion of the head may be attempted, especially in multiparas. This procedure is carried out when the cervix is dilated and soon after the membranes have ruptured. If success is not immediate, the procedure must be abandoned in favor of cesarean section without delay

MEDIAN VERTEX PRESENTATIONS: MILITARY ATTITUDE

Definition

There is neither flexion nor extension; the occiput and the brow are at the same level in the pelvis. The presenting part is the vertex. The denominator is the occiput. The presenting diameter is the occipitofrontal, which at 11.0 cm is longer than the more favorable suboccipitobregmatic of 9.5 cm. Hence the progress is slower, and arrest is a little more frequent. In many cases, the military attitude is transitory, and the head flexes as it descends. Occasionally, extension to a brow or face presentation takes place.

Diagnosis of Position: Median Vertex Presentation

Abdominal Examination

1. The long axes of the fetus and mother are parallel (Fig. 15-16A)
2. The head is at or in the pelvic inlet
3. The back is in one flank, the small parts on the opposite side
4. The breech is in the fundus
5. Since there is neither flexion nor extension, there is no marked cephalic prominence on one side or the other

Fetal Heart

The fetal heart tones are heard loudest in the lower quadrant of the mother's abdomen on the same side as the fetal back.

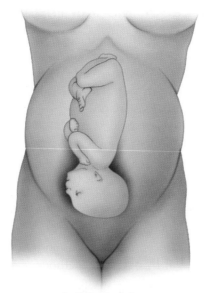

A. Abdominal view.

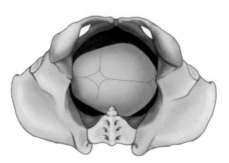

B. Vaginal view.

FIGURE 15-16. **Median vertex presentation: left occiput transverse.**

Vaginal Examination

1. The sagittal suture is felt in the transverse diameter of the pelvis, as LOT or ROT (Fig. 15-16B)

2. The two fontanels are equally easy to palpate and identify. They are at the same level in the pelvis

Mechanism of Labor: Median Vertex Presentation

Engagement takes place most often in the transverse diameter of the inlet. The head descends slowly, with the occiput and the brow at the same level (there is neither flexion nor extension) and with the sagittal suture in the transverse diameter of the pelvis until the median vertex reaches the pelvic floor. Then several terminations are possible:

1. Most often the head flexes, the occiput rotates to the anterior, and delivery takes place as an occipitoanterior position
2. The head may become arrested in the transverse diameter of the pelvis. Operative assistance is necessary for deep transverse arrest
3. The head may rotate posteriorly with or without flexion. The occiput turns into the hollow of the sacrum and the forehead to the pubis. The mechanism is that of persistent occipitoposterior positions. Delivery may be spontaneous or by operative methods
4. In rare instances, delivery can occur with the sagittal suture in the transverse diameter
5. Occasionally, the head extends, and the mechanism becomes a face or brow presentation

Prognosis: Median Vertex Presentation

Although labor is a little longer and harder than normal on the mother and child, the prognosis is reasonably good. Many cases flex and proceed to normal delivery.

Management of Median Vertex Presentation

1. Since flexion occurs so frequently, there should be no interference as long as progress is being made
2. When flexion takes place, the management is that of occipitoanterior or occipitoposterior positions
3. Cases in which the head extends are treated as face or brow presentations
4. When arrest occurs in the military attitude and the head is low in the pelvis, vaginal delivery may be attempted by flexing the head manually, rotating the occiput to the anterior, and extracting the head by forceps or vacuum (see Chapter 17)
5. When there is disproportion, when the head is high in the pelvis, or when an attempt at vaginal delivery fails, cesarean section should be performed

FACE PRESENTATION

General Considerations

Definition
The lie is longitudinal, the presentation is cephalic, the presenting part is the face, the attitude is one of complete extension, the chin (mentum, M) is the denominator and leading pole, and the presenting diameter is the submentobregmatic of 9.5 cm. In face presentations, the part between the glabella and chin presents; in brow presentations, it is the part between the glabella and bregma. However, positions intermediate to these are seen.

Incidence
The incidence is less than 1 percent (1 in 600-800) and is higher in multiparas than primigravidas. Primary face presentations are present before the onset of labor and are rare. Most face presentations are secondary, extension taking place during labor generally at the pelvic inlet. About 70 percent of face presentations are anterior or transverse, while 30 percent are posterior.

Etiology
Anything that delays engagement in flexion can contribute to the etiology of attitudes of extension. There is an association between attitudes of extension and cephalopelvic disproportion, and since this is a serious combination, the presence of a small pelvis or a large head must be ruled out with certainty. Prematurity is another etiology; as with smaller head dimensions, preterm infants can engage before conversion to vertex position. Rare causes of extension include thyroid neoplasms, which act by pushing the head back; multiple coils of cord around the neck, which prevent flexion; and spasm or shortening of the extensor muscles of the neck. Anencephalic fetuses frequently present by the face. In many cases, no cause can be found.

Anterior Face Presentations

The following descriptions apply to the left mentum anterior (LMA) presentation. The mechanism for the right mentum anterior (RMA) presentation is similar to that for LMA except that the chin, small parts, and fetal heart are on the right side, and the back and cephalic prominence are on the left.

Diagnosis of Position: LMA

Abdominal Examination

1. The long axes of the fetus and mother are parallel (Fig. 15-17)
2. The head is at the pelvis. Early in labor, the head is not engaged
3. The back is on the right side of the mother's abdomen, but since it is posterior, it is often felt indistinctly. The small parts are on the left and anterior. Extension of the spine causes the chest to be thrown out and the back to be hollowed

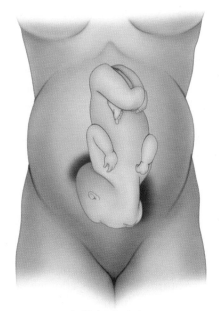

A. Abdominal view.

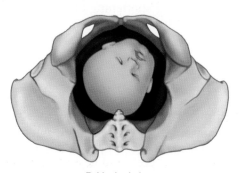

B. Vaginal view.

FIGURE 15-17. Left mentum anterior.

4. The breech is in the fundus
5. The cephalic prominence (the occiput) is on the right. An important diagnostic sign of extension attitudes is that the back and the cephalic prominence are on the same side. When flexion is present, the cephalic prominence and the back are on opposite sides
6. It must be kept in mind that in anterior face presentations, the baby's back and occiput are posterior. When the chin is posterior, on the other hand, the back and occiput are anterior

Fetal Heart. The fetal heart tones are transmitted through the anterior chest wall of the fetus and are heard loudest in the left lower quadrant of the maternal abdomen on the same side as the small parts.

Vaginal Examination

1. The clue to diagnosis is a negative finding—that is, absence of the round, even, hard vertex. In place of the dome of the skull with its identifying suture lines and fontanels, there is a softer and irregular presenting part. One suspects a face or breech presentation. Identification of the various parts of the face clinches the diagnosis. After prolonged labor, marked edema may confuse the picture
2. The long axis of the face is in the right oblique diameter of the pelvis (Fig. 15-17B)
3. The chin is in the left anterior quadrant of the maternal pelvis
4. The forehead is in the right posterior quadrant of the pelvis
5. Vaginal examination must be performed gently to avoid injury to the eyes
6. Ultrasonography can be useful for radiographic demonstration of the hyperextended head with the facial bones at or below the pelvic inlet

Late Diagnosis. Because most face presentations make good progress, the diagnosis may not be made until the face has reached the floor of the pelvis or until advance has ceased.

Mechanism of Labor: LMA

Extension. For some reason, the head does not flex. Instead, it extends (Fig. 15-18), so that in place of an LOP or ROP, there is an RMA or an LMA. The baby enters the pelvis chin first. The presenting diameter in face presentations (submentobregmatic) and in well-flexed head presentations (suboccipitobregmatic) is 9.5 cm in each case. This is one of the reasons why most anterior face presentations come to spontaneous delivery.

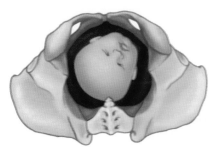

A. LMA: Onset of labor.

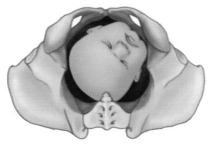

B. Extension and descent.

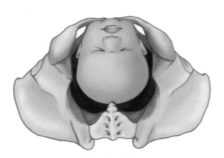

C. Vaginal view.

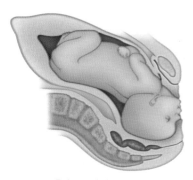

D. Lateral view.

C and D. Internal rotation: LMA to MA.

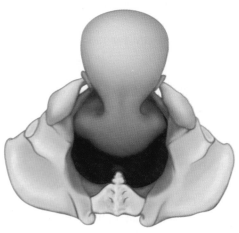

E. Flexion.

FIGURE 15-18. **A** to **D,** Mechanism of labor. **E** to **G**, Birth of the face and head by flexion. **H** and **I,** Head falls back in extension. **J** and **K,** Restitution and external rotation. LMA, left mentum anterior; LMT, left mentum transverse; MA, mentum anterior.

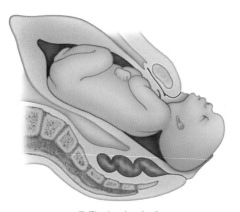

F. Flexion beginning.

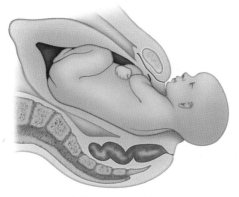

G. Flexion complete.

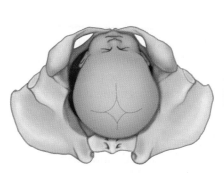

H. Vaginal view.

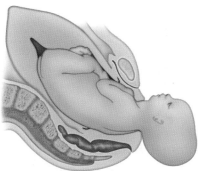

I. Lateral view.

FIGURE 15-18. *(Continued)*

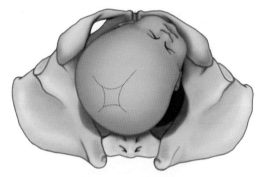

J. Restitution: MA to LMA.

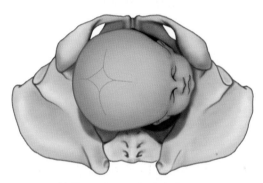

K. External rotation: LMA to LMT.

FIGURE 15-18. *(Continued)*

Descent. With the chin as the leading part, engagement takes place in the right oblique diameter of the pelvis. Descent is slower than in flexed attitudes. The face is low in the pelvis before the biparietal diameter has passed the brim. When the forward leading edge of the presenting face is felt at the level of the ischial spines, the tracheobregmatic diameter is still above the inlet.

Internal Rotation. With descent and molding, the chin reaches the pelvic floor, where it is directed downward, forward, and medially. As it rotates 45° anteriorly toward the symphysis (LMA to mentum anterior [MA]), the long axis of the face comes into the anteroposterior diameter of the pelvis (Figs. 15-18C and 18D). With further descent, the chin escapes under the symphysis. The shoulders have remained in the oblique diameter, so the neck is twisted 45°. An essential feature of internal rotation is that the chin must rotate anteriorly and under the symphysis, or spontaneous delivery is impossible. Anterior rotation does not take place until the face is well applied to the pelvic floor and may be delayed until late in labor. The attendant must not give up hope too soon.

Flexion. The head is born by flexion (Figs. 15-18E to G). The submental region at the neck impinges under the symphysis pubis. With the head pivoting around this point, the mouth, nose, orbits, forehead, vertex, and occiput are born over the perineum by flexion. The head then falls back (Figs. 15-18H and I).

Restitution. As the head is released from the vagina, the neck untwists, and the chin turns 45° back toward the original side (Fig. 15-18J).

External Rotation. The anterior shoulder reaches the pelvic floor and rotates toward the symphysis to bring the bisacromial diameter from the oblique to the anteroposterior diameter of the outlet. The chin rotates back another 45° to maintain the head in its correct relationship to the shoulders (Fig. 15-18K).

Molding. Molding (Fig. 15-19) leads to an elongation of the head in its anteroposterior diameter and flattening from above downward. The forehead and occiput protrude. The extension of the head on the trunk disappears after a few days.

FIRST STAGE OF LABOR

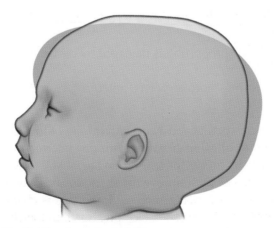

FIGURE 15-19. Molding: face presentation.

Prognosis: Anterior Face Presentations

Labor. Because the face is a poor dilator and because attitudes of extension are less favorable, labor takes longer than in normal occipitoanterior positions. The labor is conducted with this in mind. Delay takes place at the inlet, but when the face presentation and the labor are well established, steady progress is the rule. More than 90 percent of anterior face presentations deliver per vagina without complications. Figure 15-20 summarizes the mechanism of labor with the LMA presentation.

Mother. The mother has more work to do, has more pain, and receives greater lacerations than in normal positions.

Fetus. The baby does well in most cases, but the prognosis is less favorable than in normal presentations. The outlook for the child can be improved by early diagnosis, carefully conducted first and second stages of labor, and the restriction of operative vaginal deliveries to easily performed procedures. Cesarean section is preferable to complicated, difficult, and traumatic assisted vaginal deliveries. The membranes rupture early in labor, and the face takes the brunt of the punishment so that it becomes badly swollen and misshapen. Its appearance is a great worry to the parents. The edema disappears gradually, and the infant takes on a more normal appearance. Edema of the larynx may result from prolonged pressure of the hyoid region of the neck against the pubic bone. For the first 24 hours, the baby must be watched carefully to detect any difficulty in breathing.

Management of Anterior Face Presentations

1. *Disproportion*: Disproportion is managed by cesarean section

2. *Normal pelvis*: In a normal pelvis, anterior face presentations are left alone for these reasons:

   a. Most deliver spontaneously or with the aid of low forceps
   b. If conversion (flexion) is successful, the anterior face presentation is replaced by an occipitoposterior one (LMA to ROP or RMA to LOP). This does not improve the situation and may make it worse
   c. If conversion is partially successful, the face is changed to a brow presentation. In this case, a face presentation, which usually delivers spontaneously, is replaced by a brow presentation, which cannot

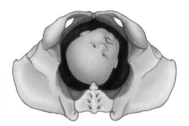

A. LMA: Onset of labor.

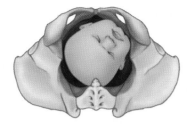

B. Extension and descent.

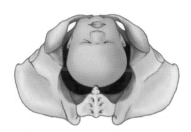

C. Internal rotation: LMA to MA.

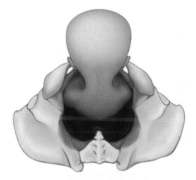

D. Flexion.

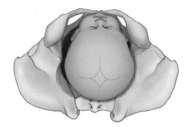

E. Extension.

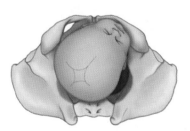

F. Restitution: MA to LMA.

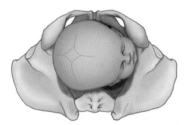

G. External rotation: LMA to LMT.

FIGURE 15-20. Summary of mechanism of labor: **left mentum anterior (LMA).**
LMT, left mentum transverse; MA, mentum anterior.

FIRST STAGE OF LABOR

3. *Arrest*:

    a. Low in the pelvis, well below the ischial spines: Extraction with low forceps

    b. High in the pelvis: Cesarean section

Transverse Face Presentations

The long axis of the face is in the transverse diameter of the pelvis, with the chin on one side and the forehead on the other (Fig. 15-21).

    The following descriptions apply to the left mentum transverse (LMT) presentation. The mechanism of labor for the right mentum transverse (RMT) presentation is the same as that for LMT except that the chin, small parts, and fetal heart are on the right, and the back and cephalic prominence are on the left.

Diagnosis of Position: LMT

Abdominal Examination

1. The long axis of the fetus is parallel to that of the mother
2. The head is at the pelvis
3. The back is on the right, toward the maternal flank. The small parts are on the left side
4. The breech is in the fundus
5. The cephalic prominence (the occiput) is on the right, the same side as the back

Fetal Heart. The fetal heart is heard loudest in the left lower quadrant of the mother's abdomen.

Vaginal Examination

1. The long axis of the face is in the transverse diameter of the pelvis
2. The chin is to the left at 3 o'clock
3. The forehead is to the right at 9 o'clock

Mechanism of Labor: LMT

A summary of the mechanism of labor for the LMT presentation is given in Figure 15-22.

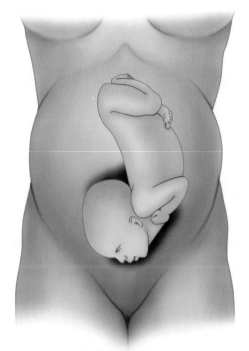

A. Abdominal view.

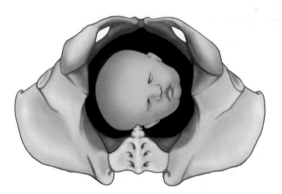

B. Vaginal view.

FIGURE 15-21.   **Left mentum transverse.**

FIRST STAGE OF LABOR

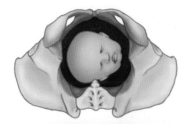

A. LMT: Onset of labor.

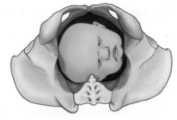

B. Descent.

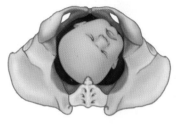

C. Internal rotation: LMT to LMA.

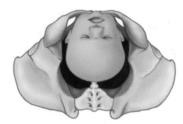

D. Internal rotation: LMA to MA.

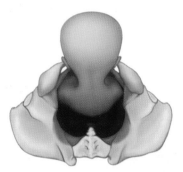

E. Birth by flexion.

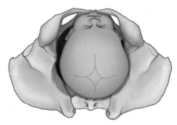

F. Extension.

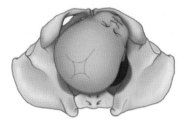

G. Restitution: MA to LMA.

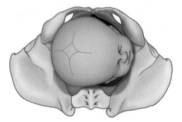

H. External rotation: LMA to LMT.

FIGURE 15-22. Mechanism of labor: left mentum transverse (LMT). LMA, left mentum anterior; MA, mentum anterior.

Extension. Extension to LMT occurs instead of flexion to ROT.

Descent. Engagement takes place in the transverse diameter of the pelvis. Descent is slow.

Internal Rotation. The chin rotates 90° anteriorly to the midline (LMT to LMA to MA). The chin comes under the symphysis.

Flexion. The submental region of the neck impinges in the subpubic angle. Birth is by flexion, after which the head falls backward.

Restitution. As the neck untwists, the head turns back 45°.

External Rotation. The shoulders turn from the oblique into the antero-posterior diameter of the pelvis, and the head rotates back another 45°.

Clinical Course of Labor and Management: LMT

1. Anterior rotation takes place in the majority of cases, LMT to LMA to MA. The treatment is the same as LMA. Delivery is spontaneous or assisted by low forceps

2. Arrest as LMT low in the pelvis

   a. Rotation to LMA manually or by forceps followed by extraction of the head by forceps
   b. If rotation is difficult or fails, cesarean section is performed

3. Arrest as LMT high in the pelvis is treated by cesarean section

Posterior Face Presentations

Some 30 percent of face presentations are posterior. Most of these rotate anteriorly. The flexed counterpart of the posterior face is the anterior occiput; thus, LMP flexes to ROA and RMP to LOA. Persistent posterior face presentations become arrested because they cannot deliver spontaneously. The descriptions here are for the left mentum posterior (LMP) presentation.

Diagnosis of Position: LMP

Abdominal Examination

1. The long axis of the fetus is parallel to the long axis of the mother (Fig. 15-23)

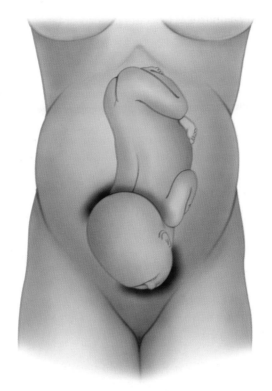

A. Abdominal view.

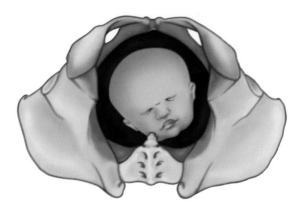

B. Vaginal view.

FIGURE 15-23. **Left mentum posterior.**

2. The head is at the pelvis
3. The back is anterior and to the right. The small parts are on the left and posterior
4. The breech is in the fundus of the uterus
5. The cephalic prominence (occiput) is to the right and anterior. It is on the same side as the back

Fetal Heart. The fetal heart tones, transmitted through the anterior shoulder, are heard loudest in the left lower quadrant of the mother's abdomen.

Vaginal Examination.

1. The long diameter of the face is in the left oblique diameter of the pelvis
2. The chin is in the left posterior quadrant of the pelvis (Fig. 15-23B)
3. The forehead is in the right anterior quadrant

Mechanism of Labor: LMP

There are two basic mechanisms:

1. Long arc rotation, with the chin rotating 135° to the anterior. About two-thirds of posterior face presentations do this and deliver spontaneously or with the aid of low forceps
2. Short arc rotation of 45° to the posterior, with the chin ending up in the hollow of the sacrum. These cases become arrested as persistent posterior face presentations

Long Arc Rotation: 135° to the Anterior

Extension. Extension to LMP (Fig. 15-24) occurs instead of flexion to ROA.

Descent. Descent is slow. The presenting part remains high while the essential molding takes place. Without extreme molding, the vertex cannot pass under the anterior part of the pelvic inlet.

Internal Rotation. The slow descent continues; the marked molding enables the chin to reach the pelvic floor, where it rotates 135° to the anterior and comes to lie under the symphysis. Since the original position was LMP, the sequence is LMP to LMT to LMA to MA in rotations of 45° between each step (Figure 15-24B to D).

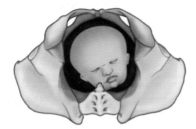

A. LMP: Descent.

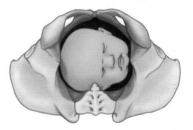

B. Internal rotation: LMP to LMT.

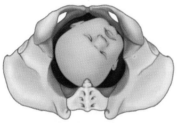

C. Internal rotation: LMT to LMA.

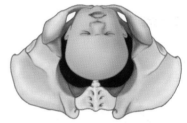

D. Internal rotation: LMA to MA.

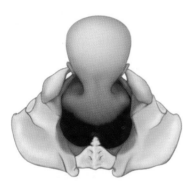

E. Birth by flexion.

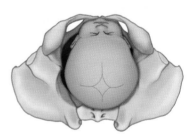

F. Head falls back in extension.

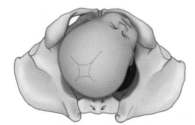

G. Restitution: MA to LMA.

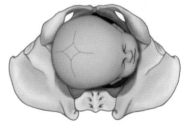

H. External rotation: LMA to LMT.

FIGURE 15-24. **Left mentum posterior (LMP): long arc rotation.** LMA, left mentum anterior; LMT, left mentum transverse; MA, mentum anterior.

Flexion. The submental area pivots under the symphysis, and the head is born by flexion. The head then falls backward.

Restitution. The chin rotates back 45° as the neck untwists.

External Rotation. With the rotation of the shoulders from the oblique into the anteroposterior diameter of the pelvis, the chin turns back another 45°.

Short Arc Rotation: 45° to the Posterior

Extension. Extension to LMP takes place (Fig. 15-25).

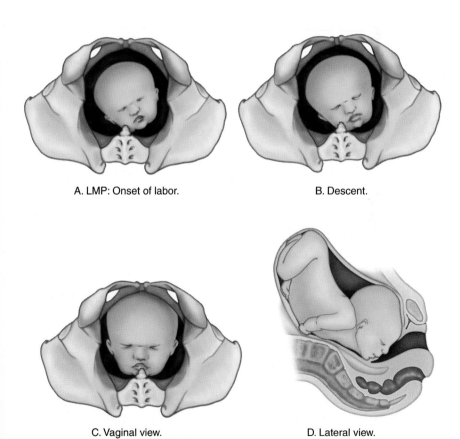

A. LMP: Onset of labor.

B. Descent.

C. Vaginal view.

D. Lateral view.

C. and D. Internal rotation: LMP to MP.

FIGURE 15-25. Left mentum posterior (LMP): short arc rotation. MP, mentum posterior.

Descent. Descent occurs with the help of extreme molding.

Internal Rotation. The chin rotates 45° posteriorly into the hollow of the sacrum (LMP to MP). Impaction follows, and the progress of labor comes to a halt. Flexion cannot take place and further advancement is not possible, except in the rare situation in which the baby is so small that the shoulders and head can enter the pelvis together.

Prognosis: Posterior Face Presentations

The prolonged labor and difficult rotation are traumatic to both the baby and mother. When the chin rotates posteriorly, the prognosis is poor unless the situation is corrected. Maternal morbidity is directly proportional to the degree of difficulty of the birth. High forceps or version and extraction carry with them the most morbid postpartum courses.

Management of Posterior Face Presentations

1. *Disproportion:* Disproportion is managed by cesarean section

2. *Trial of labor:* Since two-thirds of posterior faces rotate anteriorly and deliver spontaneously, and since internal rotation may not be completed until later in labor when the face is distending the pelvic floor, plenty of time should be allowed for the rotation to be accomplished. Interference must not be premature

3. *Persistent posterior face:* Since face presentations that have remained posterior cannot be delivered spontaneously, operative delivery is necessary

   a. Cesarean section is the modern treatment of choice, giving the best results for both the mother and child

   b. Flexion (conversion) from mentoposterior to occipitoanterior may be considered if cesarean section cannot be performed. One method of accomplishing this is by the *Thorn maneuver* (Fig. 15-26). The cervix must be fully dilated. With the vaginal hand, the operator flexes the fetal head. With the other hand, the operator pushes on the breech to flex the body. At the same time, an assistant presses against the baby's thorax or abdomen to try and jack-knife the

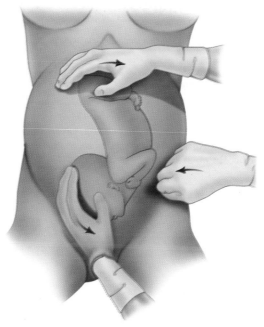

FIGURE 15-26. Thorn maneuver.

infant's body. This procedure is performed under anesthesia and must be done soon after the membranes rupture. If the amniotic fluid has drained away, the dry uterine cavity and snug fit of the uterus around the baby make it difficult or impossible to carry out this treatment. Once flexion has been accomplished, the head is pushed into the pelvis and held in place

c. Rotation to mentum anterior can sometimes be achieved by the use of forceps, but the operation is difficult and may be traumatic

Management Summary

In the setting of a normal pelvis and effective contractions, successful vaginal delivery with face presentation is usually possible. It is important to monitor fetal heart rate with external devices because internal monitoring may cause injury to the face and eyes. In the presence of pelvic inlet contraction and posterior face presentation, cesarean delivery is usually indicated.

SELECTED READING

Benedetti TJ, Lowensohn RI, Truscott AM: Face presentation at term. Obstet Gynecol 55:199, 1980

Cruikshank DP, White CA: Obstetric malpresentations: twenty years' experience. *Am J Obstet Gynecol.* 116:1097, 1973

Cunningham FG, Gant NF, Leveno KJ, et al: Abnormal labour. In: *Williams Obstetrics,* 23rd ed. New York: McGraw-Hill, 2010, pp 452-454

Duff P: Diagnosis and management of face presentation. Obstet Gynecol 57:105, 1981

Shaffer BL, Cheng YW, Vargas JE et al: Face presentation: Predictors and delivery route. Am J Obstet Gynecol 194: e10, 2006

PART III

Second Stage
of Labor

CHAPTER 16

The Second Stage of Labor

Lawrence Oppenheimer
Amanda Black

DEFINITION OF THE SECOND STAGE OF LABOR

The second stage of labor lasts from the end of the first stage, when the cervix has reached full dilatation, to the birth of the baby. This is the stage of expulsion of the fetus. The duration of the normal second stage of labor is influenced mainly by two factors: parity and the presence of an epidural. The median durations of the second stage are given in Table 16-1, but there is a large range in duration.

Second Stage in the Absence of Epidural Analgesia

In the absence of an epidural, a woman will often experience more intense and frequent contractions as she approaches full dilatation. This is sometimes referred to as *transition*. The patient should be discouraged from pushing (bearing down) before full dilatation. Breathing deeply and slowly during each contraction may help in coping with the pain. Once the head reaches the perineum, the maternal desire to bear down may become difficult to resist. The following are possible indicators of the onset of the second stage, although they are not exclusive to the second stage:

1. There is an increase in bloody show.
2. The woman wants to bear down with each contraction.
3. She feels pressure on the rectum accompanied by the desire to defecate.
4. Nausea and retching may occur as the cervix reaches full dilatation.

TABLE 16-1: DURATION OF SECOND STAGE IN MINUTES

| | Epidural | | No Epidural | |
Parity	Median	IQ Range	Median	IQ Range
0	82	45-134	45	27-76
1	36	20-77	15	10-25
2	25	14-60	11	7-20
3	23	12-53	10	5-16
≥4	22	9-30	10	5-15

IQ, interquartile range (25%-75% of the population).

The cervical dilation and station of the presenting part must be confirmed by vaginal examination.

Second Stage with Epidural Analgesia

In the presence of epidural analgesia, the duration of the second stage is approximately twice the duration of a non-epidural second stage. This is because the neurohumoral reflex of oxytocin release due to the perineal pressure of the head, which assists the urge to bear down, may be interrupted. In addition, the incidence of instrumental vaginal delivery, but not cesarean section, is also increased twofold. For this reason, it is important for the care provider to have an understanding of how to best manage the second stage under epidural.

Phases of the Second Stage of Labor

There are two phases of the second stage of labor, the passive stage and the active stage.

Passive Phase of the Second Stage

During the passive phase of the second stage, the cervix is fully dilated, but there are no voluntary or involuntary expulsive efforts. The head usually has not yet reached the pelvic floor (thus the station is +1 or higher). The rotation of the occiput to the optimal position of occipitoanterior may not yet be completed, and the head may be in an oblique or transverse position. There is usually no urge to bear down even in the absence of epidural analgesia.

Active Phase of the Second Stage

During the active (pushing) phase of the second stage, the cervix is fully dilated, and the woman begins to push either voluntarily or involuntarily. The woman may begin pushing because she experiences a strong urge to push or bear down, or she may be instructed to start pushing even though she has no urge to push, provided that the head is at or below the level of the pelvic floor (station +2 or lower) and is in the occipitoanterior position. The active phase may also commence when a woman is instructed to start pushing regardless of the head station—for instance, when the recommended time limit for the passive phase is exceeded or there are concerns about the fetal heart rate (FHR). Women with an epidural may not have a strong urge to push.

SECOND STAGE OF LABOR

Fetal Monitoring in the Second Stage of Labor

Fetal health surveillance is discussed in depth in another chapter. In the active portion of the second stage, FHR auscultation should be carried out immediately after a contraction for 1 minute at 5-minute intervals. In some instances, continuous electronic fetal monitoring may be indicated. These would include higher risk situations in which there is an increased risk of perinatal death, cerebral palsy, or neonatal encephalopathy, such as fetal growth restriction and preeclampsia, as well as when oxytocin is being used for augmentation of labor. FHR abnormalities are common in the second stage of labor but are generally well tolerated by the fetus if the FHR was normal throughout the first stage of labor. A prolonged second stage must be avoided if there are persistent FHR abnormalities, particularly when there are other risk factors that may impact the degree of fetal reserve. The maternal pulse should be palpated to ensure there is no confusion between the fetal and maternal heart rates, especially if there are decelerations or a prolonged bradycardia. One clue regarding such maternal heart rate artifacts is that the maternal pulse usually rises, showing a uniform acceleration with every contraction caused by the Valsalva maneuver associated with pushing.

Situations of particular concern include repetitive severe variable decelerations with pushing that may be associated with cord compression or a nuchal cord. This can be followed by a prolonged bradycardia as the cord tightens in the late second stage. End-stage bradycardia may also be caused by head compression. A fetus with a previously normal tracing can withstand a bradycardia for a few minutes, and if the head is crowning, it need not lead to instrumental delivery right away. Finally, attention should always be paid to the uterine contraction frequency. Too frequent contractions or hypersystole, especially when oxytocin is being used on top of the maternal Valsalva maneuver from pushing, which further diminishes uterine blood flow, can exhaust even a healthy fetus over a period of time. Following the suggested guidelines below for delaying pushing in the second stage of labor applies only in instances with ongoing evidence of fetal well-being.

MANAGMENT OF THE SECOND STAGE OF LABOR

There are very few comprehensive evidence-based clinical practice guidelines for management of the second stage of labor; however, the ideal management of the second stage of labor should maximize the probability of vaginal delivery while minimizing the risk of maternal and neonatal morbidity and mortality. Appropriate management of the second stage of labor requires recognition of its passive and active phases. The fundamental principles of care in the second stage include (1) establishing fetal and maternal well-being before any delay in pushing; (2) performing hourly vaginal assessments in the second stage by a consistent examiner to assess fetal position and station; (3) informing the primary health care provider when the cervix is fully dilated, if there is a lack of progress in any 1-hour block, and at the end of 2 hours; and (4) regularly assessing the bladder to ensure that a full bladder is not obstructing progress. There is a lack of evidence to support an absolute time limit to end the second stage with an intervention, and care providers must be aware of the benefits and risks of intervention versus continued expectant management in the second stage.

A woman does not need to start pushing as soon as the cervix is fully dilated. Studies have found that delaying maternal pushing for a maximum of up to 2 hours, particularly in primigravidas, can reduce the incidence of difficult operative vaginal deliveries. Overall, a policy of delayed rather than early pushing for women with epidural anesthesia reduces operative intervention (operative vaginal deliveries and caesarean sections) at the expense of an increased duration of second stage. Studies have found that when the second stage of labor exceeded 4 hours, fewer than one-third of these women would achieve a spontaneous vaginal birth (24% of nulliparous women with an epidural; 28% in women with an epidural). Although conclusive time limits for the active stage of pushing cannot be made because of a lack of evidence, it is known that the duration of the active (pushing) phase of the second stage is more important for the fetal and maternal condition than the total duration of the second stage of labor. Based on the best available evidence, The Ottawa Hospital has developed a second stage protocol that allows up to 4 hours total duration of the second stage in primigravidas under epidural and 3 hours for multiparas (Table 16-2). The protocol recommends to wait 2 hours before pushing in all women with epidural anesthesia who have no urge to push, or in whom the station of the presenting part is above +2, or in whom the fetus is in the occipitoposterior or occipitotransverse position. After 2 hours, the woman should be instructed to push regardless of head station. The duration of pushing within the total time frame should preferably not exceed 2 hours because the pH of the fetus will gradually fall during active pushing, although again absolute time limits cannot be stipulated because of a lack of conclusive evidence. The flow sheets contained in our protocol may be helpful for standardization of practice on birthing units.

SECOND STAGE OF LABOR

TABLE 16-2: THE OTTAWA HOSPITAL SECOND STAGE PROTOCOL

	Hour Begins			
	1	2	3	4
Primigravida, epidural	Wait	Wait	Wait/push*	Push
Primigravida, no epidural	Wait	Wait	Push	
Multigravida, epidural	Wait	Wait	Push	
Multigravida, no epidural	Wait	Push		

*Waiting for a third hour may be appropriate if the active phase is not yet reached but there is continuous progress.

A second stage using the above time parameters has been demonstrated to be safe for the mother and baby. We suggest consideration of operative vaginal delivery at the end of these time limits unless spontaneous delivery is thought to be imminent (i.e., the head is visible and there is continued progress with contractions). If that is the case, it is unnecessary to impose an absolute limit on the duration of the second stage. There are, however, some important caveats when using delayed pushing in this way:

1. It is assumed the fetus is healthy, at term, and in an uncomplicated cephalic presentation.
2. There is no uterine scar (e.g., no previous cesarean section).
3. The fetal heart, assessed by intermittent auscultation or electronic monitoring, and other tests of fetal well-being are normal and reassuring.
4. There is continued progress as evidenced by gradual descent of the head on hourly assessments.

If any of these conditions is not met or if there are concerns about fetal or maternal health, then the management should be individualized. This usually means shortening the above time parameters or earlier consideration of operative delivery.

Dystocia in the Second Stage

There is no clear consensus on what constitutes delay in the second stage of labor. In general, no change in the head station during any 1-hour interval warrants careful evaluation for dystocia. An active (pushing) phase longer than 2 hours in a primigravida or 1 hour in a multigravida warrants assessment by a health care professional trained in operative vaginal delivery unless birth is imminent. Oxytocin may be started at any time during the second stage, particularly when contractions are inadequate or there is a lack of progress. Women who are already on oxytocin at the onset of the second stage should continue to receive it. Malposition of the fetal head is a frequent cause of delay in the second stage and may be associated with infrequent or insufficient uterine contractions. Maternal positioning may be an important intervention when fetal malposition is identified. In some cases, the fetal head position may be difficult to determine. In these instances, transvaginal ultrasonography, if available, can be helpful in determining head position with great accuracy.

Second stage management should be individualized depending on the clinical situation. In some situations, it may be appropriate to allow longer for spontaneous head rotation, but in other situations, it may be preferable to shorten the timeline for waiting and pushing to avoid the additional complications of a prolonged second stage when operative delivery may be required. Caution should be exercised in the infrequent situation of failure of head descent in a multipara with an occipitoanterior presentation and strong, frequent contractions. This clinical picture may represent true cephalopelvic disproportion, in which the baby may be significantly larger than her previous delivery. In this case, allowing excessive uterine action for too long a period could lead to complications. Around 80% of multiparas under epidural analgesia will deliver within 3 hours and almost all within 90 minutes without an epidural.

Well-grown fetuses that are not compromised during the first stage of labor and are carefully monitored in the second stage seldom get into trouble from asphyxia, even when the second stage is prolonged. One should avoid a traumatic forceps or vacuum delivery just because an arbitrary time point has past. However, the decision to allow labor to continue should be based on evidence of continued progress of descent or rotation

Pushing in the Second Stage

During the second stage of labor, the expulsive powers include (1) involuntary uterine contractions, (2) voluntary efforts of the abdominal, thoracic and diaphragmatic muscles, and (3) action of the levator ani muscles. In general, the more effectively the mother bears down, the shorter the second stage. This action may be more efficient if the woman braces herself against a solid object, such as a hand bar or birthing bars. When the contraction begins, the woman takes one or two deep breaths and then holds her breath to fix the diaphragm. She then pulls on the hand bars (or on her own legs with her hands behind her knees) and at the same time bears down as hard and for as long a period as she can. In general, she should not be encouraged to push beyond the time of completion of each uterine contraction.

Although many care providers encourage pushing that incorporates a Valsalva maneuver, the use of "physiologic bearing down" instead of sustained breath holding during expulsive efforts may be equally effective. Physiologic bearing down (making several short pushes without breath-holding, the "open glottis technique"), although resulting in a slightly longer second stage, may result in improved maternal–fetal gas exchange and maternal satisfaction with the birth experience. Recent studies have concluded that spontaneous (uncoached rather than coached) pushing had no disadvantages and was associated with a maternal perception of a supportive and encouraging style of care. In general, women should be guided by their own urge to push.

Positioning in the Second Stage of Labor

There is no single correct position for delivery. Women should choose a position that is comfortable for them and enhances their pushing efforts. It has been traditional practice for women to be positioned and to push in the horizontal (dorsal), semi-Fowler's (head and back elevated at 30 degrees), or lithotomy position during the second stage of labor (Fig. 16-1A to D). Use of these positions is often dictated by interventions

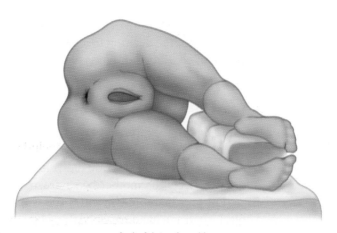

A. Left lateral position.

FIGURE 16-1. Positions for delivery.

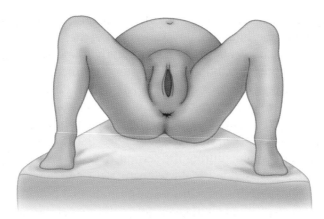

B. Dorsal position.

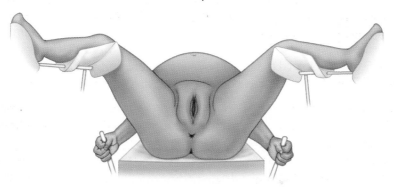

C. Lithotomy position.

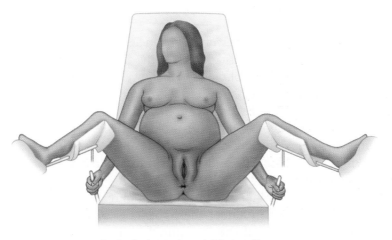

D. Back elevated: semisitting position.

FIGURE 16-1. (*Continued*)

such as epidural analgesia, electronic fetal monitoring, or intravenous lines and pumps that limit mobility. Upright or vertical positions such as squatting, semi-recumbency, standing, and upright kneeling generate up to 30 percent more intraabdominal pressure and increased anteroposterior and transverse diameters of the pelvic outlet. Positioning may be important when lack of progress is identified in the second stage. Frequent changes in position may help when fetal malposition is identified or to relieve back pain. It is recommended that women should not lie supine or semi-supine during the second stage (in which case a firm wedge should be inserted under the woman's right side to prevent supine hypotension) and should adopt any other position that is comfortable for her and enhances pushing efforts.

In women with epidural analgesia and especially in women with any degree of motor neuron blockade, appropriate positioning is important to prevent injury associated with lack of sensation, poor alignment, or unnatural positioning of joints (e.g., hyperflexion of hips). Women with epidural anaesthesia do not need to remain horizontal. More upright positions can be used when local anesthetic is combined with narcotics to minimize motor blockade.

Postural Supine Hypotension

Laboring women should avoid supine positioning. In the late stages of pregnancy, hypotension occurs when a woman lies on her back; there is rapid recovery when she turns on her side. Symptoms include nausea, shortness of breath, faintness, pallor, tachycardia, and increased femoral venous pressure.

When a pregnant, near-term woman lies on her back, the uterus bulges over the vertebral column and compresses the inferior vena cava. This leads to an increased volume of blood in the lower limbs but a decreased return to the heart, lowered pressure in the right atrium, diminished cardiac output, and hypotension. Reduced perfusion of the uterus and placenta leads to fetal hypoxia and changes in the FHR.

Supine hypotension may be exacerbated by an epidural caused by the sympathetic blockade and venous pooling in the lower body. The pregnant woman may not display any signs or symptoms, but significant impairment of uterine blood flow can result. It is important to use a wedge, preferably under the right flank or buttock, for any woman in late pregnancy if she is required to lie supine for delivery or surgery.

DELIVERY OF THE FETUS

Descent, Crowning, and Spontaneous Birth of the Head

With each contraction, the head advances and then recedes as the uterus relaxes. Each time a little ground is gained. The introitus becomes an anteroposterior slit, then an oval, and finally a circular opening (Fig. 16-2A to C). With each contraction, the perineum bulges increasingly, and the pressure of the head thins out the perineum. Feces may be forced out of the rectum. With descent, the occiput comes to lie under

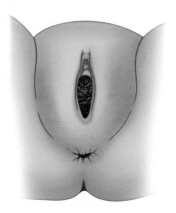

A. Anteroposterior slit.

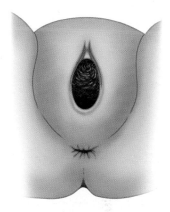

B. Oval opening.

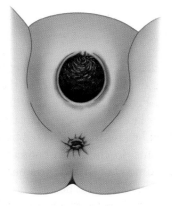

C. Circular shape.

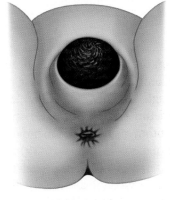

D. Crowning.

FIGURE 16-2. Dilatation of the introitus and birth of the head.

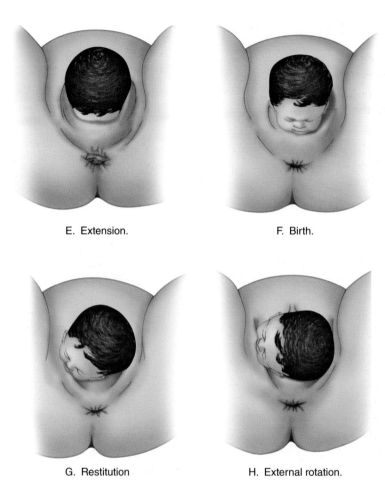

E. Extension.

F. Birth.

G. Restitution

H. External rotation.

FIGURE 16-2. (Continued)

the pubic symphysis. The head continues to advance and recede with the contractions until a strong one forces the largest diameter of the head through the vulva (*crowning*), as seen in Figure 16-2D. At this time, the perineum is very thin, and spontaneous laceration may occur. Routine episiotomy is not recommended. The fetal head is then delivered by a process of extension (Fig. 16-2E) as the bregma, forehead, nose, mouth, and chin sequentially appear over the perineum (Fig. 16-2F). The head then falls posteriorly back toward the anus. After the fetal head is out of the vagina, it restitutes (Fig. 16-2G) as the head assumes a transverse position, and external rotation takes place (Fig. 16-2H) as the shoulders move from the oblique to the anteroposterior diameter of the pelvis.

Controlled Birth of the Head

Many women can deliver their babies spontaneously without assistance. However, there are advantages to having a birth attendant present. If an unexpected complication arises, immediate action can be taken. In addition, the birth attendant is able to assist the woman so that the incidence of large and uncontrolled lacerations is reduced.

Procedures designed to encourage a slowly progressive delivery of the fetal head should be performed. Slow, gradual birth of the head reduces the incidence of lacerations. The attendant should try to avoid a sudden bursting out of the head that may lead to large lacerations that in turn may extend through the anal sphincter and into the rectum.

1. *Management of bearing-down efforts*: Correct management of the bearing-down efforts is important. The two forces responsible for birth of the child are uterine contractions and bearing-down forces. The uterine contractions are involuntary, but the bearing-down forces can be controlled. During the first part of the second stage, the patient must bear down during the uterine contractions to expedite progress. However, during the actual delivery, having the woman pant rapidly during the contractions may help to avoid a too rapid emergence of the fetal head. When the patient breathes in and out rapidly, the diaphragm moves, making it impossible for effective intraabdominal pressure to be built up, and so the power to bear down is lost.

2. *Manual pressure*: In most cases, the speed of delivery can be reduced by gentle manual pressure against the baby's head. Occasionally, the propulsive force is so great that it is impossible to try slowing the birth. The head should never be held back forcibly.

3. *Ritgen maneuver*: The objective of this maneuver is to encourage extension of the fetal head and thus expedite its birth. This procedure is performed ideally between uterine contractions. During this interval, the head can be delivered slowly, gradually, and under the attendant's control. Furthermore, the soft tissues are more relaxed, and tissue damage is less. The maneuver cannot be carried out before the occiput has come under the symphysis. It is done when the suboccipitofrontal diameter is ready to be born.

The operator's hand, covered with a towel or a pad, is placed so that the fingers are behind the maternal anus just in front of the coccyx (Fig. 16-3). The attendant's other hand is placed on the fetal occiput to exert pressure superiorly against the occiput and to help control the speed of its delivery. Extension of the fetal head is furthered by pressing against the baby's face, preferably the chin, through the rectum.

SECOND STAGE OF LABOR

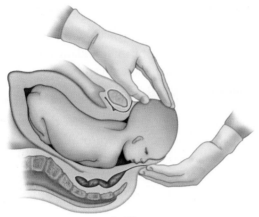

A. Ritgen maneuver.

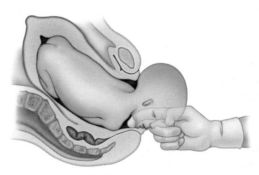

B. Hooking out of chin.

FIGURE 16-3. Birth of the head.

The bregma, forehead, and face are born in that order. The other hand is placed against the baby's occiput to control the speed of its delivery.

The alternative approach is to have the hands not actually touching the perineum but poised ready to assist with head control if needed. Studies show that the outcome in terms of perineal lacerations and pain is similar between these two methods.

4. *Episiotomy*: The routine use of episiotomy is discouraged because there is a higher incidence of extensions into the external anal sphincter. The use of episiotomy should be individualized. Usually allowing the perineum to tear spontaneously results in an easier repair with less discomfort. When an episiotomy is required because of instrumental birth or suspected fetal compromise, the recommended technique is a mediolateral episiotomy originating at the vaginal fourchette and

usually directed to the right side. The angle to the vertical axis should be between 45° and 60° at the time of the episiotomy.

After Delivery of the Head

1. The head should be supported as it restitutes and rotates externally.
2. Aspiration of mucus from the mouth and throat used to be practiced but is no longer believed to be necessary because a normal, vigorous baby will clear his or her airway spontaneously. To prevent meconium aspiration syndrome if meconium is present, a skilled attendant should be present who can suction the newborn and intubate the trachea or suction meconium from beneath the glottis (at or below the level of the vocal cords). Meconium should be suctioned out before any resuscitative measures, such as positive-pressure ventilation, are performed.
3. The region of the neck is explored for coils of umbilical cord. Nuchal cords occur in approximately 25 percent of births. If the cord is around the neck loosely, it can be slipped over the head, or the fetus may in fact be able to deliver through the loop of cord. If it is coiled around the neck tightly, it must be clamped doubly, cut between the clamps, and then unwound.

Birth of the Body and Shoulders

By the time the shoulders are ready for delivery, restitution has occurred, and external rotation is taking place. During a uterine contraction, the patient is asked to bear down. The sides of the head are grasped with two hands, and gentle downward traction is applied with the head depressed toward the rectum until the anterior shoulder appears under the pubic arch (Fig. 16-4A). The head of the baby is usually grasped with both hands on the parietal bones. When the anterior shoulder has emerged from under the symphysis pubis (Fig. 16-4B), the head is raised upward so that the posterior shoulder can be born over the perineum (Fig. 16-4C). The birth attendant merely lowers and lifts the baby's head to facilitate birth of the shoulders. He or she does not exert excessive traction because of the risk of damaging the nerve plexus in the neck. The force that actually pushes out the shoulder is provided by the bearing-down efforts of the mother if she is awake or by pressure on the fundus by an assistant if the mother is asleep.

Trunk and Lower Limbs

Once the head and shoulders have been delivered, the rest of the body usually slips out easily, often with a gush of amniotic fluid.

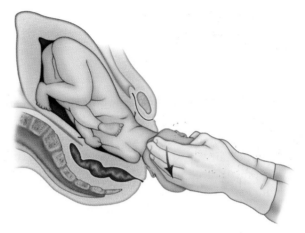

A. Lowering of fetal head.

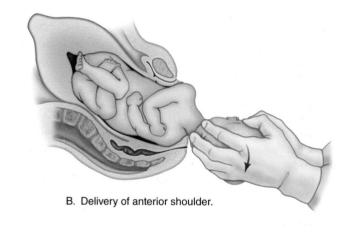

B. Delivery of anterior shoulder.

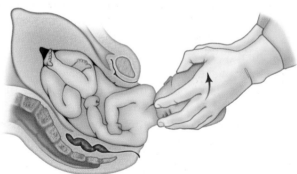

C. Delivery of posterior shoulder.

FIGURE 16-4. **Delivery of the shoulders.**

Clamping the Umbilical Cord

After delivery, the infant should be placed at or below the level of the vaginal introitus to allow for some shifting of blood from the placenta to the infant. The umbilical cord is cut between a cord clamp placed 2 to 3 cm from the fetal abdomen and another clamp. If cord clamping is delayed for up to 3 minutes, an average of 80 cc of blood may be shifted from the placenta to the infant. Benefits of this include a reduced frequency of iron deficiency in later infancy; however, there may be an increased risk of hyperbilirubinemia. In general, one may delay cord clamping while stimulating and drying off the newborn; however, a prolonged delay in cord clamping is not routinely recommended.

SELECTED READING

American College of Obstetrics and Gynecology: Operative vaginal delivery: ACOG practice bulletin No. 17. Washington, DC; 2000

Andersson O, Hellström-Westas L, Andersson D, Domellöf M: Effect of delayed versus early umbilical cord clamping on neonatal outcomes and iron status at 4 months: A randomized controlled trial. BMJ 343:d7157, 2011.

Caughey AB: Is there an upper time limit for the management of the second stage of labor? Am J Obstet Gynecol 337, 2009

Fraser WD, Marcoux S, Krauss I, Douglas J, Goulet C, Boulvain M, et al: Multicenter randomized controlled trial of delayed pushing for nulliparous women in the second stage of labor with continuous epidural analgesia. Am J Obstet Gynecol 182:1165, 2000

Menticoglou S, Manning F, Harman C, et al: Perinatal outcome in relation to the second stage: perinatal outcome in relation to second-stage duration. Am J Obstet Gynecol 173:906, 1995

McDonald SJ, Middleton P: Effect of timing of umbilical cord clamping of term infants on maternal and neonatal outcomes. Cochrane Database Syst Rev (2):CD004074, 2008

National Collaborating Centre for Women's and Children's Health: Intrapartum care: care of healthy women and their babies during childbirth. London, UK: RCOG Press; 2007

Patterson C, Saunders N St G, Wadsworth J: The characteristics of the second stage of labour in 25,069 singleton deliveries in the North West Thames Health Region, 1988. Br J Obstet Gynecol 99:377, 1992

Roberts CL, Torvaldsen S, Cameron CA, Olive E: Delayed versus early pushing in women with epidural analgesia: a systematic review and meta-analysis. Br J Obstet Gynecol 111:1333, 2004

Society of Obstetricians and Gynecologists of Canada Technical Update: Management of Meconium at Birth. No. 224, April 2009.

Society of Obstetricians and Gynecologists of Canada Clinical Practice Guideline: Fetal Health Surveillance: Antepartum and Intrapartum Consensus Guideline. No.97, September 2007.

Sprague AE, Oppenheimer L, McCabe L, Brownlee J, et al: The Ottawa Hospital's Clinical Practice Guideline for the Second Stage of Labour. J Obstet Gynaecol Can 28:769, 2006

SECOND STAGE OF LABOR

Operative Vaginal Delivery

Gihad Shabib
Amanda Black

Assisted or operative vaginal birth refers to the use of a vacuum or forceps to achieve a vaginal delivery in the second stage of labor. When the decision is being made as to whether or not a birth requires assistance, including the timing and choice of instrument, considerations must include indications and contraindications to the procedure, the maternal or fetal risks of using either instrument, the urgency of the need to expedite delivery, the experience and skills of the birth attendant, and the risks associated with the alternative choice of cesarean section. Assisted vaginal delivery should only be attempted if there is a reasonable chance of success, and a backup plan should be in place in case the attempt is not successful.

Indications for an operative vaginal birth include nonreassuring fetal status, maternal conditions that preclude Valsalva maneuvers such as congestive heart failure or cerebral vascular malformations, and inadequate progress in the second stage of labor (provided that there is adequate uterine activity and there is no evidence of cephalopelvic disproportion [CPD]).

INCIDENCE OF OPERATIVE VAGINAL DELIVERY

Between 9 and 10 percent of all deliveries in North America are assisted vaginal deliveries. The vacuum is used in 7 percent of all births, while forceps are used in only 3 percent of all births. The rate of forceps delivery is decreasing. This may be because of increased litigation, unfavorable publicity regarding forceps, decreasing family size, and improved safety of cesarean section. The decrease in forceps use and the increase in cesarean section rates may also be secondary to a decrease in the skills required to perform a forceps delivery because obstetric trainees now receive less exposure to forceps training.

OBSTETRIC FORCEPS

The obstetric forceps are instruments designed for extraction of the fetal head. Forceps cradle the parietal and malar bones of the fetal skull and apply traction to these areas as well as laterally displacing maternal tissue. There are many varieties of forceps, but the basic design and purpose are the same. They may be used to provide traction, rotation, flexion, and extension.

All forceps consist of two crossing branches. Each branch consists of four parts: the blade, shank, lock, and handle. Each blade has two curves: the cephalic curve that conforms to the shape of the fetal head and the pelvic curve that conforms to the shape of the birth canal. Some blades are fenestrated, and some are solid (Fig. 17-1A).

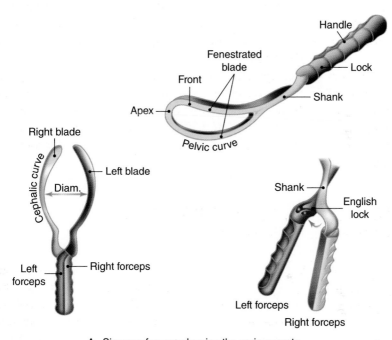

A. Simpson forceps showing the various parts.

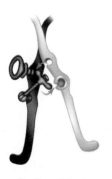

B. French lock.

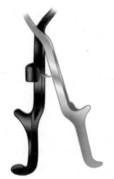

C. Sliding lock.

FIGURE 17-1. Obstetric forceps.

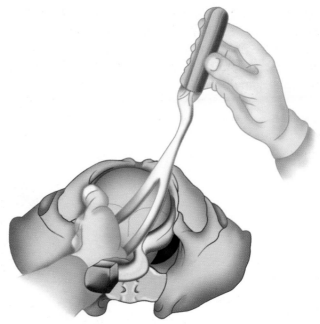

FIGURE 17-1. *(Continued)*

Parts of the Forceps

1. *Handles:* These are used to grip the forceps

2. *Lock:* This holds the forceps together. It is constructed so that the right one fits on over the left. For this reason, the left blade should usually be applied first. The main types of lock are:

   a. *The English lock* (e.g., Simpson forceps) has a shoulder and flange in each shank that fit into each other. Articulation is fixed at a given point

   b. *The French lock* (e.g., Tarnier and De Wees) has a pinion and screw. The left shank bears a pivot fitting into a notch on the right shank. After articulation, the pivot is tightened by screwing it in (Fig. 17-1B)

   c. The sliding lock (e.g., Kielland). The articulation is not fixed. This allows the shanks to move forward and backward independently so can be useful to correct an asynclitic head (common in deep transverse arrest) (Fig. 17-1C)

3. *Shank:* This connects the handle to the blade. The shanks are either parallel as in the Simpson forceps or overlapping as they are in the Tucker-McLane forceps. A short-shanked instrument such as the Wrigley's forceps can be used only when the fetal head (not the caput) is on the perineum (≥+3 station). When the head has not reached the perineum, longer shanks are needed. A single blade can be used to scoop out the head during cesarean delivery. The shank of the Piper forceps is noticeably longer to allow for ventral application to the after-coming head

4. *Blades:* These enclose the fetal head and may be solid or fenestrated. They are designed to grasp the head firmly but without excessive compression. The solid blades may cause less maternal tissue trauma, but the fenestrated blades are lighter, grip the fetal head better, and are less likely to slip. The edges are smooth to reduce damage to the soft tissues

5. *Right and left forceps:* The forcep is designated right or left depending on the side of the maternal pelvis to which it is applied. Since most forceps cross at the lock, the handle of the right forceps is held in the operator's right hand, and the right blade fits the right side of the pelvis. The left blade fits the left side of the maternal pelvis, and its handle is held in the left hand of the operator. This does not apply in Kielland forceps where there is minimal pelvic curve

6. *Curves:* The forceps have two curves. The *cephalic* curve fits the shape of the baby's head and reduces the danger of compression. The *diameter* is the widest distance between the cephalic curve of the blades (~7.5 cm). The *pelvic* curve follows the direction of the birth canal. It makes application and extraction easier, and decreases damage to the maternal tissues. The pelvic curve is very small in Kielland forceps

Types of Forceps

There are many general-duty forceps and several with specialized functions (Figs. 17-2A to E). Certain situations such as a rotational forceps or forceps for the after-coming head at breech delivery require specific forceps. New birth attendants should learn to use one instrument and become thoroughly skilled and comfortable with that instrument before learning the use of another instrument.

SECOND STAGE OF LABOR

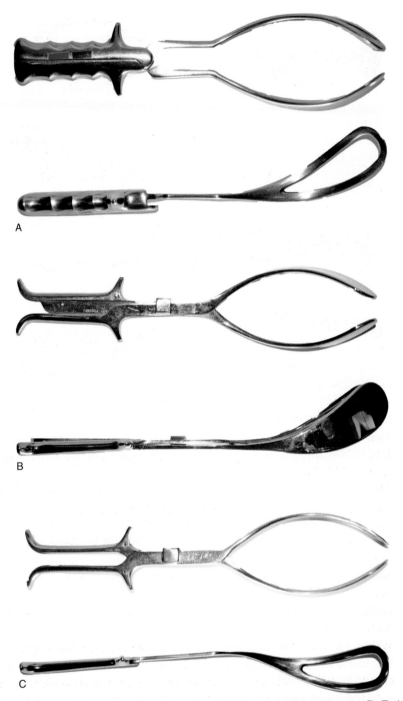

FIGURE 17-2. A, Simpson forceps. **B,** Luikart forceps. **C,** Kielland forceps. **D,** Tucker-McLane forceps. **E,** Piper forceps.

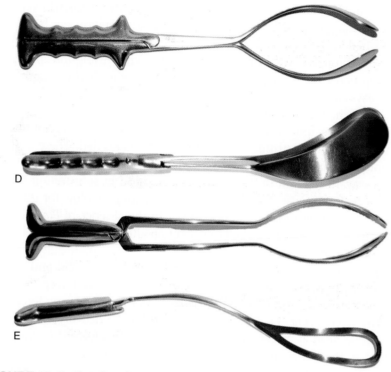

FIGURE 17-2. *(Continued)*

1. *Simpson forceps* (Fig. 17-2A): This is the most commonly used forceps. It has a cephalic and an ample pelvic curve. These forceps have a fenestrated blade and a wide straight shank in front of an English lock. The shank is straight. This is a good general-duty forceps and is used widely for direct obstetric forceps operations (when the sagittal suture is in the midline anteroposterior [AP] diameter)

2. *DeLee forceps:* This is the Simpson forceps with a few minor modifications. The shank is a little longer to keep the handle away from the anus. The handle is changed to secure lightness, a better grip, and ease of cleaning

3. *Luikart forceps* (Fig. 17-2B): This is a modified Simpson forceps with a semi-fenestrated blade

4. *Wrigley's forceps:* This is similar to Simpson forceps but has very short (or no) shanks. It can be used only when the fetal head (not the caput) is on the perineum (>+3 station) (i.e., no downward traction is required). A single blade can be used to scoop out the head during cesarean delivery

SECOND STAGE OF LABOR

5. *Kielland forceps* (Fig. 17-2C): The pelvic curve is minimal, which makes these forceps ideal for rotating the fetal head. Rotation can be accomplished simply by twisting the closed handles instead of sweeping them through a wide arc, as is necessary when using forceps with a deep pelvic curve. The sliding lock allow for simultaneous correction of asynclitism before rotation. There are knobs on the handle on the side of the minimal pelvic curve, and these should be directed toward the fetal occiput during application. Delivery can be accomplished with the same instrument; no reapplication is needed. There is also a unique perineal curve that rests on the perineal body and can aid in the downward traction in mid-forceps application in substitution for the axis-traction piece. The shanks are usually long to allow for the anterior wandering method of application. In the absence of *Piper forceps*, Kielland forceps can be used to deliver an after-coming head in breech presentation

6. *Tucker-McLane forceps* (Fig. 17-2D): The blades are solid and have a more rounded cephalic curve. Some operators use this forceps for rotation because its pelvic curve is smaller than that of Simpson forceps

7. *Piper forceps* (Fig. 17-2E): These are used for the delivery of the after-coming head at breech delivery. The blade of this forceps is similar to that of the Simpson forceps. The shank is longer and curved downward so that the handles are lower than the blades. This forceps has a prominent perineal curve, which facilitates application to the after-coming head from underneath the fetal body in breech presentations

8. *Axis-traction forceps:* These forceps are designed to direct traction efforts into the pelvic curve. A traction apparatus can be attached either to the blades at the base of the fenestrae (*Tarnier and Milne-Murray*) or to the handles (*DeWees or Barnes-Neville forceps*). In the past, they were used for difficult high and midforceps deliveries; however, they are rarely used in modern obstetrics

USE OF FORCEPS

Indications for Use of Forceps

Forceps may be used for either fetal or maternal indications. In general, an operative vaginal delivery may be indicated if there is a threat to the mother or fetus that may be relieved by delivery. When signs of distress are present and delivery can be expedited by an easy forceps delivery, this should be done as quickly as possible. On the other hand, one should avoid panicky attempts to deliver a fetus with possible anoxia because these attempts may in fact be damaging to the fetus if a difficult, traumatic, and sometimes needless forceps traction is attempted.

Fetal Indications

1. Suspicion of fetal compromise, such as nonreassuring fetal heart pattern or placental abruption
2. Fetal malpositions, such as direct occipitoposterior (OP), occipitotransverse (OT), or persistent occipitoposterior (POP)
3. After-coming head in breech vaginal delivery

Maternal Indications

1. Shortening of the second stage because of a maternal condition such as cardiac or pulmonary disease, certain neurologic conditions, spinal tap, or history of spontaneous pneumothorax
2. Maternal exhaustion as evidenced by dehydration, concentrated urine, tachycardia, fever, or lack of effective maternal effort

Prolonged Active Second Stage

Lack of progress in the second stage includes failure of descent and failure of internal rotation. After 2 hours of synchronized pushing aided by adequate uterine contractions, operative delivery should be considered if there is no other evidence of CPD. Situations that may predispose to a prolonged second stage include poor uterine contractions, minor degrees of relative disproportion, abnormal fetal position such as occiput posterior position or attitudes of extension, a rigid perineum that the advancing head cannot thin out, and a lax pelvic floor that inhibits proper rotation of the head.

Contraindications to the Use of Forceps

1. Absence of a proper indication
2. Any contraindication to vaginal delivery
3. Refusal of the patient
4. Incompletely dilated cervix
5. Unengaged or high fetal head
6. Nonvertex or brow presentation
7. Fetal coagulopathy or demineralization disorder
8. Inability to determine the presentation and fetal head position or pelvic adequacy

SECOND STAGE OF LABOR

9. CPD
10. Absence of adequate anesthesia
11. Inadequate facilities and support staff
12. Inexperienced operator

Morbidity and Mortality Associated with Forceps Delivery

Maternal Risks

Maternal risks tend to increase significantly with rotations of greater than 45° and at higher stations. Maternal risks include:

1. Lacerations of the vulva, vagina, and cervix, including third- and fourth-degree lacerations and extension of episiotomy
2. Postpartum hemorrhage secondary to lacerations and uterine atony
3. Postpartum urinary retention and bladder dysfunction. Bladder atony usually starts as sensory atony where the bladder is overdistended. This leads to motor atony with high postvoid residuals and subsequent urinary infections. Bladder rest by a Foley catheter insertion after a difficult forceps delivery followed by bladder training usually leads to a return in normal function after a few days
4. Genital tract infection
5. Anal sphincter injury and dysfunction

Fetal Risks

1. Cephalohematoma (1%)
2. Fetal facial mark
3. Fetal facial lacerations (1%)
4. Intracranial hemorrhage (0.5%)
5. Subaponeurotic hemorrhage
6. Minor external ocular trauma
7. Fetal skull fractures
8. Facial nerve palsies (0.5%)
9. Cord compression

Serious injuries to the fetus delivered by forceps consist mainly of damage to the falx cerebri, the tentorium cerebelli, and the associated venous sinuses and other vessels. Lacerations are caused by excessive force and excessive compression. These injuries are associated mainly with deliveries from the midpelvis or higher. The dangers are especially great when (1) the forceps are **poorly applied** (applied in other than the BPD), (2) the fetal head is forced downward through the least favorable diameters of the pelvis, (3) forceful rotation is made at the wrong level of the pelvis or against the fetal back, and (4) excessive force is used in other than the correct line of the axis of the pelvis.

Classification of Forceps Operations

A forceps delivery may be classified into one of four categories: outlet, low, mid, or high forceps (Fig. 17-3). Most cases fit into these categories. However, when there is extreme molding, marked asynclitism, a large caput succedaneum, or an abnormal pelvis, the operator may make the error of thinking that the station is lower than it really is. In general, high forceps deliveries are contraindicated in modern obstetrics.

Outlet forceps	• Fetal scalp is visible on the vulva without separating the labia • Fetal skull (not caput) has reached the pelvic floor (+3 station) • Fetal head is at or on the perineum • Sagittal suture is in the AP diameter (OA or OP) or rotation does not exceed 45° (LOA, ROA, LOP, ROP)
Low forceps	• Leading point of the skull is at ≥+2 station and not on the pelvic floor • A) Rotation of < 45° (LOA, ROA, LOP, ROP) • B) Rotation of > 45°
Mid forceps	• Fetal head is engaged (<1/5 palpable abdominally) • Leading point of fetal skull is >+2 station
High forceps	• Fetal head is not engaged • *Contraindicated in modern obstetrics*

Prerequisites for Forceps Delivery

1. The head must be deeply engaged in the pelvis (i.e., the vault bone must be >1 cm below the ischial spines). Assessing engagement of the bony skull in relation to the ischial spines should not be confused with caput succedaneum. Abdominal assessment using the fourth Leopold's maneuver can be used to ensure that the biparietal diameter (BPD) has passed the pelvic brim. Less than 1/5 of the head should be palpable abdominally

"If you feel the fetal head abdominally, deliver it abdominally."

SECOND STAGE OF LABOR

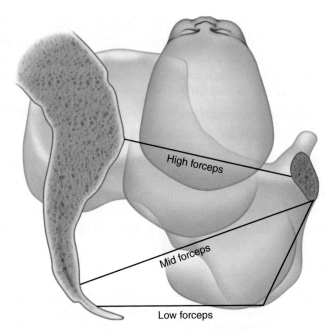

High forceps

Mid forceps

Low forceps

FIGURE 17-3. **Classification of forceps operations according to station.**

2. The fetus must present as a vertex or by the face with the mentum anterior

3. The exact position of the fetal head must be known

   a. Suspect malposition of the head if labor progress was slow or when there is a prolonged decelerative phase of labor (the cervix is 9 cm for more than 1 hour) or when there are repeated early decelerations on the fetal heart tracing. This is usually the result of vagal stimulation secondary to compression of the anterior fontanel of the deflexed head against the pelvic floor
   b. Abdominal examination (Leopold's maneuvers) can be used to diagnose OP malposition in early labor:
   • Flattening of the abdomen below the umbilicus
   • Fetal limbs may be felt over the front of the uterus
   • The fetal back is not palpated in the flank but rather laterally
   • The fetal heart is best heard on the outer third of a line between the umbilicus and anterior superior iliac spine
   c. Pelvic examination during labor: Use the fontanels and sutures to determine the position (Figs. 17-4A to C). This is not always easy

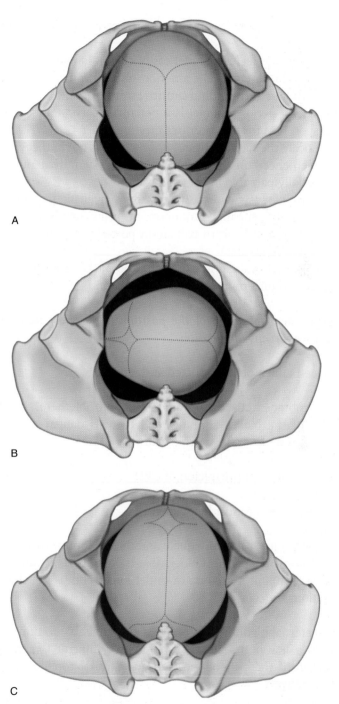

FIGURE 17-4. A, Direct occipitoanterior (OA) position. **B,** Left occipitotransverse (LOT) position. **C,** Direct occipitoposterior (OP) position.

at the end of the second stage because of the skull molding and scalp caput

- If you can feel a fontanel easily, then it is more likely to be the anterior fontanel. The anterior fontanel is merely a bony defect with four surrounding sutures meeting as an X
- The posterior fontanel is a potential space, not a palpable soft spot. Feel for three sutures meeting as a Y
- Locate the sagittal suture. If the suture is not in the AP diameter, then check for the fetal ear under the symphysis pubis. This is usually palpable in OT malposition
- Check for asynclitism. In anterior asynclitism, the sagittal suture is easily palpable (common in primigravidas). The sagittal suture is difficult to palpate in posterior asynclitism (common in multigravidas)

d. Ultrasound evaluation is a useful tool if the exact position of the head was uncertain by clinical evaluation

"Correct determination of the position is the most important step before forceps application."

4. The cervix must be fully dilated and retracted

5. The membranes must be ruptured. If they are not, there is an increased chance of the blades slipping, and there is danger of pulling the placenta away from the uterine wall

6. There should be no suspicion of CPD

7. Informed consent must be obtained

8. The woman must have adequate anesthesia. Topping up the epidural anesthesia with a perineal block dose is often used. A pudendal block may be useful for a vacuum or outlet forceps but is not sufficient for a rotational forceps

9. The maternal bladder is empty. It is also advisable to drain the bladder for a few hours after a rotational or difficult forceps delivery, especially if the patient received an epidural top up immediately before delivery

10. Adequate facilities and back-up personnel should be available

11. The operator should be fully competent and have the knowledge, experience, and skill necessary to use the instruments, recognize when to stop, and manage complications that may arise

APPLICATION OF FORCEPS

Cephalic Application

A cephalic application is made to fit the baby's head (Fig. 17-5A). An ideal cephalic application in **occipito anterior (OA) positions** is along the occipitomental diameter, with the fenestrae including the parietal bosses and the zygomotemporal arch with its tips lying over the cheeks. The convex edges are toward the face.

With this application, pressure on the head causes the least damage. Forceps marks lateral to the eyes and over the ear or the mastoid bone indicate good application. If the forceps are applied so that one blade lies over the face and the other over the occiput **(bad application)**, any degree of compression may cause fetal tentorial tears, intracranial hemorrhage, and facial soft tissue damage. This type of poor application is almost always the result of an inability to determine with certainty the exact position of the fetal head in the pelvis.

Pelvic Application

A pelvic application is made to fit the maternal pelvis (Fig. 17-5B), regardless of how the forceps grip the fetal head. Pelvic application alone is associated with a high risk of fetal injuries. The term *pelvic application* is used when:

1. The left blade is next to the left side of the pelvis
2. The right blade is on the right side of the pelvis
3. The concave margin is near the symphysis pubis
4. The convex margin is in the hollow of the sacrum
5. The diameter of the forceps is in the transverse diameter of the pelvis

Perfect Application

A perfect (cephalopelvic) application (Fig. 17-5C) is achieved when both the cephalic and pelvic requirements have been fulfilled. A perfect application is possible in direct OA positions when the occiput has already rotated to be directly under the symphysis pubis and the sagittal suture is in the AP diameter.

SECOND STAGE OF LABOR

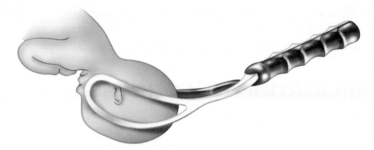

A. Cephalic application.

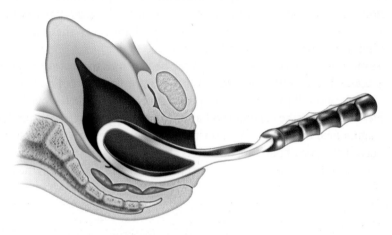

B. Pelvic application.

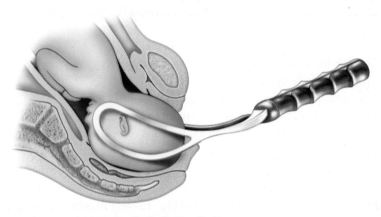

C. Perfect application.

FIGURE 17-5. **A,** Cephalic application of obstetric forceps. **B,** Pelvic application of obstetric forceps. **C,** Perfect application of obstetric forceps.

THE USES OF OBSTETRIC FORCEPS

Direct Occipitoanterior Forceps Delivery

In other than expert hands, the use of forceps should be restricted to that of direct application and traction. *Simpson* or *Tucker-McLane forceps* are useful for simple direct application and traction.

Application

1. Recheck that the prerequisite conditions and indications have been met

2. Perform a vaginal examination to accurately diagnose the position and station of the head, whether there is flexion or extension, and the presence of synclitism or asynclitism

3. Perform a *phantom application*. The locked forceps are held outside the vagina in front of the perineum in the way they are to be applied to the fetal head in the pelvis

4. The left blade is inserted first. The left blade is held in the left hand (pencil grip). At first the blade is in an almost vertical position. Gently introduce the blade into the left lower side of the pelvis (5 o'clock position) using the back of the right index and middle fingers to retract the vaginal wall laterally while the right thumb is directing the blade on the hollow of the sacrum then upward opposite to the ala of sacrum (Fig. 17-6A)

5. The handle is lowered slowly to the horizontal and toward the midline by pushing downward on the handle. This should help to complete the last part of the head rotation from left occipitoanterior (LOA) to direct OA (Fig. 17-6B)

6. The right blade is then held in the right hand, and the fingers of the left hand are inserted in the right side of the vagina between the fetal head and the vaginal wall. The right blade is gently introduced over the left forceps between the operator's fingers and the fetal head at about 7 o'clock (Fig. 17-6C). The right handle is lowered to the horizontal and toward the midline. At the same time, the blade is moved by the vaginal fingers up over the right side of the head to the occipitomental

position. The fingers of the left hand are then removed from the vagina (Fig. 17-6D)

7. Lock blades: This should be achieved without any excessive force, and the handles must never be forced together. If the blades do not lock easily, suspect a **bad application**. Remove the forceps and reevaluate the fetal head position (Fig. 17-7)

8. The application must then be checked to confirm a good application

   a. The posterior fontanel should be midway between the blades, and the lambdoid sutures should be one finger above the shanks. If this

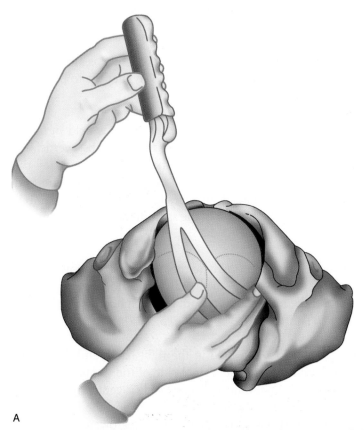

A

FIGURE 17-6. A, Insertion of left blade between fetal head and left side of pelvis. **B,** Handle of left forceps is lowered and the blade moved up over the left parietal bone. **C,** Insertion of right blade between fetal head and right side of pelvis. **D,** Handle of right forceps is lowered and the blade moved up over the right parietal bone.

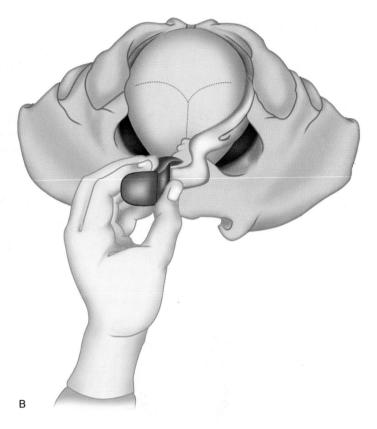

B

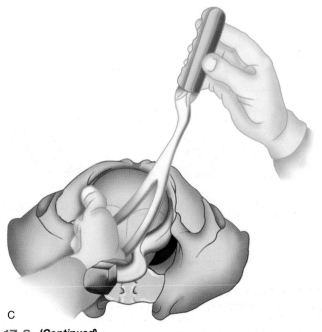

C

FIGURE 17-6. (*Continued*)

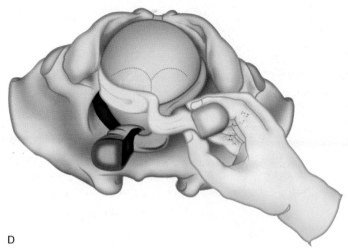

D

FIGURE 17-6. *(Continued)*

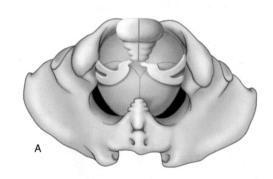

A

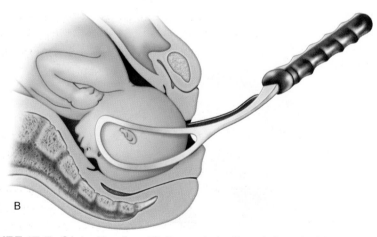

B

FIGURE 17-7. OA: Locking. **A** and **B,** Forceps locked in cephalic and pelvic application.

is too far, suspect head deflexion that would increase the risk of maternal injuries
b. The sagittal suture should be perpendicular to the plane of the shanks, and the blades should be equidistant from the sagittal suture. An asymmetrical relationship indicates that one of the blades was applied in a higher or a lower position in relation to the fetal face and subsequently increases the risks of fetal injury
c. The fenestration of the blades is barely felt and is equal. If you can easily introduce your finger, suspect a short application and a subsequent higher risk of fetal injury

Traction and Delivery

It is preferable to provide traction with each contraction, and the head should be allowed to recede in intervals between contractions. The direction of traction must be along the pelvic curvature (a backward tilted L-shape with the lower end pointed up 45°), and as the station changes during descent, so will the line of traction (Fig. 17-8A). Gentle downward traction is applied during the uterine contractions until the vault of the fetal skull is at +3 station. At that point, the direction should change to upward (Fig. 17-8B) and then toward the mother's abdomen as the head reaches the perineum and becomes visible within the vulva and the parietal bones emerge. This allows for delivery of the head by extension. This step should be undertaken very slowly to minimize maternal soft tissue trauma and perineal lacerations. Episiotomy can be used but only if it is deemed necessary. The forceps are removed when the head is crowning by a process that is the reverse of their application. The handle of the right blade is raised toward the mother's left groin, and the blade slides around the head and out of the pelvis (Fig. 17-9). Then the same is done with the left forceps by raising the handle toward the maternal right groin.

Left Occipitoanterior Forceps Delivery

The principles of forceps application with an LOA presentation are similar to those with a direct OA position with the exception that the head is rotated with the use of the forceps from an LOA to OA position. In many cases, the head may rotate spontaneously from LOA to OA as traction is applied, but if not, the operator must rotate the occiput 45° to the anterior at the same time that he or she is exerting traction (Fig. 17-10).

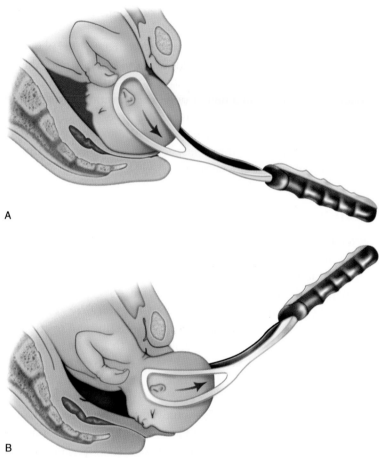

A

B

FIGURE 17-8. A, Traction is made outward and posteriorly until the nape of the neck is under the pubic symphysis. **B,** The direction of traction is changed to promote extension of the fetal head.

DIRECT OCCIPTOPOSTERIOR DELIVERY

In direct OP positions, delivering the head by direct application and traction using *Simpson* or *Tucker-McLane* forceps is possible. However, the risk of perineal trauma, including fourth-degree tears, is high as the wider part of the head, the occiput, lies against the perineum. The head is delivered in flexion. It is advisable to change the direction of traction to upward earlier than in OA presentations before the occiput fills the posterior half of the vulva.

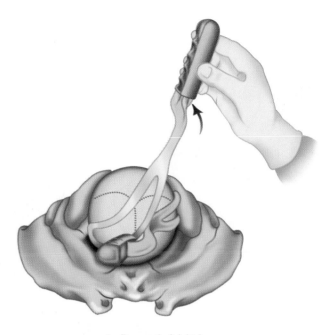

A. Removal of right forceps.

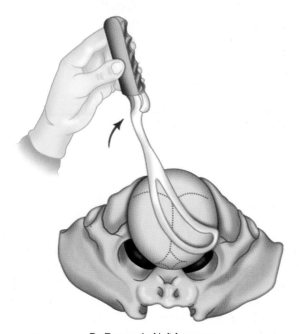

B. Removal of left forceps.

FIGURE 17-9. Removal of forceps.

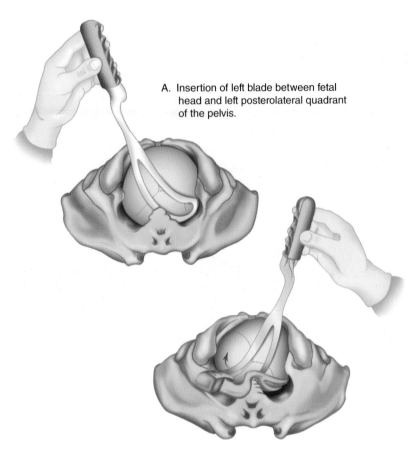

A. Insertion of left blade between fetal head and left posterolateral quadrant of the pelvis.

B. Insertion of right blade between fetal head and right posterolateral quadrant of the pelvis, followed by upward movement of the blade to right anterolateral quadrant of the pelvis.

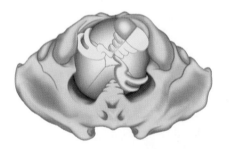

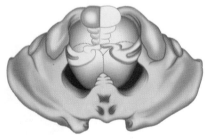

C. Locking of forceps in cephalic application.

D. Head is rotated from LOA to OA. It is now ready for extraction.

FIGURE 17-10. Application of forceps in left occiput anterior position.

Orientation and Desired Application

The cephalic application:

1. The blades of the forceps are over the parietal bones in an occipitomental application. The left blade is on the right parietal bone, and the right blade is on the left parietal bone
2. The front of the forceps (concave edges) point to the face. In an ideal cephalic application, they point to the occiput
3. The convex edges point to the occiput. In the ideal application, they point to the face

The pelvic application:

1. The diameter of the forceps is in the transverse diameter of the pelvis
2. The sides of the blades are next to the sidewalls of the pelvis, the left blade near the left side and right blade near the right side
3. The concave edges point to the pubis
4. The convex edges point to the sacrum (Fig. 17-11)

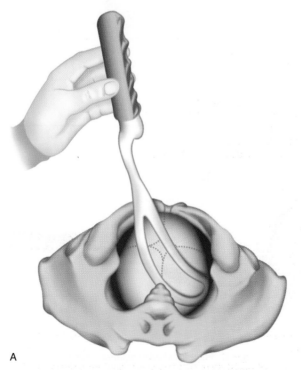

A

FIGURE 17-11. Application of forceps in the occipitoposterior position.

SECOND STAGE OF LABOR

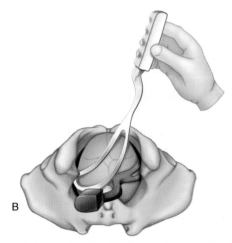

B

Handle of left blade is lowered and the blade moved up over the right parietal bone. Insertion of right blade between fetal head and right side of pelvis.

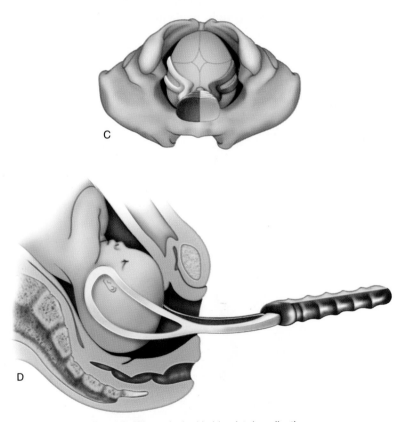

C

D

C and D. Forces locked in biparietal application.

FIGURE 17-11. *(Continued)*

Extraction of the Head

1. Traction is made outward and posteriorly until the area between the bregma and the nasion lies under the pubic arch (Fig. 17-12A)

2. Delivery is by one of two methods:

   a. The direction is changed to outward and anterior (Fig. 17-12B). As the handles of the forceps are raised, the occiput is born over the perineum by flexion. The forceps then slip off the head
   b. The direction is changed to outward and anterior until the occiput is on the perineum. The forceps are removed by raising first the right handle toward the left groin so that the blade slips around the

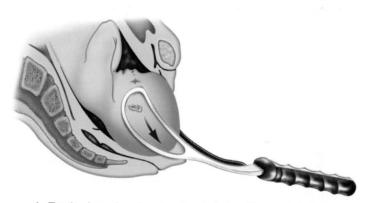

A. Traction is made outward and posteriorly until the area between the bregma and nasion lies under the pubic arch.

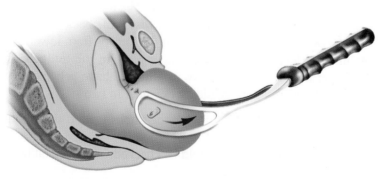

B. Traction is made outward and anteriorly to promote flexion.

FIGURE 17-12. Extraction of the fetal head in the occipitoposterior position.

SECOND STAGE OF LABOR

head and out of the vagina. Then the left handle is raised toward the right groin so that the left blade slides out. By a modified Ritgen maneuver, flexion is increased until the occiput has cleared the perineum completely

3. The head then falls back in extension. The nose, face, and chin are delivered under the pubis

4. If the head cannot be delivered as a posterior presentation without using an excessive amount of force, this method of delivery should be abandoned and an anterior rotation of the occiput carried out

Rotation in the Event of a Failed Direct OP Assisted Delivery

If the head is arrested in the midpelvis or if direct application and traction fails, a *long forceps rotation* by *Kielland* forceps can be performed by an experienced operator. On each handle of the Kielland forceps is a small knob that indicates the direction of the occiput.

1. The operator should determine the position of the fetal back (right or left)

2. Perform a phantom application where the Kielland forceps are assembled with the knobs on the handles directed downward toward the occiput. The blades are then introduced directly on each side of the head with the pelvic curve in an inversed position

3. The head is then rotated gently toward the fetal back. Forceful rotation in the opposite direction of the fetal back may violently twist the baby's neck and may result in fatal axis fracture. The rotation is counterclockwise if the back is on the left and clockwise if the back is on the right. It is advisable that the operator rotate the forceps from lower than the patient's bed level as the rotation takes place in the midpelvic plane (the upper limb of the 45° backward tilted L-shape pelvic curvature). Gentle and easy rotation should be executed in two stages

   a. From direct OP to OT, bringing the knobs toward the position of the fetal back
   b. The forceps application should be checked, and the fetal heart rate should be evaluated
   c. Then rotate OT to OA, bringing the knobs upward

ROTATIONAL FORCEPS OF HEAD FROM TRANSVERSE POSITIONS

Single Application for Rotation and Traction: Kielland Forceps

1. Kielland forceps do not have a right or left blade, so the operator uses the **phantom application** to determine the *anterior* and *posterior* blades. This is performed by holding the forceps outside the patient while directing the knobs on the shanks toward the fetal occipital bone

2. The anterior blade is applied first by guiding it into the pelvis poste-riorly (as in the direct forceps application). The operator kneels down while pushing the blade deep in the pelvis. The blade is then rotated upward and laterally around the occiput or the face (clockwise or counterclockwise) according to the position of the occiput (left occiput transverse [LOT] or right occiput transverse [ROT]). Then gently ease the blade concavity over the head in the occipitomental diameter, where it lays immediately under the symphysis pubis. This maneuver is called the *wandering method.* There are other methods of applying the anterior blade, but these are rarely used in modern obstetrics. These include:

    a. *Direct method:* The anterior blade is pushed directly below the sym-physis pubis with the concavity over the side of the head. This can cause significant damage to the urethrovesical sphincter and subse-quent stress incontinence or urinary fistulae

    b. *Classical method:* The anterior blade is introduced with its con-cavity under the symphysis pubis and pushed upward inside the uterus, above the head, and then twisted to bring the cephalic curve inward and downward over the fetal head. This maneuver has become obsolete because of the associated high risk of uterine rupture

3. The posterior blade is applied and guided directly into the hollow of the sacrum

4. The forceps handles are locked. In cases of anterior asynclitism, the handles appear unequal outside the vulva with the posterior blade seeming longer (the reverse is seen in posterior asynclitism). Using the

SECOND STAGE OF LABOR

sliding lock, the longer handle is pushed inward to bring the blades opposite to each other. This motion corrects the asynclitism and disengages the head slightly to allow for the rotation

5. The head is then rotated gently from OT to OA, bringing the knobs upward

6. If the head is low in the pelvis, rotation may bring it to the "crowning" stage. The forceps can be removed because further traction is not required. More often traction is needed and should be carried out during uterine contraction after checking the application as in the direct forceps delivery

Double Application of Forceps: "Scanzoni Maneuver"

Tucker-McLane or Simpson forceps can be applied to rotate the occiput anteriorly (Fig. 17-13). The handles should be maneuvered through a wide arc to reduce the arc of the blades and to lower the incidence and extent of vaginal lacerations (Fig. 17-14). The handles of the forceps are raised toward the opposite groin (in right occiput posterior [ROP] toward the left groin), which favors flexion of the fetal head. Without traction, the handles are carried around in a large circle so that they point first to the left groin (ROP), next toward the left thigh (ROT), then toward the left ischial tuberosity, and finally toward the anus and pelvic floor. With the wide sweep of the handles, the blades turn in a small arc and do not deviate from the same axis during the process of rotation.

At this point, the forceps are not in a suitable position to extract the head (Fig. 17-15), and adjustments are necessary. The forceps are then unlocked and removed. The right blade is removed first by depressing the handle further so that the blade slides around the head and out of the vagina (Fig. 17-16). The left blade is then removed in the same way.

A vaginal examination is performed to confirm the position. The forceps are then reapplied so that the pelvic curve of the forceps is directed anteriorly (as in a direct OA application) (Figs. 17-17A to C) and the head is extracted in the usual way. Some operators use *Kielland* forceps (or Tucker-McLane or Simpson) for rotation and then remove the blade on the left side of the pelvis to apply the left blade of a *Tucker-McLane or Simpson* forceps; then the same is repeated on the right side (Fig. 17-18). This modification, called a two-forceps maneuver, is useful to avoid rotation of the fetal head back to the transverse or posterior position.

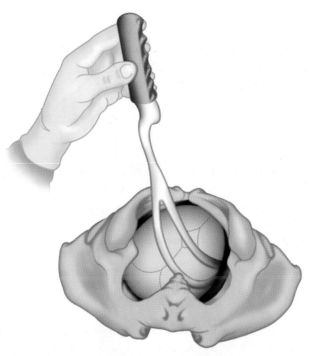

A. Insertion of left blade between fetal head and left posterolateral quadrant of pelvis.

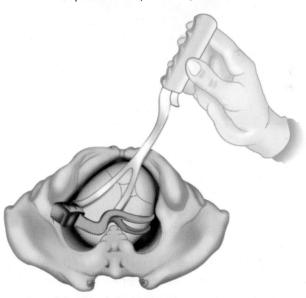

B. Handle of left blade is lowered. Insertion of right blade between fetal head and right posterolateral quadrant of pelvis, followed by upward movement of blade to right anterolateral quadrant of pelvis.

FIGURE 17-13. Application of forceps in the right occiput posterior position for the Scanzoni maneuver.

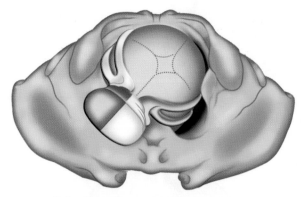

C. Locking of forceps in biparietal application.

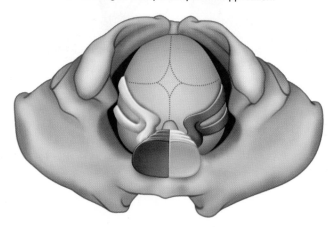

D. Posterior rotation ROP to OP (45°)

FIGURE 17-13. *(Continued)*

Forceps for After-Coming Head

Piper forceps are ideal for delivery of the after-coming head in a breech presentation. Kielland forceps can be used as a substitute.

1. After delivering the body and the appearance of the nape of the baby's neck outside the vulva, an assistant gently lifts the fetus upward. The body should not be lifted too much because the structures of the neck can be damaged by excessive stretching
2. The right hand is introduced into the vagina between the head and the left posterolateral wall of the vagina. The left blade is held in the left hand and guided into the vulva from underneath the body and around

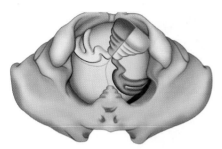

A. ROP: Head is flexed by raising the handles of the forceps.

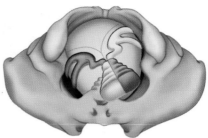

C. ROT to ROA (45°).

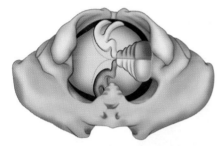

B. Anterior rotation by forceps: ROP to ROT (45°).

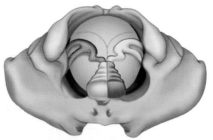

D. ROA to OA (45°).

FIGURE 17-14. Scanzoni maneuver from right occiput posterior (ROP) to occiput anterior (OA). ROA, right occiput anterior; ROT, right occiput transverse.

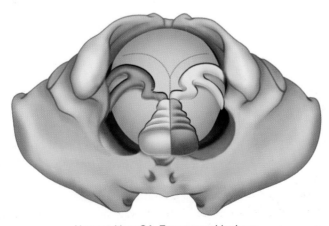

New position: OA. Forceps upside down.

FIGURE 17-15. New position: occiput anterior (OA). Forceps upside down.

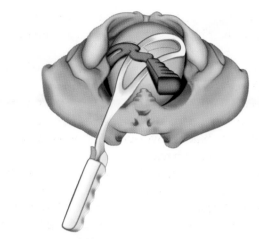

A. Removal of right blade.

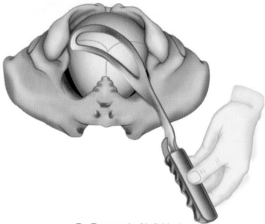

B. Removal of left blade.

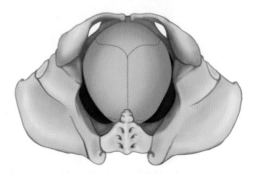

C. New position: OA

FIGURE 17-16. Scanzoni maneuver: removal of forceps. OA, occiput anterior.

the right side of the fetal face. This is a mento occipital application. The right blade is then introduced in the same manner around the left side of the fetal face

3. The handles are then locked underneath the fetal chest, and the fetal body is allowed to rest on the operator's forearms. Vaginal examination is performed to be certain that the application is correct (Fig. 17-19)

4. Traction is applied outward and posterior until the nape of the neck is in the subpubic angle. Downward traction is rarely needed to ensure complete delivery of the neck

5. After delivery of the nape, the direction of traction is changed to upward toward the mother's abdomen to deliver the head in flexion. This step should be performed very slowly to avoid sudden decompression. As the face appears, it is advisable to wipe the nose and mouth clean before delivering the occiput

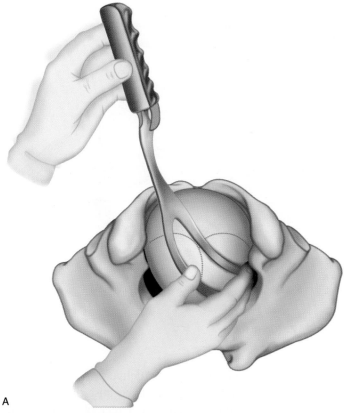

A

FIGURE 17-17. A, Reapplication of left blade between fetal head and left side of pelvis. **B,** Reapplication of right blade between fetal head and right side of pelvis. **C,** Locking of forceps in biparietal cephalic and pelvic application.

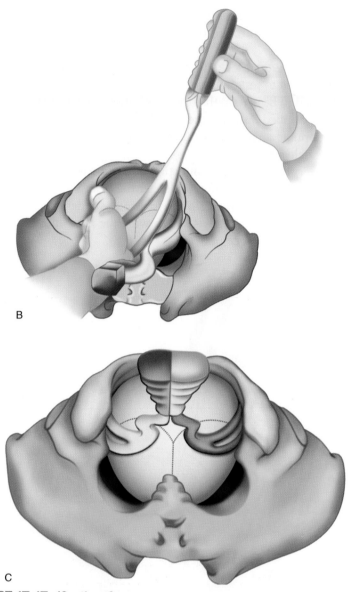

B

C

FIGURE 17-17. *(Continued)*

Some advocate an elective forceps delivery for breech deliveries for delivery of the after-coming head. This is because the forceps are applied on the parietal bone, so there is reduced chance of soft tissue trauma that may result from difficult after-coming head delivery using the jaw-flexion shoulder-traction technique.

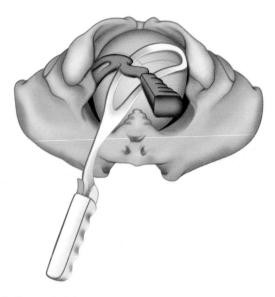

A. Removal of right Simpson forceps from left side of pelvis.

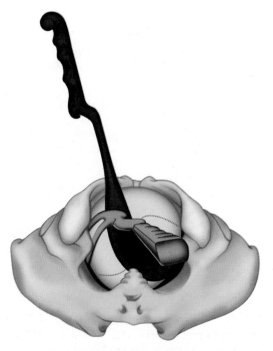

B. Insertion of left Tucker-McLane forceps between fetal head
and left side of pelvis. The left Simpson is still in place.

FIGURE 17-18. **Two-forceps maneuver.**

SECOND STAGE OF LABOR

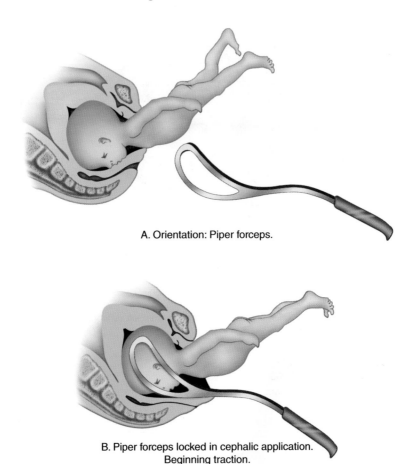

A. Orientation: Piper forceps.

B. Piper forceps locked in cephalic application.
Beginning traction.

FIGURE 17-19. **Piper forceps for delivery of the after-coming head.**

Forceps for Face Presentation

Direct Mentum Anterior

Direct mentum anterior face presentations (Fig. 17-20) can be delivered using *Simpson, Tucker-McLane, or Kielland* forceps (Fig. 17-21). The forceps blades are applied to the sides of the head along the occiptomental diameter with the pelvic curve directed toward the neck. Forceps should not be applied to mentum posterior presentations because the head is at maximum extension. Mentum transverse face presentations usually spontaneously rotate to mentum anterior positions. In rare occasions, an expert operator may attempt to rotate a mentum transverse to a mentum anterior with Kielland forceps.

In the direct mentum anterior position, the forceps are applied, and their position is verified. Then the handles of the forceps are depressed

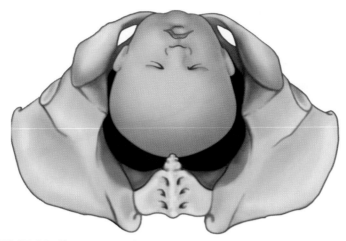

FIGURE 17-20. Face presentation, mentum anterior.

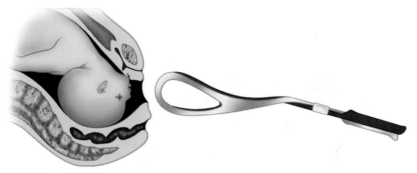

FIGURE 17-21. Face presentation phantom application.

toward the floor to deflex the head completely. Traction is made in an outward, horizontal, and slightly posterior direction until the chin appears under the symphysis pubis and the submental region of the neck impinges in the subpubic angle (Fig. 17-22). With further descent, the face and forehead appear, and the direction of traction is changed to outward and anterior (upward). This brings about both descent and flexion, and the vertex and occiput are born over the perineum.

CAUSES OF CATASTROPHIC FORCEPS

An attempt to deliver the child by forceps may fail completely or may produce a damaged baby and significant maternal lacerations. Pitfalls that contribute to making a wrong decision include the following:

SECOND STAGE OF LABOR

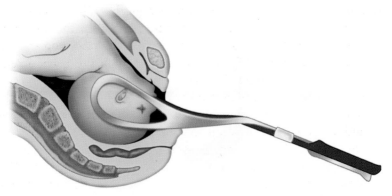

A. Locking of forceps. Beginning traction in the axis of the birth canal.

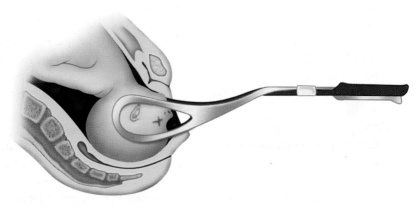

B. Horizontal traction.

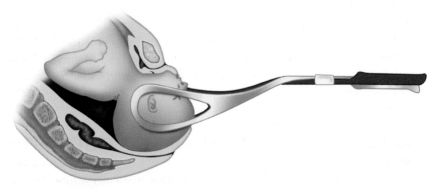

C. Delivery by flexion of the head.

FIGURE 17-22. **Forceps delivery of mentum anterior.**

1. Misunderstanding the significance and the relationship of station and the level of the BPD. Station zero means that the presenting part has reached the level of the ischial spines. In most women, when the station is zero, the BPD is at or just through the pelvic inlet. Thus, when forceps are applied at station zero, the procedure does not simply involve extracting the presenting part from the midpelvis; rather, the BPD must be pulled all the way from the inlet, through the midpelvis, and the outlet. This is a difficult and potentially dangerous procedure. On the other hand, when the station is +2 and the BPD is at or below the spines, a midforceps operation is often easy and safe. We must always consider both the station of the presenting part and the level of the BPD

2. Unrecognized disproportion caused by:
   - A small or abnormal pelvis
   - A large baby. This is particularly concerning in a multipara who had a normal delivery previously. An operative vaginal delivery in this instance may be complicated by a difficult forceps extraction, shoulder dystocia, vaginal and cervical lacerations, postpartum hemorrhage, and potentially a damaged infant. Whenever progress has ceased, the size of the baby must be reassessed before any action is taken

3. Misdiagnosis of station because of:
   - Caput succedaneum (scalp edema). In prolonged labor, the caput may be 1 to 2 cm thick, and hence the bony skull is at a correspondingly higher level in the pelvis. It is important to ascertain the station of the skull and not the edematous scalp. A large caput indicates strong contractions, great resistance, or both. A small or absent caput suggests that the contractions or the resistance of the pelvic tissues are weak
   - Molding. Excessive molding makes the head pointed by lengthening its long axis; therefore, the BPD is at a greater distance from the leading part of the skull. In these situations, engagement may not have taken place when the station is zero. Not only is the forceps operation difficult, but the pressure of the instrument on a brain already under stress increases the risk of permanent damage. Extreme molding and lack of progress are very concerning

4. Misdiagnosis of position. In descending order of importance, the steps in the use of forceps are diagnosis of position, application, and traction. It is obvious that if the exact position of the fetal head is not known, the forceps cannot be applied correctly. Difficulty in applying forceps demands a complete reevaluation of the situation, not forceful

SECOND STAGE OF LABOR

delivery. Whenever labor ceases to advance, the possibility of an abnormal position or a malpresentation (e.g., brow) must be kept in mind

5. Misdiagnosis of inefficient uterine action. The erroneous assumption that the lack of progress is the result of poor contractions leads to trouble in two ways: (1) forceps are applied too soon, and (2) an oxytocin infusion may dilate the cervix and jam the fetal head into the pelvis just far enough to encourage the performance of a misguided forceps extraction

6. Premature interference. This involves the use of forceps either before the patient is ready and the prerequisites are fulfilled or when there are no valid indications. Modern management of second stage is a good way to prevent this problem

TRIAL OF FORCEPS AND FAILED FORCEPS

All midpelvic forceps and low rotational forceps should be considered a trial of forceps. The principle of trial forceps involves the idea that after successful application of the forceps has been achieved, gentle traction is made. If the head comes down easily, then the attempt at operative vaginal delivery should be continued and the baby delivered. Episiotomy (if required) should not be done before crowning. If, on the other hand, the operator believes that an undue amount of force would be required to extract the head, the forceps are removed, and a cesarean section should be performed.

Factors predictive of a failed operative vaginal delivery include increased maternal age, higher body mass index, diabetes, presumed fetal macrosomia, OP positions of the fetal head, midpelvic procedures, induction of labor, dysfunctional labor, and prolonged labor. Operative vaginal deliveries that have a higher rate of failure should be considered a trial of instrumental delivery in the operating room setting with anesthesia present so that one can proceed immediately to cesarean section if necessary (double setup).

VACUUM EXTRACTOR

A vacuum extractor applies suction and traction to an area of the fetal scalp covered by a suction cup in order to assist maternal expulsive efforts. It is not a device for applying rotational forces, although rotation may occur with descent of the vertex. Vacuum cups can be metal, plastic, or silicone and can be rigid or soft. They are usually 50 or 60 mm in diameter. The vacuum extractor should not be considered as an easier alternative to forceps or for use by less skilled operators. It is not likely to succeed in the absence of maternal expulsive efforts, and the vacuum has been found to be more likely to fail as the instrument of delivery than forceps.

The vacuum has some advantages over forceps. It does not encroach on the space in the pelvis, reducing the incidence of damage to maternal tissues. In addition, the fetal head is not fixed by the application, so it can go through the rotations that the configurations of the birth canal require. The fetal head is allowed to find the path of least resistance.

Indications for Use of a Vacuum

The indications for vacuum-assisted vaginal delivery are much the same as those for forceps delivery. These include fetal indications, such as an atypical or abnormal fetal heart tracing, maternal indications (e.g., indications to avoid Valsalva maneuver), inadequate progress of labor, and lack of effective maternal expulsive efforts.

Contraindications to Use of a Vacuum

1. Noncephalic presentation such as face or brow presentation
2. Fetal conditions such as bleeding disorder or demineralization disorder
3. Any contraindication to vaginal birth
4. Less than 34 weeks of gestation
5. Fetal congenital anomalies such as hydrocephalus
6. Evidence of CPD
7. Dead fetus: suction and traction are not efficient in this case
8. Need for operator-applied rotation
9. An incompletely dilated cervix with an unengaged head. Note: Although it is preferable for the cervix to be fully dilated and the head to be engaged, in some circumstances with a multiparous patient, a vacuum delivery may still be performed, but only when the benefits significantly outweigh the risks and when there is no viable alternative

Previous fetal scalp sampling is not a contraindication to a vacuum-assisted delivery.

SECOND STAGE OF LABOR

Morbidity and Mortality

Many studies have reported that maternal injury is less frequent and less extensive with the use of vacuum cups compared with forceps. Potential maternal complications include cervical lacerations, severe vaginal lacerations, vaginal hematomas, and third- and fourth-degree tears.

Potential fetal complications are similar to those seen with forceps. These include fetal scalp trauma, subgaleal hemorrhage, intracranial hemorrhage, hyperbilirubinemia, and retinal hemorrhage.

1. The formation of a pronounced caput succedaneum is a part of the procedure and is seen in almost all cases. The caput usually disappears within a few hours
2. Abrasions, necrosis, and ulceration of the scalp at the site of application of the cup. The longer the cup is on, the greater the chance of scalp trauma. These should be treated by gentle cleansing and antibiotic ointments. The skin at the site of the suction must be handled carefully to avoid rubbing off the friable superficial layer
3. Cephalohematoma. This occurs in 10 to 15 percent of cases and is higher than that reported for spontaneous births and deliveries by forceps. Serious difficulties are rare, and the prognosis is good
4. Subaponeurotic or subgaleal hemorrhage may occur from beneath the galea aponeurotica layer of the scalp. Sometimes it is not evident until a couple of days after birth. The bleeding may be massive and life threatening because the subaponeurotic space is continuous across the cranium without periosteal attachments. A hematoma in this space can dissect across the cranial vault, elevating part or all of the scalp. If there is a suspicion of or increased risk for a subgaleal hemorrhage, head circumferences should be closely monitored
5. Retinal hemorrhage occurs more frequently than with spontaneous births or deliveries by forceps. There seems to be no residual damage

Prerequisites for a Vacuum-Assisted Vaginal Delivery

The same criteria as for a forceps delivery must be met before an attempt at a vacuum-assisted vaginal delivery. These include:

1. Informed consent
2. No fetal contraindications

3. Appropriate analgesia and anesthesia
4. Cervix fully dilated
5. Membranes rupture
6. Vertex presentation
7. Vertex engaged
8. Adequate uterine contractions
9. No evidence of CPD
10. Empty maternal bladder
11. Experienced operator; adequate facilities and resources available
12. Properly functioning equipment
13. Ongoing maternal and fetal assessment
14. Backup plan in place in case the procedure is unsuccessful

Application of the Vacuum and Delivery

The patient is positioned and prepared just as for a forceps delivery. The largest cup that fits is used. When soft cups are used, they are inserted by compressing the cup in an AP direction and then introducing it into the posterior fourchette while making space and protecting the maternal tissue with the opposite hand. When a hard cup is used, it is slid sideways into the vagina and then flipped onto the fetal skull. Once in the vagina, the cup is moved anteriorly to a position over the sagittal suture slightly anterior to the posterior fontanel (~1 cm) to ensure that the smallest diameter of the head will travel through the pelvis. This is called the flexion point. Verification of a good placement is then required, including ensuring that no maternal tissue is trapped between the cup and the fetal head.

Slowly, the negative pressure is pumped up until it reaches 500 to 600 mm Hg (0.6-0.8 kg/cm²). An artificial caput succedaneum, a "chignon," is formed. The vacuum pressure may be released between contractions to resting pressures of between 100 and 200 mm Hg (0.1-0.3 kg/cm²). However, there is no evidence that there is a difference in neonatal outcome if the vacuum is maintained, with or without traction, between contractions.

Traction is then applied with the right hand pulling downward on the tube or handle of the vacuum while the left hand presses on the cup and the fetal head to ensure a continuous good seal (Fig. 17-23). This produces a force in the direction of the birth canal. Traction should be synchronized with adequate uterine contraction and maximum maternal pushing effort. Traction is applied in the direction of the pelvic curve, initially downward and then upward. No rotational force should be applied,

SECOND STAGE OF LABOR

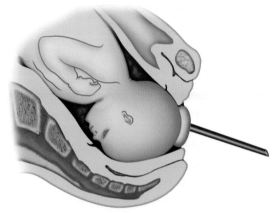

A. Traction outward and posteriorly.

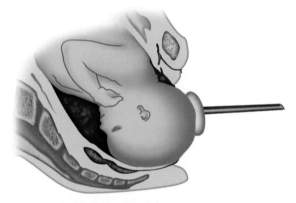

B. Traction outward and horizontally.

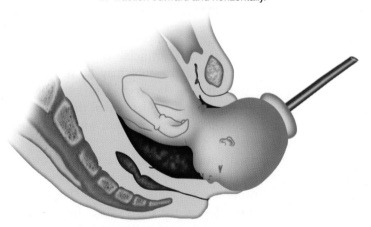

C. Traction outward and anteriorly.

FIGURE 17-23. Vacuum-assisted vaginal delivery.

but the fetal head may rotate on its own with descent. When the head is crowning, the direction of the pulling is changed to upward and toward the mother's abdomen. The left hand then moves to support the perineum. A common mistake is to extend the head prematurely, thereby increasing the diameter that must pass over the perineum and increasing the likelihood of fetal–maternal trauma and a vacuum pop-off. Rocking motions may also increase the possibility of scalp damage.

Pop-offs (i.e., when the suction cup loses it seal on the fetal head and is inadvertently pulled away by the operator) should not be considered a normal event in a vacuum-assisted vaginal delivery. Causes of pop-offs include:

1. Poor seal causing a vacuum leak
2. Excessive traction force
3. Unrecognized CPD
4. Midpelvic application
5. OP presentation
6. Deflexed attitude
7. Paramedian application
8. Improper angle of traction causing shearing
9. Impingement of maternal soft tissue

When to Abandon an Attempted Vacuum-Assisted Vaginal Delivery

It is important that the operator knows when to abandon an attempted operative vaginal delivery. The operator should abandon the procedure if any of the three circumstances occur:

1. After three pulls over three contractions with no progress or descent
2. After three pop-offs without obvious cause
3. After 20 minutes if delivery is not imminent

In these instances, the vacuum should be removed, and a different method of delivery should be considered. In most instances, this would be achieved by cesarean section, although a forceps-assisted delivery may also be considered. The risk of complications increases with the sequential use of different instruments. The following table provides a brief "ABC" mnemonic to help guide operators at a vacuum-assisted vaginal delivery.

SECOND STAGE OF LABOR

A	Address Anesthesia Assistance	• The patient • Adequate relief • Neonatal support
B	Bladder	• Empty
C	Cervix	• Fully dilated • Membranes ruptured
D	Determine	• Position, station, pelvic adequacy • Anticipate shoulder dystocia
E	Equipment	• Inspect cup, pump, tubing, pressure
F	Fontanel (posterior)	• Under or posterior to cup
G	Gentle traction	• With contractions
H	Halt	• If no progress after: Three contractions Three pop-offs 20 minutes
I	Incision	• Consider episiotomy

Adapted from Bachman J. A forceps needs to be documented in the same manner as any other operative procedure. Forceps Delivery Correspondence. J Am Acad Fam Pract 1989;29:4.

DOCUMENTATION OF AN OPERATIVE VAGINAL DELIVERY

Clear documentation is important throughout labor and birth, particularly in the case of an operative vaginal delivery. The following points should be clearly documented after an operative vaginal delivery:

1. Indication for intervention
2. Discussion with the woman of the risks, benefits, and options
3. Position and station of the fetal head as well as how it was assessed (i.e., vaginally, abdominally, or both)
4. Amount of molding and caput present
5. Assessment of maternal pelvis
6. Assessment of fetal heart and contractions
7. Number of attempts and ease of application of vacuum or forceps
8. Duration of traction and force used
9. Description of maternal and neonatal injuries

SELECTED READING

American College of Obstetricians and Gynecologists: ACOG Practice Bulletin No. 17: Operative Vaginal Delivery. Washington, DC: ACOG: 2000

Bachman J. A forceps needs to be documented in the same manner as any other operative procedure. Forceps Delivery Correspondence. J Am Acad Fam Pract 29:4, 1989

Cargill Y, MacKinnon CJ: Society of Obstetricians and Gynaecologists of Canada: Guidelines for Operative Vaginal Birth. J Obstet Gynaecol Can 148:347-353, 2004

Gei AF, Pacheco, LD: Operative vaginal deliveries: practical aspects. Obstet Gynecol Clin North Am 38: 323, 2011

Goplani S, Bennet K, Critchlow C: Factors predictive of failed operative vaginal delivery. Am J Obstet Gynecol 191: 892, 2004

Healy DL, Quinn MA, Pepperell RJ: Rotational delivery of the fetus: Kielland's forceps and two other methods compared. Br J Obstet Gynaecol, 89:501, 1982

Ingardia CJ, Cetrulo CL: Forceps—use and abuse. Clin Perinatol 8:63, 1981

Majoko F, Gardner G: Trial of instrumental delivery in theatre versus immediate caesarean section for anticipated difficult vaginal births. Cochrane DataBase Syst Rev 4:CD005545, 2008

Royal College of Obstetricians and Gynaecologists: Operative vaginal delivery. Clinical Guideline 26. http://www.rcog.org.uk/files/rcog-corp/GTG26.pdf, 2011.

Society of Obstetricians and Gynaecologists of Canada. Assisted Vaginal Birth and Vaginal Breech Birth. MORE[OB].

CHAPTER 18

Shoulder
Dystocia

Yaa Amankwah

GENERAL CONSIDERATIONS

Definition of Shoulder Dystocia

Shoulder dystocia occurs when the fetal head is delivered but the shoulders cannot be spontaneously delivered by the usual method of gentle downward traction. The fetus must be in the cephalic presentation for this term to be applicable. Shoulder dystocia happens when the fetal anterior shoulder impacts on the maternal pubic symphysis or, less commonly, the fetal posterior shoulder impacts on the maternal sacral promontory. Additional obstetric maneuvers are often required to help deliver the fetal shoulders.

Incidence of Shoulder Dystocia

The general incidence of shoulder dystocia is between 0.6 and 1.4 percent. The wide variation in incidence is a result of varied clinical scenarios used to describe shoulder dystocia. The definition of shoulder dystocia, the characteristics of the population being examined, and the consistency and accuracy of reporting such cases all affect the reported incidence. Approximately 50 percent of shoulder dystocias occur in women without risk factors.

Mechanism of Shoulder Dystocia

In most cases of normal labor and delivery, the shoulders enter the pelvis in an oblique diameter. As labor progresses, the shoulders descend and rotate the bisacromial diameter toward the anteroposterior (AP) diameter of the pelvis. By this mechanism, the anterior shoulder comes under the pubic symphysis a little to the side of the midline and is then delivered.

Impaction of the shoulders occurs when the fetus attempts to enter the pelvis with the bisacromial diameter in the AP diameter of the inlet (Fig. 18-1) instead of using one of the oblique diameters. Rarely do both shoulders impact above the pelvic brim. Usually the posterior shoulder can negotiate its way past the sacral promontory, but the anterior shoulder becomes wedged against the pubic symphysis.

CLINICAL PRESENTATION

When the anterior shoulder, or less commonly the posterior shoulder, is impacted against the symphysis pubis/sacral promontory in the AP diameter, the result is the inability of the remainder of the body to be

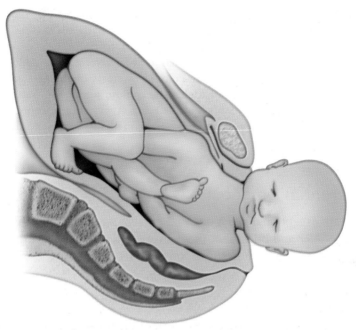

FIGURE 18-1. Shoulder dystocia: bisacromial diameter in the anteroposterior diameter of the pelvis.

delivered by the usual methods. The head remains tight against the perineum (the "turtle sign"), spontaneous restitution does not occur, and the baby does not deliver with the usual maternal effort. In 1955, Morris described the classic picture of shoulder dystocia as follows:

> The delivery of the head with or without forceps may have been quite easy, but more commonly there has been a little difficulty in completing the extension of the head. The hairy scalp slides out with reluctance. When the forehead has appeared it is necessary to press back the perineum to deliver the face. Fat cheeks eventually emerge. A double chin has to be hooked over the posterior vulval commissure, to which it remains tightly opposed. Restitution seldom occurs spontaneously, for the head seems incapable of movement as a result of friction with the girdle of contact of the vulva. On the other hand, gentle manipulation of the head sometimes results in sudden 90-degree restitution as the head adjusts itself without descent to the AP position of the shoulders.
>
> Time passes. The child's head becomes suffused. It endeavours unsuccessfully to breathe. Abdominal efforts by the mother or by her attendants produce no advance; gentle head traction is equally unavailing.

SECOND STAGE OF LABOR

Usually equanimity forsakes the attendants. They push, they pull. Alarm increases. Eventually by greater strength of muscle or by some infernal juggle the difficulty appears to be overcome, and the shoulders and trunk of a goodly child are delivered. The pallor of its body contrasts with the plum-colored cyanosis of the face, and the small quantity of freshly expelled meconium about the buttocks. It dawns upon the attendants that their anxiety was not ill-founded, the baby lies limp and voiceless, and too often remains so despite all efforts at resuscitation.

Differential Diagnosis

There are exceptional situations that prevent spontaneous delivery of the fetal shoulder and body after the delivery of the head. These are not considered "true" shoulder dystocia and include:

1. Short umbilical cord
2. Tight nuchal cord
3. Abdominal or thoracic enlargement of the infant (anasarca, abdominal or back neoplasms)
4. Locked or conjoined twins
5. Uterine constriction ring

RISK FACTORS FOR SHOULDER DYSTOCIA

Shoulder dystocia is often unpredictable and therefore cannot be prevented in the majority of cases. Most of these prenatal risk factors have extremely poor positive predictive values and therefore do not allow the obstetrician to accurately and reliably predict the occurrence of shoulder dystocia.

A greater proportion of cases occur in women without risk factors. When standard risk factors are used to predict shoulder dystocia, only 16 percent of shoulder dystocia cases with resultant infant morbidity were associated with known risk factors. The main risk factors include maternal obesity, postterm pregnancy, fetal macrosomia, maternal diabetes mellitus, and a history of previous shoulder dystocia. Multiparity, induction of labor, labor dystocia, and assisted vaginal delivery are also risk factors.

Fetal Macrosomia

Although there is a relationship between fetal size and shoulder dystocia, this is not an accurate predictor. In 48 percent of shoulder dystocia cases, infants weigh less than 4000 g at birth. Interestingly, a large proportion of infants with birth weights of 4500 g or more do not develop shoulder dystocia. In babies weighing over 4500 g, shoulder dystocia is encountered 22.6 percent of the time. Macrosomic infants tend to deposit their excess weight in the chest and abdominal regions, causing these areas to be significantly out of proportion to the head. In postterm babies, as well as babies of diabetic mothers, the size of the baby's chest and trunk can potentially increase and result in shoulder dystocia. This disproportion between the shoulder and head dimensions is much more pronounced in babies of mothers with diabetes.

Maternal Diabetes Mellitus

Fetal macrosomia in the setting of maternal diabetes increases the risk of shoulder dystocia; however, these factors combined predict only about 55 percent of shoulder dystocia cases. In addition to the disproportionately larger shoulder-to-head circumference generally noted in macrosomic infants, babies born to mothers with diabetes have more body fat, which tends to be deposited in the arms and folds of the triceps, contributing to shoulder dystocia.

Maternal Obesity

Obesity in pregnancy (prepregnancy maternal body mass index >30 kg/m^2) is associated with fetal macrosomia. In some situations, macrosomic infants may be at risk for shoulder dystocia.

Previous Shoulder Dystocia

A history of shoulder dystocia appears to be one of the most accurate predictors for recurrent shoulder dystocia. The quoted risk of recurrent shoulder dystocia from the literature ranges from 10 to 15 percent. This translates to a 10- to 20-fold risk compared with baseline. When shoulder dystocia results in injury to the fetus, the likelihood of recurrent shoulder dystocia and injury to the fetuses of subsequent pregnancies is greater. This is explained by the fact that subsequent babies tend to be larger.

SECOND STAGE OF LABOR

Other Risk Factors

Among a myriad of other factors, multiparity, postterm pregnancies, labor dystocia, and assisted vaginal deliveries are commonly linked to shoulder dystocia. It is unclear what the direct causes are in the cases above; however, fetal macrosomia is often present in these scenarios and may explain their association with shoulder dystocia.

SEQUELAE OF SHOULDER DYSTOCIA

Complications of shoulder dystocia include fetal or neonatal as well as maternal injuries. Up to 20 percent of babies will have a temporary or permanent injury. Fetal injuries include birth hypoxia or asphyxia and possible death, brachial plexus injuries, fractured clavicles and humeri, and contusions and lacerations. Maternal morbidities include lacerations of the birth canal, uterine rupture, and postpartum hemorrhage secondary to uterine atony or lacerations.

Birth Asphyxia

Birth asphyxia is the most dreaded complication of shoulder dystocia because it may result in permanent neurologic damage and even death. With each uterine contraction, large amounts of blood are transferred from the baby's trunk to his or her head. The angulation of the neck and the compression of the chest interfere with cardiac function and impair the venous return. The intracranial vascular system of the fetus cannot compensate for the excessive intravascular pressure. Compression of the umbilical cord between the baby's body and the maternal birth canal results in a further reduction of blood flow and oxygenation to the fetus. This results in increasing fetal acidosis and asphyxia. Under these conditions, anoxia develops and may be accompanied by hemorrhagic effusions. If this condition persists too long, the baby may sustain irreversible brain damage. The infant may die during the attempts at delivery or in the neonatal period. Studies suggest that after abrupt cessation of umbilical blood flow, babies not delivered within 5 to 10 minutes will have permanent neurologic damage or death. This is a result of the increasing acidosis with the umbilical artery pH declining at a rate of 0.04 units/min in the presence of total cord occlusion. In shoulder dystocia, there may be some preservation of maternal–fetal circulation and a less rapid drop in pH unless the cord has previously been clamped and cut.

This underscores the reason for not routinely cutting a nuchal cord in the presence of suspected shoulder dystocia.

Brachial Plexus Injury

Brachial plexus injury occurs after about 10 percent of all shoulder dystocia deliveries, although rates of 4 to 40 percent have been reported. It may be associated with extreme lateral traction being applied to the fetal head by the birth attendant. Brachial plexus injuries can also occur in the absence of shoulder dystocia, after breech deliveries, and in uncomplicated cesarean sections. A brachial plexus injury most commonly involves the C5 and C6 nerve roots, resulting in the classical Erb-Duchenne palsy (waiter's tip sign). When the damage involves C8 and T1, it is called Klumpke's brachial plexus palsy ("claw hand" sign). The majority of brachial plexus birth injuries are transient, and most resolve by 3 months. If there is residual impairment by the end of the first month of life, the infant should be referred for a specialist assessment. Approximately 5 to 22 percent result in some degree of permanent injury.

Fetal Fractures and Bruising

Fetal clavicle fractures occur in 10 percent of deliveries complicated by shoulder dystocia. After the delivery of the fetal head, excessive pressure may be applied to the shoulders in an attempt to complete the delivery with a resultant fracture to the clavicle. In some cases, the attendant deliberately fractures the clavicle to reduce the diameter of the fetal chest and intershoulder distance to facilitate delivery. Humeral fractures occur in approximately 4 percent of infants with shoulder dystocia deliveries. They tend to heal quickly with no long-term complications.

Bruises on the fetal body may result from pressure of the attendant's hands on the fetus while performing various maneuvers to effect delivery. Such bruises may also occur during routine deliveries that are not complicated by shoulder dystocia.

Maternal Morbidity

Shoulder dystocia can result in maternal morbidity and mortality. Complications include lacerations of the vulva, vagina, and cervix as well as episiotomy extensions. Intrapartum or postpartum hemorrhage occurs in about 25 percent of deliveries. This could be potentially life threatening and results from the genital tract lacerations, uterine atony, and rarely

SECOND STAGE OF LABOR

uterine rupture. Temporary urinary retention may occur in the postpartum period from bladder atony. This is a result of prolonged and intense pressure on the bladder from the fetal anterior shoulder. Extreme hyperflexion of the maternal legs required for maneuvers to help resolve shoulder dystocia can cause damage to the lateral femoral cutaneous nerve as well as separation of the maternal pubic symphysis.

DIAGNOSIS

Diagnosis can be made only after the head has been delivered. The following signs may then appear:

1. The fetal head delivers but restitution does not take place spontaneously. Because of friction with the vulva, the head seems incapable of movement.
2. The head recoils back against the perineum after it comes out from the vagina ("turtle sign").
3. The shoulders fail to deliver with maternal expulsive efforts and gentle downward traction from below.

MANAGEMENT OF SHOULDER DYSTOCIA

Shoulder dystocia cannot be reliably predicted; therefore, all deliveries should be considered to have the potential for a shoulder dystocia. If a woman is considered at risk for shoulder dystocia, the woman, her support person, and the birth attendant's team should prepare for a shoulder dystocia in advance of delivery of the fetal head. Preparing the team for the possibility of flattening the bed, the McRoberts maneuver, suprapubic pressure, and rolling over can increase cooperation in the event of a shoulder dystocia. In addition, a stool placed at the side of the bed corresponding to the fetal back helps to indicate to the team the location to apply oblique suprapubic pressure. Low-fidelity simulation exercises may be used to improve the aspects of teamwork that may be helpful for the management of shoulder dystocia.

As soon as shoulder dystocia is recognized, several measures have to be taken. The attendant must seek help from other health care personnel. If an obstetrician is not present, he or she should be notified to proceed to the delivery room. An anesthesia and neonatal team should also be called.

The most responsible birth attendant should be constantly informed of the time that has elapsed since delivery of the head. An effective way of ensuring this is to designate a time keeper to document the timing of events. In all instances, one should avoid pulling on the head, pushing on the fundus, panicking, and pivoting (severely angulating the fetal head using the coccyx as a fulcrum). It is important to ask the woman to stop pushing until maneuvers to relieve the obstruction are carried out.

Several obstetric maneuvers can be used to resolve shoulder dystocia, including the McRoberts maneuver, suprapubic pressure, delivery of the anterior shoulder, delivery of the posterior shoulder and arm, the Wood's corkscrew maneuver, deliberate fracture of the fetal clavicle or humerus, the Zavanelli maneuver, and maternal symphysiotomy. Delivery of the posterior shoulder appears to be associated with the highest rate of delivery compared with the other maneuvers; thus, it should be considered after the McRoberts maneuver and suprapubic pressure. The need for additional maneuvers is associated with higher rates of neonatal injury. Despite historical recommendations to perform an episiotomy at the time of a diagnosed shoulder dystocia to prevent a brachial plexus injury, the literature does not support a benefit to this practice.

McRoberts Maneuver and Suprapubic Pressure

These two maneuvers are often used simultaneously as the first steps to help resolve shoulder dystocia. About 50 to 60 percent of all shoulder dystocias resolve by using a combination of McRoberts maneuver and suprapubic pressure, thereby eliminating the need for further maneuvers.

The McRoberts maneuver involves flexing the legs sharply upon the maternal abdomen. This causes the symphysis pubis to rotate cephalad and the sacrum to be straightened, thus allowing the fetal shoulder to slide out beneath the maternal pubic bone anteriorly.

An assistant can perform suprapubic pressure (*not* fundal pressure) by applying oblique pressure just above the maternal pubic bone with the heel of their clasped hands against the posterior aspect of the shoulder to dislodge it (Mazzanti maneuver). A stool may be useful to facilitate this maneuver, particularly in the case of a shorter assistant. It is necessary to know the position of the occiput so that pressure is applied from the correct side and is most effective. Shoulder dystocia is caused by an infant's shoulders entering the pelvis in a direct AP axis instead of the physiologic oblique axis; therefore, pushing the baby's anterior shoulder to one side or the other from above can often change his or her position to the oblique, thus allowing its delivery.

SECOND STAGE OF LABOR

The birth attendant may also attempt to manually dislodge the anterior shoulder from behind the symphysis pubis. One may place a hand deep in the vagina behind the anterior shoulder and attempt to rotate the axis of the shoulders into the oblique diameter of the pelvis (Fig. 18-2). Firm traction is then applied to the fetal head, deflecting it toward the floor.

Posterior Arm and Shoulder Delivery

The fetal arm is usually flexed at the elbow, and if it is not, pressure in the antecubital fossa can assist with flexion. The hand can then be grasped and swept across the chest and delivered.

1. The hand of the operator is placed deeply into the vagina along the curvature of the sacrum and behind the posterior shoulder of the fetus. If the back of the fetus is toward the operator's right side, the left hand is used. If the back is toward the operator's left, the right hand is preferred (Fig. 18-3A).
2. The antecubital fossa of the posterior arm is located and using the pressure of a finger, an attempt is made to flex the arm in a fashion similar to the Pinard maneuver in a breech extraction.
3. The forearm is swept across the chest and face, the hand is then grasped, and the arm is extended along the fetal face and delivered (Fig. 18-3B).
4. Once this has been accomplished, the anterior shoulder delivers in most cases. If it does not, the body is rotated 180° so that the anterior shoulder is now posterior. It is then extracted by the same maneuver. This maneuver tends to increase the risk of fracturing the humerus; however, most humeral fractures heal quickly with no permanent damage. In view of this, it is worth trying this maneuver to resolve the shoulder dystocia of an infant in a life-threatening situation when the other maneuvers have not worked.

Woods' Corkscrew Maneuver

This maneuver was first described in 1943. In this maneuver, the birth attendant pushes the posterior shoulder through a 180° arc by applying pressure on the anterior surface of the posterior shoulder. The idea is to progressively rotate the posterior shoulder in a corkscrew fashion to release the opposite impacted anterior shoulder. The reverse Woods' maneuver, or Rubin maneuver, involves pushing on the posterior surface of the posterior shoulder. This flexes the shoulders across the chest and decreases the

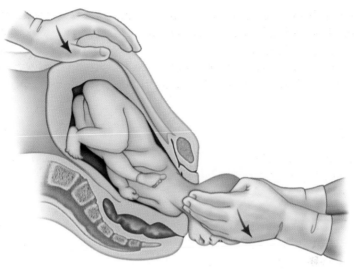

A. Basic method of delivering shoulders.

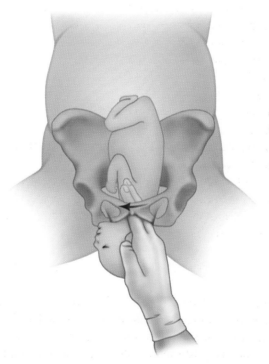

B. Shoulder dystocia: Rotation of bisacromial diameter from anteroposterior diameter pelvis into the oblique.

FIGURE 18-2. **Delivery of anterior shoulder.**

SECOND STAGE OF LABOR

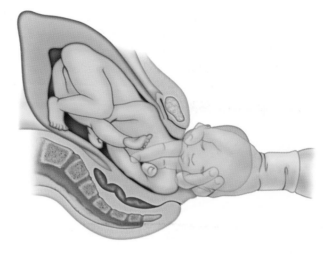

A. First step.

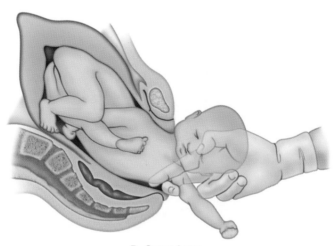

B. Second step.

FIGURE 18-3. **A** and **B,** Extraction of the posterior shoulder and arm.

distance between the shoulders, thus decreasing the dimension of the fetal chest that must fit out through the pelvis.

To perform the Woods' maneuver, the posterior shoulder must have passed the spines for this maneuver to be successful. In a situation in which the fetal head position is left occiput transverse (LOT), two fingers of the left hand are placed on the anterior aspect of the posterior shoulder.

Pressure is made against the shoulder so that it moves counterclockwise, the posterior aspect leading the way (Fig. 18-4). It is turned 180°, past 12 o'clock. In this way, the posterior shoulder is delivered under the pubic arch. The head has turned from LOT to right occiput transverse (ROT). This should result in delivery of the posterior shoulder, and the anterior shoulder should now be posterior.

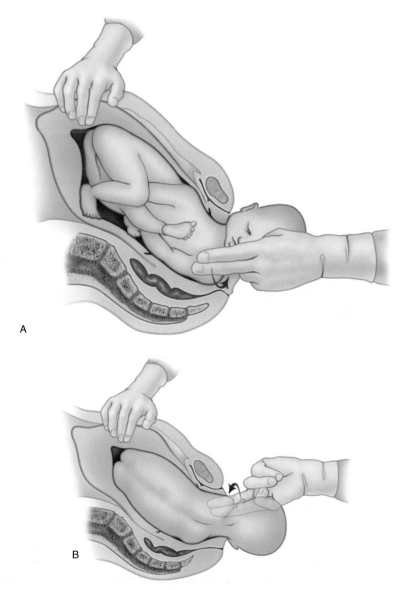

FIGURE 18-4. Woods' corkscrew maneuver.

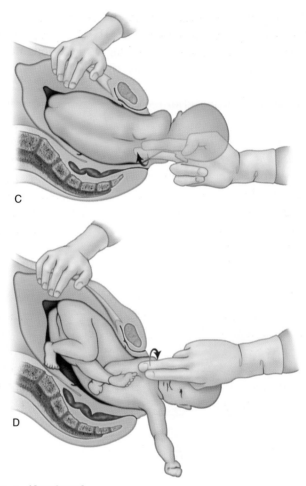

FIGURE 18-4. (*Continued*)

Fetal Clavicle Fracture

Although this maneuver is often described in shoulder dystocia literature, it is rarely performed. The fetal clavicle is a strong bone and not that easy to deliberately fracture. The fractured clavicle decreases the bisacromial diameter, facilitating resolution of the dystocia. Serious fetal consequences that may occur include damage to the lungs and major blood vessels.

Rolling Over to "All Fours" Position

Moving the mother onto all fours may increase the effective pelvic dimensions and allow the fetal position to shift, thereby freeing the impacted shoulder. With gentle downward traction on the posterior shoulder, the anterior shoulder may become more impacted (with gravity) but will facilitate the freeing up of the posterior shoulder.

Zavanelli Maneuver

This is a cephalic replacement maneuver whereby cardinal movements of labor are reversed; the head must first be rotated back to its pre-restitution position, flexed, pushed up, rotated to the transverse, and disengaged, and then a cesarean section is performed. Constant firm pressure is applied from below while the head is pushed back into the vagina. A general anesthetic is often administered in addition to tocolytics to produce uterine relaxation required for this maneuver. Cesarean delivery must be performed immediately after replacement of the head.

Symphysiotomy

This procedure is rarely performed and is usually reserved for areas with no quick access to performing cesarean sections. It involves dividing the ligaments between the right and left pubic symphyseal bones. This results in an increase in the transverse diameter of the pubis by adding about 3 cm to the circumference of the pelvis. The major risk involves potential injury to maternal soft tissues especially the bladder and urethra.

RISK MANAGEMENT

The American College of Obstetricians and Gynaecologists practice bulletin recommends performing the McRoberts Maneuver as the initial approach. Practice drills have been suggested to enhance obstetrical readiness for all the members of the team. Mnemonics are often used to plan a step-wise approach to managing shoulder dystocia. One such mnemonic is "*ALARMER*":

A—Ask for help (assistant, anaesthesia, neonatology)
L—Lift legs (McRoberts)
A—Anterior shoulder delivery (suprapubic pressure)
R—Rotate (Woods' corkscrew maneuver)
M—Manual removal of the posterior arm and shoulder
E—Episiotomy
R—Repeat steps above

SECOND STAGE OF LABOR

CONCLUSION

Shoulder dystocia is an unpredictable and often unpreventable obstetric event. Several factors have been identified in the literature as contributing to this condition, but these factors in isolation are often not strong predictors of shoulder dystocia. However, they help raise awareness of shoulder dystocia to the health care provider. All delivering personnel need to have a uniform and organized approach to handling this emergency in order to minimize risks to the mother and infant.

SELECTED READING

Acker DB, Sachs BP, Friedman EA: Risk factors for shoulder dystocia. Obstet Gynecol 66:762, 1985

American Congress of Obstetricians and Gynecologists: ACOG Practice Bulletin Number 40. Shoulder Dystocia. November 2002 (reaffirmed 2010). Obstet Gynecol 100:1045, 2002

Al Hadi M, Geary M, Byrne P, et al: Shoulder dystocia: risk factors and maternal and perinatal outcome. J Obstet Gynaecol 21:352, 2001

Bahar AM: Risk factors and fetal outcome in cases of shoulder dystocia compared with normal deliveries of a similar birth weight. Br J Obstet Gynaecol 103:868, 1996

Baskett TF, Allen AC: Perinatal implications of shoulder dystocia. Obstet Gynecol 86:14, 1995

Ecker JL, Greenberg JA, Norwitz ER, et al: Birth weight as a predictor of brachial plexus injury. Obstet Gynecol 1997; 89:643, 1997

Gherman RB: Persistent brachial plexus injury: The outcome of concern among patients with suspected fetal macrosomia. Am J Obstet Gynecol 178:195, 1998

Gherman RB: Shoulder dystocia: An evidence-based evaluation of the obstetrical nightmare. Clinic Obstet Gynecol 45:345, 2002

Gherman RB, Goodwin TM, Souter I, et al: The McRoberts' maneuver for the alleviation of shoulder dystocia: How successful is it? Am J Obstet Gynecol 176:656, 1997

Ginsberg NA, Moisidis C: How to predict recurrent shoulder dystocia. Am J Obstet Gynecol 184:1427, 2001

Grobman WA, Hornbogen A, Burke C, Costello R: Development and implementation of a team-centered shoulder dystocia protocol. Simul Healthc 5:199, 2010

Gross TL, Sokol RJ, Williams T, et al: Shoulder dystocia: a fetal-physician risk. *Am J Obstet Gynaecol* 156:1408, 1987

Hoffman MK, Bailit JL, Branch DW, et al: A comparison of obstetric maneuvers for the acute management of shoulder dystocia. Obstet Gynecol 117:1272, 2011

McFarland MB, Langer O, Piper JM, Berkus MD: Perinatal outcome and the type and number of manoeuvres in shoulder dystocia. Int J Gynecol Obstet 55:219, 1996

Morris WIC: Shoulder dystocia. J Obstet Gynaecol 62:302, 1955

Ouzounian JG, Korst LM, Ahn MO, et al: Shoulder dystocia and neonatal brain injury: Significance of the head-shoulder interval. Am J Obstet Gynecol 178:S76, 1998

Paris AE, Greenberg JA, Ecker JL, McElrath TF: Is an episiotomy necessary with a shoulder dystocia? Am J Obstet Gynecol 205: e1, 2011

Resnik R: Management of shoulder girdle dystocia. Clin Obstet Gynecol 23:559, 1980

Sheiner E, Levy A, Menes TS, et al: Maternal obesity as an independent risk factor for caesarean delivery. Paediatr Perinat Epidemiol 18:196, 2004

Smith RB, Lane C, Pearson JF: Shoulder dystocia: What happens at the next delivery? Br J Obstetric Gynecol 101:713, 1994

Society of Obstetricians and Gynaecologists of Canada: MORE^OB: Shoulder Dystocia and Umbilical Cord Prolapse, 2010. http://www.moreob.com

Stallings SP, Edwards RK, Johnson JWC: Correlation of head-to-body delivery intervals in shoulder dystocia and umbilical artery acidosis. Am J Obstet Gynecol 185:268, 2001

Wood C, Ng KH, Hounslaw D, et al: Time: an important variable in normal delivery. J Obstet Gynaecol Br Commonw 80:295, 1973

PART IV

Third Stage of Labor

CHAPTER 19

Delivery of the Placenta, Retained Placenta, and Placenta Accreta

Lawrence Oppenheimer

NORMAL PLACENTA

Size and Shape

The placenta is a round or oval disk, 20 × 15 cm in size and 1.5 to 2.0 cm thick. The weight, usually 20 percent of that of the fetus, is between 425 and 550 g.

Organization

On the uterine side, there are eight or more maternal cotyledons separated by fissures. The term *fetal cotyledon* refers to the part of the placenta that is supplied by a mainstem villus and its branches. The maternal surface is covered by a layer of decidua and fibrin, which comes away with the placenta at delivery. The fetal side is covered by membranes.

Location

Normally, the placenta is implanted in the upper part of the uterus or fundus. Occasionally, it is placed in the lower segment, and sometimes it lies over the cervix. The latter condition is termed *placenta previa* and is a cause of bleeding in the third trimester.

ABNORMALITIES OF THE PLACENTA

Succenturiate Lobe

This is an accessory lobe that is placed at some distance from the main placenta. The blood vessels that supply this lobe run over the intervening membranes and may be torn when the latter rupture or during delivery. A succenturiate lobe may be retained after birth and cause postpartum hemorrhage (PPH).

Circumvallate Placenta

The membranes are folded back on the fetal surface and insert inward on themselves. The placenta is situated outside of the chorion.

Amnion Nodosum

This is a yellow nodule, 3 to 4 cm in diameter, situated on the fetal surface of the amnion. It contains vernix, fibrin, desquamated cells, and lanugo hairs. It may form a cyst. This condition is associated with oligohydramnios.

Infarcts

Localized infarcts are common. The clinical significance is not known, but if the condition is excessive, the functional capacity of the placenta may be reduced.

Discoloration

Red staining is associated with hemorrhage. Green color is caused by meconium and may be an indication of fetal hypoxia.

Twin Placenta

In monochorionic twins the placenta forms one mass, whereas in dichorionic twins the placentas may be fused or separate.

Weight

Placentas weighing more than 600 g or less than 400 g are usually associated with an abnormal pregnancy.

DELIVERY OF THE PLACENTA

Delivery of the placenta occurs in two stages: (1) separation of the placenta from the wall of the uterus and into the lower uterine segment and/or the vagina and (2) actual expulsion of the placenta out of the birth canal. There are two approaches to delivery of the placenta, active management and physiological management. These have been compared in a number of trials, and active management is recommended because it reduces the incidence of PPH (blood loss >1000 mL) and shortens the third stage.

Active management consists of:

- Use of uterotonics
- Early cord clamping or cutting
- Controlled cord traction

Oxytocin (10 international units [IU] should be given by intramuscular injection), preferably after delivery of the fetal head or after delivery of the body. An equally effective alternative is oxytocin 5 IU plus ergot alkaloid (called Syntometrine as used commonly in the United Kingdom), although there is a higher incidence of nausea with this combination.

Separation of the Placenta

Placental separation takes place, as a rule, within 5 minutes of the end of the second stage. Signs suggesting that detachment has taken place include:

1. Gush of blood from the vagina
2. Lengthening of the umbilical cord outside the vulva
3. Rising of the uterine fundus in the abdomen as the placenta passes from the uterus into the vagina
4. Uterus becoming firm and globular

Expulsion of the Placenta

When these signs have appeared, the placenta is ready for expression. This is achieved by the Brandt-Andrews maneuver. This procedure involves exerting gentle traction on the cord by one hand while the other hand applies upward counterpressure on the uterus above the symphysis pubis. It is wise to avoid rough manipulations of the uterus before placental separation has taken place. Such actions do not hasten delivery of the placenta and may lead to excessive bleeding (Fig. 19-1). The average blood loss during the third stage is 250 to 500 mL.

Physiological Management

Women at low risk of PPH who request physiological management of the third stage should be supported in their choice. Physiological management consists of:

- No routine use of uterotonic drugs
- No clamping of the cord until pulsation has ceased
- Delivery of the placenta by maternal effort

If there is hemorrhage, failure to deliver within 1 hour of physiological management, or increased risk of PPH, then active management should be implemented. Women at higher risk of PPH include those with (1) an overdistended uterus (multiple pregnancy, polyhydramnios); (2) high parity; (3) history of previous PPH; (4) prolonged labor, especially

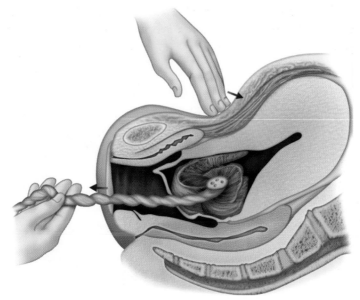

FIGURE 19-1. Expulsion of the placenta.

when associated with ineffective uterine contractions; (5) deep general anesthesia; (6) difficult operative delivery; (7) induction or augmentation of labor by oxytocin. They should be managed actively.

Delayed Cord Clamping

Early cord clamping as part of active management is associated with a reduction in PPH. Delaying clamping of the cord by at least 3 minutes or until it has stopped pulsating has been shown to reduce the incidence of anemia in the baby by giving an infusion of blood from the placenta. This benefit is particularly seen in lower income countries.

There is limited medium-level evidence from trials in high-income countries showing that delayed cord clamping reduced the incidence of anemia and increases in hyperbilirubinemia in the baby. Other longer term outcomes are reported variably. There is high-level evidence from low to middle-income countries that delayed cord clamping reduces the incidence of anemia in the baby.

Delivery of the Membranes

In most cases, as the placenta is born, the membranes peel off from the endometrium and are delivered spontaneously. Occasionally, this does

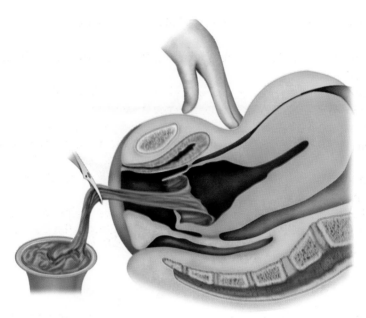

FIGURE 19-2. **Delivery of the membranes.**

not take place, and the membranes are removed by gentle traction with forceps (Fig. 19-2). Retention of small bits of membrane does not usually seem to lead to any untoward effects.

Examination of the Delivered Placenta

Examination of the delivered placenta is performed to see that no parts are missing (i.e., left in the uterus). Torn blood vessels along the edge suggest that an accessory lobe may have remained in the uterus. Some obstetricians believe that examination of the placenta does not ensure that fragments have not been left behind, and they explore the uterine cavity manually after each delivery. Even with the best efforts, retained products, usually manifested by delayed PPH, will occur in about 1 percent.

Delayed Separation and Delivery of the Placenta

The third stage of labor is diagnosed as prolonged if not completed within 30 minutes of the birth of the baby with active management and 60 minutes with physiological management.

Retention of the placenta in utero falls into four groups:

1. *Separated but retained:* There is failure of the forces that normally expel the placenta
2. *Separated but incarcerated:* An hourglass constriction of the uterus, or cervical spasm, traps the placenta in the uterus
3. *Adherent but separable:* In this situation, the placenta fails to separate from the uterine wall. The causes include failure of the normal contraction and retraction of the third stage, an anatomic defect in the uterus, and an abnormality of the decidua, which prevents formation of the normal decidual plane of cleavage
4. *Adherent and inseparable:* Here are the varying degrees of placenta accreta. The normal decidua is absent, and the chorionic villi are attached directly to and through the myometrium (see later in this chapter)

Manual Removal of the Placenta

Current practice is to remove the placenta manually if it does not deliver within 30 to 60 minutes after the birth of the baby, provided bleeding is not excessive. If hemorrhage is profuse, the placenta must be removed immediately. An intravenous infusion is set up, and blood is made available. Anesthesia is necessary. The procedure is carried out under aseptic conditions.

The uterus is steadied by one hand holding the fundus through the maternal abdomen and applying downward counterpressure (Fig. 19-3). The other hand is inserted into the vagina and through the cervix into the uterine cavity. The placenta is reached by following the umbilical cord. If the placenta has separated, it is grasped and removed. The uterus is then explored to be sure that nothing has been left.

If the placenta is still adherent to the uterine wall, it must be separated. First some part of the margin of attachment is identified and the fingers inserted between the placenta and the wall of the uterus. The back of the hand is kept in contact with the uterine wall. The fingers are forced gently between the placenta and uterus, and as progress is made, they are spread apart. In this way, the line of cleavage is extended, the placenta is separated from the uterine wall, and it is then extracted. Oxytocics are given to ensure good uterine contraction and retraction.

Manual Exploration of the Uterus

Manual exploration of the uterus for tears or retained products is required if there is PPH not responsive to therapy. Lacerations of the uterus and cervix should also be excluded by careful inspection.

THIRD STAGE OF LABOR

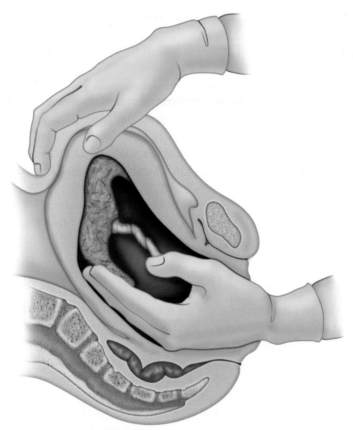

FIGURE 19-3. Manual removal of the placenta.

PLACENTA ACCRETA

Placenta accreta is defined as the abnormal adherence, either in whole or in part, of the afterbirth to the underlying uterine wall. The placental villi adhere to, invade into, or penetrate through the myometrium.

Pathology

Normally, the decidua basalis lies between the myometrium and the placenta (Fig. 19-4A). The plane of cleavage for placental separation is in the spongy layer of the decidua basalis. In placenta accreta, the decidua basalis is partially or completely absent (Fig. 19-4B), so that the placenta is attached directly to the myometrium. The villi may remain superficial to the uterine muscle or may penetrate it deeply. This condition is caused by a defect in the decidua rather than by any abnormal invasive properties of the trophoblast.

In the superficial area of the myometrium, a large number of venous channels develop just beneath the placenta. Rupture of these sinuses by forceful extraction of the placenta is the source of the profuse hemorrhage that occurs.

Classification

1. *Accreta:* The placenta is adherent to the myometrium. There is no line of cleavage

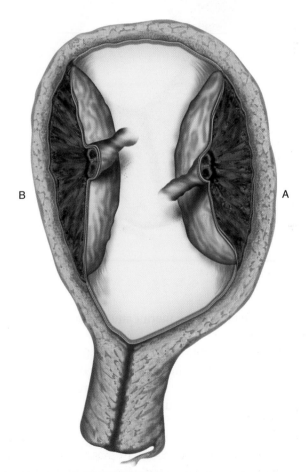

FIGURE 19-4. Uteroplacental relationships. A, Normal: decidua separates the placenta from the myometrium. **B,** Placenta accreta: absence of the decidua. **C,** Placenta increta: villi penetrate the myometrium. **D,** Placenta percreta: villi extend through the uterine wall.

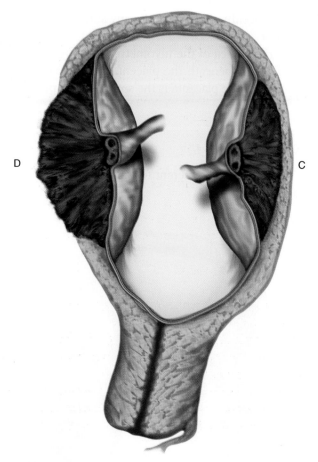

FIGURE 19-4. *(Continued)*

2. *Increta:* The villi penetrate the uterine muscle but not its full thickness (Fig. 19-4C)
3. Percreta: The villi penetrate the wall of the uterus and perforate the serosa (Fig. 19-4D). Intraperitoneal bleeding occurs frequently. Occasionally, the uterus is ruptured. The villi may grow into the cavity of the bladder and cause gross hematuria

Incidence

The incidence of placenta accrete is rising because of the increasing cesarean section rate. The approximate incidence currently is around 1 per 2000.

Etiology

By far, the most important predisposing factors are the combination of placenta previa and previous cesarean section. Because the decidua of the lower segment is less abundant than that in the fundus, a placenta implanted near the cervix may be abnormally adherent, especially where there has been disruption of the lower segment by previous surgery. In this situation, there is a 25 percent risk of accreta with one prior cesarean section and 40 percent with two prior cesarean sections. A history of any uterine surgery, curettage, or previous manual removal of placenta or cornual pregnancy is significant. Placenta accreta is rare in primigravidas.

The underlying condition that appears to be common to all causal conditions is a deficiency of the endometrium and the decidua:

1. The decidua overlying the scar of a previous cesarean section is often deficient
2. In women who have placenta previa, the decidua of the lower uterine segment is relatively poorly developed
3. The decidua of the uterine cornu is usually hypoplastic
4. With increasing age and parity, there is, in many women, a progressive inadequacy of decidua
5. Previous curettage or manual removal of placenta may not be an etiologic factor so much as an indication that an abnormal adherence of the placenta was the reason for the procedure being necessary

Clinical Picture

After Vaginal delivery

1. *Retained placenta*: This is the main and presenting feature. Manual attempts to remove the placenta may demonstrate no plane of cleavage between the placenta and the uterus
2. *PPH*: The amount of bleeding depends on the degree of placental attachment. In complete placenta accreta, there may be no bleeding. In the partial variety, bleeding takes place from the uterine vessels underlying the detached area, and the adherent portion prevents the uterus from retracting properly. Often the bleeding is precipitated by the obstetrician as he or she attempts manual removal of the placenta. Blood loss with attempted removal of placenta accreta can be extreme

3. *Uterine inversion*: This is a rare but serious complication. This may occur spontaneously but is more often the result of attempts to remove the placenta

4. *Rupture of the uterus*: This may occur during too vigorous attempts to extract the afterbirth

Placenta Previa Accreta

The presence of placenta previa significantly increases the risk of placenta accreta, particularly with a prior cesarean section as discussed earlier. Accreta may be suspected during cesarean section for previa because of the presence of abnormal vascularity on the surface of the uterus, or with percreta, there may be visible placental tissue extruding through the uterus. If abnormal placentation is suspected, it is best to avoid incising the lower segment by performing a classical cesarean section. Once the baby has been delivered, the placenta should be left undisturbed and the situation assessed.

Management Options

1. *Hysterectomy:* This is generally preferred by patients in whom further childbearing is not desired, or in unstable patients where there is ongoing bleeding. Blood should be available and expertise in tying off the internal iliac arteries in the most difficult cases. Unless there is doubt about the diagnosis, no attempt should be made to remove the placenta because profuse hemorrhage can result. If there is extensive invasion of the lower segment by accreta, one strategy in deciding whether to embark on a challenging hysterectomy in stable patients is to attempt to reflect the bladder. If this proves very difficult because of abnormal vascularity, conservative management can still be followed. If bladder involvement is suspected preoperatively, cystoscopy may be helpful in planning

2. *Conservative management:* This may be indicated in patients who do not have significant bleeding from the placental site and in whom preservation of fertility is preferred or when the surgical expertise to perform a difficult hysterectomy is not available. The umbilical cord is trimmed and ligated, and the whole placenta left in situ (or any retained pieces where a partial removal of placenta has been performed). Methotrexate has been used postoperatively to shrink the placenta but is probably unnecessary and ineffective. Angiographic uterine artery embolization (UAE), if available, may be a useful adjunct to prevent hemorrhage. In about 80 percent of cases, conservative management

with uterine preservation will be successful. The placenta takes up to 6 months or more to be completely reabsorbed. Successful pregnancies after both conservative management and UAE have been reported

Prenatal Diagnosis

Ultrasonography is reasonably accurate at diagnosing placenta accreta. The ultrasonic features include multiple placental lakes or vascular lacunae and a loss of the normal hypolucent zone between the placenta and uterine wall. A lack of ultrasonic features of accreta does not exclude the diagnosis with certainty, especially with a high-risk situation of previa and a prior cesarean section. Magnetic resonance imaging may be a useful adjunct for prenatal diagnosis. If accreta is suspected, delivery may be planned accordingly.

SELECTED READING

National Collaborating Centre for Women's and Children's Health Intrapartum Care: Care of Healthy Women and Their Babies During Childbirth. RCOG Press, 2007.

Royal College of Obstetricians and Gynaecologists: Placenta Praevia, Placenta Praevia Accreta and Vasa Praevia: Diagnosis and Management. Green Top Guideline No. 27, January 2011

Society of Obstetricians and Gynecologists of Canada Clinical Practice Guideline: Diagnosis and Management of Placenta Previa. No. 198, March 2007.

Timmermans S, van Hof AC, Duvekot JJ: Conservative management of abnormally invasive placentation. Obstet Gynecol Surv 62(8):529-539, 2007

THIRD STAGE OF LABOR

CHAPTER 20

Postpartum Hemorrhage

Glenn D. Posner

The term *postpartum hemorrhage* (PPH), in its wider meaning, includes all bleeding after the birth of a baby—before, during, and after the delivery of the placenta. By definition, loss of more than 500 mL of blood during the first 24 hours constitutes PPH. After 24 hours, it is called late PPH. The incidence of PPH worldwide is about 5 percent and is a major contributor to maternal mortality.

During normal delivery, an average of 200 mL of blood is lost. Episiotomy raises this figure by 100 mL and sometimes more. Pregnant women have an increased amount of blood and fluid, enabling the healthy patient to lose 500 mL without serious effect. To a patient with anemia, however, an even smaller amount of bleeding can be dangerous.

CLINICAL FEATURES

Clinical Picture

The clinical picture is one of continuing bleeding and gradual deterioration. The pulse becomes rapid and weak; the blood pressure falls; the patient turns pale and cold; and there is shortness of breath, air hunger, sweating, and finally coma and death. A treacherous feature of the situation is that because of compensatory vascular mechanisms, the pulse and blood pressure may show only moderate changes for some time. Then suddenly the compensatory function can no longer be maintained, the pulse rises quickly, the blood pressure drops suddenly, and the patient is in hypovolemic shock. The uterine cavity can fill up with a considerable amount of blood, which is lost to the patient even though the external hemorrhage may not be alarming.

Danger of Postpartum Hemorrhage

The danger of PPH is twofold. First, the resultant anemia weakens the patient, lowers her resistance, and predisposes to puerperal infection. Second, if the loss of blood is not arrested, death will be the final result.

Studies of Maternal Deaths

Studies of maternal deaths show that women have died from continuous bleeding of amounts that at the time were not alarming. It is not the sudden gush that kills, but the steady trickle. In a large series of cases, Beacham found that the average interval between delivery and death was

THIRD STAGE OF LABOR

5 hours, 20 minutes. No woman died within 1 hour, 30 minutes of giving birth. This suggests that there is adequate time for effective therapy if the patient has been observed carefully, the diagnosis made early, and proper treatment instituted.

ETIOLOGY

The causes of PPH fall into four main groups.

Uterine Atony

The control of postpartum bleeding is by contraction and retraction of the myometrial fibers. This causes kinking of the blood vessels, cutting off flow to the placental site. Failure of this mechanism, resulting from disordered myometrial function, is called *uterine atony* and is the main cause of PPH. Although the occasional case of postpartum uterine atony is completely unexpected, in many instances, the presence of predisposing factors alerts the observant physician to the possibility of trouble.

1. *Uterine dysfunction*: Primary uterine atony is an intrinsic dysfunction of the uterus
2. *Mismanagement of the placental stage*: The most common error is to try to hurry the third stage. Kneading and squeezing the uterus interfere with the physiologic mechanism of placental detachment and may cause partial placental separation with resultant bleeding
3. *Anesthesia*: Deep and prolonged inhalation anesthesia can cause uterine atony. There is excessive relaxation of the myometrium and failure of contraction and retraction, resulting in uterine atony and PPH
4. *Ineffective uterine action*: Ineffective uterine action during the first two stages of labor is likely to be followed by poor contraction and retraction during the third stage
5. *Overdistention of the uterus*: A uterus that has been overdistended by conditions such as a large baby, multiple pregnancy, and polyhydramnios has a tendency to contract poorly
6. *Exhaustion from prolonged labor*: Not only is a tired uterus likely to contract weakly after delivery of the baby, but a severely fatigued mother is less able to stand loss of blood
7. *Grandmultiparity*: A uterus that has borne many children is prone to inefficient action during all stages of labor

8. *Myomas of the uterus*: By interfering with proper contraction and retraction, uterine myomas predispose to hemorrhage
9. *Operative deliveries*: These include operative procedures such as ventouse and forceps deliveries, especially those that involve version and extraction

Trauma and Lacerations

Considerable bleeding can take place from tears sustained during normal and operative deliveries. The birth canal should be inspected after each delivery so that the sources of bleeding can be controlled.

Sites of hemorrhage include:

1. Episiotomy: Blood loss may reach 200 mL. When arterioles or large varicose veins are cut or torn, the amount of blood lost can be considerably more. Hence, bleeding vessels should be clamped immediately to conserve blood
2. Vulva, vagina, and cervix
3. Ruptured uterus
4. Uterine inversion
5. Puerperal hematomas

In addition, other factors operate to cause an excessive loss of blood where there is trauma to the birth canal. These include:

1. Prolonged interval between performance of the episiotomy and delivery of the child
2. Undue delay from birth of the baby to repair of the episiotomy
3. Failure to secure a bleeding vessel at the apex of the episiotomy
4. Neglecting to inspect the upper vagina and cervix
5. Failure to appreciate the possibility of multiple sites of injury
6. Undue reliance on oxytocic agents accompanied by too long a delay in exploring the uterus

Retained Placenta

Retention in the uterus of part or the entire placenta interferes with contraction and retraction, keeps the blood sinuses open, and leads to PPH. Once part of the placenta has separated from the uterine wall, there is bleeding from that area. The part of the placenta that is still attached prevents proper retraction, and bleeding goes on until the rest of the organ has separated and is expelled.

Retention of the whole placenta, part of it, a succenturiate lobe, a single cotyledon, or a fragment of placenta can cause postpartum bleeding. In some cases, there is placenta accreta. There is no correlation between the amount of placenta retained and the severity of the hemorrhage. The important consideration is the degree of adherence.

Bleeding Disorders

Any of the hemorrhagic diseases (blood dyscrasias) can affect pregnant women and occasionally are responsible for PPH.

Disseminated intravascular coagulation (DIC) may follow abruptio placentae, prolonged retention in utero of a dead fetus, and amniotic fluid embolism. One etiologic theory postulates that thromboplastic material arising from the degeneration and autolysis of the decidua and placenta may enter the maternal circulation and give rise to intravascular coagulation and loss of circulating fibrinogen. The condition, a failure of the clotting mechanism, causes bleeding that cannot be arrested by the measures usually used to control hemorrhage.

INVESTIGATION

1. To obtain a reasonable idea of the amount of blood lost, an estimate is made and the figure doubled
2. The uterine fundus is palpated frequently to make certain it is not filling up with blood
3. The uterine cavity is explored both for placental remnants and for uterine rupture
4. The vulva, vagina, and cervix are examined carefully for lacerations
5. The pulse and blood pressure are measured and recorded
6. A sample of blood is observed for clotting, and blood work is sent for a complete blood count as well as a type and screen

TREATMENT

Prophylaxis

1. Every pregnant woman should know her blood group and Rh status

2. Antepartum anemia is treated

THIRD STAGE OF LABOR

3. Certain patients are susceptible to and certain conditions predispose to PPH. These include:

   a. Multiparity
   b. History of PPH or manual removal of the placenta
   c. Abruptio placentae
   d. Placenta previa
   e. Multiple pregnancy
   f. Polyhydramnios
   g. Intrauterine death with prolonged retention of a dead fetus
   h. Prolonged labor
   i. Difficult operative vaginal delivery
   j. Version and extraction
   k. Breech extraction
   l. Cesarean section

4. When uterine atony is anticipated, an intravenous infusion is set up before the delivery, and oxytocin is added to ensure good uterine contractions. This is continued for at least 1 hour postpartum

5. Excessive and prolonged inhalatory anesthesia should be avoided

6. As long as the child is in good condition and there is no need for rapid extraction, the body is delivered slowly. This facilitates placental separation and permits the uterus to retract sufficiently to control bleeding from the placental site

7. Once the placenta has separated, it should be expelled

8. Squeezing or kneading the uterus before the placenta has separated can be traumatic and harmful

9. Careful postpartum observation of the patient is made, and the uterine fundus is palpated to prevent its filling with blood. The patient remains in the delivery room for at least 1 hour postpartum

10. Fibrinogen studies are done in cases of placental abruption and retained dead fetus

11. When hemorrhage is anticipated, adequate amounts of blood should be cross-matched and available

Supportive Measures

1. The key to successful treatment is the transfusion of blood. The amount must be adequate to replace at least the amount lost. Usually a minimum of 1 L is needed, and it is given quickly. When response to blood replacement is not satisfactory, the following conditions must be considered:

   a. Continued unappreciated ooze
   b. Bleeding into an atonic uterus
   c. Silent filling of the vagina
   d. Bleeding behind and into a uterine pack
   e. Hematoma formation
   f. Intraperitoneal bleeding as with ruptured uterus
   g. DIC

2. Until blood is available, plasma expanders are used

3. If the blood pressure is falling, the foot of the table is elevated

4. General anesthesia should be discontinued and oxygen given by facemask

5. Warmth is provided by blankets or intraoperative warming units (e.g., Bair Hugger)

6. Morphine is given by hypodermic injection

7. If bleeding continues, the coagulation factors of the blood must be measured and deficiencies corrected

Placental Bleeding

Active management of the third stage of labor is recommended. This includes any interventions designed to assist in expulsion of the placenta and the prevention of excessive blood loss. In the presence of excessive bleeding associated with the third stage, no time should be wasted. Manual removal of the placenta is carried out immediately and oxytocics given. The uterus should not be manhandled in efforts to squeeze out the placenta.

Uterine Atony

Uterine Massage
The uterine fundus is massaged through the abdomen.

Uterine Exploration
Manual exploration of the uterus is carried out, and blood clots and fragments of placenta and membrane are removed. Examination under anesthesia along with dilatation and curettage in the operating room may be necessary.

Lacerations
The cervix, vagina, and vulva are examined for lacerations.

Uterine Compression
Bimanual compression of the uterus (Fig. 20-1) is a valuable method of controlling uterine atonic bleeding. One hand is placed in the vagina

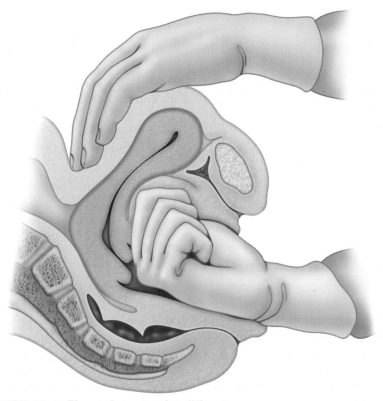

FIGURE 20-1. Bimanual compression of the uterus.

against the anterior wall of the uterus. Pressure is exerted against the posterior aspect of the uterus by the other hand through the abdomen. With a rotatory motion, the uterus is compressed and massaged between the two hands. This provides twice the amount of uterine stimulation that can be achieved by abdominal massage alone. In addition, compression of the venous sinuses can be effected and the flow of blood reduced. As part of this procedure, the atonic uterus is elevated, anteverted, and anteflexed.

Oxytocin

Oxytocin can be given intramuscularly, and 10 units IM is the recommended dose and route for uncomplicated vaginal deliveries. Alternatively, an intravenous drip containing 20 to 40 units of oxytocin in 1 L of fluid can be run at a speed sufficient to keep the uterus contracted, often 150 to 500 cc/hr. Oxytocin can also be given as an intravenous bolus of 5 to 10 units over 1 to 2 minutes. Rapid infusions of high doses of oxytocin should be avoided in hypotensive patients.

Carbetocin

Carbetocin is a long-acting oxytocin that has been shown to decrease the need for uterine massage for uterine atony. The recommended dose of carbetocin is 100 µg given either intravenously or intramuscularly slowly (over 1 minute). The use of carbetocin for prevention of PPH after uneventful low-risk vaginal delivery is not warranted, but its use has been advocated to reduce blood loss at the time of elective cesarean section or in patients with risk factors for PPH.

When first-line therapy with oxytocics is insufficient, there are several more pharmacologic interventions in the armamentarium.

Ergometrine

The first pure ergot alkaloid, ergotamine, was isolated in 1920. Later, another active alkaloid was discovered and named ergometrine (ergonovine). Only the latter is used in obstetrics. It has no adrenergic blocking action, and the emetic and cardiovascular effects are less than those of ergotamine. These are powerful ecbolic agents, exciting a tonic contraction of the myometrium. The maximum effect is during labor and the puerperium. They are never used during the first and second stages of labor. Ergometrine 0.125 or 0.25 mg is given intravenously and/or 0.5 mg intramuscularly.

Undesirable effects include hypertension, tachycardia, headache, and nausea and vomiting. The ergot alkaloids should not be used in

THIRD STAGE OF LABOR

hypertensive patients, in women with cardiac disease, and in HIV-positive patients taking protease inhibitors.

Prostaglandin

Prostaglandins are 20-carbon carboxylic acids that are formed enzymatically from polyunsaturated essential fatty acids. Most organs are capable of synthesizing prostaglandins, as well as metabolizing them to less active compounds. On the basis of their structure, prostaglandins are divided into four groups, namely E, F, A, and B. Three of the E group and three of the F group are primary compounds. The other eight are metabolites of the parent six. Thirteen of the 14 known prostaglandins occur in humans.

First isolated from the seminal fluid, these substances are distributed widely in all mammalian tissues. Their exact mode of action is not known, but prostaglandins are thought to be part of the mechanism that controls transmission in the sympathetic nervous system. Two generalized activities are apparent: (1) alteration of smooth muscle contractility and (2) modulation of hormonal activity. How an organ will respond depends on the (1) specific prostaglandin, (2) dose, (3) route of administration, and (4) hormonal or drug environment. Prostaglandins are metabolized rapidly, and their systemic effects are of short duration.

Prostaglandins produce a wide variety of physiologic responses. Both E and F have profoundly stimulating effects on the myometrium. In adequate dosage, they can initiate labor at any stage of pregnancy. Prostaglandins can be given intravenously, intramuscularly, intravaginally, and directly into the myometrium. The latter technique will control PPH when other methods fail.

Adverse reactions include:

1. Gastrointestinal symptoms, including nausea, vomiting, and diarrhea, occur in half of patients. In most cases, these effects are short in duration and not severe
2. A syndrome of bronchial constriction (asthma attack) with tachycardia, vasovagal effects, and alterations in blood pressure may take place. If this occurs, the drug is discontinued and supportive therapy instituted. The vital signs return to normal within a few minutes, probably because the drug is metabolized rapidly
3. Hyperpyrexia occurs occasionally

Contraindications to prostaglandins include asthma, cardiovascular disease, and hypertension.

Prostaglandins appear to be involved in postpartum hemostasis by means of their versatile biologic properties, including the function of platelets; vasoactive effects; and, especially, myometrial stimulation. These drugs have a powerful effect on uterine contractility. PPH resulting from uterine atony has been treated by intramuscular injections of prostaglandin $F_{2\alpha}$ ($PGF_{2\alpha}$; Carboprost or Hemabate) and direct intramyometrial injection of $PGF_{2\alpha}$. The latter technique is the most effective. The dose is 1 mg administered transabdominally into the myometrium (1 cc of Hemabate diluted in 9 cc of sterile saline can be injected suprapubically after emptying the bladder). A transvaginal approach has also been used using the same dose. A sustained uterine contraction develops rapidly, and bleeding is reduced within 2 to 3 minutes. Side effects include nausea and hypertension, both of which are controlled easily. Care must be taken to avoid direct intravenous injection. In patients who have asthma or hypertension, a test dose of 0.25 mg should be tried before giving the full amount (Fig. 20-2). Misoprostol

THIRD STAGE OF LABOR

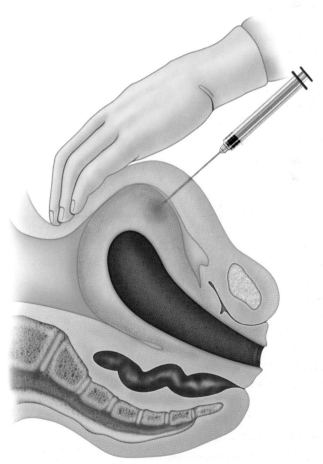

FIGURE 20-2. Transabdominal intramyometrial injection of prostaglandin.

or Cytotec is a synthetic prostaglandin E1 (PGE1) analogue that has been studied and used for labor induction as well as both prevention and treatment of PPH. Misoprostol is a tablet that can be administered orally, sublingually, vaginally, or rectally. The typical dose is 600 to 800 µg orally, sublingually, or rectally. Misoprostol is especially suited to management of the third stage of labor when other medications are not available for reasons of cost, storage, or difficulty of administration.

When PPH is refractory to medical management, compressive techniques and surgical intervention become necessary.

Uterine Packing

Packing the uterine cavity is a controversial subject (Fig. 20-3). Most authorities condemn its use because the procedure is unphysiologic. Up to this point, attempts had been made to empty the uterus; now it is to be filled. It is unlikely that a uterus that does not respond to powerful oxytocic drugs will be stimulated to contract by a gauze pack. It is impossible to pack an atonic uterus so tightly that the blood sinuses are closed off. The uterus simply balloons and fills up with more blood. Thus, the packing

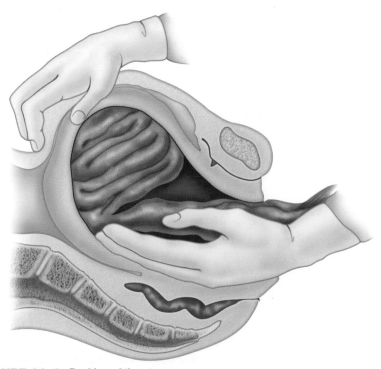

FIGURE 20-3. Packing of the uterus.

not only does no good but is also dangerous in that it leads to a false sense of security by obscuring the flow of blood. Ten yards of 3-inch packing gauze absorbs 1000 mL of blood. Furthermore, packing favors infection.

Despite these antipacking arguments, many obstetricians believe that it is worth trying to control bleeding by this method before more radical measures are used. The patient must be observed carefully. Deterioration of the vital signs, ballooning of the uterus, and continuation of the bleeding are signs that the pack is ineffective and must be removed. Packing must be done properly. One or two 5- or 10-yard rolls of gauze are needed. With one hand on the abdomen, the operator steadies the uterine fundus while the pack is pushed through the cervix and into the cavity of the uterus with the fingers of the other hand. The gauze is placed first into one corner of the uterus and then the other, coming down the cavity from side to side. The uterus must be packed tightly. Then the vagina is packed. A large, firm pad is placed on the abdomen above the uterus, and a tight abdominal and perineal binder is applied. The gauze packing is removed in 12 hours.

Beyond the use of gauze, internal uterine compression using tamponade balloons (Bakri SOS tamponade balloon catheter) have become popular (Fig. 20-4). Several commercially available silicon models are on the

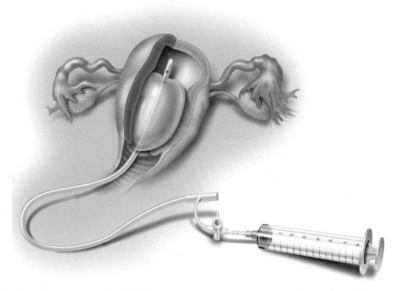

FIGURE 20-4. **The Bakri SOS tamponade balloon catheter deployed within the uterus.**

THIRD STAGE OF LABOR

market, although regular Foley catheters and Sengstaken-Blakemore tubes can be used as well. Essentially, the balloon is inserted into the uterus and inflated with a large volume of water or saline (250-500 cc). The balloon is kept in place by packing the vagina with gauze and slowly deflated 8 to 48 hours later. The use of a device with a secondary port that drains any blood accumulating above the balloon allows caregivers to monitor ongoing bleeding. Of note, the Bakri balloon can also be inserted at the time of a cesarean section in situations of uterine atony or to tamponade the lower uterine segment in the case of bleeding from a low placental implantation site. When inserted at the time of laparotomy, the inflation channel is pushed into the vagina from above.

Uterine Compression Sutures

When uterine atony is the culprit and laparotomy is performed to control the hemorrhage, consideration can be given to external compression sutures, as popularized by B-lynch and Cho. In these uterus-sparing techniques, relatively large, braided, absorbable sutures (such as #2 Polysorb or Vicryl) are used to bind the uterus and force compression of the bleeding sinuses. In the B-lynch technique, the goal is to create a pair of "overalls" for the uterus to compress it (Fig. 20-5). In the Cho or

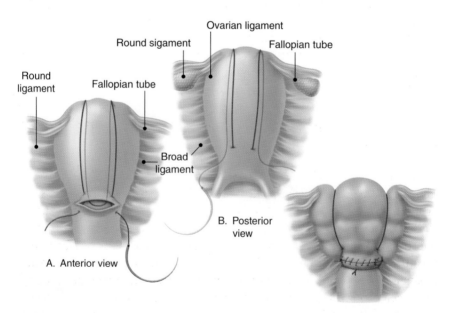

FIGURE 20-5. B-Lynch technique for uterine compression sutures.

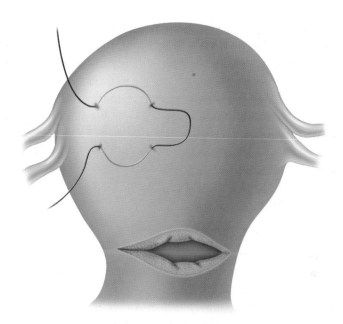

FIGURE 20-6. Cho technique for uterine compression sutures.

"square-suture" technique, areas of posterior and anterior myometrium are sutured together to force compression (Fig. 20-6).

If neither external nor internal compression is adequate to control hemorrhage, techniques aimed at reducing the blood flow to the uterus are next in line.

Compression of the Aorta
In thin women, compression of the aorta against the spine may slow down the bleeding.

Embolization of Pelvic Arteries
This technique can be used instead of, or after failure of, hysterectomy or ligation of the internal iliac artery for the treatment of pelvic hemorrhage. Under radiologic angiographic control, a polyethylene catheter is introduced into the aorta via the right femoral artery. Each internal iliac artery is catheterized and occluded with small (2-3 mm) fragments of Gelfoam. In situations of pelvic hemorrhage other than that caused by uterine atony, the specific bleeding vessel can be identified and selectively embolized. The procedure can be carried out in less than 2 hours and imposes little additional morbidity and no mortality. An advantage over internal iliac

THIRD STAGE OF LABOR

ligation is that the distal blood vessels are occluded, so that bleeding from reconstituted distal vessels is rare. In addition, the uterus is retained, and further childbearing is possible.

Ligation of Uterine Arteries

Since most of the uterine blood is supplied by the uterine arteries, their ligation can control PPH. The collateral supply is sufficient to maintain the viability of the organ. The abdomen is opened, the uterus is elevated by the surgeon's hand, and the area of the uterine vessels is exposed. Using a large needle and absorbable suture (#1 Vicryl or Chromic Catgut), the suture is placed through the myometrium of the lower segment of the uterus 2 to 3 cm medial to the vessels. It is brought out through the avascular area of the broad ligament. A substantial amount of myometrium is included in the suture to occlude some of the inferior coronary branches of the uterine artery. In most cases, the uterine vein is also ligated, but the hypertrophied ovarian veins drain the uterus adequately. The vessels are ligated but not divided. Recanalization will take place in most cases. The uterus becomes blanched with a pink hue, and bleeding subsides. Subsequent menstruation and pregnancy are unaffected. Transvaginal ligation of the uterine arteries is a blind and hazardous procedure that is not recommended. Subsequent pregnancy has been successful after uterine artery ligation.

Ligation of Internal Iliac Arteries

This procedure may be performed in any situation associated with uncontrollable pelvic bleeding (Fig. 20-7). The collateral circulation is so extensive that the pelvic arterial system is never deprived of blood, and no necrosis of any of the pelvic tissue takes place. Entry into the abdomen is made by a midline or transverse incision. First the common iliac artery and its bifurcation into the external and internal iliac arteries is palpated and visualized through the posterior peritoneum. The bifurcation feels like the letter Y. The branch coming off at right angles is the internal iliac artery; it courses medially and posteriorly. The continuing branch is the external iliac artery. It is essential that these two branches be identified positively. If the external iliac artery is ligated by accident, loss of the lower limb may result. The ureter lies anterior to the vessels and crosses the common iliac artery from lateral to medial at a point just proximal to the bifurcation. It must be identified to prevent its being damaged.

The posterior peritoneum is tented and incised in a longitudinal direction, beginning proximal to the bifurcation of the common iliac artery

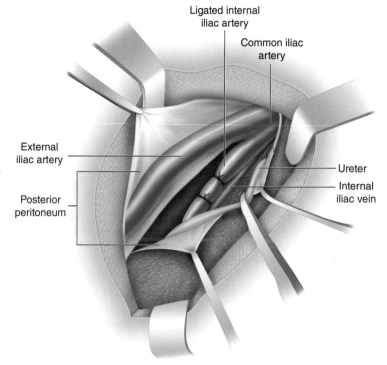

FIGURE 20-7. Ligation of the internal iliac artery.

and extending caudad for 4 to 6 cm. The incision is lateral to the ureter. The ureter is located on the medial peritoneal flap and usually remains attached to it. The external and internal iliac arteries must be re-identified to avoid any error. Care is taken to avoid injury to the veins. The internal iliac artery is elevated from the vein gently and with care to avoid damage to the vein. Two no. 2-0 silk sutures are placed beneath the artery and tied firmly but gently. The artery is not transected. If possible, identification and ligation of only the anterior branch of the internal iliac artery is ideal because it will spare potential devascularization of muscles supplied by the posterior branch. The peritoneum is closed with interrupted 3-0 catgut or similar suture; a continuous suture might kink the ureter. The procedure is repeated on the contralateral side.

Hysterectomy

If the bleeding continues, the abdomen must be opened and hysterectomy performed. Deaths after and during hysterectomy have been reported;

these resulted from delaying the operation until the patient was nearly moribund. Performed in time, hysterectomy is effective and lifesaving.

Lacerations

1. Rupture of the uterus necessitates laparotomy with either repair of the tear or hysterectomy
2. Lacerations of the cervix, vagina, and vulva are repaired and the bleeding controlled with figure-8 sutures
3. In some cases, the bleeding from the vaginal tears cannot be controlled with sutures. Where there are large varicosities, each passage of the needle through the tissue seems to provoke fresh bleeding. In such cases, the vagina should be packed firmly with gauze that is left in for 24 hours

PITUITARY INSUFFICIENCY

The profound hypotension that may result from PPH has a particular effect on the blood supply to the anterior pituitary gland. In 1937, Sheehan described insufficiency of the anterior lobe of the pituitary gland in women of childbearing age. Symptoms include:

1. Mammary involution and failure to lactate
2. Weakness and lethargy
3. Hypersensitivity to cold
4. Diminished sweating
5. Excessive involution of the uterus
6. Atrophy of the external genitalia
7. Amenorrhea or oligomenorrhea
8. Loss of body hair, including the pubic area
9. Absence of menopausal symptoms
10. Later signs of failure of the thyroid and adrenal glands may appear

The condition is initiated by severe shock, the result of massive hemorrhage. The pituitary gland undergoes ischemia followed by necrosis. From 5 to 99 percent of the anterior lobe may be affected. As long as 10 percent of the gland is left in a functioning state, the patient will retain reasonably normal glandular function. In severe cases, death may occur. In less acute situations, the patient can live for years in a subnormal state, and the resulting immunocompromise may lead to infection.

The exact nature of the vascular disturbance is not known. Possible conditions include:

1. Arterial spasm
2. Interruption of the portal circulation of the pituitary
3. Coagulation in the capillaries
4. Venous thrombosis
5. DIC

LATE POSTPARTUM HEMORRHAGE

Late PPH is the loss of 500 mL of blood after the first 24 hours but within 6 weeks. Although most of these episodes occur by the 21st day, the majority take place between the fourth and ninth postpartum days. The incidence is around 1 percent.

Non-uterine Bleeding

In a few cases, the origin is the cervix, vagina, or vulva. Local infection leads to sloughing of sutures and dissolution of thrombi, with hemorrhage at the site of the episiotomy or lacerations. The amount of blood lost depends on the size of the vessels. Treatment includes cleaning out infected debris; suturing bleeding points; and if necessary, pressure packing the vagina. Blood transfusion is given as needed.

Uterine Bleeding

Etiology

1. Retained fragments of placenta
2. Intrauterine infection
3. Subinvolution of the uterus and the placental site
4. Uterine myoma, especially when submucous

Mechanism of Bleeding

The exact sequence of events is not known, but some type of subinvolution is present. Three probable factors are (1) late detachment of thrombi at the placental site with reopening of the vascular sinuses; (2) abnormalities in the separation of the decidua vera; and (3) intrauterine infection, leading to dissolution of the thromboses in the vessels. The basic mechanism is similar regardless of whether placental tissue has been retained.

Clinical Picture
The amount of bleeding varies. Most of these patients require hospitalization and many need blood transfusion; hemorrhagic shock can occur.

Treatment

1. Oxytocics are given
2. If bleeding continues, curettage is performed carefully, so as not to perforate the soft uterus. In many cases, no placental tissue is found, the histologic examination showing organized blood clot, decidual tissue, or fragments of muscle. The results of curettage are satisfactory regardless of whether placenta was present. Removal of the inflamed tissue with its superficial bleeding vessels permits the uterus to contract around the deeper, healthier vessels, thus producing more effective hemostasis
3. Blood is replaced by transfusion
4. Antibiotics are given to control infection
5. Repeat curettage may be necessary
6. If all other treatment fails, hysterectomy is performed

ETIOLOGY OF SHOCK IN OBSTETRICS

Direct Obstetric Causes

Placental Site

1. Spontaneous abortion
2. Placenta previa
3. Abruptio placentae
4. Retained placenta
5. Postpartum uterine atony

Trauma

1. Lacerations of the vagina and vulva
2. Uterine rupture
3. Uterine inversion

Extraperitoneal

1. Broad ligament hematoma
2. Paravertebral hematoma

Intraperitoneal

1. Ectopic pregnancy

Related Obstetric Conditions

1. Embolism

   a. Thrombotic
   b. Amniotic
   c. Air

2. Eclampsia

3. Septic shock

4. Neurogenic shock

5. Anesthetic complications

   a. Aspiration of gastric fluid
   b. Extended spinal or regional block

6. Drug reactions

Nonobstetric Conditions

1. Cardiac (e.g., myocardial infarct)

2. Respiratory (e.g., spontaneous pneumothorax)

3. Cerebrovascular accidents

4. Abdominal causes

   a. Ruptured spleen
   b. Torsion or rupture of ovarian cyst
   c. Perforated peptic ulcer
   d. Acute pancreatitis

SELECTED READING

Bakri YN, Amri A, Abdul Jabbar F: Tamponade-balloon for obstetrical bleeding. Int J Gynaecol Obstet 74:139, 2001

B-Lynch C, Coker A, Lawal AH, Abu J, Cowen MJ: The B-Lynch surgical technique for the control of massive postpartum haemorrhage: An alternative to hysterectomy? Five cases reported. Br J Obstet Gynaecol 104:372, 1997

Cho JH, Jun HS, Lee CN: Hemostatic suturing technique for uterine bleeding during cesarean delivery. Obstet Gynecol 96:129, 2000

Leduc D, Senikas V, Lalonde AB, et al: Active management of the third stage of labour: Prevention and treatment of postpartum hemorrhage. J Obstet Gynaecol Can 31:980, 2009

O'Leary JL, O'Leary JA: Uterine artery ligation for control of post cesarean section hemorrhage. Obstet Gynecol 43:849, 1974

Pais SO, Glickman M, Schwartz P, et al: Embolization of pelvic arteries for control of postpartum hemorrhage. Obstet Gynecol 55:754, 1980

CHAPTER 21

Episiotomy, Lacerations, Uterine Rupture, and Inversion

Ramadan El Sugy

EPISIOTOMY

An episiotomy (perineotomy) is an incision into the perineum to enlarge the space at the outlet, thereby facilitating the birth of the child.

Maternal Benefits

1. A straight incision is simpler to repair and heals better than a jagged, uncontrolled laceration
2. The structures in front are protected as well as those in the rear. By increasing the room available posteriorly, there is less stretching of and less damage to the anterior vaginal wall, bladder, urethra, and periclitoral tissues
3. The second stage of labor is shortened

Fetal Benefits

Proposed fetal benefits of episiotomy include cranial protection, especially for premature infants, reduced perinatal asphyxia, less fetal distress, better APGAR scores, less fetal acidosis, and reduced complications from shoulder dystocia. Episiotomy may be useful to facilitate the management of shoulder dystocia.

Indications

1. Prophylactic: To preserve the integrity of the pelvic floor

2. Arrest of progress by a resistant perineum

    a. Thick and heavily muscled tissue
    b. Operative scars
    c. Previous well-repaired episiotomy

3. To obviate uncontrolled tears, including extension into the rectum

    a. When the perineum is short with little room between the back of the vagina and the front of the rectum
    b. When large lacerations seem inevitable

4. Fetal reasons

    a. Premature and infirm babies
    b. Large infants
    c. Abnormal positions such as occipitoposteriors, face presentations, and breeches

d. Fetal distress, where there is need for rapid delivery of the baby and dilatation of the perineum cannot be awaited

e. Operative vaginal delivery

f. Shoulder dystocia

Current data and clinical opinion suggest that there are insufficient objective evidence-based criteria to recommend episiotomy, especially routine use of episiotomy, and that clinical judgment remains the best guide for use of this procedure.

Timing of Episiotomy

There is a proper time to make the episiotomy. When made too late, the procedure fails to prevent lacerations and to protect the pelvic floor. When made too soon, the incision leads to needless loss of blood. The episiotomy is made when the perineum is bulging, when a 3- to 4-cm diameter of fetal scalp is visible during a contraction, and when the presenting part will be delivered with the next three or four contractions. In this way, lacerations are avoided, overstretching of the pelvic floor is prevented, and excessive bleeding is obviated.

There are three types of episiotomy: (1) midline; (2) mediolateral, left or right; and (3) lateral episiotomy, which is no longer used (Fig. 21-1A).

Midline Episiotomy

Technique

In making the incision, two fingers are placed in the vagina between the fetal head and the perineum. Outward pressure is made on the perineum, away from the fetus, to avoid injury to the baby. The scissors are placed so that one blade lies against the vaginal mucosa and the other on the skin. The incision is made in the midline from the fourchette almost to but not through the external fibers of the anal sphincter (Fig. 21-1B). The cut is in the central tendinous portion of the perineal body to which are attached the bulbocavernosus muscle in front, the superficial transverse perineal and part of the levator ani muscles at the sides, and the anal sphincter behind (Fig. 21-1B). This is an excellent anatomic incision.

Advantages

1. The muscle belly is not cut

2. It is easy to make and easy to repair

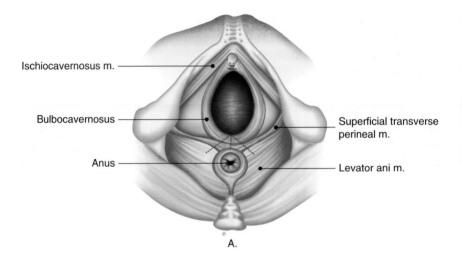

Ischiocavernosus m.

Bulbocavernosus

Superficial transverse perineal m.

Anus

Levator ani m.

A.

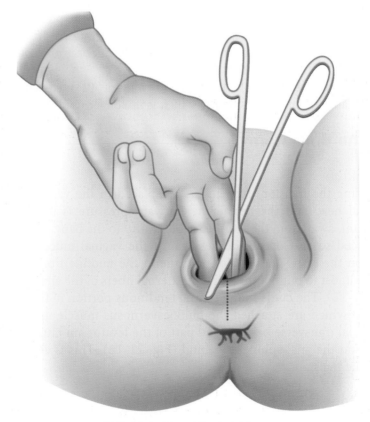

B. Incision of the midline episiotomy.

FIGURE 21-1. Midline episiotomy.

3. The structural results are excellent
4. Bleeding is less than with other incisions
5. Postoperative pain is minimal
6. Healing is superior, and dehiscence is rare

Disadvantages

The one drawback is that if there is extension of the incision as the head is being born, the anal sphincter is torn and the rectum entered. Although most bowel injuries heal well if repaired properly, this complication should be avoided. Median episiotomies are not ideal in the following situations:

1. Short perineum
2. Large baby
3. Abnormal positions and presentations
4. Difficult operative deliveries

Repair

Since in most cases the third stage is completed soon after the birth of the child, the repair of the episiotomy is performed after the placenta is delivered, the uterus contracted, and the cervix and vagina found to be uninjured. Not only are intrauterine procedures, such as manual removal of the placenta, and intravaginal procedures more difficult to perform after the episiotomy has been closed, but the repair may be broken down.

Except for the subcuticular layer, a medium, round needle is used. In the deep tissues, a cutting edge needle may lacerate a blood vessel and cause a hematoma. Our preference is for a minimally reactive, absorbable polyglycolic acid suture.

First the vaginal mucosa is sewn together (Fig. 21-2A). The procedure is begun at the top of the incision, the first bite being taken a little above the apex to include any retracted blood vessel. The suture is tied, leaving one end long. The edges of the wound are then approximated but not strangulated using a simple continuous or a lock stitch to assure hemostasis. Each bite includes the mucous membrane of the vagina and the tissue between the vagina and rectum. This reduces bleeding, eliminates dead space, and makes for better healing. The repair is carried past the hymenal ring to the skin edges. The last two bites include the subcutaneous tissue at the base of the episiotomy but do not come through the skin. This end of the continuous suture may be tied, or it may be left untied and held with a hemostat.

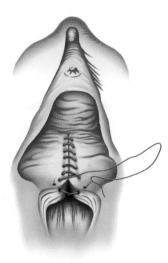

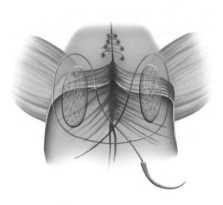

A. Closure of the vaginal mucosa
by a continuous suture.

B. The crown suture, reuniting the
divided bulbocavernous muscle.

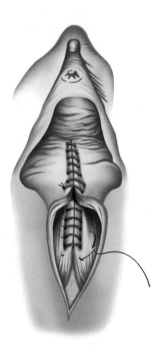

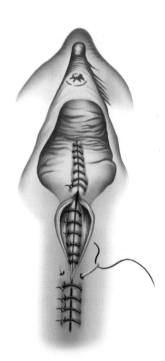

C. Drawing together the perineal muscles
and fascia with interrupted sutures.

D. Approximation of the skin edges
with interrupted sutures.

FIGURE 21-2. Repair of a midline episiotomy.

The second stitch near the base of the wound is the crown suture (Fig. 21-2B). The needle passes under the skin deeply enough to catch and bring together the separated and retracted ends of the bulbocavernosus muscle and fascia. The crown suture is important: If these tissues are approximated too tightly, coitus is painful, and if too loose, the introitus gapes.

Next the transverse perineal and levator ani muscles and fascia are approximated in the midline anterior to the rectum with three or four interrupted sutures (Fig. 21-2C). One layer is enough in most cases.

Finally, the incision is closed by one of several methods:

1. The skin edges are united by interrupted, or mattress, sutures that pass through the skin and subcutaneous tissue. These are tied loosely to prevent strangulation as postpartum swelling takes place (Fig. 21-2D)
2. The skin edges are approximated using a continuous subcuticular stitch on a small cutting needle, starting at the lower end of the incision. The first bite is taken in the subcuticular tissue just under but not through the skin, going from side to side until the base (upper end) of the wound is reached. There it is tied separately, or if the suture used to repair the vaginal mucosa has been left untied, this suture and the subcuticular one are tied together. This completes the repair (Fig. 21-3D)

Aftercare

Aftercare of the episiotomy is essentially a matter of cleanliness. The perineum is cleaned with a mildly antiseptic solution after each urination and bowel evacuation. We recommend the use of sitz baths and an analgesic such as ibuprofen. Heat, as from a hair dryer, may be used to dry the area and to reduce the swelling. Daily showers and washing with mild soap and water are excellent ways of keeping the perineum clean and free from irritating discharges. If a woman has excessive pain in the days after a repair, she should be examined immediately because pain is a frequent sign of infection in the perineal area. After repair of episiotomy, we include several weeks of therapy with a stool softener, such as docusate sodium, to minimize the potential for repair breakdown from straining during defecation.

Mediolateral Episiotomy

When a large episiotomy is needed, or when there is danger of rectal involvement, the mediolateral variety is advised. Included here are patients with short perineums, contracted outlets, large babies, face-to-pubis

deliveries, attitudes of extension, breech births, and midforceps operations. It maximizes perineal space for delivery while reducing the likelihood of third- or fourth-degree extension. Reported disadvantages of the
mediolateral procedure include difficulty of repair, greater blood loss, and
possibly more early postpartum discomfort.

Technique

The incision is made from the midline of the posterior fourchette toward
the ischial tuberosity, far enough laterally to avoid the anal sphincter. The
average episiotomy is about 4 cm long and may reach the fatty tissues
of the ischiorectal fossa. Whether it is placed on the left or right side is
unimportant.

The following structures are cut:

1. Skin and subcutaneous tissue
2. Bulbocavernosus muscle and fascia
3. Transverse perineal muscle
4. Levator ani muscle and fascia. The extent to which this structure is
   involved is determined by the length and depth of the incision

Repair

The technique is essentially the same as for the median perineotomy. The
vaginal mucosa is repaired starting at the apex and brings together the
mucous membrane and the underlying supporting tissue (Fig. 21-3A).
The crown suture is placed carefully (Fig. 21-3B).

The muscles and fascia that were cut are approximated with interrupted sutures (Fig. 21-3C). The tissues on the medial side tend to retract,
and care must be taken not to enter the rectum. Some operators prefer
to place these sutures, leaving them untied, before the vaginal mucosa
is repaired. In many patients, a single layer of four or five stitches is
sufficient. When the wound is deep or when there is much bleeding, two
layers may be necessary, one in the muscles, and one to bring together the
overlying fascia. The skin edges are joined by a subcuticular stitch beginning at the apex (Fig. 21-3D) or by interrupted sutures through skin and
subcutaneous tissue.

Disruption of Episiotomy: Infection

Etiology

Similar to incisions in other parts of the body, an episiotomy may dehisce.
Predisposing factors include:

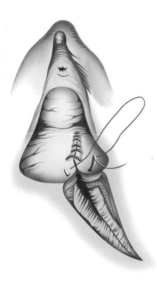

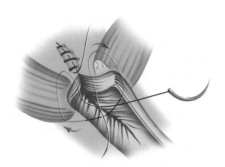

A. Closure of the vaginal mucosa
by a continuous suture.

B. The crown suture.

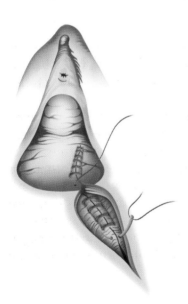

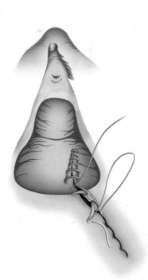

C. Drawing together the perineal
muscles and fascia with interrupted
sutures.

D. Approximation of the skin
edges with a continuous
subcuticular suture.

FIGURE 21-3. **Repair of a left mediolateral episiotomy.**

1. Poor healing powers:

   a. Nutritional deficiencies
   b. Anemia
   c. Exhaustion after a long and difficult labor
   d. Avascular scarred tissue

2. Failure of technique:

   a. Careless approximation of the wound
   b. Incomplete hemostasis leading to hematoma formation
   c. Failure to obliterate dead space

3. Devitalization of tissue:

   a. Use of crushing instruments
   b. Strangulation of tissue by tying sutures too tightly
   c. Use of too heavy catgut

4. Infection:

   a. Infected lochia in puerperal sepsis
   b. Poor technique and neglect of aseptic standards
   c. Proximity of the rectum
   d. Extension of the incision into or passage of the needle through the bowel
   e. Sepsis in a hematoma
   f. Improper postpartum cleanliness

Clinical Course

The episiotomy becomes extremely painful, tender, swollen, red, and indurated. The patient may or may not have fever. Sometimes there is a discharge from the incision. In most cases, infections are localized and may resolve with perineal wound care. In rare cases, an abscess may form, which will result in either the need for disruption of the repair to allow for evacuation of the abscess or spontaneous breakdown of the repair. In extreme cases, infections such as necrotizing fasciitis can cause maternal death if not effectively evaluated and treated.

Management of Disruption

Supportive Management. The area is kept clean and free from irritating discharge and debris by warm sitz baths twice daily for 20 minutes.

After this, the perineum is lamped for 30 minutes. The wound granulates in and heals from the deep layers up. The patient may go home at the usual time and continue the treatment there. Unless there has been damage to the rectum, this management has always been successful in the author's experience. This expectant management with perineal care allows for spontaneous healing to occur over a period of several weeks. The wound heals well, no aftereffects are noted, and prolonged hospitalization is avoided.

Secondary Repair. Supportive treatment is carried on until the area is clean. This takes 5 to 6 days. Then the patient is anesthetized, the devitalized tissue debrided, and the episiotomy repaired.

In the author's experience supportive therapy alone has given the best results and is the simplest to carry out.

A late complication of an infected episiotomy is a rectovaginal fistula. This results from an unrecognized tear of the rectum or from a suture being passed through the rectal wall and left there.

LACERATIONS OF THE PERINEUM

Many women have tears of the perineum during the birth of the first child. In about half the cases, these tears are extensive. Lacerations must be repaired carefully.

Maternal causes include:

1. Precipitate, uncontrolled, or unattended delivery (the most frequent cause)
2. The patient's inability to stop bearing down
3. Hastening the delivery by excessive fundal pressure
4. Edema and friability of the perineum
5. Vulvar varicosities weakening the tissue
6. Narrow pubic arch with outlet contraction, forcing the head posteriorly
7. Extension of episiotomy

Fetal factors are:

1. Large baby
2. Abnormal positions of the head (e.g., occipitoposterior and face presentations)

3. Breech deliveries
4. Difficult forceps extractions
5. Shoulder dystocia
6. Congenital anomalies, such as hydrocephaly

Classification of Perineal Lacerations

First-Degree Tear
First-degree tear involves the vaginal mucosa, the fourchette, or the skin of the perineum just below it.

Repair. These tears are small and are repaired as simply as possible. The aim is reapproximation of the divided tissue and hemostasis. In the average case, a few interrupted sutures through the vaginal mucosa, the fourchette, and the skin of the perineum are enough. If bleeding is profuse, figure-8 stitches may be used. Interrupted sutures, loosely tied, are best for the skin because they cause less tension and less discomfort to the patient.

Second-Degree Tear
Second-degree lacerations are deeper. They are mainly in the midline and extend through the perineal body. Often the transverse perineal muscle is torn, and the rent may go down to but not through the anal sphincter. Usually the tear extends upward along the vaginal mucosa and the sub-mucosal tissue. This gives the laceration a doubly triangular appearance with the base at the fourchette, one apex in the vagina, and the other near the rectum.

Repair. Repair of second-degree lacerations is in layers:

1. Interrupted, continuous, or lock stitches are used to approximate the edges of the vaginal mucosa and submucosa (Fig. 21-4A)
2. The deep muscles of the perineal body are sewn together with interrupted sutures (Fig. 21-4B)
3. A running subcuticular suture or interrupted sutures, loosely tied, bring together the skin edges (Fig. 21-4C)

Third-Degree Tear
Third-degree tears extend through the perineal body, the transverse perineal muscle, and the anal sphincter. In partial third-degree tears, only the

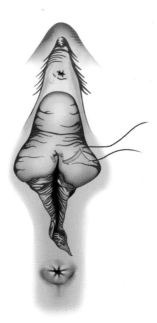

A. Closure of the rent in the vaginal mucosa with a continuous suture.

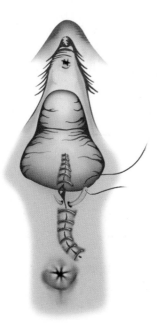

B. Drawing together the perineal muscles and fascia with interrupted sutures.

C. Closure of the skin edges with interrupted sutures tied loosely.

FIGURE 21-4. Repair of a second-degree perineal laceration.

rectal sphincter is torn; in complete tears, the rectal sphincter is severed, and the laceration extends up the anterior rectal wall for a variable distance. Some authors refer to this as a fourth-degree tear.

Repair of Complete Tear. Complete third-degree tear (Fig. 21-5A) is repaired in layers:

1. The anterior wall of the rectum is repaired with fine 000 or 0000 chromic catgut on a fused needle. Starting at the apex, interrupted sutures are placed submucosally so that the serosa, muscularis, and submucosa of the rectum are apposed (Fig. 21-5B). Some authors advise that the knot be tied in the lumen of the bowel. Others approximate the edges of the rectum with a continuous suture going through all layers. This part of the repair must be performed meticulously
2. The line of repair is oversewn by bringing together the perirectal fascia and the fascia of the rectovaginal septum. Interrupted or continuous sutures are used
3. The torn ends of the rectal sphincter (which have retracted) are identified, grasped with Allis forceps, and approximated with interrupted sutures or two figure-8 sutures (Figs. 21-5C and D)
4. The vaginal mucosa is then repaired as in a midline episiotomy, with continuous or interrupted sutures
5. The perineal muscles are sewn together with interrupted stitches
6. The skin edges are sewn together with a continuous subcuticular suture or loosely tied interrupted sutures

Repair of Partial Tear. Repair of partial third-degree tear is similar to that of the complete variety except that the rectal wall is intact and the repair starts with reapproximation of the torn ends of the rectal sphincter.

Aftercare. Aftercare of third-degree tears includes:

1. General perineal asepsis
2. The use of sitz baths
3. An analgesic such as ibuprofen
4. Low-residue diet
5. Encouragement of soft bowel movements with mild laxatives
6. A suppository or carefully given enema is prescribed on the fifth or sixth day if the bowels have not moved

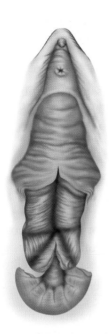

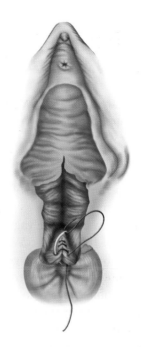

A. Torn and retracted ends of the rectal sphincter, laceration of the anterior wall of the rectum, and the torn vagina and perineum.

B. Closing the tear in the anterior wall of the rectum with interrupted sutures tied in the lumen.

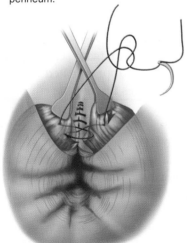

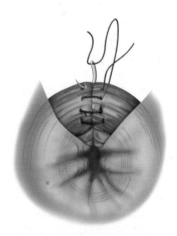

C. Retracted ends of the rectal sphincter are grasped with Allis forceps, and the first figure-8 suture is being placed.

D. Reunion of torn rectal sphincter completed with two figure-8 sutures.

FIGURE 21-5. Repair of a third-degree laceration (complete tear).

LACERATIONS OF ANTERIOR VULVA AND LOWER ANTERIOR VAGINAL WALL

Various areas may be involved. Superficial tears are not serious, but with deep tears, the bleeding may be profuse.

Locations of Lacerations

1. Tissue on either side of the urethra
2. Labia minora
3. Lateral walls of the vagina
4. Area of the clitoris: With deep tears, the corpora cavernosa may be torn. Because of the general vascularity of this structure, as well as the presence of the deep and dorsal blood vessels of the clitoris, these lacerations are accompanied by severe bleeding
5. Urethra under the pubic arch
6. Bladder: The bladder is close to the anterior vaginal wall and may be damaged. Vesicovaginal fistula can occur. The main causes of fistula are prolonged labor with pressure necrosis of the wall of the bladder and instrumental damage during difficult deliveries

Repair of Lacerations

Superficial small lacerations do not need repair in many cases. When the legs are brought together, the torn edges are approximated and heal spontaneously. Larger tears should have the edges brought together with interrupted sutures to promote healing.

Deep lacerations must be repaired. Profuse bleeding is controlled best by figure-8 sutures placed to include and shut off the torn and bleeding vessels. Unfortunately, in many cases, the lacerated area is the site of varicosities, and passage of the needle through the tissue provokes fresh bleeding. If sutures do not stop the bleeding, a firm pack should be applied against the bleeding site and the hemorrhage controlled by tamponade.

Often the area of bleeding is *near the urethra,* and when the periclitoral region is involved, the hemorrhage can be excessive. Repair is difficult because of the proximity of the urethra. To prevent damaging the urethra, a catheter should be inserted to guide the needle away from it (Fig. 21-6).

Tears of the *urethra and bladder* are repaired in three layers to approximate the bladder mucosa, bladder wall, and anterior wall of the vagina. An indwelling catheter should be inserted into the bladder for drainage.

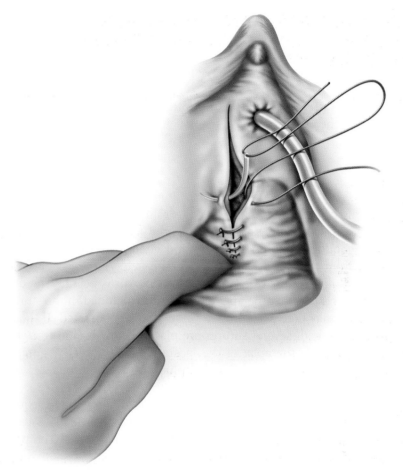

FIGURE 21-6. Anterior paraurethral laceration: placing of fine interrupted sutures. A catheter is in the urethra.

LACERATIONS OF UPPER VAGINA

These lacerations may take place during spontaneous delivery but are more common with operative deliveries and are associated with a variety of conditions. Predisposing factors include congenital anomalies of the vagina; a small or infantile vagina; loss of tissue elasticity in elderly primigravidas; scar tissue after the use of caustic substances in attempting to induce abortions; and unhealthy tissues, which tear like wet blotting paper.

Forceps rotation and extractions after deep transverse arrest, persistent occipitoposteriors, or face presentations often cause vaginal tears. The fact that these malpositions are frequently associated with small or male-type pelves aggravates the situation and increases the incidence and extent of the lacerations. During rotation, the edge of the blades may shear off the vaginal mucosa. Improper traction tends to overstretch the tissues and may result in a large tear. A large infant increases the danger of extensive lacerations.

The majority of vaginal tears are longitudinal and extend in the sulci along the columns of the vagina. In many cases, the lacerations are bilateral.

Technique of Repair

Lacerations of the upper vagina bleed profusely; the bleeding must be controlled as soon as possible. Because the tear is often high and out of sight, good exposure, good light, and good assistance are essential. Bleeding from the uterus may obscure the field. The placenta should be removed and oxytocics given before the repair is begun. The operator must be certain that the apex of the tear is included in the suture or hemorrhage may take place from a vessel that has retracted. If the apex cannot be reached, several sutures are placed below it, and traction on these then expose the apex of the laceration (Fig. 21-7). Figure 21-8 sutures are preferable if bleeding is profuse, or a continuous lock stitch may be used.

In some instances, the sutures do not control the bleeding adequately. The vagina should be packed tightly with a 5-yard gauze. This reduces the oozing and helps prevent the formation of hematomas. The pack is removed in 24 hours.

VESICOVAGINAL FISTULA

A fistula is an abnormal communication between two or more organs. One variety is formed between the vagina and the urinary tract—the urethra, bladder, or ureter. The classic clinical symptom of a urinary tract fistula is the painless and almost continuous loss of urine, usually from the vagina. A fistula may be confirmed by placing a tampon in the vagina and instilling a dilute solution of methylene blue dye into the urinary bladder.

Fistulas occur: (1) during childbirth, (2) during surgery, or (3) as a complication of cancer and radiation therapy. Because of improved obstetrics, most fistulas are associated with surgery, but they do occur in association with parturition in the following ways:

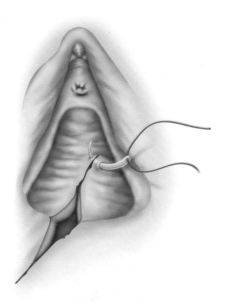

A. Introduction of first suture at highest point visible.

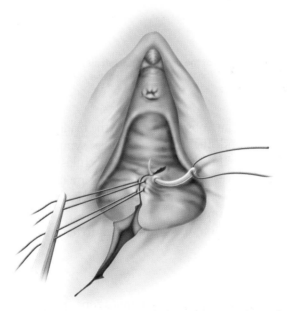

B. Traction on first suture exposes apex of the laceration and
enables top suture to be placed. The remainder of the vaginal
laceration is closed with continuous or interrupted sutures.

FIGURE 21-7. **Right mediolateral episiotomy with a high left vaginal sulcus tear.**

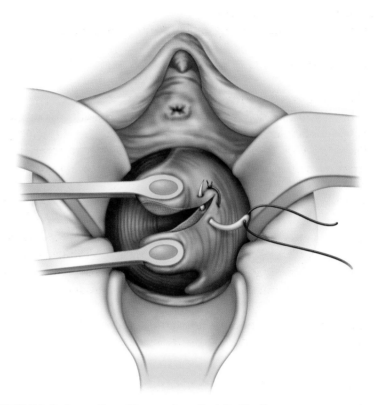

FIGURE 21-8. Laceration of the cervix on the left side. The uppermost suture is placed just above the apex of the tear. The laceration is being closed with interrupted sutures. Figure-8 sutures may be used.

1. During prolonged and obstructed labor, the bladder is trapped between the fetal head and the maternal pubic symphysis. The resulting ischemic necrosis and slough results in fistulas of varying sizes. The proximal urethra, vesical neck, and trigone are involved
2. Direct injury can occur during a difficult forceps delivery. Usually the trigone and urethra are damaged
3. During cesarean section, the bladder and ureter may be cut or torn

Management

As with most other postoperative complications, preventive medicine is paramount. Prevention of fistula formation include:

1. Optimum operative technique
2. Emptying of the urinary bladder

3. Adequate exposure of the site
4. Sharp dissection made along tissue planes with proper traction and countertraction
5. Adequate hemostasis

If the injury is recognized, an immediate two- or three-layer repair should be performed followed by continuous bladder drainage for 10 days. The principles for a successful operation include adequate exposure, dissection, and mobilization of each tissue layer; excision of the fistulous tract; closure of each layer without tension on the suture line; and excellent hemostasis with closure of the dead space.

When the damage is not recognized or if repair is not possible, continuous bladder drainage is instituted. Sometimes spontaneous closure of the fistula takes place. If the fistula persists, active treatment is delayed for 2 to 3 months to allow the edema to subside, the slough to separate, and a new circulation to be established. Repair of the fistula is then carried out. However, the loss of urine from the vagina causes considerable distress to these women, and it is difficult for them to carry on. With the use of new techniques for repair and antibiotics to control infection, early correction of the problem has been carried out with success.

RECTOVAGINAL FISTULA

This is an opening between the rectum and the vagina. The patient notices the passage of air from the vagina and an irritating vaginal discharge.

Most of these occur as the result of an unsuccessful repair of a third- or fourth-degree lacerations. The sphincter, or part of it, heals, but the area above the sphincter breaks down. A low rectovaginal fistula is the result. Occasionally, a stitch in the apex of the episiotomy enters the rectum. Most of these cause no trouble. Occasionally, healing does not take place, and a fistula develops. Treatment is by surgical repair.

HEMATOMAS

Vulva and Vagina

Puerperal Hematoma

1. *Vulvar:* The bleeding is limited to the vulvar tissue and is readily apparent

2. *Vulvovaginal*: The hematoma involves the paravaginal tissue and the vulva, perineum, or ischiorectal fossa. The extent of the bleeding is only partially revealed on inspection of the vulva
3. *Vaginal or concealed*: The hematoma is confined to the paravaginal tissue and is not visible externally
4. *Supravaginal or subperitoneal*: The bleeding occurs above the pelvic fascia and is retroperitoneal or intraligamentous

These result from rupture of the blood vessels, especially veins, under the skin of the external genitals and beneath the vaginal mucosa. The causal trauma occurs during delivery or repair. In rare cases, the accident takes place during pregnancy or very early labor, in which case a large hematoma can obstruct progress. Damage to a blood vessel may lead to its necrosis, and the hematoma may not become manifest for several days.

Most hematomas are small and are located just beneath the skin of the perineum. Although they cause pain and skin discoloration, they are not important. Because the blood is absorbed spontaneously, no treatment is required beyond ordinary perineal care.

Rupture of the vessels under the vaginal mucosa is serious because large amounts of blood can collect in the loose submucosal tissues. Many vaginal hematomas contain more than 0.5 L of blood by the time the diagnosis is made. The mass may be so large that it occludes the lumen of the vagina, and pressure on the rectum is intense. When bleeding occurs at the base of the ligament, the blood may extend in the retroperitoneal space even as far as the kidneys.

Many hematomas occur after easy spontaneous deliveries as well as in association with traumatic deliveries. The hematoma often is located on the side opposite the episiotomy. Stretching of the deep tissues can result in rupture of a deep vessel without visible external bleeding. Varicosities play a predisposing role. The possibility of a coagulation defect must be considered. Failure to achieve perfect hemostasis is an important etiologic factor.

Diagnosis

The diagnosis is made within 12 hours of delivery. Classically, the patient's complaints of pain are dismissed as being part of the usual postpartum perineal discomfort. After a time, it is realized that the pain is out of proportion to that associated with the ordinary trauma of delivery. Sedatives and analgesics do not alleviate the pain. Careful examination of the vulva and vagina reveals the swelling, discoloration, extreme tenderness, rectal pressure, and large fluctuant mass palpable per rectum or vaginam.

When large amounts of blood have been lost from the general circulation, patients have pallor, tachycardia, hypotension, and even shock. If the hematoma is high and ruptures into the peritoneal cavity, sudden extreme shock may occur, and the patient may die.

Treatment

Active treatment is not needed for small hematomas and those that are not getting larger. The area should be kept clean; and since tissue necrosis may be followed by infection, antimicrobial agents are prescribed.

Big hematomas and those that are enlarging require surgical therapy. The wound is opened; the blood clots are evacuated; and if bleeding points can be found, they are ligated. The area is packed with sterile gauze, and a counter pack is placed in the vagina. This is left in situ for 24 to 48 hours. Antibiotics are given, blood transfusion is used as needed, and the patient is observed carefully for fresh bleeding. An indwelling catheter should be placed.

Because there is a tendency for the bleeding to recur and the hematoma to reform, careful observation is necessary. Most patients do well, but several weeks pass before the wound heals and the perineum looks normal.

Broad Ligament

The danger of broad ligament hematomas is that they can rupture into the general peritoneal cavity and cause sudden and extreme shock.

Diagnosis

The diagnosis is made by vaginal examination. Rupture of the lower uterine segment must be ruled out. If the hematoma is large, the uterus is pushed to the opposite side.

Treatment

Treatment depends on the degree of bleeding. Conservative therapy consists of bed rest, antibiotics, blood transfusion, and observation. Serial blood counts are done.

In the event of continued bleeding or progressive anemia, surgical intervention is carried out. The abdomen is opened, and the blood clots are evacuated. When possible, the bleeding points are tied off, care being taken to avoid the ureter. An extraperitoneal drain may be inserted. In older women, hysterectomy is considered, and this operation may also be necessary in young women to control the situation.

LACERATIONS OF THE CERVIX

As a result of its dilatation, superficial lacerations of the cervix occur during almost every confinement. They are partly responsible for the bloody show. These small tears heal spontaneously and require no treatment.

Deep lacerations, on the other hand, can cause severe hemorrhage and shock to the extent of endangering the life of the patient. This is particularly so when the laceration extends into the lower uterine segment, where the large uterine vessels may be involved. The lacerations may be unilateral or bilateral. The most common sites are at the sides of the cervix, at 3 or 9 o'clock.

Etiology

The etiology of deep lacerations includes precipitate labor, a rigid or scarred cervix, the forceful delivery of the child through an undilated cervix, breech extraction, and a large baby.

Diagnosis

The diagnosis is made by careful inspection. We believe that the cervix and vagina should be inspected after every delivery. Some obstetricians do not agree. There is no question, however, that this examination must be made after all difficult confinements and whenever bleeding is excessive. Ring forceps are used to grasp the lips of the cervix so that the whole circumference can be visualized.

Repair

Repair of cervical tears is important. The cervix is exposed with a vaginal speculum or with retractors. An assistant is invaluable. Ring forceps are placed on each side of the laceration. Interrupted or figure-8 sutures are placed starting at the apex and are tied just tightly enough to control the bleeding and to approximate the tissues. Care must be taken not to include the ring of the forceps in the stitch. It is important that the first stitch be placed a little above the apex (Fig. 21-8) to catch any vessel that may have retracted. If the tear is high, there is danger of injury to the ureter. When the tear has extended into the lower uterine segment or into the broad ligament, repair from below may be impossible and laparotomy necessary.

Careful repair of the torn cervix is important, not only to control bleeding, but also as prophylaxis against scarring, erosions, and chronic ascending infections. Lacerations more than 1 cm in length warrant treatment.

DÜHRSSEN CERVICAL INCISIONS

Incisions of the cervix are used to facilitate immediate delivery when the cervix is fully effaced but not completely dilated. This procedure is used rarely today, the incidence being under 1 percent and being needed more often in primigravidas.

Reasons why this procedure is used so seldom today include the following:

1. The use of the intravenous oxytocin drip has reduced the incidence of failure of cervical dilatation
2. The increased safety of cesarean section has steered obstetricians away from incising the cervix
3. It is realized that nondilatation of the cervix may be an indication of disproportion
4. In the presence of fetal distress, cervical incisions and midforceps may be more than the baby can stand

Indications

Dührssen incisions may be necessary to relieve cervical head entrapment in vaginal breech delivery. However, extension of the incision can occur into the lower segment of the uterus, and the operator must be equipped to deal with this complication.

Technique

The cervix is grasped with ring forceps, and the incisions are made between them at 2, 6, and 10 o'clock (Fig. 21-9). These are extended to the junction of the cervix and vaginal wall. When the three incisions have been made, the diameter of the cervix is equivalent to full dilatation.

Because the bladder is pulled upward as effacement takes place, its dissection from the anterior vaginal wall is not required.

Appropriate measures for delivery of the infant are then carried out. The incisions are repaired with continuous, interrupted, or figure-8 sutures. Although there is rarely much bleeding, preparations to

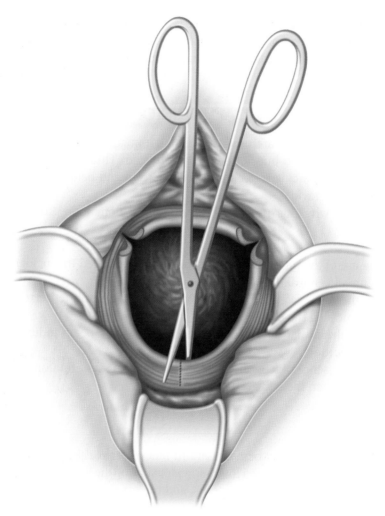

FIGURE 21-9. Dührssen cervical incisions at 2, 6, and 10 o'clock.

treat hemorrhage should be at hand. Most cervices heal well, and future pregnancies deliver normally.

ANNULAR DETACHMENT OF THE CERVIX

The anterior lip of the cervix may be compressed between the fetal head and the pubic symphysis. If this situation continues for a long time, edema, local anemia, anoxia, and even necrosis may develop. Rarely, an entire ring of cervix undergoes anoxic necrosis, and a section of the vaginal part of the cervix comes away. This is known as annular detachment of the cervix. Because the prolonged pressure has caused the blood vessels to thrombose, excessive bleeding from the cervix is unusual.

Etiology

1. Seventy-five percent of cases occur in primigravidas
2. Prolonged labor is almost always the rule
3. There is often a history of early rupture of the membranes
4. The fetal head is low in the pelvis
5. The cervix is well effaced and often quite thin. It is the external os that does not dilate. Several observers have reported that the cervix feels rigid to palpation during the first stage of labor
6. The uterine contractions are strong and efficient

Mechanism

The myometrial contractions press the presenting part against the thinned out, rigid external os; in addition, the retracting upper segment of the uterus pulls the cervix upward. This double action leads to poor circulation in the cervix, anoxia, and necrosis. A tear starts at the cervicovaginal junction, and a line of cleavage develops and continues until the separation is complete. The characteristic doughnut-shaped ring of tissue becomes detached when the cervix is about 3 to 5 cm dilated. Gross histologic examinations have revealed these cervices to be no different from the normal term organ.

Clinical Picture

The clinical picture is one of good labor obstructed by an unyielding external os. In almost every case, the fetus is delivered without difficulty once the cervical obstruction is overcome. Annular detachment is the result of true cervical dystocia.

Treatment

Because the vessels are thrombosed, serious bleeding from the stump is rare. No active treatment is needed. The rare maternal death occurs either from sepsis or from uterine bleeding associated with prolonged labor and postpartum uterine atony. Any hemorrhage that originates in the cervix must be controlled by figure-8 sutures.

Prevention

Prevention is achieved by recognizing the situation before the actual detachment takes place. When the cervix is effaced and thin, cervical incisions are indicated; delivery usually follows. If the situation is not right for the cervical incisions, cesarean section must be done.

Prognosis

Many women avoid future pregnancy. Stenosis and hematometra have been recorded. Several subsequent gestations have been delivered vaginally with no difficulty, and there have been one elective cesarean section and one abortion from an incompetent os reported.

RUPTURE OF THE UTERUS

Rupture of the uterus is a dangerous complication of pregnancy. It is responsible for 5 percent of maternal deaths in the United States and Canada and is an even greater hazard in underdeveloped countries. *The most common cause of uterine rupture is separation of a previous cesarean section scar.*

Incidence

The reported incidence in Canada is 0.075 percent. Recent publications suggest that the number of uterine ruptures is increasing and blame this fact on (1) more frequent use of cesarean section, leaving a scarred uterus for the next pregnancy; (2) careless administration of oxytocic drugs; (3) inadequate professional care during labor; and (4) poor management of labor and delivery (i.e., nonrecognition of an obstructed labor).

Types of Rupture

1. *The rupture is complete* when all the layers of the uterus are involved and there is a direct communication between the uterine and abdominal cavities. This is the common variety
2. *An incomplete rupture* includes the whole myometrium; the peritoneum covering the uterus remains intact

3. *A third variety* may occur. In this instance, the serosa and part of the external myometrium are torn, but the laceration does not extend into the cavity. A severe intraperitoneal hemorrhage may take place without the condition being diagnosed. This situation should be suspected when there are signs of an intraabdominal catastrophe during or after labor but no uterine defect is detectable on manual exploration of the uterine cavity

Site and Time of Rupture

Tears that take place during pregnancy are more often in the upper segment of the uterus at the site of previous operation or injury. During labor, the rupture is usually in the lower segment. The longer the labor, the more thinned out the lower segment and the greater the danger of rupture. The tear may extend into the uterine vessels and cause profuse hemorrhage. Tears in the anterior or posterior walls of the uterus usually extend transversely or obliquely. In the region of the broad ligament, the laceration runs longitudinally up the sides of the uterus.

It may occur during pregnancy, normal labor, or difficult labor, or it may follow labor. Most ruptures take place at or near term. Those happening before the onset of labor are usually dehiscences of cesarean section scars.

Classification

Spontaneous Rupture of the Normal Uterus
These accidents occur during labor, are more common in the lower segment of the uterus, and are the result of mismanagement and neglect. Etiologic factors include:

1. Multiparity
2. Cephalopelvic disproportion
3. Abnormal presentation (brow, breech, transverse lie)
4. Improper use of oxytocin
5. Uterine anomalies

Traumatic Rupture
This is caused by ill-advised and poorly executed operative vaginal deliveries. The incidence is decreasing. Etiologic factors include:

1. Version and extraction
2. Difficult forceps operations

3. Forceful breech extraction
4. Craniotomy
5. Excessive manual pressure on the fundus of the uterus
6. Manual dilatation of the cervix

Postcesarean Rupture

This is the most common variety seen today. It may occur before or during labor. Upper segment scars rupture more often than lower segment incisions. Although hysterograms done 3 months after operation may give an indication as to whether good healing has taken place, there is no accurate way of predicting the behavior of a uterine scar. All cesarean section scars present a hazard.

Rupture After Trauma Other Than Cesarean

The danger is that often the damage is not recognized, and the accident comes as a surprise. Included in this group are:

1. Previous myomectomy
2. Too vigorous curettage
3. Perforation during curettage
4. Cervical laceration
5. Manual removal of an adherent placenta
6. Placenta percreta
7. Endometritis and myometritis
8. Hydatidiform mole
9. Cornual resection for ectopic pregnancy
10. Hysterotomy
11. Amniocentesis during the pregnancy may lead to a weakened area in the myometrium

Silent Bloodless Dehiscence of a Previous Cesarean Scar

This is a complication of lower segment cesarean sections. Part or all of the incision may be involved. Usually the peritoneum over the scar is intact. Many of these windows are areas not of current rupture but of failure of the original incision to heal. This complication is in no way as serious as true uterine rupture. Features of this complication include:

1. Usually diagnosed during repeat cesarean section, being unsuspected before operation
2. No hemorrhage at the site of dehiscence

3. No shock
4. Hysterectomy not necessary
5. No fetal death
6. No maternal mortality

Clinical Picture

The clinical picture of uterine rupture is variable in that it depends on many factors:

1. Time of occurrence (pregnancy, early or late labor)
2. Cause of the rupture
3. Degree of the rupture (complete or incomplete)
4. Position of the rupture
5. Extent of the rupture
6. Amount of intraperitoneal spill
7. Size of the blood vessels involved and the amount of bleeding
8. Complete or partial extrusion of the fetus and placenta from the uterus
9. Degree of retraction of the myometrium
10. General condition of the patient

On a clinical basis, rupture of the uterus may be divided into four groups.

1. *Silent or quiet rupture*: The accident occurs without (initially) the usual signs and symptoms. The diagnosis is difficult and often delayed. Nothing dramatic happens, but the observant attendant notices a rising pulse rate, pallor, and perhaps slight vaginal bleeding. The patient complains of some pain. The contractions may go on, but the cervix fails to dilate. This type is usually associated with the scar of a previous cesarean section
2. *Usual variety*: The picture develops over a period of a few hours. The signs and symptoms include abdominal pain, vomiting, faintness, vaginal bleeding, rapid pulse rate, pallor, tenderness on palpation, and absence of the fetal heart. These features may have arisen during pregnancy or labor. If the diagnosis is not made, hypotension and shock supervene
3. *Violent rupture*: It is apparent almost immediately that a serious accident has taken place. Usually a hard uterine contraction is followed by the sensation of something having given way and a sharp pain in the lower abdomen. Often the contractions cease, there is a change in

the character of the pain, and the patient becomes anxious. The fetus can be palpated easily and feels close to the examining fingers. The presenting part is no longer at the pelvic brim and can be moved freely. Sometimes the uterus and fetus can be palpated in different parts of the abdomen. Fetal movements cease, and the fetal heart is not heard. The symptoms and signs of shock appear soon, and complete collapse may occur

4. *Rupture with delayed diagnosis:* Here the condition is not diagnosed until the patient is in a process of gradual deterioration. Unexplained anemia leads to careful investigation, a palpable hematoma develops in the broad ligament, signs of peritoneal irritation appear, or the patient goes into shock (either gradually or suddenly as when a hematoma in the broad ligament ruptures). Sometimes the diagnosis is made only at autopsy

Diagnosis

The diagnosis is made easily when the classic picture is present or when the rupture is catastrophic. In atypical cases, the diagnosis may be difficult. A high index of suspicion is important. In all difficult deliveries, whenever there is unexplained shock or postpartum bleeding, the interior of the cavity should be explored manually and the lower segment searched for tears.

Palpatory findings, as described in the previous section, may be pathognomonic. The fetal heartbeat is absent in most cases. A radiograph of the abdomen may demonstrate the fetus lying in the peritoneal cavity surrounded by the intestines with the shadow of the uterus to one side.

Treatment

Treatment must be prompt and in keeping with the patient's condition. Laparotomy is performed, and the bleeding is controlled as quickly as possible. Aortic compression (by the hand or by using a special instrument) is useful in reducing the bleeding until the situation can be evaluated. Most patients are critically ill and are unable to stand prolonged surgery.

In many cases, total hysterectomy may be required. If the patient is in poor condition, rapid subtotal hysterectomy may be performed. If, however, the tear has extended into the cervix, the bleeding will not be controlled by subtotal hysterectomy. In such cases, if it cannot be removed, the cervix must be sutured carefully to tie off all bleeding points.

In young women and in those who desire more children, treatment may be limited to repair of the tear. This should be done only when the uterine musculature can be so reconstituted as to ensure a reasonable degree of success and safety for a future pregnancy. In repairing the laceration, the edges of the wound are freshened and the tissues approximated carefully in two or three layers. As supportive treatment blood must be replaced rapidly. Subsequent fertility is impaired, and the reported rate of recurrent rupture is between 4 and 19 percent.

Maternal Mortality

Maternal deaths from rupture are uncommon. In 2.5 million women who gave birth in Canada between 1991 and 2001, there were 1898 cases of uterine rupture, and four of these—0.2 percent—resulted in maternal death.

Spontaneous rupture of the uterus is responsible for the largest number of deaths followed by the traumatic variety. The amount of hemorrhage is greatest in these types. The lowest death rate is associated with postcesarean ruptures, probably because these patients are observed so carefully during labor.

The main causes of death are shock and blood loss (usually over 1000 mL). Sepsis and paralytic ileus are contributory factors.

The prognosis for the mother depends on (1) prompt diagnosis and treatment, the interval between rupture and surgery being important; (2) the amount of hemorrhage and the availability of blood; (3) whether infection sets in; and (4) the type and site of the rupture.

The mortality rate is lower today because of:

1. Early diagnosis
2. Immediate laparotomy
3. Blood transfusion
4. Antibiotics
5. Reduction or elimination of traumatic vaginal operative deliveries
6. Better management of prolonged or obstructed labor

Fetal Mortality

Fetal mortality is high, ranging from 30 to 85 percent. Most fetuses die from separation of the placenta. There is a reduction of blood supply available to the fetus after the uterus has ruptured. Probably the prolonged labor before rupture plays a part in causing fetal hypoxia. Many of these

THIRD STAGE OF LABOR

babies are premature. The highest mortality rate is associated with fundal rupture in which the fetus has been extruded into the abdominal cavity.

Pregnancy After Rupture of the Uterus

Ritchie reported 28 patients who had 36 pregnancies after repair of a ruptured uterus. Repeat rupture occurred in 13 percent, with two maternal deaths. The risk of repeat rupture is:

1. Least when the scar is confined to the lower segment
2. Greater if the scar extends into the upper segment
3. Greatest in women whose original rupture occurred after classic cesarean section

Management

Cesarean section should be performed before the scar is subjected to stress.

1. Scar in lower segment: cesarean section at 39 weeks
2. Scar in upper segment: cesarean section at 36 weeks

INVERSION OF THE UTERUS

Uterine inversion is a turning inside out of the uterus. In the extreme case, the doctor may see the purplish endometrium, with the placenta often still attached. In the severe situation, the patient may be bleeding profusely, hypotensive, and sometimes pulseless. The reported incidence ranges from one in 100,000 to one in 5000 deliveries. It occurs rarely in the nongravid uterus in association with a pedunculated submucous myoma. The rate of maternal mortality rate varies between 0 and 18 percent, depending on diagnosis and management.

Hippocrates (460-370 BC) recognized uterine inversion, and Avicenna (980-1037 AD) described uterine inversion and prolapse, but it is chiefly since the time of Ambroise Paré in the 16th century that a true understanding of uterine inversion exists.

Etiology

The disorder's mechanism is not understood completely. It is believed to be related to an abnormality of the myometrium. Some inversions are spontaneous and tend to recur at subsequent deliveries; however, it occurs more often in primigravidas.

Many are caused by improper obstetric manipulations, but they may take place after normal or abnormal labor. Most often inversion is a catastrophe of the third stage of labor.

Predisposing Factors

1. Abnormalities of the uterus and its contents

   a. Adherent placenta
   b. Short umbilical cord
   c. Congenital anomalies
   d. Weakness of uterine wall at the placental site
   e. Fundal implantation of the placenta
   f. Neoplasm of the uterus

2. Functional conditions of the uterus

   a. Relaxation of the myometrium
   b. Disturbance of the contractile mechanism

Exciting Causes

1. Manual removal of the placenta

2. Increase in abdominal pressure

   a. Coughing
   b. Sneezing

3. Mismanagement of third stage of labor

   a. Improper fundal pressure
   b. Traction on the cord
   c. Injudicious use of oxytocics

Classification

Classification on the basis of stage is as follows:

1. *Acute*, occurring immediately after birth of the baby or placenta before there is contraction of the cervical ring

2. *Subacute,* beginning when contraction of the cervix becomes established
3. *Chronic,* present for more than 4 weeks

Classification on the basis of degree includes three types:

1. *Incomplete,* when the fundus is not beyond the internal os of the cervix
2. *Complete,* when the fundus protrudes through the external os of the cervix
3. *Prolapse,* in which the fundus protrudes through the vulva

Pathology

The following sequence of events may take place, especially if the diagnosis is not made:

1. Acute inversion
2. Contraction of the cervical ring and lower segment of the uterus around the encircled portion of the uterus
3. Edema
4. Reduction of blood supply
5. Gangrene and necrosis
6. Sloughing

Clinical Picture

Sometimes the symptoms are minor so the diagnosis is not made, or the condition is recognized but treatment is not carried out at the time. These are the chronic inversions. Those that cause shock and require immediate therapy are the acute ones.

In the typical case, after the birth of the infant, traction on the cord, in an effort to deliver the placenta, leads to its advancement, but if the patient is awake, there is a good deal of pain. Finally, with continued traction on the cord, the placenta is delivered, but it is attached to a bluish-gray mass that fills the vaginal outlet. This is the interior of the uterine fundus. If the diagnosis is made and replacement accomplished quickly, the patient will remain in good condition and bleeding will not be excessive.

In a different situation, the placenta is delivered with some difficulty by fundal pressure and traction on the umbilical cord. As the episiotomy is being repaired, the physician notes that bleeding is profuse. The uterus cannot be felt by the nurse as he or she tries to massage it. On vaginal examination, the cervix cannot be located. Instead, a grayish mass, oozing blood, fills the vagina. Rapid diagnosis and deinversion of the uterus will avoid blood loss, trauma, and shock. The latter will take place if the diagnosis is not made.

When the inversion is complete, the diagnosis is easy. Partial inversions may fool the observer. Classically, shock is greater than expected for the amount of bleeding. The extreme shock is probably caused by tension on the nerves of the broad ligament, which are drawn through the cervical ring, and by irritation of the peritoneum. Whenever shock is out of proportion to hemorrhage, the accoucheur should think of uterine inversion. The placenta may have separated or may remain attached. The hemorrhage may be excessive or minimal.

Diagnosis

1. High index of suspicion
2. Absence of uterine fundus on abdominal examination
3. Vaginal examination
4. Uterine rupture must be excluded

Prophylaxis

1. No attempt should be made to deliver the placenta until it has separated
2. To deliver the placenta, the Brandt maneuver is safer than the Credé method of expression by fundal pressure or by traction on the cord
3. Routine exploration of the postpartum uterus will detect a uterine inversion in its incomplete stage before it has descended through the vaginal introitus

Treatment of Acute Inversion

The aim of treatment is to replace the uterus as soon as possible. The patient should be cross-matched and blood given as necessary. Replacement of the uterus must not be delayed until shock has been treated because the latter may not be overcome as long as the uterus remains inverted.

In most cases, the placenta will have been delivered. If it is still attached, it can be removed manually or replaced with the fundus, whichever is easier. On the one hand, attempts to remove the placenta before the uterine replacement may lead to profuse bleeding. On the other hand, if the placenta has been removed, correction of the inversion will be easier because the mass that has to be replaced is smaller.

Technique of Replacement

The patient is anesthetized. In the first step of the procedure, the uterus is grasped so that the inverted fundus lies in the palm of the hand with the fingers placed near the uterocervical junction (Fig. 21-10). As pressure is exerted on the uterus, it gradually returns into the vagina. In the second step (Fig. 21-10B), the uterus is lifted out of the pelvis and held in the abdominal cavity above the level of the umbilicus. This stretches and tautens the uterine ligaments. As the uterine ligaments are placed under tension, the resultant pressure widens the cervical ring and then pulls the fundus through it. In this way, the uterus is replaced to its normal position. Success may not be immediate, and it may take 3 to 5 minutes until the uterine fundus recedes from the palm of the hand.

Treatment of Subacute Inversion

Once the cervix has contracted, immediate replacement of the uterus is no longer feasible.

1. The vagina is packed with 2-inch gauze without replacing the uterus, pushing the cervix into the abdominal cavity. A Foley catheter is inserted into the bladder
2. The patient is treated for shock, and blood transfusion is given in the amount lost
3. Antibiotics may be used
4. During the next 48 hours, fluids and electrolytes are infused in an attempt at restoring the patient to a condition suitable for surgery. At the same time, it is hoped that some uterine involution will take place
5. Laparotomy is carried out and the inversion corrected by a combined abdominovaginal operation, as for chronic inversion

Treatment of Chronic Inversion

Spinelli Procedure

Using the vaginal approach, the contracted cervical ring is incised anteriorly, so that the fundus of the uterus can be pushed back into place.

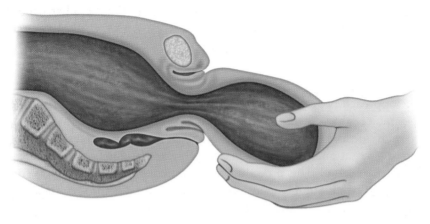

A

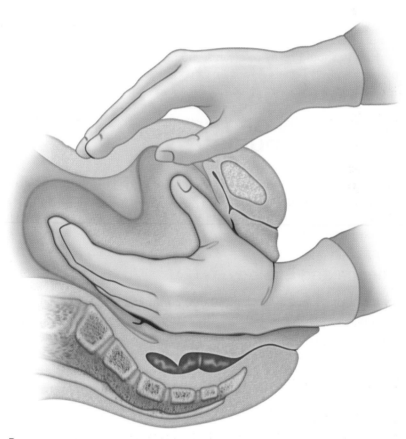

B

FIGURE 21-10. **Replacement of the inverted uterus. A,** Step 1. **B,** Step 2.

Haultain Procedure

Laparotomy is performed. The cervical ring is incised posteriorly, and the uterine fundus is drawn up.

Huntington Procedure

The approach is per abdominal incision. The surface of the uterus inside the crater is grasped with Allis forceps about 2 cm below the inversion cup on each side and upward traction exerted. As the uterus comes up through the ring, additional forceps are placed below the original ones and further traction is exerted. This procedure is continued until the inversion is completely reversed. Simultaneous pressure on the fundus through the vagina by an assistant may make the procedure easier.

Prognosis

The reported rate of recurrence is greater than 40 percent. Some authorities believe that further pregnancy should be avoided. It is probable that subsequent delivery should be by cesarean section. However, this does not obviate the problem entirely because inversion can occur even during cesarean section.

SEPARATION OF THE SYMPHYSIS PUBIS

During pregnancy, relaxation and weakening of the pelvic joints take place. This begins during the first half of pregnancy and reaches a maximum in the seventh month. Return to normal begins after delivery and is complete by the sixth month.

Incidence and Etiology

This varies from 1 in 250 to 1 in 30,000 confinements. Minor degrees of separation take place, but because the symptoms are minimal, the diagnosis is not made, and spontaneous correction follows. This accident may occur during labor or in the second half of pregnancy.

Rupture of the pubic symphysis occurs in patients with excessive relaxation of the pelvic joints. Precipitating factors include:

1. Tumultuous labor
2. Difficult forceps extractions
3. Cephalopelvic disproportion

4. Excessive abduction of the thighs at delivery
5. Any condition that might place sudden and excessive pressure on the pubic symphysis

Many cases occur after spontaneous delivery.

Pathology

There is an actual tear of the ligaments connecting the pubic bones. The rupture is usually incomplete, and a fibrocartilagenous bridge remains. Hemorrhage and edema are present. Arthritis and osteomyelitis are possible complications.

Clinical Picture and Diagnosis

The onset of symptoms is usually sudden but may not be noted until the patient tries to walk. At the time of rupture, the patient may experience a bursting feeling, or a cracking noise may be heard.

Motion of the symphysis (as by moving the legs) causes great pain. If the patient can walk, she does so with a waddling gait.

There is a marked tenderness of the pubic symphysis. Edema and ecchymosis are present frequently. A gaping defect in the joint is often palpable. Walking or pressure causes motion of the loose joint.

The diagnosis is made by the symptoms and signs. Radiography helps, but the degree of separation seen on radiologic study may not be proportional to the clinical manifestations. To be considered pathologic, the separation seen on radiographs should be greater than 1 cm.

Management of symptomatic separation must be directed at relieving the patient's discomfort and compensating for her disability. Treatment is governed by the severity of the condition. Analgesia is essential.

Some patients require prolonged bed rest, with a tight corset or peritrochanteric belt to keep the separated bones as nearly apposed as possible. The local injection of Novocain may help. While in hospital, the patient should sleep with a bed board under the mattress; she should also use a trapeze to pull herself to a sitting position so as not to strain her pelvis.

When the rupture is minor, early ambulation is permissible. When the problem is more severe, crutches should be used. Support is needed for 6 weeks. The patient must limit her use of stairs.

Surgical intervention is indicated rarely. When necessary, fusions may be carried out, often supplemented by bone grafts, bolts, and crossed wires.

SELECTED READING

ACOG Practice Bulletin, Number 71, April 2006—Episiotomy

Bodner-Adler B, Bodner K, Kaider A, Wagenbichler P, Leodolter S, Husslein P, et al: Risk factors for third-degree perineal tears in vaginal delivery, with an analysis of episiotomy types. J Reprod Med 46:752, 2004

Harris BA: Acute puerperal inversion of the uterus. Clin Obstet Gynecol 27:134, 1984

Hartmann K, Viswanathan M, Palmieri R, Gartlehner G, Thorp J, Lohr KN: Outcomes of routine episiotomy: A systematic review. JAMA 293:2141, 2005

Lee WK, Baggish MS, Lashgari M: Acute inversion of the uterus. Obstet Gynecol 51:144, 1978

Leeman L, Spearman M, Rogers R: Repair of obstetric perineal lacerations. Am Fam Physician 68:1585, 2003

Ritchie EA: Pregnancy after rupture of the pregnant uterus. J Obstet Gynecol Brit Commonw 78:642, 1971

Schrinsky DC, Benson RC: Rupture of the pregnant uterus: A review. Obstet Gynecol Surv 33:217, 1978

Shiono P, Klebanoff MA, Carey JC: Midline episiotomies: More harm than good? Obstet Gynecol 75:765, 1990

Spaulding LB, Gallup DG: Current concepts of management of rupture of the gravid uterus. Obstet Gynecol 54:437, 1979

Thacker SB, Banta HD: Benefits and risks of episiotomy: An interpretive view of the English language literature, 1860-1980. Obstet Gynecol Survey 38:322, 1983

Watson O, Besch N, Bowes WA: Management of acute and subacute puerperal inversion of the uterus. Obstet Gynecol 55:12, 1980

PART V

Complicated Labor

Cesarean Section

Darine El-Chaar

Cesarean section is an operation by which a child is delivered through an incision in the abdominal wall and the uterus. The first professional cesarean section was performed in the United States in 1827. Before 1800, cesarean section was performed rarely and was usually fatal. In London and Edinburgh in 1877, of 35 cesareans performed, 33 resulted in the death of the mother. By 1877, there had been 71 cesarean section operations in the United States. The mortality rate was 52 percent, mainly because of infection and hemorrhage.

FREQUENCY OF CESAREAN SECTION

The rate of cesarean section has risen steadily from an incidence of 3 to 4 percent 25 years ago to the present 25 to 30 percent. Not only has the operation become safer for the mother, but the number of infants damaged by prolonged labor and traumatic vaginal operations has been reduced. In addition, concern for the quality of life and the intellectual development of the child has widened the indications for cesarean section.

The largest increase in the use of cesarean section is in those cases described as having "dystocia." Although conditions such as disproportion, malpresentation, and incoordinate uterine action are included in this group, in many instances, the exact diagnosis is not made, and the diagnosis of "dystocia" represents slow progress in labor from whatever cause. The use of cesarean section for these patients is part of a more aggressive management of poor progress in labor and the abandonment of difficult midforceps operations.

Although it appears clear that the replacement of high forceps and difficult midforceps operations by cesarean section has reduced the perinatal morbidity and mortality in this area, the available evidence does not support the contention that the great expansion in the rates of cesarean section for other indications has contributed significantly to the reduction in the rates of perinatal mortality in recent years. Certainly, the more frequent use of cesarean section has led to an increase in the rate of maternal morbidity. Higher rates of repeat cesarean sections are a cause for complications with placental anomalies in subsequent pregnancies.

INDICATIONS FOR CESAREAN SECTION

Indications for cesarean section are absolute or relative. Any condition that makes delivery via the birth canal impossible is an absolute indication for abdominal delivery. Among these are extreme degrees of pelvic contraction and neoplasms blocking the passage. With a relative indication, vaginal birth is possible, but the conditions are such that cesarean section is safer for the mother, the child, or both.

Pelvic Contraction and Dystocia

1. Fetopelvic disproportion
2. Malpresentation and malposition
3. Uterine dysfunction
4. Soft tissue dystocia
5. Neoplasms
6. Failure to progress
7. Previous shoulder dystocia

Previous Uterine Surgery

1. Cesarean section
2. Hysterotomy
3. Myomectomy
4. Cervical suture

Hemorrhage

1. Placenta previa or vasa previa
2. Abruptio placentae

Toxemia of Pregnancy

1. Preeclampsia and eclampsia
2. Hypertension
3. Renal disease

Fetal Indications

1. Fetal distress
2. Previous fetal death or damage
3. Prolapse of the umbilical cord
4. Placental insufficiency (IUGR)
5. Maternal diabetes
6. Rhesus incompatibility
7. Postmaternal death
8. Maternal genital herpes
9. Prevent vertical transmission of HIV infection

COMPLICATED LABOR

Miscellaneous

1. Elderly primigravida
2. Previous vaginal repair or pelvic surgery
3. Congenital uterine anomaly
4. Poor obstetric history
5. Failed forceps or vacuum
6. Elective cesarean: cesarean delivery on maternal request

Pelvic Contractions and Mechanical Dystocia

Fetopelvic Disproportion

Fetopelvic disproportion includes a contracted pelvis, an overgrown fetus, or a relative disparity between the size of the baby and that of the pelvis. Contributing to the problem of disproportion are the shape of the pelvis, the presentation of the fetus and its ability to mold and engage, the dilatability of the cervix, and the effectiveness of the uterine contractions.

Malposition and Malpresentation

These abnormalities may make cesarean section necessary when a baby in normal position could be born per vagina. A great part of the increased incidence of cesarean section in this group is associated with breech presentation. Today more than half of babies in breech presentation are born by cesarean section. Recent guidelines are now encouraging breech delivery with specific criteria, but it is not yet routinely implemented given obstetrician inexperience with breech delivery for the past 10 years.

Uterine Dysfunction

Uterine dysfunction includes incoordinate uterine action, inertia, constriction ring, and inability of the cervix to dilate. Labor is prolonged, and progress may cease altogether. These conditions are often associated with disproportion and malpresentations.

Soft Tissue Dystocia

Soft tissue dystocia may prevent or make normal birth difficult. This includes such conditions as scars in the genital tract, cervical rigidity from injury or surgery, and atresia or stenosis of the vagina. Forceful vaginal delivery results in large lacerations and hemorrhage.

Neoplasms

Neoplasms that block the pelvis make normal delivery impossible. Invasive cancer of the cervix diagnosed during the third trimester of pregnancy is treated by cesarean section followed by radiation therapy, radical surgery, or both. Benign growth such as fibroids could also pose a problem.

Failure to Progress

This group includes such conditions as cephalopelvic disproportion, ineffective uterine contractions, a poor pelvis, a large baby, and deflexion of the fetal head. Often an exact diagnosis cannot be made and is academic in any case. The decision in favor of cesarean section is made on the failure of the labor to achieve cervical dilatation and/or fetal descent regardless of the etiology.

Previous Uterine Surgery

Cesarean Section

In 1916, E.B. Cragin expressed the opinion that in women who had had a previous cesarean section, the risk of uterine rupture was so high and the consequences of such an accident so costly that a repeat cesarean section should be performed before the onset of labor. His dictum, "Once a cesarean, always a cesarean," has been observed for many years, but the concept is being reevaluated because of the increasing incidence of cesarean section, the high rate of maternal morbidity with abdominal delivery, and the lower risk of rupture when the original incision was transverse and confined to the lower segment of the uterus. Under certain conditions, a trial of labor is permissible for women who have had a cesarean section. When successful, maternal morbidity, length of stay in hospital, and period of convalescence are reduced. The faster recovery enables the woman to participate earlier in the care of the infant, herself, and her family. Recent data suggest that about half the women who have had a delivery by cesarean section can have a trial of labor in future pregnancies (see Chapter 23).

Hysterotomy

Pregnancy in a uterus in which a previous gestation was terminated by hysterotomy is attended by danger of uterine rupture. The risk is similar to that of classical cesarean section. Hysterotomy should be avoided whenever possible, keeping in mind that the next pregnancy might necessitate cesarean section.

Extensive Myomectomy

Myomectomy in the past is an indication for cesarean section only if the operation was extensive, the myometrium disorganized, and the incision extended into the endometrial cavity. The previous removal of pedunculated or subserous fibromyomas does not call for cesarean section.

Cervical Cerclage

In some cases when there has been a cervical suture or repair of an incompetent os, cesarean section is necessary if the cerclage was performed abdominally, either by laparotomy or by a laparoscopic approach.

Hemorrhage

Placenta Previa

Cesarean section in all cases of central and many cases of marginal placenta previa has reduced both fetal and maternal mortality. Cesarean section is also indicated in suspected vasa previa in patients with a history of a low-lying placenta.

Abruptio Placentae

Abruptio placentae occurring before or during early labor may be treated by rupture of the membranes and oxytocin drip. When the hemorrhage is severe, the cervix hard and closed, or uteroplacental apoplexy suspected, cesarean section may be necessary to save the baby, control hemorrhage, prevent disseminated intravascular coagulation, and observe the condition of the uterus and its ability to contract and control the bleeding. In some cases, hysterectomy is necessary.

Toxemia of Pregnancy

These states must be considered:

1. Preeclampsia and eclampsia
2. Essential hypertension
3. Chronic nephritis

Toxemia of pregnancy may require termination of the pregnancy before term. In most cases, induction of labor is the method of choice. When the cervix is not ripe and induction would be difficult, cesarean section is sometimes preferable.

Fetal Indications

ABNORMAL FETAL HEART RATE (FHR) Fetal distress, severe bradycardia, irregularity of the FHR, or late patterns of deceleration sometimes necessitates emergency cesarean section. The rate of cesarean section is high in monitored patients. This is not surprising since the main indications for monitoring are those that predispose to fetal hypoxia. However, fetal distress is not the prime reason for increasing the rate of cesarean section. Problems associated with dystocia are the main indications for abdominal delivery. A new indication for cesarean section is described as fetal intolerance of labor. This is seen in patients who have desultory labors. Stimulation by oxytocin may result in abnormalities of the FHR. Often an emergency cesarean section is performed, but a normal baby with no evidence of asphyxia is delivered.

PREVIOUS FETAL DEATH OR DAMAGE Especially in older women who have had an intrapartum death or a child with birth injuries, cesarean section may be elected.

PROLAPSE OF THE UMBILICAL CORD Prolapse of the umbilical cord in the presence of an undilated cervix is managed best by cesarean section, provided the baby is in good condition.

PLACENTAL INSUFFICIENCY In cases of intrauterine growth restriction or postterm pregnancy, when clinical examinations and various tests suggest that the baby is in jeopardy, delivery may be necessary. If induction is not feasible or fails, cesarean section is indicated. There is an increased ability of pediatricians to resuscitate small babies and, when the need exists, cesarean section may offer these infants the best chance for survival and a good chance for normal development.

MATERNAL DIABETES Fetuses of diabetic mothers are inclined to be larger than normal, which can lead to difficult labor and delivery. Although these infants are large, they behave like premature infants and do not withstand well the rigors of a long labor. Death during labor and the postnatal period is common. In addition, there is an increased risk of stillbirth with maternal diabetes. Because of these dangers to the fetus and because a high proportion of pregnant women with diabetes develop toxemia, the pregnancy may require termination before term. When conditions are favorable and a rapid and easy labor is anticipated, induction of labor can be carried out. However, if there are urgent reasons for immediate delivery, if induction fails, or if good progress in labor is not made, cesarean section should be performed.

RHESUS INCOMPATIBILITY When a fetus is becoming progressively damaged by the antibodies of a sensitized Rh-negative mother and when induction and delivery per vagina would be difficult, the pregnancy may be terminated by cesarean section in selected cases for fetal salvage.

COMPLICATED LABOR

POSTMORTEM CESAREAN SECTION Postmortem cesarean sections were performed in Rome as early as 715 BC, when Numa Pompilius decreed that if a pregnant woman died, the fetus was to be cut out of her abdomen. The intent of the decree was not to save the life of the infant but to obviate his or her being buried with the mother. In 237 BC, the first reported infant who survived postmortem cesarean section was Scipio Africanus. He grew up to become the Roman General who defeated Hannibal. Some 15 percent of infants born in these circumstances are in good condition. Their survival depends on how soon they are delivered, their maturity, the nature and duration of the maternal illness, the performance of cardiopulmonary resuscitation on the mother, and the availability of neonatal intensive care.

HERPES VIRUS INFECTION OF THE GENITAL TRACT This is a cause of serious, often fatal, infection of the newborn infant. When genital herpes infection is present at term, the risk of clinically apparent infection in the infant delivered per vagina has been estimated at being between 40 and 60 percent. In about half of these, the infection will be severe or fatal. Herpes infection in the newborn is almost always acquired from the mother's infected birth canal, either as an ascending infection after the membranes have ruptured or during passage through the vagina. In the latter situation, there is contamination of the child's eyes, scalp, skin, umbilical cord, and upper respiratory tract. The possibility of transplacental transmission is small, certainly far less important than direct contact during labor and delivery. The greatest hazard to the baby exists when the primary genital infection occurred 2 to 4 weeks before delivery. The risk of fetal infection at term is greater during primary genital herpes infection than during recurrent genital herpes. Often it is difficult to distinguish between these two. Fetuses at risk receive some maternal antibodies transplacentally, and this may play some part in limiting infection.

All women with known recurrent genital HSV infection should be offered acyclovir or valacyclovir suppression at 36 weeks' gestation to decrease the risk of clinical lesions and viral shedding at the time of delivery and therefore decrease the need for cesarean section.

Cesarean section is indicated for women with prodrome symptoms or clinically suspicious cases of genital herpes infection at the time of labor. Although the risk of fetal infection is higher when the membranes have been ruptured for 4 to 6 hours, cesarean section should be performed in all cases of proven or strongly suspicious cases of herpes infection regardless of the duration of labor or the length of time that the membranes have been ruptured.

Breast feeding by infected mothers is permissible, provided that direct contact between the infant and infected areas in the mother is avoided. Nursing is prohibited when herpetic lesions are present on the breast.

HIV INFECTION The available evidence regarding the prophylactic role of cesarean section in preventing vertical transmission of HIV to the neonate applies only to women who have not received optimal antiretroviral therapy.

Miscellaneous

ELDERLY PRIMIGRAVIDITY Elderly primigravidity is difficult to define. Although the age varies from 35 to 40 years, other factors are equally important. These include the presence or absence of a good lower uterine segment, elasticity or rigidity of the cervix and the soft tissues of the birth canal, ease of becoming pregnant, number of abortions, fetal presentation, and coordination of the uterine powers. When all of these points are favorable, vaginal delivery should be considered. When the adverse factors are present, cesarean section may be the wiser and safer procedure.

PREVIOUS VAGINAL REPAIR Fear that vaginal delivery will cause a recurrence of cystocele, rectocele, and uterine prolapse may lead to an elective cesarean section. A history of pelvic surgery for fistulas because of inflammatory bowel disease may be an indication for cesarean section.

CONGENITAL UTERINE ANOMALY Not only does an abnormal uterus often function badly, but in the case of anomalies such as a bicornuate uterus, one horn may block the passage of the baby from the other. In such cases, cesarean section must be performed.

POOR OBSTETRIC HISTORY When a previous delivery has been difficult and traumatic with extensive injury to the cervix, vagina, and perineum or when the baby has been injured, cesarean section may be selected for subsequent births.

FAILED INSTRUMENTAL ASSISTED VAGINAL DELIVERY Failed forceps or failed vacuum delivery is an indication for cesarean section. It is wiser to turn to abdominal delivery than to drag a baby through the pelvis by force.

ELECTIVE CESAREAN SECTION OR CESAREAN DELIVERY ON MATERNAL REQUEST This is a controversial topic where some women prefer a cesarean delivery. The reasons for this include avoiding pelvic floor injury, fear of labor, convenience, and perceived reduced risk to the fetus. The National Institutes of Health held a conference on this subject, and insufficient data are available to permit recommendations currently. The conclusions drawn to date are that more research is required in this area and that cesarean section should be performed after 39 weeks of gestation and should be avoided in women desiring several children because of the risk of placental invasion in future pregnancies.

COMPLICATED LABOR

TYPES OF CESAREAN SECTION

Position of the Patient on the Operating Table

The practice of placing a wedge under the patient's right hip to tilt her to her left side at the time of cesarean section is well established. This permits the uterus and its contents to fall away from the inferior vena cava and the aorta. The return circulation from the patient's lower extremities to the right heart is improved, supine hypotension is prevented, and good placental perfusion is maintained. When difficult delivery of an impacted head (e.g., after failed forceps or vacuum or after prolonged second stage) or excessive bleeding is anticipated (e.g., placenta previa or accreta), the legs may be placed in Yellowfin stirrups to allow for abduction and enhanced surgical site access to the lower pelvis and vagina.

Skin Incisions

Vertical Incision

The skin incision used for cesarean section in an acute emergency is the midline, vertical, hypogastric incision, extending from the symphysis pubis to the umbilicus and above the umbilicus when necessary. The advantages of this approach are that it provides excellent exposure, and entry into the abdominal cavity can be made rapidly. In cases of acute fetal distress, when time is of paramount importance, the vertical incision is the one of choice.

Transverse Incision

The Pfannenstiel transverse suprasymphyseal incision is the most commonly used. The incision in the skin is semilunar just above the pubic hairline, the angles inclined slightly upward toward the anteriorsuperior iliac crests. This incision has several advantages. The cosmetic result is far better than the vertical incision, and the scar is narrow and often is partly hidden by the hair on the mons pubis. The abdominal wall, postoperatively, is stronger because of the perpendicular relationship between the incisions in the fascia, the muscles, and the peritoneum and because there is less side-to-side tension on the scar. Postoperative pain is reduced, and the patient can be active much sooner. The risk of dehiscence is low. The disadvantages of the Pfannenstiel incision are that the exposure may not be as good as with a vertical incision and the fact that the procedure is time consuming and should not be used when an acute emergency exists.

Uterine Incisions

Lower Segment of Uterus: Transverse Incision

Because it permits safe abdominal delivery even when performed late in labor and even when the uterine cavity is infected, the lower segment transverse incision (Fig. 22-1A) has revolutionized obstetric practice in the following respects:

1. It has resulted in the concepts of trial of labor, trial of oxytocin stimulation, and trial forceps
2. The need for traumatic forceps delivery has been virtually eliminated
3. The indications for cesarean section have been widened
4. Maternal morbidity and mortality rates are lower than with upper segment procedures
5. The uterus is left with a stronger scar

The lower uterine segment transverse incision is the procedure of choice. The abdomen is opened and the uterus exposed. The vesicouterine fold of peritoneum (bladder flap), which lies near the junction of the upper and lower uterine segments, is identified and incised transversely; it is dissected off the lower segment and, with the bladder, is pushed

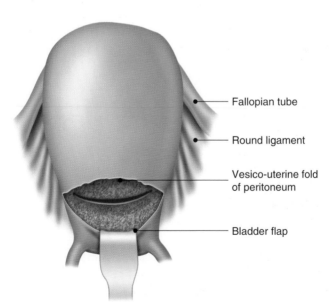

Fallopian tube

Round ligament

Vesico-uterine fold of peritoneum

Bladder flap

A. Lower segment transverse incision.

FIGURE 22-1. Cesarean section incisions.

COMPLICATED LABOR

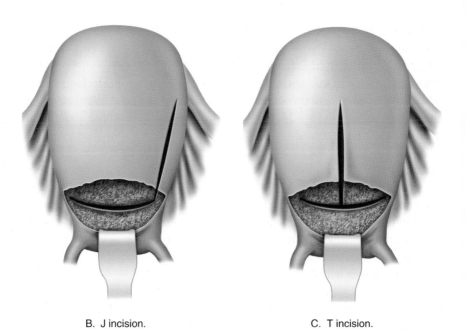

B. J incision.

C. T incision.

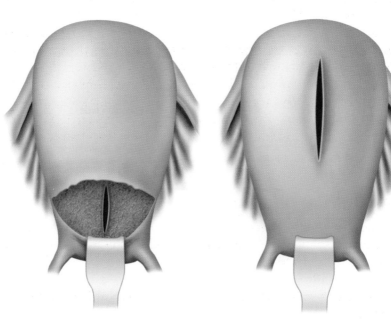

D. Lower segment vertical incision.

E. Classical (upper segment vertical) incision.

FIGURE 22-1. *(Continued)*

downward and retracted out of the way. A small transverse incision is made in the lower segment of the uterus and is extended laterally with the fingers or with bandage scissors, stopping short of the area of the uterine vessels. It is important to make a higher incision on the uterus in women with advanced or complete cervical dilatation in order to minimize lateral extension and to avoid bladder injury because it can be higher and in some cases almost to the level of the umbilicus. To avoid injury to the fetus by the sharp blade of the scalpel, this incision can be made easily by the scalpel handle. The fetal head, which in most cases lies under the incision, is extracted or expressed, followed by the body and then the placenta and membranes. The head is delivered by gently elevating it and directing it through the incision; this is assisted with transabdominal fundal pressure. In some cases, a vacuum or forceps device may be used to assist in delivery of the head.

Fundal pressure should be initiated after delivery to reduce bleeding and to aid in delivery of the placenta. The uterine incision should be clamped with ring forceps or Green-Armytage clamps to reduce vigorous bleeding until the incision is closed. The transverse incision is closed with a single or double layer of continuous #0 or #1 absorbable suture. Traditionally, the bladder flap of peritoneum is sewn back to the wall of the uterus above the incision so that this area is covered completely and isolated from the general peritoneal cavity. Many trials have suggested that omission of this step causes no further complications postoperatively and is not associated with increased adhesion formation. The abdomen is closed in layers after proper inspection to control bleeding. The closure of parietal peritoneum is not necessary because it has not shown to be of added benefit. The subcutaneous tissue is closed if it is more than 2 cm in thickness to prevent wound disruption; studies have found this to be superior to placing a subcutaneous drain (see Chapter 24).

Advantages

1. The incision is in the lower segment of the uterus. However, one must be certain it is in the thin lower segment and not in the inferior part of the muscular upper segment

2. The muscle is split laterally instead of being cut; this leads to less bleeding

3. Incision into the placenta is rare

COMPLICATED LABOR

4. The head is usually under the incision and is extracted easily

5. The thin muscle layer of the lower segment is easier to reapproximate than the thick upper segment

6. Rupture of the transverse scar in a subsequent pregnancy poses only a small threat to the mother and fetus

   a. The incidence of rupture is lower
   b. This accident occurs rarely before term. Hence, the patient is in the hospital under close observation at the onset of active labour
   c. The loss of blood from the less vascular lower segment is less than from the corpus
   d. Rupture of the low transverse incision is followed only rarely by expulsion of the fetus or by a separation of the placenta, so that there is a chance to save the baby

Disadvantages

1. If the incision extends too far laterally, as may occur if the baby is very big, the uterine vessels can be torn, causing profuse hemorrhage
2. The procedure is not advisable when there is an abnormality in the lower segment, such as fibroids or extensive varicosities
3. Previous surgery or dense adhesions that prevent easy access to the lower segment make the operation tedious
4. When the lower segment is not well formed, the transverse operation is difficult to perform
5. Sometimes the bladder is adherent to a previous scar, and it may be injured
6. On rare occasions, because of a narrow lower uterine segment or a large baby, the infant cannot be delivered through the transverse incision. To make more room, a J-shaped (Fig. 22-1B) or a T-shaped (Fig. 22-1C) extension is necessary. These should be avoided if possible because they have a weakening effect on the uterus. Future deliveries should be by repeat cesarean section

Lower Segment of Uterus: Vertical Incision

The exposure is the same as with the transverse incision. The vertical incision (Fig. 22-1D) is made with the scalpel and is enlarged with blunt scissors to avoid injury to the baby.

The vertical incision has an advantage in that it can be carried upward when necessary. This may be needed when the baby is large, when the lower segment is poorly formed such as in extreme prematurity, when there is a fetal malposition such as transverse lie, or when there is fetal anomaly such as conjoined twins. Some obstetricians prefer this incision for placenta previa.

One of the main disadvantages is that because the muscle is cut, there is increased bleeding from the incised edges of the thicker muscle in this part of the uterus. The uterus is usually closed in two to three layers to obtain excellent hemostasis; often, too, the incision extends inadvertently into the upper segment, and the value of a completely retroperitoneal closure is lost. Future deliveries should be by repeat cesarean section as the vertical incision weakens the uterine muscle and the risk of uterine rupture is increased compared to that of a transverse incision.

Classical Cesarean Section: Upper Segment of Uterus

A longitudinal midline incision (Fig. 22-1E) is made with the scalpel into the anterior wall of the uterus and is enlarged upward and downward with blunt-nosed scissors. A classical upper segment vertical uterine incision is performed for the same indications as a lower segment vertical incision, but a larger opening is required. Technical difficulty in exposing the lower segment or wanting to avoid the lower segment due to placenta accreta or previa are other indications for the upper segment procedure. The fetus and placenta are removed, and the uterus is closed in three layers. In modern times, a classical incision is rarely indicated. Future deliveries should be by repeat cesarean section as the vertical incision weakens the uterine muscle and the risk of uterine rupture is increased compared to that of a transverse incision.

Indications

1. Difficulty in exposing the lower uterine segment
   a. Large blood vessels on the anterior wall
   b. High and adherent bladder
   c. Myoma in the lower segment

2. Impacted transverse lie (back down transverse)

3. Some cases of anterior placenta previa or accreta

4. Certain uterine malformations

5. Massive maternal obesity

6. Preterm infant with underdeveloped lower uterine segment

COMPLICATED LABOR

Disadvantages

1. Thick myometrium is cut, large sinuses are opened, and bleeding is profuse
2. The baby is often extracted as a breech with greater aspiration of amniotic fluid
3. If the placenta is attached to the anterior wall of the uterus, the incision cuts into it and may lead to dangerous loss of blood from the fetal circulation
4. The incision lies uncovered in the general peritoneal cavity, and there is greater chance of seepage of infected uterine contents with resultant peritonitis
5. There is a higher incidence of adhesion formation of abdominal contents to the line of closure in the uterus
6. There is a higher incidence of uterine rupture in subsequent pregnancies

MORTALITY AND MORBIDITY AFTER CESAREAN SECTION

Maternal Mortality

The maternal mortality rate from cesarean section in the Western world continues to drop steadily. In 2008, the mortality rate for cesareans sections in the United States was 2.2 per 100,000 cesarean deliveries. It is misleading to directly compare the mortality rates of vaginal and cesarean deliveries. Women with adverse medical conditions, or higher risk pregnancies, often require a cesarean section, which can alter the mortality rates.

Factors That Add to the Risk

1. Maternal age older than 35 years
2. Grand multiparity
3. Obesity, body mass index (BMI) >30
4. Prolonged labor
5. Prolonged period of ruptured membranes
6. Numerous vaginal examinations
7. Low socioeconomic status

Causes of Maternal Death

1. Hemorrhage
2. Infection

3. Anesthesia
4. Pulmonary embolism
5. Renal failure after prolonged hypotension
6. Intestinal obstruction and paralytic ileus
7. Heart failure
8. Preeclampsia
9. Rupture of uterine scar
10. Miscellaneous causes not related to the operation (e.g., cancer)

Reasons for a Decline in Mortality Rate

1. Adequate blood transfusion
2. Use of antimicrobial drugs
3. Improved surgical methods
4. Better anesthetic techniques and specially trained anesthesiologists
5. The realization that patients with heart disease do better with vaginal delivery than with cesarean section
6. Basic treatment of preeclampsia by medical rather than by surgical methods
7. Alternative medical treatment of massive hemorrhage

Maternal Morbidity

Cesarean section is associated with significant maternal morbidity. Patients undergoing cesarean section develop operative and/or postoperative complications, some of which are serious and potentially lethal. It must be accepted that cesarean section is a major operation with the attendant risks.

Serious Complications

1. *Hemorrhage from*

   a. Uterine atony
   b. Extension of uterine incision
   c. Difficulty removing the placenta
   d. Hematoma of the broad ligament

2. *Infection*

   a. Genital tract (endometritis)
   b. Incision
   c. Urinary tract
   d. Lungs and upper respiratory tract
   e. Pelvic abscess

3. *Venous thromboembolic events and thrombophlebitis*

4. *Damage to the urinary tract,* with or without the formation of a fistula, occurs in less than 1 percent of cesarean sections. Most important is the recognition of the injury at the time it happens. Those that are discovered during the operation can be repaired immediately, and the return of normal function is likely. Late diagnosis necessitates a second operation and considerable discomfort in the interim. Postoperative pain in the flank after a difficult cesarean section with much bleeding calls for an intravenous pyelogram

   a. Bladder injury is caused mainly during the development of the bladder flap over the lower uterine segment and the displacement of the bladder caudally. In repeat cesarean section, adhesions and scar tissue from the previous operation may make the dissection difficult. Defects in the bladder caused by accidental entry are repaired with a double layer of 3-0 absorbable or delayed-absorbable suture. Drainage of the bladder is continued for 7 to 10 days. In most of these cases, when the injury is recognized and repaired, healing takes place.

   A rare complication of cesarean section is a vesicouterine fistula. This condition occurs during the performance of a low cesarean section when unrecognized injury to the bladder takes place or the bladder is included in the closure of the uterine incision. The fistula is between the bladder and the uterus at the site of the incision for the cesarean section. These patients have incontinence, the urine passing from the bladder into the uterus and thence through the cervix into the vagina. Urinary infection may develop. Investigation: (1) Methylene blue dye instilled in the bladder enters the vagina. (2) Cystoscopy reveals the site of the fistula and determines the relationship of the fistula to the ureteral orifices. (3) An intravenous or a retrograde pyelogram will evaluate the upper urinary tract.

   Because a number of these conditions will undergo spontaneous closure, a trial of conservative management is reasonable. This consists of continuous drainage of the bladder by urethral catheter and antibiotics to prevent infection. If this management fails, surgical closure of the fistula is performed. An abdominal approach is preferred. Early repair has been carried out successfully. It is probably advisable to wait, however, until uterine involution has taken place

b. Ureteral injury is caused by extension of the transverse incision in the lower uterine segment or the vagina and during attempts to control profuse bleeding in the broad ligament. The ureter may be cut, crushed, tied, or devitalized. If there is suspicion that a ureter has been injured, the bladder may be opened and the ureteral orifices inspected. One way of diagnosis is to inject 10 mL of indigo carmine intravenously and observe the efflux of blue urine from the ureters, indicating that they are intact. Or the dye may be seen in the surrounding tissue, suggesting that the ureter has been cut. If recognized, repair should be carried out immediately

5. *Intestinal complications*

a. Lacerations should be repaired immediately by a double-layer of 3-0 absorbable or delayed-absorbable suture. A general surgeon should be consulted for the injury subject to availability

b. Obstruction may be paralytic or mechanical. Volvulus accounts for some 25 percent of intestinal obstruction associated with pregnancy. The sigmoid is the most common site. Volvulus of the transverse colon, the small bowel, or the cecum occurs less frequently. The diagnosis of intestinal obstruction in post–cesarean section patients is difficult and is often delayed. The treatment is surgical

6. *Inadvertent vaginal incision* during cesarean section. The patient at risk is a parturient whose cervix is fully dilated and who has been pushing in the second stage of labor for some time. The operator, thinking he or she is making the incision in the thinned-out lower uterine segment, makes the incision into the vagina. Possible complications include injury to the bladder or ureter, vesical fistula, laceration of adjacent ligamentous structures, and hemorrhage. Management requires meticulous hemostasis, careful search for tears in the bladder, and anatomic closure of the vagina. The problem can be avoided by making the incision in the lower uterine segment above the reflection of the vesicouterine peritoneum.

Prevention of Infection

Along with the rise in the rates of cesarean section there has been an increase in the incidence of maternal febrile morbidity, infections of the endometrium and wound, and prolonged hospitalization. Maternal febrile morbidity is defined as a temperature of 100.4°F (38°C) or above occurring on any 2 of the first 10 days postpartum, exclusive of the first

COMPLICATED LABOR

24 hours. It is more common after cesarean section than after normal delivery, the incidence being anywhere between 5 and 20 percent. Antimicrobials, blood transfusions, better surgical technique, use of the lower segment operation, and improved anesthesia have all contributed to the significant decrease in post–cesarean section maternal morbidity. Preoperative administration of a broad-spectrum antibiotic 30 minutes before the skin incision has been consistently shown to significantly reduce the risk of maternal postoperative infection. This is true for both high-risk laboring patients and for patients undergoing elective cesarean delivery. There is no evidence to support the delay of antibiotics until delivery of the infant.

Antibiotic of Choice. When used prophylactically, a single antibiotic with broad-spectrum coverage against most pelvic pathogens appears to be as effective as a combination of two or more drugs and would be associated with fewer side effects. The most commonly used antibiotic is a single dose of 1 to 2 g (based on BMI) of a beta-lactam drug, either cephalosporin or extended-spectrum penicillin.

Fetal Mortality

Fetal mortality associated with cesarean section is higher than that of vaginal delivery. Some of the reasons follow.

1. Conditions such as toxemia of pregnancy, erythroblastosis, and placenta previa that require treatment by cesarean section result in premature, small infants

2. Iatrogenic prematurity. On occasion, the performance of an elective cesarean section on a date determined entirely by the menstrual history has led to the birth of a premature infant. In some cases, respiratory distress syndrome developed, and occasionally the baby died. It is important, therefore, that an accurate assessment of fetal gestational age be made before the pregnancy is terminated. Elective cesarean delivery in uncomplicated pregnancies should be scheduled at or after 39 weeks of gestational age to reduce the complications of iatrogenic prematurity. Certain situations may be exempted from this rule based on examination of risks and benefits

   Methods of achieving assessment of gestational age include:
   a. Clinical parameters, including the date of the onset of the last menstrual period, uterine size at the first prenatal visit, date of quickening,

date when the fetal heart tones were first heard using an ordinary fetal stethoscope, and date of an early positive pregnancy test result, taken in combination, correlate well with the gestational age of the fetus

b. Ultrasonography. Measurement of the crown–rump length between the 8th and 14th weeks of gestation permits dating to within ± 5 days, and by measurement of the biparietal diameter between 15 and 25 weeks, dating is possible to ± 10 days. Serial ultrasonic scans will narrow the spread

c. Amniocentesis with measurement of the lecithin-sphingomyelin (L/S) ratio in the amniotic fluid is an accurate way of determining fetal pulmonary maturity. It is, however, an invasive technique and carries a small risk. For this reason, many physicians restrict its use to situations in which other methods of determining the maturity of the fetus leave serious doubt

3. Although respiratory complications such as atelectasis and hyaline membrane disease and the respiratory distress syndrome are more common in premature infants, the incidence is higher when the premature baby is born by cesarean section

4. Conditions such as placenta previa, abruptio placentae, diabetes, preeclampsia, eclampsia, essential hypertension, chronic nephritis, and prolapse of the umbilical cord result in babies whose general condition and powers of resistance and recuperation are low. When these conditions need treatment by cesarean section, fetal mortality is increased

There has been a decline in the mortality rate of infants born both by cesarean section and by vaginal delivery. The great majority of fetal deaths are associated with prematurity. On the one hand, cesarean section has reduced the number of babies damaged by traumatic vaginal procedures. On the other hand, a number of babies are born alive who have congenital defects incompatible with continuing a reasonable existence.

Cesarean Hysterectomy

This is the performance of a cesarean section followed by removal of the uterus. Whenever possible, total hysterectomy should be performed. However, because the subtotal operation is easier and can be done more quickly, it is the procedure of choice when there has been profuse hemorrhage and the patient is in shock or when she is in poor condition for other reasons. In such cases, the aim is to finish the operation as rapidly as possible. The incidence of peripartum hysterectomy is about 0.4 to 0.8 percent of all deliveries.

Indications

1. Hemorrhage from uterine atony after failure of conservative therapy
2. Uncontrollable hemorrhage in certain cases of placenta previa and abruptio placentae
3. Placenta accreta
4. Gross multiple fibromyomas
5. Certain cases of cancer of the cervix or ovary
6. Rupture of the uterus that is not repairable
7. Severe chorioamnionitis. There is danger of the peritoneal cavity becoming infected both when the uterus is incised and from the seepage through the incision after it has been repaired. In such cases, and especially if future childbearing is not an issue, it may be safer to remove the infected uterus *if adequate antimicrobial therapy cannot be given*
8. Defective uterine scar
9. Extension of incision into the uterine vessels resulting in bleeding that cannot be stopped by ligature

Complications

1. Morbidity rate of 20 percent
2. Increased loss of blood and higher rate of blood transfusion
3. The incidence of damage to the urinary tract and the intestines is higher than with cesarean section or hysterectomy alone
4. Psychological trauma because of the loss of the uterus
5. Maternal mortality. If the conditions that create the need for cesarean hysterectomy are eliminated, the mortality rate is not higher than that from cesarean section or hysterectomy alone
6. Postoperative hemorrhage. There is a significant danger of this complication occurring. About 1 percent of patients require reoperation in the immediate postoperative period for the control of intraperitoneal bleeding

SELECTED READING

Alinovi V, Herzberg FP, Yannopoulos D, et al: Cecal volvulus following cesarean section. Obstet Gynecol 55:131, 1980

American College of Obstetricians and Gynecologists: Use of Prophylactic Antibiotics in Labor and Delivery. Washington, DC: American College of Obstetricians and Gynecologists. ACOG Practice Bulletin no. 120, 2011

Bryan B, Strickler RC: Inadvertent primary vaginal incision during cesarean section. Can J Surg 23:581, 1980

Buckspan MB, Simha S, Klotz PG: Vesicouterine fistula: A rare complication of cesarean section. Obstet Gynecol 62:645, 1983

Chervenak FA, Shamsi HH: Is amniocentesis necessary before elective repeat cesarean section? Obstet Gynecol 60:305, 1982

Cunningham FG, Gant NF, Leveno KJ, et al: Cesarean delivery and peripartum hysterectomy. In: *Williams Obstetrics*, 23rd ed. New York: McGraw-Hill, 2009

DePace NL, Betesh JS, Kotler MN: "Postmortem" cesarean section with recovery of both mother and offspring. JAMA 248:971, 1982

Eisenkop SM, Richman R, Platt LD, et al: Urinary tract injury during cesarean section. Obstet Gynecol 60:591, 1982

Lavin JP, Stephens RJ, Miodovnik M: Vaginal delivery in patients with a prior cesarean section. Obstet Gynecol 59:135, 1982

Ledger WJ: Management of postpartum cesarean section morbidity. Clin Obstet Gynecol 23:621, 1980

O'Driscoll K, Foley M: Correlation of decrease in perinatal mortality and increase in cesarean section rates. Obstet Gynecol 61:1, 1983

Park RC, Duff WP: Role of cesarean hysterectomy in modern obstetric practice. Clin Obstet Gynecol 23:601, 1980

Perkins RP: Role of extraperitoneal cesarean section. Clin Obstet Gynecol 23:583, 1980

Rayburn, WF: Prophylactic antibiotics during cesarean section: An overview of prior clinical investigations. Clin Perinatol 10:461, 1983

Society of Obstetricians and Gynaecologists of Canada: Antibiotic Prophylaxis in Obstetric Procedures. Clinical Practice Guideline No. 247. Ottawa, ON: Society of Obstetricians and Gynaecologists of Canada, September 2010.

Sullivan SA, Smith T, Chang E, Hulsey T, Vandorsten JP, Soper D: Administration of cefazolin prior to skin incision is superior to cefazolin at cord clamping in preventing postcesarean infectious morbidity: A randomized, controlled trial. Am J Obstet Gynecol 196:455.e 1–5, 2007

Wallace RL, Eglinton GS, Yonekura ML, Wallace TM: Extraperitoneal cesarean section: A surgical form of infection prevention? Am J Obstet Gynecol 148:172, 1984

COMPLICATED LABOR

Trial of Labor After Previous Cesarean Section

Darine El-Chaar

Vaginal birth after cesarean (VBAC) was first reported in 1923 when Schell described the successful vaginal delivery of 34 infants to 23 mothers who had previous cesarean sections. A trial of labor (TOL) after cesarean section should be considered in every woman presenting for care, discussing the risks and benefits of VBAC while planning the birth. The success rate of TOL ranges from 50 to 86 percent.

The decision for a TOL after cesarean section is made together by the patient and her care provider, given appropriate setting for trial of VBAC. This discussion based on the indications should be well documented in the prenatal record.

PREREQUISITES

1. A previous lower segment transverse incision with no extension as documented by the hospital record and the operative note
2. The previous indication for cesarean section no longer exists
3. Cephalic presentation
4. No disproportion
5. No previous uterine rupture
6. Expectation of a normal labor and delivery
7. No medical or obstetric complications
8. Readily available blood, operating facilities, and in-house anesthesia
9. Patient understands and accepts the risks

CONTRAINDICATIONS

1. More than one previous cesarean section
2. Previous fundal or lower segment vertical incision or a T-shaped extension
3. Previous hysterotomy or myomectomy entering the uterine cavity
4. Previous uterine rupture
5. Unknown incision
6. Advice by the surgeon who did the first operation against a TOL
7. Abnormal presentation, such as brow, breech, or transverse lie
8. Placenta previa
9. Contracted pelvis or disproportion
10. Recurring indication
11. Urgent medical or obstetric indication for delivery

12. Unavailability of blood or refusal of patient to accept blood transfusion

13. Operating room away from the delivery suite; inability to perform immediate cesarean section

14. Patient's refusal to undergo a TOL

GUIDELINES FOR MANAGEMENT

1. Ideally, the onset of labor is spontaneous

2. The patient should come to hospital immediately if:

a. She thinks that labor has begun

b. The membranes have ruptured

c. There is vaginal bleeding

3. Upon admission to the hospital:

a. The maternal–fetal status is evaluated

b. An intravenous infusion is set up

c. Blood is cross-matched and available

d. Electronic fetal monitoring is established

4. During labor:

a. The fetal heart is monitored by continuous electronic fetal monitoring

b. The uterine contractions are assessed by an electronic system or by a hand on the abdomen almost continually. Placement of an intrauterine pressure catheter can also be considered

c. Maternal vital signs are checked every 15 minutes

d. The patient is never left unattended

e. The physician must be on the labor floor at all times

f. Labor should progress normally

5. Although the use of oxytocin to stimulate labor is not contraindicated, it must be used with great care and only in selected cases. There is insufficient evidence about the safety of prostaglandins in TOL after cesarean section

6. If labor induction is indicated, mechanical methods using amniotomy or Foley catheters are preferable

7. Misoprostol is contraindicated for cervical ripening with previous cesarean section. All prostaglandin agents are associated with an increased risk of uterine rupture

8. There has been concern that epidural block might mask the symptoms and signs of impending or actual rupture of the uterus. This does not appear to be justified, however, and epidural block is recommended in case of emergency surgery or intervention

9. Delivery should be spontaneous or by low forceps or vacuum. Difficult vaginal operations are contraindicated

10. After the delivery, the cavity of the uterus is explored for evidence of rupture only in cases when signs or symptoms are suggestive of uterine rupture

11. The TOL continues until vaginal delivery occurs or cesarean section is performed

12. The main indications for discontinuing the TOL and performing cesarean section are:
    a. Arrest of progress
    b. Atypical or abnormal fetal heart rate pattern
    c. Suspicion of uterine dehiscence or uterine rupture

SIGNS OF UTERINE RUPTURE

Uterine rupture is the complete separation of myometrium and can be also associated with expulsion of fetal parts. This is a situation that requires an immediate cesarean section. The most common presentation of a uterine rupture is an abnormal fetal heart rate. Other signs are decrease in strength of contractions, loss of presenting part on digital examination, abdominal pain outside of contractions, vaginal bleeding, hematuria, or maternal instability.

RESULTS AND SAFETY

Recent meta-analysis and reviews indicated that properly conducted vaginal delivery after cesarean section in a previous pregnancy is relatively safe.

1. The incidence of uterine rupture ranged from 0.2 to 1.5 percent. The risk increases with vertical incision and T-shaped incision. The risk of rupture decreases with each successful VBAC

2. Rates of maternal deaths reported due to uterine rupture are very slim to nonexistent

3. Perinatal mortality associated with uterine rupture ranged from 0.02 to 0.58 percent

4. Approximately 70 to 80 percent of patients whose indication for the first cesarean section is nonrecurring can be expected to safely deliver vaginally. This rate is reduced in patients whose prior cesarean section was performed for cephalopelvic disproportion

5. Patients with a previous vaginal delivery seem to have a better prognosis for successful vaginal birth than those without a previous vaginal delivery

6. A classic cesarean section scar increases the probability of uterine rupture in a subsequent pregnancy, the rupture is more likely to be complete, and the incidence of fetal death is higher

7. A TOL is highly acceptable to most patients

OTHER CONSIDERATIONS

1. Data suggest that a TOL in patients with more than one previous cesarean may be successful but is associated with a higher risk of rupture

2. External cephalic version is not contraindicated with previous cesarean section

3. Multiple gestation is not a contraindication for TOL after cesarean section

4. Neither diabetes nor fetal macrosomia are a contraindication for TOL after cesarean

5. It is recommended that the interval between trial of vaginal birth and cesarean section be more than 24 months because there is an increased risk of rupture with a shorter interval

6. Induction of labor for postdates is not contraindicated, however, mechanical methods of induction of labor are preferred

7. A double layer closure of the uterus is associated with a lower risk of uterine rupture in a TOL after cesarean

8. Obesity is associated with a lower success rate of VBAC (see Chapter 24)

COMPLICATED LABOR

SELECTED READING

American College of Obstetricians and Gynecologists: Vaginal birth after previous cesarean delivery. Washington (DC): American College of Obstetricians and Gynecologists; 2010 Aug. 14 p. (ACOG practice bulletin; no. 115).

Cahill A, Stamilio DM, Paré E, Peipert JP, Stevens EJ, Nelson DB, et al: Vaginal birth after cesarean (VBAC) attempt in twin pregnancies: is it safe? Am J Obstet Gynecol 193:1050, 2005

Chauhan SP, Martin JN Jr, Henrichs CE, Morrison JC, Magann EF: Maternal and perinatal complications with uterine rupture in 142,075 patients who attempted vaginal birth after cesarean delivery: A review of the literature. Am J Obstet Gynecol 189:408, 2003

Macones GA, Peipert J, Nelson DB, Odibo A, Stevens EJ, Stamilio DM, et al: Maternal complications with vaginal birth after cesarean delivery: a multicenter study. Am J Obstet Gynecol 193:1656, 2005

Society of Obstetricians and Gynaecologists of Canada: Vaginal birth after previous Caesarean birth. Clinical Practice Guideline No. 155. Ottawa, ON: SOGC; February 2005

CHAPTER 24

Obesity in Pregnancy

Darine El-Chaar

Rates of obesity are continuing to rise dramatically in developed countries, including an increased prevalence of morbid obesity (body mass index [BMI] >35). This trend has led to a concurrent increase in health concerns for women of reproductive age, and it is now well established that weight gain and obesity cause major comorbidities in pregnancy that contribute to adverse maternal and neonatal outcomes.

DEFINITION OF OBESITY

The Institute of Medicine recommends use of BMI to classify maternal weight groups, using prepregnancy height and weight. According to the classification by the World Health Organization, obesity is defined as a BMI above 29 kg/m^2. Other definitions of obesity found in the literature include women who are 110% to 120% of their ideal body weight or weigh more than 91 kg (200 lb).

WEIGHT GAIN IN PREGNANCY

To reduce risk and complications of weight gain in pregnancy, women should set pregnancy weight goals according to Table 24-1.

TABLE 24-1: PREGNANCY WEIGHT GAIN ACCORDING TO BMI

	BMI (kg/m^2)	Weight Gain (kg)	Weight Gain (lb)
Underweight	<18.5	12.5-18	28-40
Normal weight	18.5-24.9	11.5-16	25-35
Overweight	25.0-34.9	7-11.5	15-25
Obese	>30	5-9	11-20

BMI, body mass index.
Adapted from: Weight Gain During Pregnancy: Re-examining the Guidelines. Institute of Medicine (US) and National Research Council (US) Committee to Reexamine IOM Pregnancy Weight Guidelines, Rasmussen KM, Yaktine AL (Eds), National Academies Press (US), 2009.

ABNORMALITIES OF LABOR

Obese mothers have an increased incidence of medical complications, such as hypertension and diabetes mellitus. Obese mothers also have a higher rate of predisposing medical issues, which is what contributes to a higher rate of labor induction in this group.

There is still conflicting and limited studies on labor characteristics in obese gravid women. The best evidence suggests that obese women have longer labors. In a cohort study of nulliparous women, as maternal weight increased, the rate of cervical dilatation decreased, and the induction to delivery interval was longer. Increased duration of labor does not seem to be due to maternal poor expulsive efforts. A recent study showed that obese nulliparous women were found to have a higher rate of cesarean section in the first but not the second stage of labor. Therefore, pushing out the baby is not the issue, but getting to the second stage is.

Furthermore, numerous studies have associated obesity in pregnancy with higher rates of cesarean sections. The underlying mechanism leading to increased cesarean delivery rates in obese patients remains unclear. However, data suggest that decreased uterine contractility and higher induction rates in obese women may contribute to this phenomenon. There is also an increased rate of elective cesarean section because of adverse maternal outcomes, fetal macrosomia, or a scheduled repeat surgery given history of previous cesarean. Observational research has consistently reported that vaginal birth after cesarean section is decreased in obese pregnant women. Obstetricians may also be reluctant to perform operative vaginal delivery on obese patients given the increased risk of shoulder dystocia caused by macrosomia, which is often seen in infants of obese mothers.

FETAL GROWTH AND NEONATAL OUTCOME

The mean birthweight of infants born to obese mothers is greater. The incidence of macrosomia (>4000 g) in obese women is almost twice that of nonobese women. Fetal macrosomia is associated with an increased risk of shoulder dystocia, malpresentation, and hemorrhage and higher degree perineal and vaginal lacerations. The incidence of low birthweight babies (<2500 g) in obese women is reduced by half.

Maternal obesity has been associated with an increase in congenital anomalies, specifically neural tube defects. Perinatal outcomes are also affected, with an increased risk in stillbirth with a higher prepregnancy BMI.

COMPLICATED LABOR

CESAREAN SECTION IN OBESE WOMEN

Meta-analysis studies have shown that obesity increases the risk of both elective and emergency cesarean delivery. Major surgery of any type in the obese patient is associated with an increase of intra and postoperative complications. In pregnancy, there are special concerns, such as emergency delivery, prolonged operative time, increased blood loss, wound infection and endomyometritis, and thromboembolism. The procedure should be performed without delay if obstetric indications are present.

Care of the Skin

Preoperative care of the skin including cleansing and local therapy of intertrigo is important.

Prophylactic Antibiotics

The incidence of wound infection is high. Obesity increases the risk of serious maternal sepsis after cesarean section. Hence, prophylactic antibiotics should be prescribed for these patients in higher dose according to their current weight.

Thromboprophylaxis

The incidence of thrombosis and embolism is higher in obese patients. Reasons for this include prolonged operative time and the postoperative period of immobilization. Low-dose heparin may reduce the danger of thrombus formation and is indicated in massively obese women who undergo cesarean section. Subcutaneous injection of heparin, low-molecular-weight heparin, or dalteparin in appropriate doses are among the choices available based on institution preference; they should be administered until the patient is fully ambulatory. This prophylactic dose is not associated with increased maternal bleeding.

Anesthesia

Because of the increased incidence of medical problems including chronic hypertension, preeclampsia, coronary artery disease, diabetes mellitus, and pulmonary insufficiency, anesthesia in obese patients may be difficult. Consultation with the anesthetist should, when possible, be obtained well before the operation.

Respiratory Function

In obese women, total respiratory compliance is reduced because of a heavy chest wall and increased abdominal pressure on the diaphragm. The amount of work needed to breathe is increased. The residual volume and functional residual capacity are lower.

Choice of Anesthesia

Emergency Cesarean Section. In this situation, general anesthesia may be best given time involvement in regional anesthesia.

Nonemergency Cesarean Section. Because of the reduction in respiratory function, regional anesthesia does offer certain advantages and is the preferred choice, even though placing the catheter may be difficult in obese women. Techniques to improve successful regional anesthesia in obese women are being developed using ultrasound guidance.

Abdominal Wall Incisions

Pfannenstiel (Transverse) Incision

The transverse incision is demanded by patients because of the cosmetic result. It is performed after the panniculus has been retracted cephalad.

Advantages.

1. Once the panniculus has been retracted, the amount of subcutaneous adipose tissue is less than in nonobese patients
2. The closure is more secure because the abdominal muscles tend to pull together the sides of the incision
3. Postoperative pain is less than with the vertical incision, and this facilitates early mobility and deep breathing
4. As a rule, transverse incisions heal well

Disadvantages

1. The area of the transverse incision is warm and moist, is difficult to clean, there is a high growth of bacteria, and intertrigo is common
2. Delivery of a large baby may be difficult
3. The vertical incision can be enlarged to make more room; the transverse incision cannot
4. Retraction of the panniculus may have an adverse effect on maternal cardiovascular functions. However, there is no clear evidence of this
5. The transverse incision takes longer

Vertical Incision

1. Low
2. High, periumbilical

These carry the same advantages and disadvantages except that in the upper abdomen, the layer of subcutaneous tissue that has to be cut is much less. The lower uterine segment can be reached with either incision.

Advantages. Speed: It takes less time to enter the abdominal cavity.

Disadvantages

1. There is an increased risk of dehiscence compared with the transverse incision
2. There is more pain
3. The patient is less mobile

Closure of the Incision
Special attention is needed in obese patients.

Transverse Incision. The standard layered closure is adequate.

Midline Vertical Incision. Some surgeons advocate a layered closure with the addition of through-and-through retention sutures. Others prefer the use of internal retention sutures of the Smead-Jones variety (Fig. 24-1).

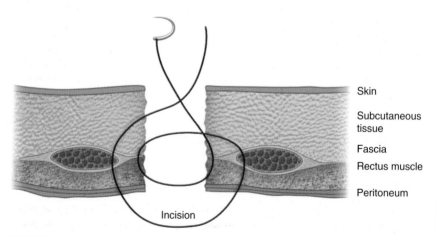

FIGURE 24-1. Smead-Jones closure.

Subcutaneous Tissue. The placing of surgical drains at the time of closure is sometimes important in obese patients. This can be accomplished by a Hemovac drain placed through a small puncture wound lateral to the incision and extending the suction catheter the entire length of the incision above the fascia. Another method is to lay a small Penrose drain in the subcutaneous layer, making it exit through one end of the incision, and removing it in 24 hours. This ensures that serum and liquefied adipose tissue, good culture media, are removed from the wound. Studies looking at the benefit of a drain have not found an improvement in wound infections and complications. However, recent studies have also initiated the practice of closing the subcutaneous tissue, when it is thicker than 2 cm, with interrupted absorbable sutures to reduce the risk of seromas and hematomas. This has been shown to improve outcomes.

Postoperative Complications

1. Longer postoperative recovery period
2. Wound infection
3. Wound dehiscence
4. Atelectasis
5. Pulmonary embolism or deep venous thrombosis
6. Increased maternal morbidity and mortality rates

SELECTED READING

Chauhan SP, Magann EF, Carroll CS, Barrilleaux PS, Scardo JA, Martin JN Jr: Mode of delivery for the morbidly obese with prior cesarean delivery: Vaginal versus repeat cesarean section. Am J Obstet Gynecol 185:349, 2001

Crane JM, White J, Murphy P, Burrage L, Hutchens D: The effect of gestational weight gain by body mass index on maternal and neonatal outcomes. J Obstet Gynaecol 31:28, 2009

Davies GA, Maxwell C, McLeod L, Gagnon R, Basso M, Bos H, et al: SOGC Clinical Practice Guidelines: Obesity in pregnancy. Int J Gynaecol Obstet 110:167, 2010

Fyfe EM, Anderson NH, North RA, Chan EH, Taylor RS, Dekker GA, McCowan LM: Risk of first-stage and second-stage cesarean delivery by maternal body mass index among nulliparous women in labor at term. Obstet Gynecol 117:1315, 2011

Gross TL: Operative considerations in the obese pregnant patient. Clin Perinatol 10:411, 1983

Institute of Medicine, National Research Council: Weight Gain During Pregnancy: Reexamining the Guidelines. Washington, DC: National Academies Press, 2009

Kore S, Vyavaharkar M, Akolekar R, Toke A, Ambiye V: Comparison of closure of subcutaneous tissue versus non-closure in relation to wound disruption after abdominal hysterectomy in obese patients. J Postgrad Med 46:26, 2000

COMPLICATED LABOR

Robinson HE, O'Connell CM, Joseph KS, McLeod NL: Maternal outcomes in pregnancies complicated by obesity. Obstet Gynecol 106:1357, 2005

Vahratian A, Zhang J, Troendle JF, Sciscione AC, Hoffman MK: Labor progression and risk of cesarean delivery in electively induced nulliparas. Obstet Gynecol 105:698, 2005

Weiss JL, Malone FD, Emig D, Ball RH, Nyberg DA, Comstock CH, Saade G, et al: Obesity, obstetric complications and cesarean delivery rate—a population-based screening study. Am J Obstet Gynecol 190:1091, 2004

World Health Organization: BMI Classification. *http://apps.who.int/bmi/index.jsp?introPage=intro_3.html,* 2012

CHAPTER 25

Breech Presentation

Jessica Dy
Darine El-Chaar

GENERAL CONSIDERATIONS

Definition

Breech presentation is a longitudinal lie with a variation in polarity. The fetal pelvis is the leading pole. The denominator is the sacrum. A right sacrum anterior (RSA) is a breech presentation where the fetal sacrum is in the right anterior quadrant of the mother's pelvis and the bitrochanteric diameter of the fetus is in the right oblique diameter of the pelvis (Fig. 25-1).

Incidence

Breech presentation at delivery occurs in 3 to 4 percent of pregnancies. However, before 28 weeks of gestation, the incidence is about 25 percent. As term gestation approaches, the incidence decreases. In most cases, the fetus converts to the cephalic presentation by 34 weeks of gestation.

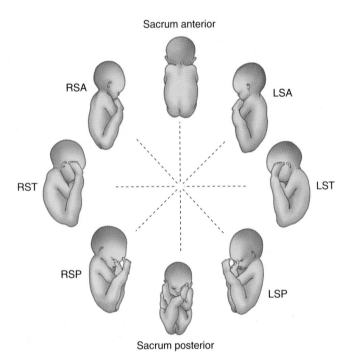

FIGURE 25-1. Positions of breech presentation. LSA, left sacrum anterior; LSP, left sacrum posterior; LST, left sacrum transverse; RSA, right sacrum anterior; RSP, right sacrum posterior; RST, right sacrum transverse.

Etiology

As term approaches, the uterine cavity, in most cases, accommodates the fetus best in a longitudinal lie with a cephalic presentation. In many cases of breech presentation, no reason for the malpresentation can be found and, by exclusion, the cause is ascribed to chance. Some women deliver all their children as breeches, suggesting that the pelvis is so shaped that the breech fits better than the head.

Breech presentation is more common at the end of the second trimester than near term; hence, fetal prematurity is associated frequently with this presentation.

Maternal Factors

Factors that influence the occurrence of breech presentation include (1) the uterine relaxation associated with high parity; (2) polyhydramnios, in which the excessive amount of amniotic fluid makes it easier for the fetus to change position; (3) oligohydramnios, in which, because of the small amount of fluid, the fetus is trapped in the position assumed in the second trimester; (4) uterine anomalies; (5) neoplasms, such as leiomyomata of the myometrium; (6) while contracted pelvis is an uncommon cause of breech presentation, anything that interferes with the entry of the fetal head into the pelvis may play a part in the etiology of breech presentation.

Placental Factors

Placental site: There is some evidence that implantation of the placenta in either cornual-fundal region tends to promote breech presentation. There is a positive association of breech with placenta previa.

Fetal Factors

Fetal factors that influence the occurrence of breech presentation include multiple pregnancy, hydrocephaly, anencephaly, chromosomal anomalies, and intrauterine fetal death.

Notes and Comments

1. The patient commonly feels fetal movements in the lower abdomen and may complain of painful kicking against the rectum, vagina, and bladder
2. Engagement before the onset of labor is uncommon. The patient rarely experiences lightening

COMPLICATED LABOR

3. The uneven fit of breech to pelvis predisposes to early rupture of the membranes, with a danger of umbilical cord prolapse. The incidence of the latter, which is 4 to 5 percent, is higher with footling breeches. It is wise, therefore, when the bag of waters breaks to make a sterile vaginal examination to determine the exact state of the cervix and to make certain that the cord has not prolapsed

4. In theory, the breech is a poor dilator in comparison with the well-flexed head, and labor, descent, and cervical dilatation are believed to take longer. Although this is true in some cases, the mean duration of labor of 9.2 hours in primigravidas and 6.1 hours in multiparas suggests that in the majority of cases, labor is not prolonged

5. In frank breeches, the baby's lower limbs, which are flexed at the hips and extended at the knees, lie anterior to and against the baby's abdomen. This has the effect of a splint and by decreasing the maneuverability of the baby may result in delay or arrest of progress

6. On the one hand, a frank breech has the disadvantage of a large and less maneuverable presenting part and may have difficulty passing through the pelvis. On the other hand, it dilates the soft parts to the greatest degree and makes the most room for the head. The small footling breech slips through the pelvis easily but makes less provision for the after-coming head

7. One of the dangers to a fetus in breech presentation is that the largest and least compressible diameter comes last

8. There is an added risk in premature infants because the head is relatively larger in proportion to the rest of the body than in full-term babies. Thus, although the small body slips through with no difficulty, it does not dilate the soft parts sufficiently to allow the head to pass easily

9. Because the posterior segment of the pelvis is roomier than the anterior segment, the posterior parts of the baby are usually born first

10. Because of the rapid passage of the head through the pelvis, there is no time for molding to take place. The fetal head is round and symmetrical

11. A baby that lies in utero as a frank breech lies with his or her hips flexed and the feet near his or her face for some time after birth

12. The external genitalia are edematous

13. The passage of meconium in a breech presentation does not have the same significance of fetal distress as in vertex presentation. The meconium is squeezed out of the intestine by the uterine contractions pressing the lower part of the baby's body against the pelvis

CLASSIFICATION

There are four types of breech presentation:

1. *Complete*: Flexion at the thighs and knees (Fig. 25-2A)
2. *Frank*: Flexion at the thighs; extension at the knees. This is the most common variety and includes almost two-thirds of breech presentations (Fig. 25-2B)
3. *Footling*: Single or double with extension at thighs and knees. The foot is the presenting part (Fig. 25-2C)

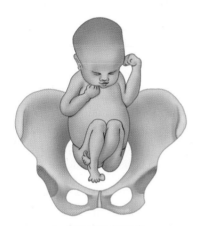

A. Complete breech.

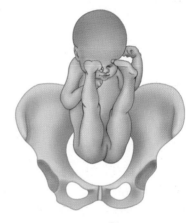

B. Frank breech.

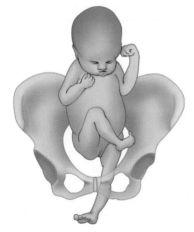

C. Footling breech.

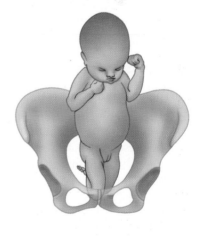

D. Kneeling breech.

FIGURE 25-2. Attitudes of breech presentation.

4. *Kneeling*: Single or double with extension at the thighs and flexion at the knees. The knee is the presenting part (Fig. 25-2D)

RIGHT SACRUM ANTERIOR

Diagnosis of Position

Abdominal Examination

1. The lie is longitudinal (Fig. 25-3A)
2. A soft, irregular mass lies over the pelvis and does not feel like the head. One suspects breech. In a frank breech, the muscles of the thighs are drawn taut over the underlying bones, giving an impression of hardness not unlike the head and leading to diagnostic errors
3. The back is on the right near the midline. The small parts are on the left, away from the midline, and posterior
4. The head is felt in the fundus of the uterus. If the head is under the liver or the ribs, it may be difficult to palpate. The head is harder and more globular than the breech, and sometimes it can be balloted. Whenever a ballotable mass is felt in the fundus, a breech presentation should be suspected
5. There is no cephalic prominence, and the breech is not ballotable

Fetal Heart

The fetal heart tones are heard loudest at or above the umbilicus and on the same side as the back. In RSA the fetal heart is heard best in the right upper quadrant of the maternal abdomen. Sometimes the fetal heart is heard below the umbilicus; hence, the diagnosis made by palpation should not be changed because of the location of the fetal heart.

Vaginal Examination

1. The presenting part is high
2. The smooth, regular, hard head with its suture lines and fontanels is absent. This negative finding suggests a malpresentation
3. The presenting part is soft and irregular. The anal orifice and the ischial tuberosities are in a straight line (Fig. 25-3B). The breech may be confused with a face
4. Sometimes in frank breeches the sacrum is pulled down and is felt by the examining finger. It may be mistaken for the head because of its bony hardness
5. The sacrum is in the right anterior quadrant of the pelvis, and the bitrochanteric diameter is in the right oblique
6. Sometimes a foot is felt and must be distinguished from a hand

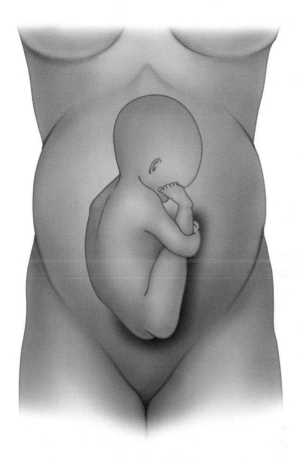

A. Abdominal view.

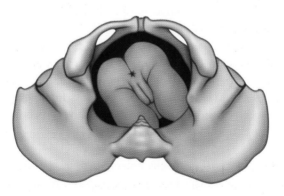

B. Vaginal view.

FIGURE 25-3. Right sacrum anterior.

Ultrasonography

This is an important tool in the management of breech presentation, especially in the following areas: (1) confirmation of the clinical diagnosis; (2) diagnosis of hyperextension of the fetal head; (3) evaluation of the size of the fetal head; (4) estimation of fetal weight; (5) diagnosis of major congenital anomalies, such as hydrocephaly, anencephaly, spina bifida. If ultrasound is not available, cesarean delivery is recommended.

MECHANISMS OF LABOR: BREECH PRESENTATIONS

Cephalic and breech presentations are similar to triangles. When the head presents, the base of the triangle leads the way: The largest and most unyielding part of the baby comes first, and the parts that follow are progressively smaller. When the breech presents, on the other hand, the apex of the triangle comes first, and the succeeding parts are progressively bigger, with the relatively large head being last. In cases of cephalopelvic disproportion, by the time it is realized that the head is too big for the mother's pelvis, the rest of the baby has been born, and vaginal delivery must be carried on, with sad results for the baby.

In breech presentations, there are three mechanisms of labor: (1) the buttocks and lower limbs, (2) the shoulders and arms, and (3) the head.

Mechanism of Labor: RSA

Buttocks and Lower Limbs

Descent. Engagement has been achieved when the bitrochanteric diameter has passed through the inlet of the pelvis. In RSA, the sacrum is in the right anterior quadrant of the maternal pelvis, and the bitrochanteric diameter is in the right oblique diameter of the pelvis (Figs. 25-4A and B). Because the breech is a less efficient dilator than the head, descent is slow, and the breech may remain high until labor has been in progress for some time. In many instances, the breech does not come down until the cervix is fully dilated and the membranes are ruptured.

Flexion. To facilitate passage of the breech through the pelvis, lateral flexion takes place at the waist. The anterior hip becomes the leading part. When the breech is frank, the baby's legs act as a splint along the body

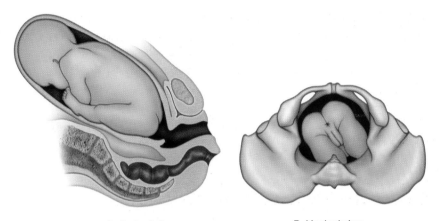

A. Lateral view.   B. Vaginal view.

FIGURE 25-4. **Right sacrum anterior: onset of labor.**

and, by reducing lateral flexion and maneuverability, may prevent descent into the pelvis.

Internal Rotation of Breech. The anterior hip meets the resistance of the pelvic floor and rotates forward, downward, and toward the midline (Figs. 25-5A and B). The bitrochanteric diameter rotates 45° from the right oblique diameter of the pelvis to the anteroposterior (AP). The sacrum turns away from the midline, from the right anterior quadrant to the right transverse (RSA to RST).

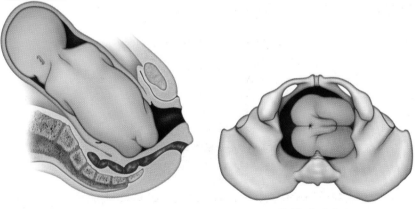

A. Lateral view.   B. Vaginal view.

FIGURE 25-5. **Descent and internal rotation of the buttocks.**

Birth of the Buttocks by Lateral Flexion. The anterior hip impinges under the pubic symphysis, lateral flexion occurs, and the posterior hip rises and is born over the perineum. The buttocks then fall toward the anus, and the anterior hip slips out under the symphysis (Fig. 25-6).

Shoulders and Arms

Engagement. Engagement of the shoulders takes place in the right oblique diameter of the pelvis as the sacrum rotates RST to RSA (Fig. 25-7A).

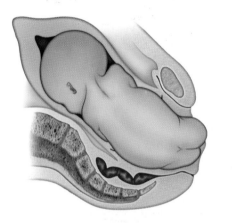
A. Breech crowning.

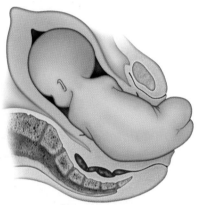
B. Birth of posterior buttock.

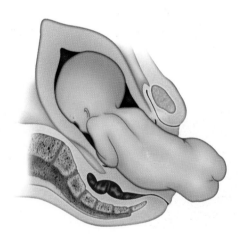
C. Birth of anterior buttock.

FIGURE 25-6. Birth of the buttocks.

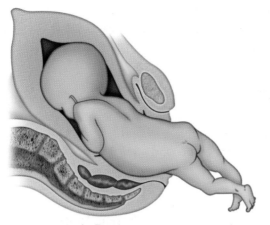

A. Feet born; shoulders engaging.

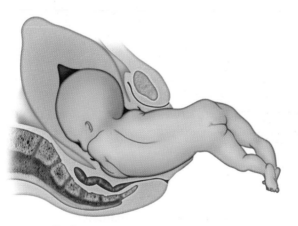

B. Descent and internal rotation of shoulders.

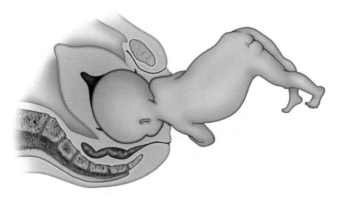

C. Posterior shoulder born; head has entered the pelvis.

FIGURE 25-7. **Birth of the shoulders.**

Internal Rotation of the Shoulders. The anterior shoulder rotates under the symphysis, and the bisacromial diameter turns 45° from the right oblique to the AP diameter of the outlet. The sacrum goes along, RSA to RST (Fig. 25-7B).

Birth of Shoulders by Lateral Flexion. The anterior shoulder impinges under the symphysis, and the posterior shoulder and arm are born over the perineum as the baby's body is lifted upward (Fig. 25-7C). The baby is then lowered, and the anterior shoulder and arms pass out under the symphysis.

Head

Descent and Engagement. When the shoulders are at the outlet, the head is entering the pelvis (Fig. 25-8A). It enters the pelvis with the sagittal suture in the left oblique diameter. The occiput is in the right anterior quadrant of the pelvis.

Flexion. Flexion of the head takes place just as in any other presentation. It is important that flexion is maintained.

Internal Rotation. The head strikes the pelvic floor and rotates internally so that it comes to the outlet with the sagittal suture in the AP diameter, the brow in the hollow of the sacrum, and the occiput under the symphysis (Fig. 25-8B). The sacrum rotates toward the pubis so that the back is anterior.

Birth of the Head by Flexion. The diameters are the same as in occipitoanterior positions but in reverse order. The nape of the neck pivots under the symphysis and the chin, mouth, nose, forehead, bregma, and occiput are born over the perineum by a movement of flexion (Fig. 25-8C).

Mechanism of Labor: Sacrum Directly Anterior

Descent
Engagement takes place with the bitrochanteric diameter in the transverse diameter of the inlet. The sacrum is directly anterior behind the symphysis pubis (SA).

Flexion
Flexion is the same as in RSA.

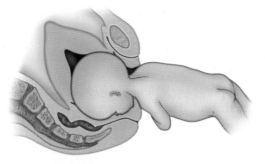

A. Anterior shoulder born, descent of head.

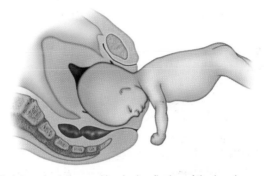

B. Internal rotation and beginning flexion of the head.

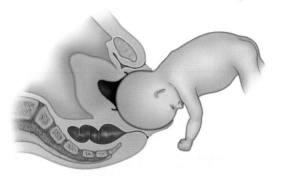

C. Flexion of the head complete.

FIGURE 25-8. **Birth of the head.**

Internal Rotation

The bitrochanteric diameter rotates 90° from the transverse diameter of the pelvis to the AP. The sacrum turns away from the midline to the transverse (SA to RST). The rest of the mechanism of labor is the same as in RSA.

Mechanism of Labor: Sacrum Posterior

In rare cases, the sacrum and head rotate posteriorly so that the occiput is in the hollow of the sacrum and the face is behind the pubis. If the head is flexed (Fig. 25-9A), delivery occurs with the occiput posterior. The nasion pivots in the subpubic angle, and the nape of the neck, occiput, and vertex roll over the perineum. The face then emerges from behind the pubis. This method of delivery is helped by lifting up the child's body.

If the head is extended (Fig. 25-9B), the chin impinges behind the pubis and the submental area of the neck pivots in the subpubic angle. For delivery to take place, the infant's body must be raised by the accoucheur so that the occiput, vertex, and forehead can pass over the perineum in that order.

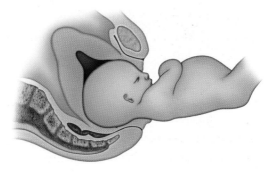

A. Head flexed.

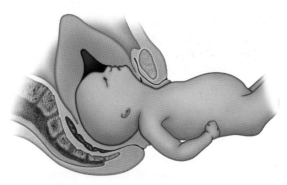

B. Head extended.

FIGURE 25-9. Arrest of the head: sacrum posterior.

Delivery of the head from this position can be difficult. The best management of this complication lies in its prevention. Once the breech has been born, any tendency for the sacrum to rotate posteriorly must be restrained by the attendant and the breech encouraged to turn with the sacrum anteriorly toward the symphysis pubis.

Mechanism of Labor in Footling and Kneeling Breech

The mechanism of labor is the same as has been described in RSA with the difference being that in complete and frank breech presentations, the buttocks form the leading part. In footling presentations, it is one or both feet, and in kneeling breeches, it is the knees.

PROGNOSIS: BREECH PRESENTATIONS

Mother

When spontaneous delivery takes place, the maternal prognosis is good. Genital tract lacerations and hemorrhage may be caused by excessively rapid and forceful delivery of the baby through a pelvis that is too small or in which the soft parts have not been dilated sufficiently.

Fetus

The fetal mortality and morbidity rates associated with vaginal delivery of full-term breech presentations are three times those of cephalic presentations. The worst prognosis is in premature breeches. The risk is highest in double footling presentations and lowest when the breech is frank. Factors influencing perinatal mortality and morbidity include (1) prematurity, (2) congenital abnormalities, (3) prolapse of the umbilical cord, (4) fetal asphyxia from other causes, and (5) fetal injury. Intracranial hemorrhage, more common with breech than with cephalic presentations, is a major cause of fetal mortality. Sometimes the unmolded head has to pass rapidly and with difficulty through a borderline pelvis.

Prolapse of the umbilical cord is more common than in cephalic presentation, especially when the presentation is footling and when the mother is multiparous. Frank breech has the lowest incidence.

The danger of injury is as great in multiparas as in primigravidas. In difficult deliveries, the risk of damage to the baby is 20 percent; in easy births, it is 3.5 percent. The fetal outcome is worse when the diagnosis is not made before the onset of labor.

Significant long-term major morbidity affecting the central nervous system are increased in breeches born per vagina. These include cerebral palsy, epilepsy, mental retardation, and hemiplegia.

Time of Death
About 15 percent of fetal deaths occur during labor. The remainder are divided more or less equally between fetal death in utero before the onset of labor, congenital anomalies incompatible with life, and neonatal death.

Causes of Death or Damage to the Baby

1. Prematurity is the major etiologic factor in the perinatal morbidity and mortality of infants presenting breech. The risk of death during labor is much higher for premature fetuses in breech than cephalic presentation

2. Congenital malformation. The incidence of anomalies among fetuses presenting by the breech is twice that seen in cephalic presentations, 6.3 versus 2.4 percent. Known fetal disorders associated with breech presentation include congenital dislocation of the hip, hydrocephaly, anencephaly, and meningomyelocele, as well as some less common anomalies

3. Asphyxia

   a. Prolonged compression of the umbilical cord between the pelvis and the after-coming head
   b. Actual prolapse of the cord
   c. Aspiration of amniotic fluid and vaginal contents caused by active breathing before the head has been born
   d. Prolonged and hard labor

4. Injury to the brain and skull

   a. The after-coming head passes through the pelvis rapidly. Instead of gradual molding taking place over several hours, rapid and sometimes excessive compression and decompression occur within a few minutes. The ligaments of the brain are subjected to sudden and marked stretching, with the risk of laceration and intracranial hemorrhage. Injury to the brain may follow delivery through an incompletely dilated cervix or through a pelvis whose adequacy has been estimated incorrectly
   b. Minute hemorrhages

c. Fractures of the skull
d. Minimal brain dysfunction. One study has reported that the frequency of learning and motor defects is higher in infants delivered vaginally as breech presentations than in infants delivered as cephalic presentations. These include difficulties in reading and writing and disturbances in hearing, sight, and speech. It is not known whether the basic etiologic factor is anoxia or trauma. Unfortunately, this study has not matched a number of important variables, and a cause-and-effect relationship has not been proved. A study in the Netherlands of the neurologic status of children born by vaginal delivery involving 256 cases and matched controls found that significant differences between the study and control groups existed only for minor neurologic dysfunctions. The conclusion reached was that the main danger of breech presentation lies in the associated complications of the pregnancy rather than the mode of delivery. Outcomes for children at 2-year follow-up in the Term Breech Trial published in 2007 showed that there was no difference between the planned cesarean delivery group and the planned vaginal delivery group

5. Damage resulting from difficult delivery

   a. Fractures of the neck, humerus, clavicle, or femur
   b. Cervical and brachial plexus paralyses
   c. Rupture of the liver caused by grasping the baby too tightly around the abdomen while extracting him or her
   d. Damage to fetal adrenal glands
   e. Injury to the spinal cord
   f. Traumatized pharynx caused by the obstetrician putting his or her finger in the baby's mouth to aid delivery
   g. Damage to abdominal organs. The baby should be grasped by the hips and not the trunk

6. Size of the baby

   a. Large babies, over 4000 g, may be too big for the mother's pelvis
   b. Premature babies have small bodies in relation to their heads. A little breech is not a good dilator and fails to make room for the head. Fetal weight less than 2500 g is not recommended for trial of vaginal delivery

7. Rupture of membranes. It has been shown that the fetal mortality rate is significantly higher if the interval from rupture of the membranes to delivery is prolonged

COMPLICATED LABOR

INVESTIGATION OF BREECH PRESENTATION AT TERM

Ultrasound Examination

An ultrasound should be performed before the onset of labor in the setting of a breech presentation. If ultrasound is not available, cesarean section is recommended for confirmed breech presentations.

1. Confirm the presentation and diagnose the type of breech presentation—frank, complete, or footling
2. Diagnose any congenital fetal anomalies
3. Assess fetal attitude—flexion or extension. Rule out hyperextension of the fetal head
4. Estimate the fetal weight
5. Measure the biparietal diameter of the fetal head and the abdominal and thoracic girth
6. Compare the biparietal diameter of the fetal head and the measurements of the maternal pelvis
7. Localize the placenta and rule out placenta previa

MANAGEMENT OF BREECH PRESENTATION DURING LATE PREGNANCY

External Cephalic Version

Recent studies on outcomes of randomized controlled trials of external cephalic version (ECV) or no ECV have shown that there is a significant reduction of noncephalic births and cesarean section. There was also no significant effect on perinatal mortality. It is therefore recommended that all women with a breech presentation should be offered an ECV. This should be performed at or beyond 36 weeks' gestation.

Timing

Delay of ECV to after 36 weeks of gestation has advantages: (1) Fewer procedures are necessary because spontaneous version will occur in a number of cases, even in late pregnancy. (2) Reversion to the original presentation is rare. (3) If fetal complications develop during the procedure that necessitate immediate delivery, the child will be mature. (4) Contraindications to ECV, such as intrauterine growth restriction (IUGR), may become evident only in the later stage of the pregnancy.

In some circumstances, ECV can be offered in labor.

Prerequisites

1. Singleton pregnancy
2. No contraindication to labor and vaginal delivery
3. Normal fetal well-being
4. Normal amniotic fluid
5. Position confirmed before ECV
6. Facilities available for immediate cesarean section

Contraindications

1. Absolute

    a. Any contraindication to labor
    b. Antepartum hemorrhage
    c. Some major fetal anomalies
    d. Multiple gestation
    e. Ruptured membranes

2. Relative

    a. Oligohydramnios
    b. Hyperextension of the fetal head
    c. Two or more previous cesarean sections
    d. Morbid obesity
    e. Active labor
    f. Uterine anomalies

Procedure

1. Consent should be obtained from the patient before the procedure. The procedure is performed in a setting where immediate intervention, including a cesarean section, can be accessible
2. A nonstress test and biophysical profile are preformed before the procedure to ensure fetal well-being. An ultrasound is also performed to confirm position
3. The abdomen is usually lubricated to facilitate the version. The first attempt is usually made using the forward roll technique. With each hand on one of the fetal poles, the buttocks are elevated from the pelvis

COMPLICATED LABOR

and moved laterally. The breech is then guided toward the fundus, with simultaneous direction of the head toward the pelvis. Another technique, if this unsuccessful, is the backward flip

4. In some cases, uterine relaxation is considered. Nitroglycerin, terbutaline, and ritodrine have been used in ECV in the same doses as for treating uterine hyperstimulation in labor

5. The procedure must be performed gently without excessive force because there is the risk of placental separation or damage to the fetus. Version may be unsuccessful and the procedure abandoned. The procedure should also be abandoned if the patient is uncomfortable or there are fetal heart rate (FHR) abnormalities. In cases in which the presentation has been changed to cephalic, most fetuses will remain in the new position, but in some instances, recurrence to the original presentation may take place

6. A nonstress test is repeated for at least 20 minutes after attempted ECV, regardless if successful or not. It is important to administer Rh immunoglobulin in unsensitized Rh-negative women

Risks of External Cephalic Version

1. Abruption
2. Rupture of membrane and possibility of cord prolapse
3. Labor or preterm labor
4. FHR abnormalities
5. Alloimmunization or fetomaternal hemorrhage
6. Twofold increase in intrapartum cesarean delivery despite ECV

MANAGEMENT OF DELIVERY OF BREECH PRESENTATION

Classification of Breech Births

Vaginal Delivery

1. *Spontaneous breech delivery*: The entire infant is expelled by the natural forces of the mother with no assistance other than support of the baby as he or she is being born
2. *Assisted breech (or partial breech extraction)*: The infant is delivered by the natural forces as far as the umbilicus. The remainder of the baby is extracted by the attendant. In normal cases, we believe this to be the best method

3. *Total breech extraction*: The entire body of the infant is extracted by the attendant

Cesarean Section

It must be pointed out that delivery of a breech by cesarean section takes skill. Infants may be injured during the procedure. The incision must be adequate in length so there is no difficulty with the head. If the lower uterine segment is not well developed, as is often the case in preterm situations, a low vertical incision, which can be extended easily, may be preferable.

Elective Cesarean Section

The following factors are unfavorable for safe vaginal delivery, and cesarean section may be best.

1. Poor obstetrical histories, such as a difficult delivery or a damaged baby
2. Contracted, borderline, or abnormal pelvis
3. Placental insufficiency, including IUGR, diabetes mellitus, and hypertensive disorders
4. Preterm rupture of the membranes or preterm labor
5. Placenta previa of any degree
6. Prolapse of the umbilical cord, especially in footling breeches
7. Small baby (<2500 g)
8. Large baby (>4000 g)
9. Hyperextension of the fetal head
10. Footling breech. The limbs and pelvis of the footling breech deliver easily but do not dilate the maternal soft parts sufficiently to make room for the after-coming head. This may make delivery of the head difficult, especially in premature infants

Elective Cesarean Section

Because no clinical or ultrasonographic assessment can guarantee a safe and easy birth of the after-coming head, many obstetricians believe that all infants presenting in breech should be delivered by cesarean section. Today many infants in breech presentation are delivered abdominally without a trial of labor.

Although maternal mortality due to cesarean delivery is rare, the overall morbidity associated with cesarean delivery is twofold higher compared with vaginal delivery. Furthermore, definite proof of the superiority of cesarean section over vaginal delivery is difficult to obtain.

The Term Breech Trial, published in 2000, was a multicenter trial in which women with a breech singleton pregnancy were randomized to a planned cesarean or a planned vaginal birth. The results of the trial showed the rate of perinatal or neonatal mortality or serious neonatal morbidity to be 1.6 percent in planned cesarean group and 5 percent in planned vaginal birth group.

The PREsentation et MODe d'Accouchement (PREMODA) study results were published in 2006 by Goffinet et al. Their study published prospective observational data from centers in France and Belgium for a total of 8105 women. A cesarean section was planned in 69 percent of these women, and a trial of labor was attempted in 31 percent of women. Of the 2526 women undergoing a trial of labor for breech presentation, 71 percent delivered vaginally. This study found no difference in perinatal or serious neonatal morbidity for either planned cesarean birth or trial of labor.

It is evident that, when the fetus is normal, cesarean section will reduce markedly, if not eliminate entirely, fetal death during delivery. At the same time, there is evidence that with proper selection of cases and meticulous management during labor and as long as indications for abdominal delivery are wide and include all unfavorable situations of even the mildest degree, many term breeches can be delivered vaginally and safely.

The controversy as to how to deliver breeches has not been settled.

Trial of Labor

Criteria.　The criteria for consideration of vaginal delivery are:

1. Frank or complete breech
2. Term gestational age of 36 to 42 weeks
3. Estimated fetal weight between 2500 and 4000 g
4. Flexed or neutral fetal head
5. Adequate maternal pelvis
6. No maternal or fetal indication for cesarean section

Conditions.　The trial of labor is carried out under the following conditions, with the understanding that any deviation from the normal is an indication for cesarean section.

1. The FHR is monitored continuously
2. The progress of labor is observed meticulously
3. Progressive cervical dilatation must take place

4. Adequate descent of the breech must occur
5. No heroic vaginal procedures are performed
6. The patient must be prepared and ready for cesarean section. The organization of the delivery room suite, the nurses, the anesthetist, and the obstetrician must allow the immediate performance of cesarean section if the need arises
7. Induction of labor is not recommended for breech presentation
8. A trained professional in neonatal resuscitation should be in attendance at time of delivery
9. An experienced obstetrician in vaginal breech delivery should be present at delivery

Management of Labor and Delivery in the Progressing Case

First Stage of Labor

1. Because most breech presentations that meet criteria for a trial of labor progress to successful vaginal delivery, observant expectancy, supportive therapy, and absence of interference are the procedures of choice
2. The patient may be ambulatory if the breech is well applied against the dilated cervix
3. It is best to maintain intact membranes until the cervical dilatation is far advanced. Too frequent vaginal or rectal examinations or any procedure that might contribute to premature rupture of the bag of waters should be avoided
4. When the membranes do rupture, vaginal examination is done to rule out prolapse of the umbilical cord and to determine the exact condition of the cervix
5. Meconium is no cause for alarm as long as the fetal heart is normal
6. An intravenous infusion of crystalloid solution (normal saline or Ringer lactate) should be instituted
7. Fetal well-being should be monitored using continuous electronic fetal monitoring
8. Progress of labor should be well documented. When progress is slow, oxytocin augmentation should be used with caution in cases of inadequate uterine contractions (e.g., caused by epidural anesthesia). If progress is less than 0.5 cm/hr or if there is no progress in 2 hours despite adequate uterine contractions, cesarean section should be performed

Second Stage of Labor

Once the cervix is fully dilated, the passive second stage may last up to 90 minutes. This allows the breech to descend into the lower pelvis. If delivery is not imminent after active pushing for 60 minutes, cesarean section should be performed.

When the breech begins to distend the perineum, the patient may be in a semi-supine or be in a hands and knees position to assist with the delivery. The semi-supine position is the best position in which to assist the birth and to handle complications. The patient's bladder should be emptied.

Assisted Breech. The fetal heart is checked frequently. As long as the baby is in good condition, spontaneous delivery is awaited. Fetal maneuvers should be used only after spontaneous delivery to the umbilicus. Premature traction on the baby, especially between contractions, must be avoided because it can lead to deflexion of the head and extension of the arms above or behind the head. It is important that the patient bear down with each contraction, and she must be encouraged to do so. Once the body has been born, the head is out of the upper contracting part of the uterus and in the lower segment, the cervix, or the upper vagina. Because these organs do not have the power to expel the head, its descent and delivery must be effected by the voluntary action of the abdominal muscles, with the attendant exerting suprapubic pressure.

Our experience has been that in normally progressing cases, the best results are obtained by a policy of:

1. No interference (except episiotomy) until the body is born to the umbilicus. This permits the cervix to become not only fully dilated but also paralyzed, an important factor in minimizing dystocia with the after-coming head
2. Hard bearing down and expulsive efforts by the mother during contractions
3. The maintenance of suprapubic pressure during descent to aid delivery and to keep the head in flexion

There are good reasons for using this technique:

1. It has proved successful
2. It is safe. There is less trauma to the baby
3. Flexion of the head is maintained
4. The danger of extension of the arms above the head is reduced

5. There is less chance of the cervix clamping down around the baby's head or neck

Anesthesia. A pudendal block or perineal infiltration permits episiotomy without pain and facilitates delivery by relaxing the muscles. In addition, with each contraction, the patient takes several breaths of an anesthetic vapor. This acts as an analgesic, eases the pain, and helps her to bear down more efficiently. Adequate anesthesia is best obtained by an epidural.

Necessary Equipment. The procedure requires that certain equipment be at hand.

1. A warm, dry towel to be wrapped around the baby's body as soon as he or she is sufficiently born. The purposes of this are:
   a. To reduce the stimulating effect of cold air on the baby in the hope that respiration does not begin while the head is in the pelvis, resulting in aspiration of amniotic fluid or vaginal contents
   b. To make it easier to hold the slippery baby

2. Piper forceps for the after-coming head if it does not deliver easily with assistance

3. Equipment for resuscitation of the infant ready for immediate use

4. Ability to perform an emergency cesarean section

Delivery of Breech

1. The patient is encouraged to bear down with the contractions but must rest between them
2. As long as there is no fetal or maternal distress, spontaneous delivery to the umbilicus is awaited. Up to this point, there is no urgency, and the operator should not interfere
3. Once the umbilicus has been delivered, time becomes an important factor, and the remainder of the birth is expedited gently and skillfully. A free airway to the mouth should be available within 3 to 5 minutes to obviate anoxic brain damage
4. The legs usually deliver spontaneously; if not they are easily extracted. Do not extract the legs until the popliteal fossae are visible (Pinard's maneuver)

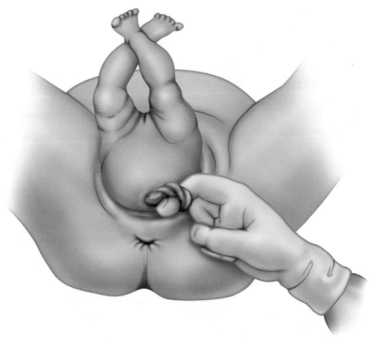

FIGURE 25-10. Delivery of the cord. Loop of umbilical cord being pulled down.

5. The baby is covered with a warm towel, and the body is supported
6. A loop of umbilical cord is pulled down (Fig. 25-10) to minimize traction on it in case it is caught between the head and the pelvic wall. At the same time, it is palpated for pulsations

Delivery of the Shoulders and Arms

1. The assistant exerts suprapubic pressure on the head to maintain its flexion
2. The operator depresses the buttocks and delivers the body to the anterior scapula so that the anterior shoulder comes under the symphysis
3. To deliver the anterior arm, the accoucheur passes his or her hand up the baby's back, over the shoulder, and down the chest, thus sweeping the arm and hand out under the pubis with his or her finger (Loveset maneuver; Fig. 25-11A)
4. The baby is raised so that the posterior scapula and then the posterior arm are born over the perineum by the same maneuver (Fig. 25-11B)
5. Some obstetricians deliver the posterior arm first

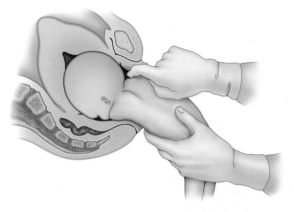

A. Extraction of anterior arm.

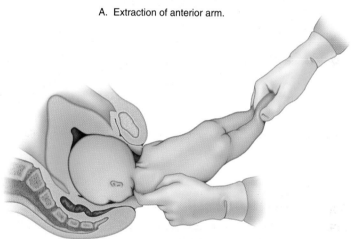

B. Extraction of posterior arm.

FIGURE 25-11. Delivery of the arms and shoulders.

Delivery of the Head

1. In almost every case, the back turns anteriorly spontaneously. This must be encouraged so that the head rotates the occiput to the pubis and the face toward the sacrum. Rarely, there is a tendency for the back to turn posteriorly. The obstetrician must counteract this and rotate the back anteriorly to prevent the head's rotating face to pubis, a serious and always avoidable complication

2. Once the back has rotated anteriorly and the fetal head is in the AP diameter of the pelvis, the body is lowered so that the occiput appears under the symphysis and the nape of the neck pivots there (Fig. 25-12A)

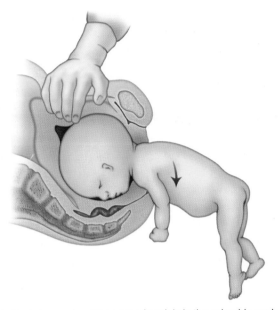

A. Body lowered so that nape of neck is in the subpubic angle. Assistant maintains flexion of the head.

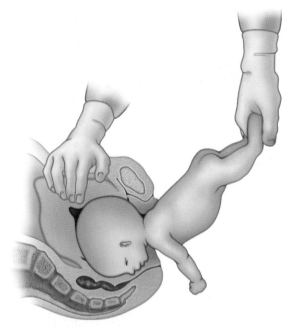

B. Kristellar maneuver; Head born in flexion.

FIGURE 25-12. Delivery of the head.

3. At the same time, the assistant maintains suprapubic pressure to guide the head through the pelvis and to keep it flexed

4. The body is then raised gently so that there is slight extension at the neck

5. Then by further suprapubic pressure (Kristellar maneuver, also known as Bracht maneuver) the head is delivered in flexion—the chin, mouth, nose, forehead, bregma, and vertex being born, in that order, over the perineum (Fig. 25-12B)

6. The speed of delivery of the after-coming head must be considered. The rapid passage of the head through the pelvis causes sudden compression and decompression of the cranial contents. In the extreme, the ligaments of the brain tear, leading to hemorrhage, cerebral damage, and death. On the other hand, too slow delivery of the head results in asphyxia, which may also be fatal. Experience teaches the middle road—slow enough to prevent injury to the brain and sufficiently rapid to avoid asphyxia

ARREST IN BREECH PRESENTATION

Most babies who present by the breech are born spontaneously or with the help of, but not interference from, the attendant. The Kristellar/Bracht maneuver (suprapubic pressure) is all that is needed to deliver the after-coming head. However, progress may cease, and active interference then becomes mandatory. Arrest may take place at the head, neck, shoulders and arms, or buttocks.

Arrest of the Head

Sometimes the body, shoulders, and arms are born, but the bearing-down efforts of the mother and the Kristellar/Bracht maneuver are not successful in delivering the head. When the head is arrested, several measures are available to extract it.

Wigand-Martin Maneuver

The body of the baby is placed on the arm of the operator with the middle finger of the hand of that arm placed in the baby's mouth and the index and ring fingers on the malar bones (Fig. 25-13A). The purpose of the finger in the mouth is not for traction but to encourage and maintain

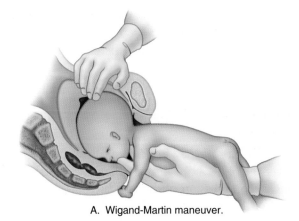

A. Wigand-Martin maneuver.

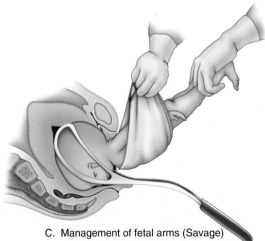

B. Mauriceau-Smellie-Veit maneuver.

C. Management of fetal arms (Savage)
as Piper forceps are applied.

FIGURE 25-13. Different maneuvers for arrest of the head.

flexion. With the other hand, the obstetrician exerts suprapubic pressure on the head through the mother's abdomen.

Mauriceau-Smellie-Veit Maneuver

The position is the same as the Wigand-Martin maneuver, with one finger in the baby's mouth and two on the malar bones. The difference is that the accoucheur places his or her other hand astride the baby's shoulders and produces traction in this way (Fig. 25-13B). The efficiency of this procedure is increased by an assistant's applying suprapubic pressure on the fetal head while the operator is performing the Mauriceau maneuver.

Piper Forceps on the After-Coming Head

With the exception of simple suprapubic pressure, the best method of delivering the after-coming head is by the use of the Piper forceps. In contrast to maneuvers in which traction on the head is applied through the neck, the forceps exert traction directly on the head, thereby avoiding damage to structures in the baby's neck.

Although any type of forceps can be used for this procedure, the Piper forceps, which was designed especially for this operation, is best. The handles are depressed below the arch of the shanks, the pelvic curve is reduced, and the shanks are long and curved. These features make this instrument easier to apply to the after-coming head.

Orientation

Vaginal Examination

1. The long axis of the head is in the AP diameter of the pelvis
2. The occiput is anterior
3. The face is posterior

Orientation and Desired Application

1. The cephalic application is biparietal and mentooccipital, with the front of the forceps (concave edges) toward the occiput and the convex edges toward the face
2. The pelvic application is good, with the diameter of the forceps in the transverse diameter of the pelvis, the concave edges pointing toward

COMPLICATED LABOR

the pubis, and the convex edges toward the sacrum. The sides of the blades are next to the side walls of the pelvis

Application of Forceps

1. The baby's feet are grasped by an assistant, and the body is raised (Fig. 25-13C). Care must be taken not to elevate the body too much for fear of damage to the sternomastoid muscles. The lower and upper limbs and the umbilical cord are kept out of the way. A good way to keep the arms out of the way is to use a folded towel as described by Savage
2. The handle of the left blade is grasped in the left hand
3. The right hand is introduced between the head and the left postero-lateral wall of the vagina
4. The left blade is then inserted between the head and the fingers into a mentooccipital application
5. The fingers are removed from the vagina, and the handle is steadied by an assistant
6. The handle of the right blade is grasped with the right hand
7. The left hand is introduced between the head and the right postero-lateral wall of the vagina
8. The right blade is introduced between the head and the fingers into a mentooccipital application
9. The fingers are removed from the vagina
10. The forceps are locked (Fig. 25-14), and vaginal examination is made to be certain that the application is correct

Extraction of the Head

1. Traction is outward and posterior until the nape of the neck is in the subpubic angle
2. The direction is then changed to outward and anterior, and the face and forehead are born over the perineum in flexion
3. An episiotomy should be used

Airway

When there is delay in delivery of the head and one is waiting for help or instruments, an ordinary vaginal retractor can be used temporarily to clear an airway in the vagina to the baby's mouth (Fig. 25-15). The retractor is placed in the vagina and pressure exerted posteriorly. The vaginal contents are sponged out so that air can get to the baby if he or she breathes.

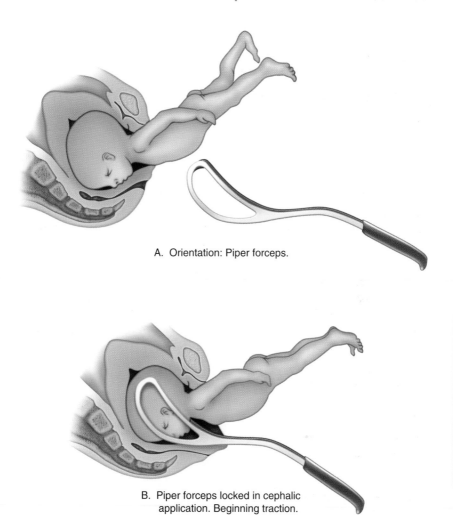

A. Orientation: Piper forceps.

B. Piper forceps locked in cephalic
application. Beginning traction.

FIGURE 25-14. **Piper forceps for delivery of an after-coming head.**

Chin-to-Pubis Rotation

Anterior rotation of the chin is rare and occurs usually as part of posterior rotation of the back. The preferred management is as follows: (1) Institute deep anesthesia. (2) Cease all traction. (3) Dislodge the chin from behind the pubis. (4) Rotate the face posteriorly and the back anteriorly. (5) Flex the chin. (6) Effect engagement by suprapubic pressure. (7) Deliver the head with Piper forceps.

When this technique fails, the Prague maneuver (Fig. 25-16) may be used. Here the fingers are placed over the shoulders, and outward and upward traction is made. The legs are grasped with the other hand, and

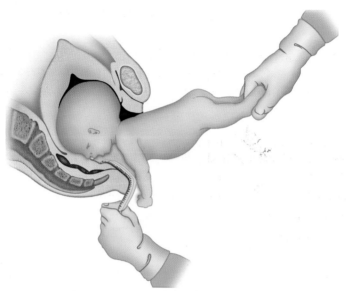

FIGURE 25-15. Vaginal retractor providing airway to the baby's mouth and nose.

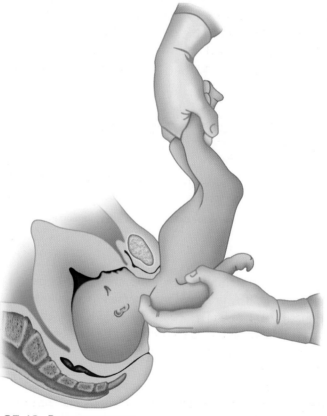

FIGURE 25-16. Prague maneuver.

the body is swung over the mother's abdomen. With this procedure, the occiput is born over the perineum. Because this method carries with it the danger of overstretching or breaking the infant's neck, it is used rarely.

Embryotomy
When delivery of the head is not accomplished within a reasonable time, the baby may die. If he or she does perish, the mother's welfare alone should be considered. To save her from needless injury, reduction of the size of the child's head by perforation of the skull is preferable to extraction by brute force.

Arrest of the Neck

Occasionally, the cervix, which has opened sufficiently to allow the trunk and shoulders to be born, clamps down around the baby's neck, trapping the head in the uterus. The possibility of this happening is greater with premature delivery, when the body has not yet developed its adipose tissue and is a poor dilating wedge. This dangerous situation calls for rapid action to break the spasm of the previously dilated cervix. This is accomplished by a single bold incision of the cervix with the scissors. The resultant relaxation of the spasm permits the head to be born.

Arrest of the Shoulders and Arms

Extended Arms
The arms are simply extended over the baby's head (Fig. 25-17A).

Nuchal Arms
There is extension at the shoulder and flexion at the elbow so that the forearm is trapped behind the fetal head (Fig. 25-17B). One or both arms may be affected.

Prophylaxis
One method of reducing the incidence of this complication is to resist the temptation of pulling on the baby's legs to speed delivery, especially when the uterus is in a relaxed state.

Simple Extraction
When this problem occurs, an attempt should be made first to deliver the arms by sweeping them over the chest in the usual way. This succeeds in

most cases of simple extension and in some instances of nuchal arms when the upper limb is not jammed tightly behind the head.

Rotation of the Body

If extraction fails in the case of a nuchal arm, the baby's body is rotated in the direction to which the hand is pointing (Fig. 25-17C). This dislodges the arm from behind the head, and its delivery is then usually possible as described above (Fig. 25-17D). If both arms are nuchal, the body is rotated in one direction to free the first arm, which is then extracted, and then in the opposite direction to free the other arm.

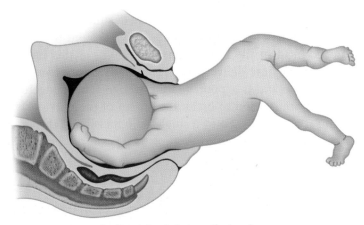

A. Arm extended above the head.

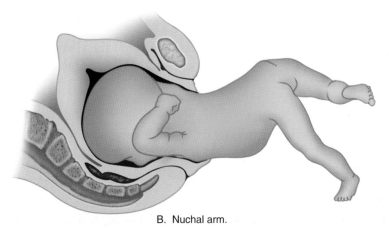

B. Nuchal arm.

FIGURE 25-17. Extended and nuchal arms.

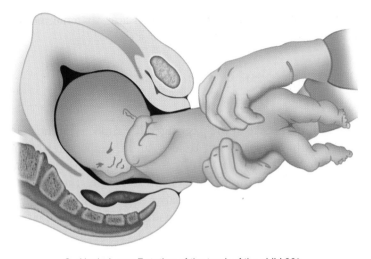

C. Nuchal arm: Rotation of the trunk of the child 90°
in the direction in which the hand is pointing.

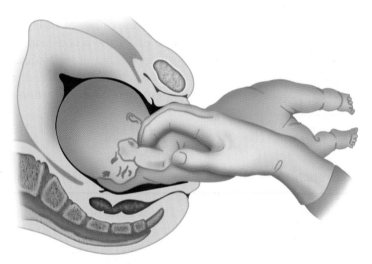

D. Nuchal arm: Hand introduced into the uterus to flex
and bring down the nuchal arm.

FIGURE 25-17. (*Continued*)

Fracture

In the rare instance when rotation fails, the humerus or clavicle must be
fractured. This can be done directly, or it can be effected by simply pulling
on the arm until it breaks. Once this occurs, delivery can be accomplished.
Because the fracture usually heals rapidly and well and because the choice

may be between a dead baby and a broken arm, extreme measures are justified.

Failure of Descent of the Breech

Etiology

In any situation, the size of the passenger, the capacity of the pelvis, the dilatability of the maternal soft tissues, and the character of the uterine contractions all play a part in determining whether spontaneous delivery takes place. In frank breech presentation, there is an added factor—the splinting effect of the baby's legs across its abdomen can reduce the maneuverability of the fetus to such an extent that progress is arrested.

Disproportion

In the presence of good uterine contractions, nondescent of the breech is an indication not for hasty interference but for the most careful reassessment. Keeping in mind the fact that one of the causes of breech presentation is a large head that cannot engage easily, the accoucheur must be assured not of the general capacity of the pelvis but of its adequacy with respect to that particular baby. When a breech fails to descend, despite good contractions, disproportion is present, and cesarean section should be performed.

Decomposition

Flexed Breech. If cesarean section cannot be performed, progress and descent can be expedited by reducing the bulk of the breech, an operation known as decomposition. This is done by bringing down the legs, both whenever possible. When there is flexion at the hips and the knees, the feet can be reached easily. The hand is placed in the uterus, the membranes are ruptured, and a foot is grasped and brought down (Fig. 25-18A). Be sure it is not a hand. The same is done with the other foot. The position has been changed to a footling breech, and labor proceeds.

Frank Breech: Pinard Maneuver. If the breech is frank (flexion at the hips and extension at the knees), it may be impossible to reach the feet because they are high in the uterus near the baby's face. In such a situation and when cesarean section cannot be carried out, the Pinard maneuver is performed under anesthesia (Figs. 25-18B and C). With a hand in the

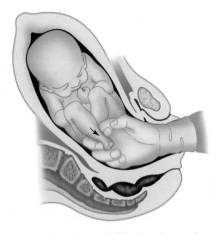

A. Decomposition of breech: Bringing down a foot and leg.

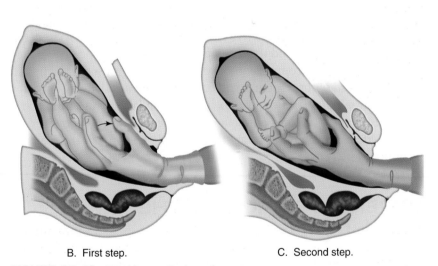

B. First step.

C. Second step.

FIGURE 25-18. Breaking up the breech.

uterus, pressure is made by the fingers against the popliteal fossa in a backward and outward direction. This brings about sufficient flexion of the knee so that the foot can be grasped and delivered. When possible, both feet should be brought down. Unless there are urgent indications for immediate extraction of the infant, labor is allowed to carry on as for a footling breech.

BREECH EXTRACTION

This operation is the immediate vaginal extraction of the baby when signs of fetal distress demand delivery without delay and urgent cesarean section is not available. This is also used in delivery of a second twin in breech presentation. In general, total breech extraction in term singleton breech fetuses is *not* appropriate.

Prerequisites

Certain conditions must be present before this procedure may be performed. (1) The pelvis must be ample, with no disproportion. (2) The cervix must be fully dilated. (3) The bladder and rectum should be empty. (4) Expert and deep anesthesia is essential. (5) Good assistance is mandatory. (6) Neonatal resuscitation is ready.

Procedure

The patient is placed in the lithotomy position, the bladder catheterized, and anesthesia administered. As described in a previous section, the breech is decomposed, and the legs are brought down. The feet are pulled down if the breech is complete; the Pinard maneuver is used if the breech is frank. Instead of the patient going on to spontaneous delivery, the baby is extracted rapidly. Traction from below and fundal pressure from above are substituted for uterine contractions, but the maneuvers for delivery of the shoulders, arms, and head are those already set forth in the management of arrested cases.

HYPEREXTENSION OF THE FETAL HEAD

Hyperextension of the fetal head (Fig. 25-19) is seen most commonly in face presentation but also occurs with transverse lie and breech presentation. In the latter, it is a serious problem.

Etiology

1. Spasm or congenital shortening of the extensor muscles of the neck
2. Umbilical cord around the neck
3. Congenital tumors of the fetal neck

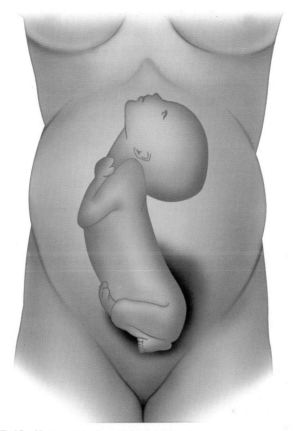

FIGURE 25-19. Hyperextension of the fetal head.

4. Fetal malformations
5. Uterine anomalies
6. Tumors in the placental site

Diagnosis

The diagnosis is made by ultrasound examination; the appearance is characteristic. When the head presents, it is that of a face presentation. When the breech presents, the appearance has been described as a "star-gazing breech." In transverse lie, the condition is seen as a "flying fetus."

Fetal Danger

There is a definite risk of damage to the lower cervical spinal cord of the fetus during vaginal delivery. The mechanisms by which the injury is caused include (1) excessive longitudinal stretching of the spinal cord, (2) extreme flexion of the neck during delivery, and (3) marked torsion. The resulting lesion is partial or complete laceration of the cervical spinal cord, occasional tears in the dura, and epidural hemorrhage. The latter is the most common manifestation and is associated with varying degrees of damage to the cord, brain stem, nerve roots, and meninges. Dislocation or fracture of the vertebrae is rare. In the vast majority of cases, the injury is caused by the sudden flexion of the head as it descends through the vagina. However, occasionally, the damage may occur during pregnancy as a result of the malposition of the fetus.

Fetal Prognosis

In a collected series of 73 cases, the perinatal mortality rate was 13.7 percent in babies delivered vaginally in contrast to no deaths in those born by cesarean section. Medullary or vertebral injury occurred in 20.6 percent of babies born per vaginam and in 5.7 percent delivered by cesarean section. Meningeal hemorrhage was found in 6.9 percent of children born vaginally, but none was noted after cesarean section. In another series of 814 breech presentations, there were 33 hyperextended heads, an incidence of 7.4 percent. All 33 infants survived. Follow-up for 2 to 4 years revealed neurologic sequelae in 5 of the 26 children born vaginally, but none in the 7 delivered by cesarean section.

A cesarean section should be performed when the fetal head is extended.

SELECTED READING

American College of Obstetricians and Gynecologists: ACOG Committee Opinion No. 340, Mode of term singleton breech delivery. Obstet Gynecol 108:235, 2006

Ben-Meir A, Erez Y, Sela HY, Shveiky D, Tsafrir A, Ezra Y: Prognostic parameters for successful external cephalic version. J Matern Fetal Neonatal Med 21:660, 2008

Collea JV: The intrapartum management of breech presentation. Clin Perinatol 8:173,1981

Collea JV, Chein C, Quilligan EJ: The randomized management of term frank breech presentation: A study of 208 cases. Am J Obstet Gynecol 137:235, 1980

Cox C, Kendall AC, Hommers M: Changed prognosis of breech-presenting low birthweight infants. Br J Obstet Gynaecol 89:881, 1982

Cunningham FG, Gant NF, Leveno KJ, et al: Breech presentation and delivery. In: Williams Obstetrics, 23rd ed. New York: McGraw-Hill, 2009.

Effer SB, Saigal S, Rand C, et al: Effect of delivery method on outcomes in the very low-birth weight breech infant: Is the improved survival related to cesarean section or other perinatal care maneuvers? Am J Obstet Gynecol 145:123, 1983

Faber-Nijholt R, Huisjes HJ, Touwen BCL, Fidler VJ: Neurological follow-up of 281 children born in breech presentation: A controlled study. Br Med J 286:9, 1983

Fall O, Nilsson BA: External cephalic version in breech presentation under tocolysis. Obstet Gynecol 53:712, 1979

Gimovsky ML, Wallace RL, Schiffrin BS, Paul RH: Randomized management of the non-frank breech presentation at term: A preliminary report. Am J Obstet Gynecol 146:34, 1983

Goffinet F, Carayol M, Foidart JM, Alexander S, Uzan S, Subtil D, et al: PREMODA Study Group. Is planned vaginal delivery for breech presentation at term still an option? Results of an observational prospective survey in France and Belgium. Am J Obstet Gynecol 194:1002, 2006

Green JE, McLean F, Smith LP, Usher R: Has an increased cesarean section rate for term breech delivery reduced the incidence of birth asphyxia, trauma, and death? Am J Obstet Gynecol 143:643,1982

Hannah ME, Hannah WJ, Hewson SA, Hodnett ED, Saigal S, Willan AR, et al: Planned cesarean section versus planned vaginal birth for breech presentation at term: a randomised multicentre trial. Lancet 356:1375, 2000

Hofmeyr GJ: Effect of external cephalic version in late pregnancy on breech presentation and cesarean section: A controlled trial. Br J Obstet Gynaecol 90:392, 1983

Ridley WJ, Jackson P, Stewart JH, Boyle P: Role of antenatal radiography in the management of breech deliveries. Br J Obstet Gynaecol 89:342, 1982

Royal College of Obstetricians and Gynaecologists: RCOG Green Top Guidelines: The management of breech presentation. Guideline no. 20b. London: Royal College of Obstetricians and Gynaecologists, December 2006.

Society of Obstetricians and Gynaecologists of Canada: Vaginal Delivery of Breech Presentation. Clinical Practice Guideline No. 226. Ottawa, ON: Society of Obstetricians and Gynaecologists of Canada, June 2009.

Westgren M, Grundsell I, Ingemarsson A, et al: Hyperextension of the fetal head in breech presentation: A study with long-term follow-up. Br J Obstet Gynaecol 88:101, 1981

Whyte H, Hannah ME, Saigal S, Hannah W, Hewson S, Amankwah K, et al: Outcomes of children at 2 years after planned cesarean birth versus planned vaginal birth for breech presentation at term: The International Randomized Term Breech Trial. Am J Obstet Gynecol 191:864, 2004

COMPLICATED LABOR

Transverse Lie

George Tawagi

CHAPTER 26

GENERAL CONSIDERATIONS

Definition

When the long axes of mother and fetus are at right angles to one another, a transverse lie is present. Because the shoulder is placed so frequently in the brim of the inlet, this malposition is often referred to as the shoulder presentation. The baby may lie directly across the maternal abdomen (Fig. 26-1) or may lie obliquely with the head or breech in the iliac fossa (Figs. 26-2A and B). Usually the breech is at a higher level than the head. The denominator is the scapula (Sc); the situation of the head determines whether the position is left or right, and that of the back indicates whether it is anterior or posterior. Thus, LScP means that the lie is transverse, the head is on the mother's left side, and the baby's back is posterior. The part that actually lies over the pelvic brim may be the shoulder, back, abdomen, ribs, or flank. This is a serious malposition whose management must not be left to nature.

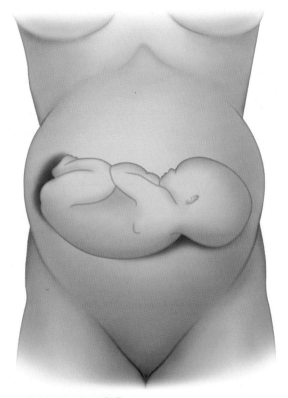

FIGURE 26-1. Transverse lie: LScP.

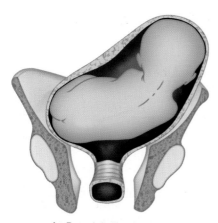 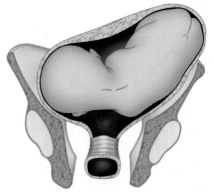

A. Breech in iliac fossa.   B. Head in iliac fossa.

FIGURE 26-2. Oblique lie.

Incidence

The incidence of transverse lie is around 1:500. The incidence is higher before term (as high as 1 in 50 at 32 weeks' gestation).

Etiology

This abnormality is more common in multiparas than primigravidas because of the laxness of the uterine and abdominal muscles. Similar condition in which there is relatively excess space for the fetus are polyhydramnios and prematurity. Other causes include anything that prevents engagement of the head or the breech, such as placenta previa; an obstructing neoplasm; multiple pregnancies; fetal anomalies; fetopelvic disproportion; contracted pelvis; and uterine abnormalities such as uterus subseptus, uterus arcuatus, and uterus bicornis. In many instances, no etiologic factor can be determined, and we assume that the malposition is accidental. The head happens to be out of the lower uterine segment when labor starts, and the shoulder is pushed into the pelvic brim.

DIAGNOSIS OF POSITION: TRANSVERSE LIE

Abdominal Examination

1. The appearance of the abdomen is asymmetrical
2. The long axis of the fetus is across the mother's abdomen

3. The uterine fundus is lower than expected for the period of gestation. It has been described as a squat uterus. Its upper limit is near the umbilicus, and it is wider than usual
4. Palpation of the upper and lower poles of the uterus reveals neither the head nor the breech
5. The head can be felt in one maternal flank. The buttocks are on the other side

Fetal Heart

The fetal heart is heard best below the umbilicus and has no diagnostic significance regarding position.

Vaginal Examination

The most important finding is a negative one—neither the head nor the breech can be felt by the examining finger. The presenting part is high. In some cases, one may actually feel the shoulder, a hand, the rib cage, or the back. Because of the poor fit of the presenting part to the pelvis, the bag of waters may hang into the vagina.

Ultrasonography

Ultrasonic examination will confirm the diagnosis and can detect certain abnormalities in the fetus or the presence of a maternal pelvic mass.

X-ray

When ultrasonography is unavailable, the fetal presentation can be established by a flat plate radiograph of the abdomen.

MECHANISM OF LABOR: TRANSVERSE LIE

Except in severely premature fetuses (in which a transverse lie may deliver vaginally), a persistent transverse lie cannot deliver spontaneously, and if uncorrected, impaction takes place (Fig. 26-3A). The shoulder is jammed into the pelvis, the head and breech stay above the inlet, the neck becomes stretched, and progress is arrested.

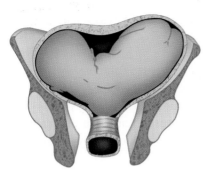

A. Impacted shoulder.

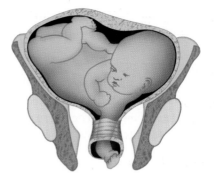

B. Prolapsed arm.

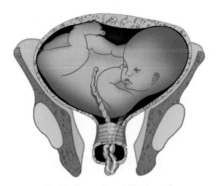

C. Prolapsed umbilical cord.

FIGURE 26-3. Complications.

COMPLICATED LABOR

Spontaneous Version

Spontaneous version takes place occasionally, more often with oblique than with transverse lies. Before or shortly after the onset of labor, the lie changes to a longitudinal one (cephalic or breech), and labor proceeds in the new position. Unfortunately, the chance of spontaneous version occurring is small, too small to warrant more than a very short delay in instituting corrective measures.

Neglected Transverse Lie

Neglected transverse lie results from misdiagnosis or improper treatment. At first, the contractions are of poor quality, and the cervix dilates slowly. Because of the irregularity of the presenting part, the membranes rupture early, and the amniotic fluid escapes rapidly. As the labor pains become stronger, the fetal shoulder is forced into the pelvis, the uterus molds itself around the baby, a state of impaction ensues, and progress is halted. From this impasse, there is one of two outcomes:

1. *Uterine rupture:* Labor goes on. The upper part of the uterus becomes shorter and thicker, and the lower segment becomes progressively more stretched and thinned until it ruptures
2. *Uterine inertia:* The uterus becomes exhausted, and the contractions cease. Intrauterine sepsis sets in and may be followed by generalized infection

In either event, fetal death is certain and maternal mortality possible. Transverse lies must not be neglected!

Complications

Because the presenting part does not fill the inlet, the membranes tend to rupture early and may be followed by prolapse of a fetal arm or the umbilical cord (Figs. 26-3B and C). Both are serious complications necessitating immediate action.

PROGNOSIS: TRANSVERSE LIE

The prognosis depends on the management. With early diagnosis and proper treatment, the outcome is favorable. Neglect leads to the death of almost all infants and puts the mother in serious danger.

MANAGEMENT OF TRANSVERSE LIE

Management Before Labor

1. Careful abdominal, pelvic, ultrasonographic, and, if necessary, radiologic examinations are performed to confirm the diagnosis and to rule out fetal and pelvic abnormalities
2. Shoulder presentations that are diagnosed before term should be managed expectantly because there is a good chance that the malposition will correct itself. If the patient is not at term but the cervix is significantly dilated, hospitalization should be considered because of the incidence of cord prolapse if spontaneous rupture of membranes occurs
3. If the patient is at or near term, external version to a breech or preferably a cephalic presentation should be attempted

Management During Early Labor

In early labor, external version may also be attempted, and if successful, the new presentation is maintained by a tight abdominal binder until it is fixed in the pelvis.

Management of Patient in Good Labor: Persistent Transverse Lie

Cesarean Section

Cesarean section is the treatment of choice. It is safest for both mother and child. It is safest for the mother even in the case of a dead fetus. Because of the exceedingly high morbidity and mortality rates for both the mother and fetus, there is no role for internal podalic version and extraction in the management of transverse lie in singleton gestation. In some instances, extraction of the infant through a transverse lower segment incision may be difficult, and a vertical incision in the lower segment, which can be extended upward if necessary, is preferred by many obstetricians.

Management of Neglected Transverse Lie

This is an obstetric emergency.

Typically, there has been prolonged labor. The lower uterine segment is very thin (or possibly ruptured). Fetal impaction has taken place. An intrauterine infection is present. The fetus is in distress or dead.

Management under these circumstances is difficult.

1. Cesarean section and intensive therapy with antibiotics are carried out even if the baby is dead
2. If infection is severe and widespread, hysterectomy may be necessary after the cesarean section
3. Internal podalic version and extraction or desperate destructive operations on the fetus should not be considered because they carry a grave risk of uterine rupture

CONCLUSION

Transverse lies at term after failure of external version are treated best by cesarean section. They must never be neglected or left to nature.

CHAPTER 27

Compound Presentations

George Tawagi

PROLAPSE OF HAND AND ARM OR FOOT AND LEG

Definition

A presentation is compound when there is prolapse of one or more of the limbs along with the head or the breech, both entering the pelvis at the same time. Footling breech or shoulder presentations are not included in this group. Associated prolapse of the umbilical cord occurs in 15 to 20 percent of cases.

Incidence

Easily detectable compound presentations occur probably once in 500 to 1000 confinements. It is impossible to establish the exact incidence because:

1. Spontaneous correction occurs frequently, and examination late in labor cannot provide the diagnosis
2. Minor degrees of prolapse are detected only by early and careful vaginal examination

Classification of Compound Presentation

1. Cephalic presentation with prolapse of:
   a. Upper limb (arm–hand), one or both
   b. Lower limb (leg–foot), one or both
   c. Arm and leg together

2. Breech presentation with prolapse of the hand or arm

By far the most frequent combination is that of the head with the hand (Fig. 27-1) or arm. In contrast, the head–foot and breech–arm groups are uncommon, about equally so. Prolapse of both hand and foot alongside the head is rare. All combinations may be complicated by prolapse of the umbilical cord, which then becomes the major problem.

Etiology

The etiology of compound presentation includes all conditions that prevent complete filling and occlusion of the pelvic inlet by the presenting

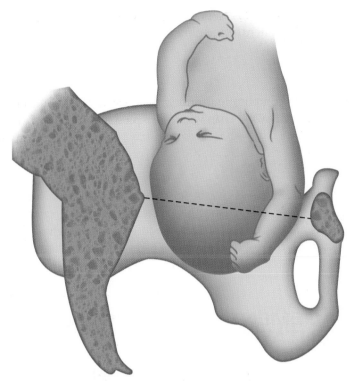

FIGURE 27-1. Compound presentation: head and hand.

part. The most common causal factor is prematurity. Others include high presenting part with ruptured membranes, polyhydramnios, multiparity, a contracted pelvis, pelvic masses, and twins. It is also more common with inductions of labor involving floating presenting parts. Another predisposing factor is external cephalic version. During the process of external version, a fetal limb (commonly the hand–arm, but occasionally the foot) can become "trapped" before the fetal head and thus become the presenting part when labor ensues.

Diagnosis

Diagnosis is made by vaginal examination, and in many cases, the condition is not noted until labor is well advanced and the cervix is fully dilated.
    The condition is suspected when:

1. There is delay of progress in the active phase of labor
2. Engagement fails to occur

3. The fetal head remains high and deviated from the midline during labor, especially after the membranes rupture

Prognosis

In the absence of complications and with conservative management, the results should be no worse than with other presentations.

Mechanism of Labor

The mechanism of labor is that of the main presenting part. Because the diameter is increased, the chance of arrested progress is greater. In many cases, labor is not obstructed, and the leading part is brought down to the outlet. If dystocia occurs, the baby remains high, and operative treatment is needed.

MANAGEMENT OF COMPOUND PRESENTATIONS

The best treatment for compound presentations (in the absence of complications such as prolapse of the cord) is masterful inactivity.

Progressing Case

In most cases, as the cervix becomes fully dilated and the presenting part descends, the prolapsed arm or leg rises out of the pelvis, allowing labor to proceed normally. Rarely, the baby might also deliver with the arm or hand alongside the head. Hence, as long as progress is being made, there should be no interference.

Arrest of Progress

1. *Reposition of the prolapsed part*: In a normal pelvis, if progress is arrested, the arm or leg should be replaced, under anesthesia, and the head pushed into the pelvis. This is done by gently pushing the small part upward into the uterine cavity while simultaneously applying fundal pressure to effect descent of the vertex or breech. If the head is very low in the pelvis and the cervix is fully dilated, the use of a vacuum pump can be attempted

2. *Cesarean section*: If there is cephalopelvic disproportion, reposition is not feasible or is unsuccessful, or there is some other condition that militates against vaginal delivery, cesarean section should be performed

3. *Internal podalic version and extraction*: This procedure carries with it the danger of uterine rupture and fetal death. Hence, it should not be used in the management of compound presentations

Prolapse of the Cord

In 13 to 23 percent of cases, the compound presentation is complicated by prolapse of the umbilical cord. This then becomes the major and urgent problem, and treatment is directed primarily to it (see Chapter 28).

COMPLICATED LABOR

The Umbilical Cord

Yvonne Cargill

THE NORMAL UMBILICAL CORD

The umbilical cord links the fetus to the placenta and is the fetal lifeline. The cord is between 30 and 60 cm in length, the average being 50 cm. It is covered on the outside by amnion, which blends with the fetal skin at the umbilicus. On the inside of the cord is the thick myxomatous Wharton jelly. Through the jelly, protected by it, run the umbilical vessels, one vein and two arteries, in a spiral arrangement. The circulation is the reverse of the adult in that the vein carries the oxygenated blood to the fetus, and the arteries bring venous blood back to the placenta.

The fetal surface of the placenta is covered by amniotic membrane, under which course the large blood vessels, branches of the umbilical vein and arteries. Normally the cord inserts into the center of the placenta.

ABNORMALITIES OF THE UMBILICAL CORD

Length

Cords have been reported to measure as short as 0 cm and as long as 104 cm.

1. A short cord may result in delay in descent of the fetus, fetal distress, and separation of the placenta from the wall of the uterus, inversion of the uterus, and rupture leading to hemorrhage and possible fetal exsanguination
2. A long cord is subject to entanglement, knotting, encirclement of the fetus, and prolapse
3. When the cord is absent, the fetus is attached directly to the placenta at the umbilicus. Body stalk anomaly is seen accompanying the absent cord. Amniotic band syndrome is associated with the pathogenesis
4. It appears that the length of the umbilical cord is determined at least partly by the amount of amniotic fluid present in the first and second trimesters of pregnancy and on the mobility of the fetus. If there is oligohydramnios, amniotic bands, or limitation of fetal movement for any reason, the umbilical cord will not develop to an average length

Single Umbilical Artery

This occurs in 1 percent of single births and in 7 to 14 percent of multiple pregnancies. If isolated, there is a 15 percent risk of intrauterine growth restriction (IUGR) in the pregnancy. If other anomalies are present, there is a 50 percent aneuploidy risk. There is no association with trisomy 21.

Umbilical Cord Cyst

There is a 2 percent prevalence of umbilical cord cyst. Most often these are a transient finding in the first trimester. If they are transient, they have a very good prognosis. They may be associated with trisomy 13 and 18, and they have a poorer prognosis if they are multiple.

Umbilical Vessel Aneurysm

An umbilical vein varix is present if the vein measures more than 9 mm in diameter. This is usually seen in the intraabdominal portion of the vein. Umbilical vein dilatation may be the first manifestation of increased venous pressure and should prompt a workup for other signs and possible etiologies.

An umbilical artery aneurysm is seen near the placental end of the cord. Pulsed Doppler will confirm its arterial origin. If other anomalies are present, trisomy 18 is common.

Both umbilical artery and vein aneurysms are associated with interruption of the umbilical cord flow, fetal compromise, and death. Venous compromise is a result of thrombosis. Umbilical artery aneurysms that expand can compress the umbilical vein, leading to hypoxia and death.

Velamentous Cord Insertion

In this case, the vessels of the cord break up into branches before reaching the placenta so that the cord inserts into the membranes rather than the placental disc. The result is that large vessels course under the membrane and are unprotected by Wharton jelly. This is associated with fetal growth abnormalities, cord separation, and fetal bleeding, resulting in fetal death and retained placenta.

Vasa Previa

In this situation, the velamentous vessels lie over the cervix in front of the presenting part. Rupture happens when the membranes rupture during or before labor. This leads to fetal bleeding, which can be fatal within a few minutes.

The diagnosis can be made by ultrasound. These patients do not have any symptoms, therefore a high index of suspicion is required. Vasa previa is more common but not exclusive to low-lying placentas with velamentous cord insertion. Color Doppler can be used to demonstrate the umbilical vessels crossing the cervical os.

When this diagnosis is made, preterm delivery by cesarean section is advised at about 34 weeks' gestation because of the high fetal death rate with rupture of membranes in this situation.

CORD ENTANGLEMENTS

The most common variety of cord entanglement is the umbilical cord around the fetal neck. As many as nine loops of cord around the neck have been reported. A single loop of cord is present in 21 percent of deliveries. Two loops are present in 2.5 percent and three loops in 0.2 percent of normal deliveries.

It is unclear if nuchal cord is associated with a statistically increased risk of perinatal adverse outcome. A positive relationship has been found in some studies between nuchal cords and fetal demise, impaired fetal growth, meconium in the amniotic fluid, abnormal fetal heart rate, operative delivery, umbilical artery acidemia, and neurodevelopmental abnormalities.

Cord entanglement is most common in the monoamniotic twins. The stillbirth rate is 50 percent. Delivery is recommended by cesarean section at 34 weeks' gestation.

KNOTS OF THE CORD

True Knot

Occasionally, a true knot of the umbilical cord is noted after delivery. This complication can occur when there is a long cord, large amounts of amniotic fluid, a small infant, or an overactive fetus or as a result of external version. In many instances, the knot is formed when a loop of cord is slipped over the infant's head or shoulders during delivery.

Rarely is the knot pulled tightly enough to cause the death of the fetus from restriction of the circulation in the cord. The umbilical vessels, protected by the thick myxomatous Wharton jelly, are rarely occluded completely. The fetal mortality rate associated with true knots is low.

In these cases, there is a flattening or dissipation of Wharton jelly and venous congestion distal to the knot, as well as partially or completely occlusive vascular thrombi.

False Knots

The blood vessels are longer than the cord. Often they are folded on themselves and produce nodulations on the surface of the cord. These have been termed *false knots.*

PROLAPSE OF THE UMBILICAL CORD

In this situation, the umbilical cord lies beside or below the presenting part. Although an infrequent complication (0.3-0.6%), its significance is disproportionately great because of the high fetal mortality rate.

Compression of the umbilical cord between the presenting part and the maternal pelvis reduces or cuts off the blood supply to the fetus and, if uncorrected, leads to death of the fetus.

Classification of Prolapsed Cord

1. *Umbilical cord presentation (funic presentation):* The cord is seen on ultrasound or palpated on pelvic examination below the fetal presenting part. The fetal membranes are intact
2. *Umbilical cord prolapse:* The membranes are ruptured, and the cord is palpated below the fetal presenting part (Fig. 28-1)
3. *Occult cord prolapse:* The cord is not palpable but is being compressed by the presenting part. This diagnosis can only be made during cesarean section

Risk Factors for Cord Prolapse

Malpresentation is the most commonly present risk factor for cord prolapse. Footling breech presentation is the presentation with the highest incidence of cord prolapse. Prematurity and the second twin are other fetal risk factors for cord prolapse.

Maternal factors include a narrow pelvis, preventing descent of the fetal presenting part and multiparity.

A long cord, a low-lying placenta, and polyhydramnios also increase the risk of cord prolapse.

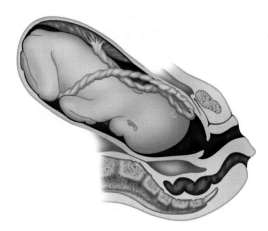

A. Cord prolapsed at the inlet.

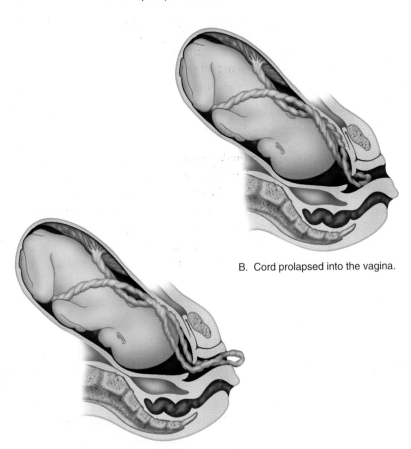

B. Cord prolapsed into the vagina.

C. Cord prolapsed through the introitus.

FIGURE 28-1. Prolapsed umbilical cord.

Many obstetric interventions can be associated with cord prolapse. The most common intervention is artificial rupture of membranes with a presenting part that is not fixed in the pelvis. Any intervention that could dislodge the presenting part, including insertion of a scalp electrode, insertion of an intrauterine pressure catheter, scalp pH sampling, manual fetal rotation, or vacuum or forceps delivery, may lead to cord prolapse if the presenting part is lifted from the pelvis.

Signs of Cord Prolapse

The first sign of cord prolapse is most often bradycardia or prolonged variable decelerations. When these occur, a digital examination should be performed to rule out cord prolapse.

The only other presentation is feeling or seeing the cord in the vagina or protruding out of the introitus.

Management of Cord Prolapse

The outcome of cord prolapse is related to the length of time between the cord prolapse and delivery. In most cases, the safest and most rapid method of delivery is a cesarean section.

While preparing for a cesarean section, the following temporary measures maybe appropriate:

1. Maternal Trendelenburg or knee–chest positioning and manual disimpaction of the fetal head by manual pressure in the maternal vagina
2. Replacing the cord above the fetal presenting part. This is often very difficult because the woman is usually in labor and there is a risk of further compromising the cord circulation
3. Tocolysis
4. Vaginal delivery may be an option if the cervix is fully dilated. This may particularly be an option for a second twin

UMBILICAL CORD DOPPLER

Umbilical cord Doppler is the test of fetal well-being with the most research to support its use. It is most often found to be abnormal in fetus with IUGR in the early third trimester. Normally, there is forward flow in the umbilical artery throughout the fetal cardiac cycle. The ratio of the peak systolic flow to the diastolic flow is less than 3 after 30 weeks.

COMPLICATED LABOR

Absent end-diastolic flow and reverse diastolic flow are associated with IUGR, oligohydramnios, and stillbirth. Reverse end-diastolic flow in the umbilical artery is associated with fetal demise in 1 to 7 days. After 30 weeks, if reverse end-diastolic flow is present, delivery is recommended usually by cesarean section.

SELECTED READING

Clare NM, Hayashi R, Khodr G: Intrauterine death from umbilical cord hematoma. Arch Pathol Lab Med 103:46, 1979

Katz Z, Lancet M, Borenstein R: Management of labor with umbilical cord prolapse. Am J Obstet Gynecol 142:239, 1982

Multiple Pregnancy

Karen Fung Kee Fung

CHAPTER 29

INCIDENCE

In 1895, Hellin described a mathematically simple rule for estimation of the rates of twinning and conception of higher order multiples in the general population. This rule, which has been widely cited and accepted, proposes the following rates of multiple pregnancy:

Twins	1:89
Triplets	$1:89^2$
Quadruplets	$1:89^3$
Quintuplets	$1:89^4$

Several authors have attempted to refine this law, which has been demonstrated to be inexact, especially when higher order multiples and older mothers are concerned. The explosion in reproductive technologies, the societal trend of delayed childbearing, and the observation of an increase in spontaneous twinning on the multiple birth rate also render this law mostly of historic interest.

Since the 1970s, there has been a phenomenal rise in twinning rates by about 80 percent in some countries. France, for example, reports rates of approximately 17 in 1000 live births. In 2006 in the United States, twins comprised approximately 32 in 1000 live births. Triplet and higher order multiple births had demonstrated similar trends until the later 1990s with a leveling off after that time, likely because of better control of reproductive cycles. The estimated contribution of reproductive technologies to the multiple birth rates is dramatic, increasing the twin birth rate 20-fold and the triplet and quadruplet rate 400-fold. Approximately two-thirds of this increase is attributed to infertility treatment and the remaining third to the trend of delayed childbearing.

Although the etiology of multiple pregnancy is unknown in most cases, it is recognized that excessive gonadotropic stimulation leading to superovulation is a factor in dizygous twinning. This phenomenon is evident in older mothers up to approximately age 37 years.

Whatever the etiology, the impact of the multiples epidemic reverberates throughout the health care system in terms of health care costs and suboptimal perinatal outcome. In the patient census of any tertiary level neonatal unit, multiples are overrepresented. It has been estimated that the annual cost of caring for multiples born prematurely after in vitro fertilization is in excess of $1 billion U.S. annually or $52,000 per infant.

Morbidity and mortality figures among multiples are also staggering. Population-based studies have reported the stillbirth and neonatal mortality rates in twins in the order of 18 in 100 births and 23 in 1000, respectively. Survival rates among multiples are also not uniformly distributed, and the effects of chorionicity on survival are both sobering and profound. Rates of fetal loss are substantially higher in monochorionic twins (44.4 in 1000 stillbirths rates) than dichorionic twins (12.2 in 1000 births; relative risk [RR], 3.6) and neonatal losses (32.4 in 1000 monochorionic vs. 21.4 in 1000 dichorionic; RR, 1.5) in dichorionic twins. The prospective risk of stillbirth was higher in monochorionic at all gestational ages and highest before 28 weeks of gestation. Survival rates decline dramatically as the number of fetal occupants of the uterus rises, and triplet loss rates of 93 to 203 in 1000 live births have been reported.

VANISHING TWIN

It is well recognized that not all twin conceptions will result in delivery of two babies. There is a high spontaneous loss rate of one twin in early pregnancy, a phenomenon referred to as a "vanishing" twin. Studies of twin pregnancy resulting from assisted reproductive technologies (ART) demonstrate that approximately 10 to 15 percent of singleton births begin as twin gestations. Early first-trimester loss of one twin may result in vaginal bleeding and symptoms of spontaneous abortion without significant maternal morbidity. Second-trimester death of one fetus in the twin pair can lead to compression and resorption of the fetus with the development of a "fetus papyraceus." The dead fetus becomes wafer-thin, blanches, and resembles old parchment (papyrus). The diagnosis of fetus papyraceus is usually evident at delivery when examination of the placenta reveals the outline of the pale, paper-like fetus on the fetal surface of the placenta between the membrane layers.

PHYSIOLOGY OF TWINNING

Nature has provided us with several biologically diverse types of twins based on the number of ova fertilized at conception and the timing of cleavage of the embryo.

The true incidence of double- versus single-ovum twins can be established following careful assignment of gender, histologic examination of the placenta and membranes, and detailed DNA analysis of umbilical cord blood. This is beyond the scope of care offered in most institutions. In centers where the zygosity of twins was well established by these methods, the frequency of dizygotic twins was found to be 71.0 percent and monozygotic twins was 29.0 percent. The latter group can be further divided into single-ovum twins having a single placenta (i.e., monozygotic, monochorionic twins) (72 percent) versus single-ovum twins with two placentas (i.e., monozygotic, dichorionic twins) (27.9 percent).

Dizygous: Double Ovum

In binovular twinning (Figs. 29-1A and B), two fetuses develop from the fertilization of two ova liberated during the same menstrual cycle. The incidence of spontaneous double-ovum twins is influenced by heredity, race, maternal age, and parity. Each twin has his or her own placenta, chorion, and amniotic sac. When the ova are implanted near each other, the two placentas may seem to fuse; however, the circulations remain completely separate. These children are dizygotic twins or in lay vernacular, "fraternal" twins. They resemble each other only to the extent that siblings of the same age would. They may be of different sexes and sometimes look entirely dissimilar. Weinberg's rule states that the number of dizygous twins in any population is twice the number of twins of different sex; the remainder are monozygous. Dizygous twinning is the result of multiple ovulations, which may be caused by high levels of gonadotropic hormones overstimulating the ovaries. The artificial induction of ovulation greatly increases the chance of multiple pregnancy.

Monozygous: Single Ovum

Uniovular or monozygous twins are commonly referred to as "identical" twins in lay vernacular. They represent complete cleavage of the blastodermic vesicle. There is one egg fertilized by a single sperm, and therefore the offspring arise from the same germ plasm. The frequency of single-ovum twinning is independent of heredity, race, maternal age, and parity and is constant the world over. The pathophysiological explanation for this twinning phenomenon is unknown. Placental sharing in monozygous twins contributes to the high morbidity figures seen in this twin category compared with dichorionic counterparts. By virtue of their biology and common origin, the offspring are of the same gender and appearance. In 99 percent of cases, there are one placenta, one chorion, and two amniotic sacs. Placental examination demonstrates vascular anastomoses between the arteries and veins of both fetuses in every case. These communications are usually

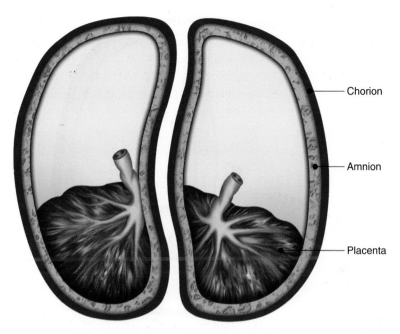

A. Separate dichorionic diamniotic placentae.

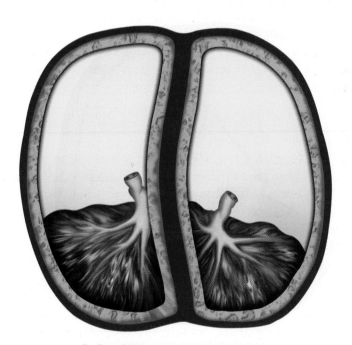

B. Fused dichorionic diamniotic placentae.

FIGURE 29-1. Placenta and membranes in twin pregnancy.

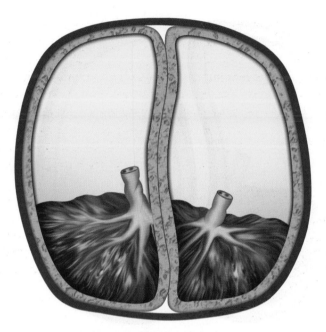

C. Monochorionic diamniotic placentae.

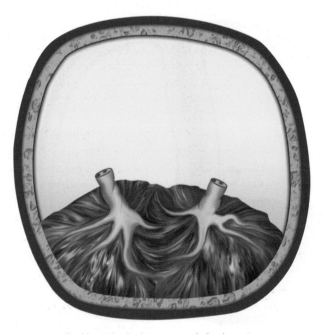

D. Monochorionic monoamniotic placentae.

FIGURE 29-1. *(Continued)*

balanced, leading to bidirectional blood flow between the fetuses. The development of unbalanced, unidirectional anastomoses in some fetuses give rise to disproportionate blood flow between twins and growth and fluid discordance or hemodynamic compromise in one or both twins. In 1 percent of monozygous twins, late splitting of the inner cell mass may result in twins with a single placenta, chorion, and amnion, and containment of the twins within the same amniotic sac provides opportunity for adverse events such as entanglement of the umbilical cords. Rarer still, incomplete division of the inner cell mass results in conjoined twins, which may share viscera or other body structures.

Not only is the survival rate of both monozygotic twins some 10 percent lower than for the dizygotic variety, but the incidence of congenital anomalies in monozygotic twins is also greater than in dizygotic twins. Because of shared genetics, the twins may have the same malformation; however, the unique hemodynamics that may arise within individuals that share a placenta may lead to unique anomalies between co-twins, both congenital and acquired.

PLACENTATION IN MONOZYGOUS TWINS

Despite the uncertainty concerning the physiological mechanisms underlying cleavage of the fertilized ovum or inner cell mass into two genetically identical individuals, it is well recognized that the timing of this event in early embryonic life influences placentation in twins and ultimately, morbidity.

1. *Dichorionic diamniotic twins*: In this case, the division occurs at the blastomere stage, no later than 2 to 3 days after fertilization. The inner cell mass has not yet been delineated. Separate embryos develop, undistinguishable at birth from dizygous twins. Each twin has his or her own chorion, amnion, and placenta. The latter may be separate or fused depending on the site of implantation (Figs. 29-1A and B)
2. *Monochorionic diamniotic twins*: The split takes place at the blastocyst stage between 4 and 6 days. The inner cell mass, which has been formed, divides in two. The placenta has one chorion but two amnions. Each twin lies in his or her own sac (Fig. 29-1C)
3. *Monochorionic monoamniotic twins*: The division takes place in the primitive germ disc at between 7 and 13 days. The amnion has already formed. The twins lie in the same amniotic sac. Monoamniotic twins are rare (Fig. 29-1D)

4. *Conjoined twins—monochorionic monoamniotic*: After the primitive streak of the embryo has appeared and the cells of the germ disc have assumed an axial arrangement (around 14 days), complete separation does not occur, and conjoined twins can develop

ESTABLISHING ZYGOSITY IN TWINS

One of the most frequently asked questions by parents expecting the birth of twins is whether the twins are "identical," that is, arising from a single fertilized ovum. Even for the obstetric caregiver, the answer to the question may be qualified. The most reliable gross morphologic marker of twin zygosity that would refute this diagnosis is discordant fetal gender. Fetuses of opposite phenotypic gender are by definition dizygous. Identical, uniovular twins are of concordant gender but may have one or two chorionic sacs. Only when there is a single chorionic sac can zygosity be proven. Thus, twins with one chorion are always monozygous. Twins of the same sex with two chorionic sacs may be monozygous or dizygous, and no examination of the placenta or membranes can establish the true status. In 80 percent of twins, zygosity can be demonstrated at birth by examination of the placental membranes. In the remainder, study of the blood types and morphologic features of the infants may be necessary. Confirmation of zygosity is achieved through DNA and human leukocyte antigen testing of the fetuses, but this is rarely carried out in routine practice.

SPECIAL COMPLICATIONS IN MONOCHORIONIC TWINS

Twins sharing a placenta with a single chorion are disproportionally represented in twin morbidity and mortality figures. This unique arrangement of vascular sharing can give rise to several fascinating structural and hemodynamic derangements and conditions peculiar to monochorionic twins.

Twin Transfusion Syndrome

This condition affects approximately 15 percent of monochorionic twins. The basic pathophysiology is an imbalance in the circulation between the fetuses secondary to unbalanced, intraplacental anastomoses. These vascular connections are primarily of the arteriovenous kind and hence are unidirectional in nature. Clinical manifestations of this condition result from the altered hemodynamics such that one fetus, the donor, becomes progressively anemic and hypovolemic, with oliguria and growth restriction, and the recipient becomes plethoric, polycythemic, and polyuric ("polyoli syndrome"). Cardiac compromise in the recipient fetus in the form of cardiogenic fetal hydrops, cardiomyopathy, or outflow tract obstruction may ensue. Pulmonary hypoplasia caused by prolonged oligo- or anhydramnios may be lethal in the donor. Preterm labor is a frequent feature, usually secondary to overdistension of the uterus from the polyhydramnios. The natural history of this disorder is known: perinatal loss of one or both fetuses may be as high as 80 to 90 percent after second-trimester diagnosis in the absence of fetal treatment.

Management includes (1) fetoscopic laser coagulation of anastomotic vessels, (2) serial amnioreduction, and (3) septostomy. Laser therapy is the preferred treatment because it directly addresses the pathophysiology behind this condition and has been found in randomized controlled trials to lead to improved short-term neurologic outcome in survivors.

Twin Reversed Arterial Perfusion Sequence

Twin reversed arterial perfusion sequence (TRAP), or "acardiac twin," is encountered in one in 35,000 pregnancies. Direct arterial anastomoses between the structurally normal fetus and the co-twin result in retrograde perfusion of deoxygenated blood from the umbilical artery of the normal "pump" twin toward the anomalous or "perfused" twin. A broad spectrum of reduction defects arise dependent on the degree of perfusion by the pump twin. The anomalous fetus will have a rudimentary or absent cardiac structures and is totally dependent on the pump twin. The mortality rate for the perfused twin is 100 percent, and mortality figures suggest that up to 50 percent of the normal, "pump" twins survive. Neurodevelopmental disability has been reported in survivors. Polyhydramnios is a common finding and is linked to the high incidence of preterm birth in this condition. Fetal cardiac failure and hydrops may be precipitated in the pump fetus from cardiac overload because the normal twin's heart does the work of two. Conservative management has been recommended when the perfused twin's fetal mass is small (<50% of the pump twin). Fetal therapy is offered when the perfused twin is large or rapidly growing or has developed hydrops. Treatment involves eliminating the blood flow to the perfused twin through cord occlusion or intrafetal radiofrequency ablation of blood flow to the anomalous twin. In approximately 33 percent of cases, spontaneous death to the perfused twin will occur before the time of planned fetal intervention at 16 to 18 weeks.

COMPLICATED LABOR

CONJOINED TWINS

Conjoined twins are uniovular twins in whom the embryonic area has failed to split completely and the two individuals remain attached. "Siamese" twins are one variety.

Incidence

The incidence is from 1:50,000 to 1:60,000 births. Approximately 70 percent are female.

Etiology

Because these fetuses originate from a single ovum, they are monovular, monozygotic, and monoamniotic with the same sex and chromosomal pattern. The basic defect is thought to be an incomplete, delayed fission of the inner cell mass, which takes place after the 14th day following fertilization. The precise etiology of conjoined twins is not known, but the same influences are responsible as those that cause monozygotic twinning.

Classification

The numerous phenotypes of conjoined twins fall into two main categories. The first is diplopagus (*Duplicatas completa*). In this group, there is equal or nearly equal and symmetrical duplication of structures. The second group is heteropagus (*Duplicatas incompleta*). In this group, only part of the anatomic structure of the fetus is duplicated. One component is smaller and dependent on the other.

The most frequently encountered anatomical arrangements include:

1. Conjoining at the level of the midtorso: 73 percent of all conjoined twins

    a. Thoracopagus: joined at the chest (40%)
    b. Xiphopagus or omphalopagus: joined at the anterior abdominal wall from the xiphisternum to the level of the umbilicus (23%)

2. Conjoining of the lower torso: 23 percent of all conjoined twins

    a. Pygopagus: joined at the buttocks (18%)
    b. Ischiopagus: joined at the ischium (6%)

3. Conjoining of the upper torso: 4 percent of conjoined twins

   a. Craniopagus—joined at the head (4 percent)

Diagnosis

The antepartum diagnosis of conjoined twins is important in that it will:

1. Define anatomical variations that will inform parental counseling
2. Facilitate timely and appropriate referral to other tertiary care services and health professionals such as maternal fetal medicine specialists, pediatric surgeons, geneticists, psychologists, and so on
3. Afford the parents the option of termination of pregnancy should they wish to interrupt the pregnancy
4. Enable the creation of a comprehensive delivery plan that will minimize maternal morbidity
5. Improve the survival of the fetus or fetuses

Before the use of ultrasonography in routine obstetric care, it was rare for conjoined twins to be discovered before the time of delivery. Most cases were diagnosed only in the second stage of labor, when obstruction had taken place. Gray-scale and color Doppler ultrasound has changed all that. Antenatal diagnosis of conjoined twins has been made as early as 7 weeks by endovaginal sonography. False-positive diagnoses are possible before 10 weeks because monoamniotic twins in a single sac can falsely appear conjoined.

In all multiple pregnancies, the possibility of conjoined twins should be considered and investigated. Suspicion-provoking factors include:

1. Polyhydramnios is found in 50 percent of cases of conjoined twins
2. The finding of a single fetal heart in a multiple pregnancy
3. A lack of engagement when the lie is longitudinal
4. A similar parallel lie (vertex–vertex, breech–breech)
5. An abnormal fetal attitude

Methods of Diagnosis

Two-dimensional imaging of fetal structure is the main diagnosis of this condition. Color Doppler and three-dimensional imaging provide additional insight into shared blood supply and surface anatomy.

1. *Ultrasonography*: Diagnostic criteria include:

a. Demonstration of a continuous nonseparated external skin contour
b. The body parts of the twins are on the same level and imaged in the same sonar plane
c. There is no change in the relative positions of the twins to one another on successive scans
d. Recognition of a face-to-face relationship in the case of thoracopagus twins
e. The demonstration of a single placenta. Real-time scanning is of value in assessing fetal movement and in identifying individual structures, such as the heart

2. *Magnetic resonance imaging (MRI)*: Magnetic resonance imaging is a valuable adjunct tool to obstetric ultrasound when used in investigation of the complex anatomical arrangement characteristic of conjoined twins. MRI provides the advantage of exquisite anatomic detail and enhanced tissue contrast to highlight the extent of fetal anomalies and shared organs.

   During labor, fortunately, intrapartum diagnosis of conjoined twins is a rare event given the implementation of a routine, second-trimester dating sonogram as a standard of modern obstetric care. However, dystocia or malpresentation in a known or suspected twin pregnancy may arouse a clinical suspicion of conjoined twins, locked twins, or congenital anomalies in the rare circumstances when ultrasound has not been performed. Because conjoined twins always develop within a single amniotic sac, palpation of a second sac after the rupture of the first will rule out conjoined twins. On the other hand, multiple fetal limbs close to each other, failure of traction to deliver the first twin in the second stage of labor, and an inability to move one twin without moving the other all suggest conjoined twins. When vaginal examination reveals a bridge of tissue between the fetuses, the diagnosis is confirmed

3. *Fetal echocardiography*: Fetal echocardiography also provides detailed structural and functional assessment of the fetal heart

4. *X-ray*: This modality may play a minor role in diagnosing cases with bony fusion of the fetal skeleton(s). Diagnostic criteria include:

   a. The fetal heads are at the same level and in the same body plane
   b. The spines are in unusually close proximity
   c. The spines are extended

d. The fetuses do not change position relative to each other after movement, manipulation, or the passage of time. Unless there is a bony fusion, the radiographic diagnosis is unreliable, and radiography has been largely replaced by ultrasonography

Management

The decision as to whether delivery should proceed per vaginam or by cesarean section is based on the following factors:

1. The possibility of the infants' survival: In most cases, this cannot be predicted accurately. However, when serious anomalies, such as anencephaly, are present, the answer is clear. More accurate methods of diagnosis and improved surgical techniques and care have increased the chances for survival of conjoined twins as separate individuals. In all cases, therefore, the welfare of the infants is of paramount importance

2. The gestational age and size of the infants: In most reported cases, the combined weight is less than 5000 g; often the combined weight does not exceed that of a normal infant. The small size is the result of the frequent occurrence of preterm labor and delivery

3. The extent and location of the union: In many cases, the union is sufficiently flexible that enough movement is possible to allow vaginal delivery with or without manipulation or by forceps. Extensive bony fusion may preclude movement, and vaginal delivery is impossible

4. Fetal presentation: Abnormal presentations, such as breech and transverse lie, occur frequently

5. The possibility of surgical separation

6. The attitudes of the parents

Method of Delivery

1. *Cesarean section*: This procedure offers the best chance for fetal survival, obviates damage to the mother by a difficult vaginal delivery, and is considered to be the method of choice for delivery when the diagnosis of conjoined twins has been made during the pregnancy. Elective cesarean section is performed when fetal maturity has been attained. Even in cases of fetal death, especially when the fetuses are large, cesarean section is advisable to avoid maternal injury. During cesarean section, the choice of uterine incision is determined by fetal presentation and lie with the goal of achieving maximum exposure. A lower segment vertical incision that allows upward extension if required may be preferable

2. *Vaginal delivery*: If the pregnancy is previable, the point and type of union permit mobility, and if the infants are dead, vaginal delivery can be effected without serious injury to the mother. However, dystocia is common, and manipulations such as forceps extraction or traction on the head, legs, or buttocks are necessary
3. *Destructive operations*: When part of the fetus has been born and complete delivery is not possible, a destructive operation may be the only alternative. Such procedures may include evisceration and amputation of parts of the body. Early diagnosis and careful anatomical mapping of the shared viscera and limbs with liberal use of cesarean section would obviate the need for such destructive procedures

Selective Intrauterine Growth Restriction

Despite similar genetics and intrauterine environment, fetal weights may vary significantly between co-twins in a monochorionic twin pair. Intertwin differences in estimated fetal weights of more than 25 percent may be found in up to 20 percent of all monochorionic twins. Such significant growth discordance may predict poor fetal outcome. Approximately 10 to 15 percent of these twins may also manifest intrauterine growth restriction (IUGR), having an estimated fetal weight below the 10th percentile. Large growth discordance and low fetal weight in one member of a monochorionic twin pair is known as "selective" IUGR (sIUGR) and carries a guarded fetal prognosis. The consequences of concern in sIUGR are intrauterine fetal death of the smaller fetus and fetal demise of both twins with the concomitant risk of ischemic brain damage in the survivor secondary to exsanguination into the dead or dying fetus through functional vascular anastomoses.

Three types of sIUGR are recognized, characterized by the pattern of arterial flow in the umbilical cord of the smaller fetus on Doppler ultrasound examination. Type 1 displays normal forward flow in the umbilical artery of the affected twin throughout systole and diastole, type 2 shows persistently absent or reversed umbilical artery flow, and type 3 demonstrates intermittently absent end diastolic flow. Fetal outcome deteriorates with increasing type. Fetal therapy by cord occlusion or laser photocoagulation of communicating vessels is reserved for advanced disease (type 2 or 3), and delivery is usually accomplished before term.

Monoamniotic Twins

Because the fetuses are not separated by membranes in monoamnionic twins, there is a great possibility of knotting, tangling, and strangulation of the umbilical cords. The resultant anoxia may lead to fetal death. In the absence of prenatal diagnosis of this condition and intense fetal surveillance, the prognosis for monoamniotic twins is known to be poor, with only 50 percent survival of both twins. Routine use of antenatal ultrasound has lead to earlier diagnosis of this condition, allowing for more informed parental counseling and management planning. The finding of entangled umbilical cords is the *sine que non* of diagnosis, found in almost all cases on antenatal ultrasound. Fetal surveillance remains problematic, however, because entangled cords may strangulate at any time during the pregnancy. Modern management of this condition consists of intense, multimodality methods of fetal assessment, including (1) biophysical profile testing on ultrasound, and (2) frequent use of nonstress testing to rule out signs of cord compression and fetal compromise. Early delivery by cesarean section is carried out (≥32 weeks) after priming of the immature fetal lungs by administration of maternal glucocorticoids to accelerate lung maturity. With a policy of aggressive fetal surveillance and early operative delivery by cesarean section at 32 to 35 weeks, the survival rates in this condition have been improved above that usually quoted in early literature.

Multifetal Reduction in Twins and Higher Order Pregnancies

Occupation of the uterus by more than one fetus at a time places the pregnancy at high risk of adverse outcome. Many parents, faced with the prospect of a very preterm birth or high cerebral palsy rates in multifetal pregnancies, may choose to reduce the multiple pregnancy to twins or singletons. Multifetal pregnancy reduction (MFPR) is carried out by intracardiac injection of potassium chloride into one or more late first-trimester fetuses. Overall loss rates of 5 percent are reported. Reduction of multiples in this fashion is associated with lower rates of fetal loss, prematurity, mortality, and morbidity for the surviving infants.

In Utero Death of a Co-twin

Fortunately, 97 percent of twin births reaching viability results in the birth of two live-born infants. Intrauterine fetal death of one co-twin occurs in about 2.5 percent of twins, and loss of both fetuses happens in 0.6 percent of twin gestations. Generally, despite enhanced fetal surveillance, the prospective rate of unexpected fetal death is higher among monochorionic twins, reaching one in 23 in some large series. In many cases, the etiology is unknown, although late-onset twin–twin transfusion has been implicated in some

COMPLICATED LABOR

cases. The median gestational age of intrauterine fetal death of a co-twin is around 34 weeks.

In cases of dichorionic placentation, the death of one member of a twin pair has little physical effect on the mother or the viable fetus. Death of a co-twin in a monochorionic twin pair may be a more ominous event, leading to a 20 percent risk of significant neurodevelopmental morbidity for the survivor. Severe fetal anemia or exsanguination in the survivor through intraplacental vascular anastomoses may lead to hypoxia and decreased brain perfusion. Hypoxic brain lesions, including porencephalic cysts, periventricular leukomalacia, and cerebral and cerebellar infarcts, may result. Thrombotic or ischemic events may occur elsewhere in the survivor after death of a co-twin, leading to renal cortical necrosis, bowel atresias, or aplasia cutis. The timing of the in utero demise of the monochorionic co-twin also influences the outcome. First-trimester loss of a co-twin usually carries a more favorable prognosis than demise occurring in the second or third trimesters. In cases of twin–twin transfusion syndrome, in utero death of a recipient twin is associated with a higher rate of intracranial lesions in the surviving donor than if the donor had in utero loss.

Antenatal detection of destructive brain lesions in twins may not be obvious until several weeks after in utero demise of a co-twin. Ultrasonography remains less sensitive than MRI in detecting subtle, early ischemic changes in the brain. Ventriculomegaly may be the only sonographic sign of underlying damage. Because of the immediacy of damage caused by hypoperfusion of the brain of the surviving fetus, a better perinatal outcome is not assured by shortening the interval between death of one twin and delivery of the other.

Preventive strategies such as early delivery of monochorionic twins between 32 and 34 weeks of gestation has been proposed to reduce the risk of in utero death of a co-twin (after administration of antenatal steroids to accelerate lung maturity). It is estimated that 23 monochorionic pregnancies would need to be delivered at this stage of pregnancy to prevent one intrauterine fetal death.

Twins Discordant for Fetal Structural or Chromosomal Anomaly

Although the incidence of fetal anomalies is substantially higher in multiples, both members of the twin pair may not be concordant for the anomaly, even when they originate from a single fertilized ovum. Several postzygotic events may arise in the early embryonic period that may give rise to both subtle differences among monochorionic twin pair, such as "mirror image" differences or lateral asymmetry or major anomalies that are not shared by both fetuses. Even karyotypically identical monochorionic twins may have different phenotypes because of differences in allocation of blastomeres or other genetic or epigenetic phenomena.

In fetuses discordant for an abnormality of structure or chromosomes, selective reduction of the affected fetus may be offered. Accurate assignment of chorionicity is vital if selective reduction is being considered. For dichorionic twins, intracardiac administration of KCl effects cardiac asystole in the anomalous fetus. This approach is contraindicated in monochorionic twin gestations, however, because of the intertwin vascular anastomoses within the single placental bed, which could lead to passage of the potassium solution into the unaffected fetus or exsanguination of the survivor into the dying, anomalous fetus. In these single-placental pregnancies, a surgical approach is often taken to completely occlude the umbilical cord vessels of the affected fetus, often using bipolar cord cauterization, laser cord coagulation, radiofrequency ablation, or fetoscopic cord occlusion. Survival of the unaffected fetus of the twin pair after selective reduction is in the order of 70 to 80 percent.

DIAGNOSIS OF MULTIPLE PREGNANCY

1. Suggestive findings

   a. Familial history
   b. Hyperemesis gravidarum
   c. The uterus and abdomen seem larger than expected for the period of amenorrhea

2. Positive signs

   a. Ultrasonography demonstrates the presence of two embryos
   b. Palpation of two heads or two breeches
   c. Two fetal hearts auscultated at the same time differing in rate by at least 10 beats/min

EFFECTS OF MULTIPLE PREGNANCY

Maternal Effects

1. Because the volume of the intrauterine contents is large, the center of gravity is shifted even more than in a singleton pregnancy, and

COMPLICATED LABOR

symptoms of discomfort and fatigue are frequent. Pressure against the diaphragm may lead to dyspnea

2. The mechanical and metabolic loads increase with the multiplicity of the pregnancy

3. Polyhydramnios, an excessive amount of amniotic fluid, is more common than in single pregnancies

4. The incidence of preeclampsia (23%) and gestational diabetes (69%) is increased over that of mothers of singletons

5. Anemia is prevalent (36%)

6. An additional weight gain of 35 to 45 pounds is to be expected because of the presence of more than one fetus, enhanced placental and maternal blood volume, and polyhydramnios

7. Increased risk of cholestasis of pregnancy

8. Multiple pregnancy is an independent risk factor for acute fatty liver disease

9. Pulmonary edema secondary to volume overload is more common

Fetal Effects

1. Although the individual child is smaller than average, the combined weight of the babies is larger than that of a single child. Low birth weight is common, with more than 50 percent of twins having a birth weight less than 2500 g. This is primarily because of the propensity for preterm birth in twins and twin-specific growth issues as outlined above. Even in a twin appropriately grown for gestational age, the second twin, on average, is about 80 g less than his or her co-twin

2. The combination of small babies and large amounts of amniotic fluid leads to an increased incidence of malpresentation and operative delivery

3. Fetal mortality is increased in twin pregnancy to four times that of singletons. Although malpresentations and congenital abnormalities play a part, the major cause of death is prematurity. Whereas approximately 10 percent of singletons are born prematurely, about 50 percent of twins and 88 percent of triplets are born before 37 weeks' gestation

4. The risk to the second twin is greater than to the first. Reasons include:

   a. Greater incidence of operative deliveries
   b. Too long an interval between the birth of the first and second twins

c. Reduction of the uterine capacity after the birth of the first baby: This may alter the placental hemodynamics and result in fetal anoxia

d. The second twin occupies a less favorable position in the actively contracting upper uterine segment

e. There is an increased incidence of malpresentation in the second twin

5. The least possible delay should be permitted between delivery of the infants. After the first is born, the mother is given oxygen to breathe in an effort to prevent anoxia of the second twin. The greater loss of the second twin is the result of death in the neonatal period rather than before or during labor

6. Congenital malformations, particularly cardiovascular defects, are more common in twins than in singletons, and twin fetuses with congenital anomalies are more likely to die of these anomalies than their singleton counterparts

7. In multiple pregnancies of higher fetal order, these complications are even more pronounced. Fetal outcome decreases with increasing fetal order because of the reasons cited above

Effects on Labor

1. Overstretching of the uterus by the large combined weights of the babies, two placentas, and copious amniotic fluid leads to the following:

a. Preterm labor occurs, on average, 3 weeks before term

b. Early rupture of the membranes is frequent (4%) and is one cause of premature labor

c. Most twin labors are satisfactory. Sometimes the overlengthened uterine muscles produce weak and inefficient contractions, resulting in slow progress

d. The increased incidence and danger of postpartum hemorrhage must be kept in mind (19%) and planned for

e. Malpresentations are common

f. Umbilical cord prolapse is caused by rupture of the membranes with the gushing out of large amounts of fluid, especially with the second twin

g. Multiple pregnancy accelerates the problem of cervical incompetence and can result in effacement and dilatation as early as the first trimester

2. In 80 percent of cases, the second twin is born within 30 minutes of the first

3. The two babies are born first and then the two placentas

4. The combinations of presentations (Fig. 29-2) are, in descending order of frequency:

   a. Two vertices (most common and most favorable presentation)
   b. Vertex and breech
   c. Two breeches
   d. Vertex and transverse lie
   e. Breech and transverse lie
   f. Both in the transverse lie

MANAGEMENT OF MULTIPLE PREGNANCY

Management During Pregnancy

Principles of antepartum management of twin pregnancy include the following:

1. Early diagnosis enables the parents to make preparations for more than one child and alerts the doctor to anticipate the problems of multiple pregnancy. The two main complications, premature labor and pre-eclampsia, call for special care during the prenatal period
2. Early establishment of chorionicity
3. Consideration of aneuploidy screening
4. Prenatal vitamin supplementation
5. Enhanced prenatal visits for early detection of preterm labor, preeclampsia, and IUGR
6. If the babies have attained a good size, the patient may resume her activities gradually

Delivery Planning For Multiple Pregnancy

Mode of Delivery

Factors influencing mode of delivery in twins are multiple and include (1) presentation (2) estimated fetal weight, (3) gestational age, (4) skill

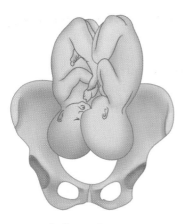

A. Two vertexes.

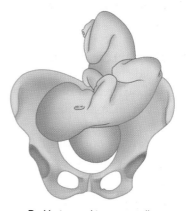

D. Vertex and transverse lie.

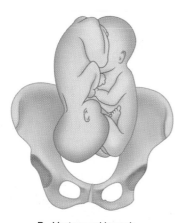

B. Vertex and breech.

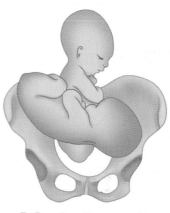

E. Breech and transverse lie.

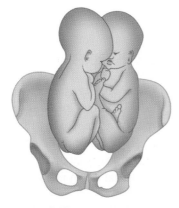

C. Two breeches.

FIGURE 29-2. Twin presentations.

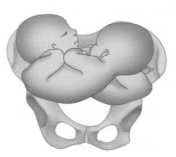

F. Two transverse lies.

COMPLICATED LABOR

of the operator, (5) previous operative delivery, (6) whether the patient is participating in a randomized controlled trial of the same, and possibly (7) chorionicity.

With this multitude of influences, it is not surprising that planned vaginal delivery of viable twins occurs in less than 50 percent of all twins. Overall, when trial of labor is offered to twins, it can be expected to be successful in approximately 77 percent of cases.

Despite both fetuses presenting by the vertex, in only about 53 percent of cases will both twins deliver vaginally. Another 43 percent of vertex–vertex twins will delivery by cesarean section, and the remainder will result on a combined delivery in which the presenting twin is delivered vaginally and the second twin by cesarean section.

Various clinical practice guidelines have suggested that estimated fetal weight be used to plan mode of delivery in twins. When fetal weight is estimated to be less than 1500 g, a liberal policy of cesarean section is suggested even when both fetuses are in vertex presentation.

Rates of emergency delivery of the second twin by cesarean section after successful vaginal delivery of the presenting twin appears to be highly influenced by fetal weight as well. Cesarean section rates of approximately 5.7 percent have been reported in larger second twins (>2500 g) in contrast to rates of about 11.3 percent in second twins weighing less than 1500 g. The highest mortality rates of second twins occur in the setting of combined delivery in which the first twin has been born vaginally and the second twin by cesarean section. These observations, along with concerns for higher maternal morbidity rates after emergency versus elective cesarean delivery, have raised questions about the optimal delivery route for all twins, and multicenter, international randomized trials are ongoing to answer this question.

Timing of Delivery

Not only is the optimal route of delivery of twins controversial, but the optimal timing of delivery also remains in question. Neonatal respiratory morbidity rates are lowest when elective delivery is completed at or beyond 37 completed weeks. Controversy stems from reports of increased stillbirth and early neonatal death rates when twin pregnancy is prolonged. In Australia, the lowest composite neonatal mortality and morbidity rates are seen when twin delivery is accomplished at 37 weeks and increases thereafter, but Canada and Japan report lowest rates of perinatal death in twins delivered at 38 weeks. Prospective risk of perinatal death in twins is such that it is reasonable to consider delivery of twins by 38 weeks. These figures do not take into consideration the influence of chorionicity on twin outcome. The risks of late fetal loss in monochorionic twin gestations are such that perinatal centers in the United Kingdom advocate elective delivery of these twins at 36 to 37 weeks and delivery of dichorionic twins approximately 1 to 2 weeks later.

It must be remembered, however, that if elective cesarean section of twins is performed at 35 weeks or later but before 37 weeks, respiratory morbidity is in the order of 5 percent, and patients should be counseled regarding the risks.

Intrapartum Management

Preparation for a planned twin delivery is a team sport involving collaboration and effective communication of various health professionals. Essential elements of room setup include the following:

1. Presence of experienced obstetrical personnel skilled in operative management of twins
2. Availability of accurate fetal and maternal monitoring systems
3. Duplicate sets of instruments
4. Oxytocin infusion set
5. Immediate availability of anesthesia support
6. Adequate pediatric personnel skilled in resuscitative measures
7. Portable ultrasound scanner
8. Rapid availability of blood products

Conduct of Delivery of Twins

1. Accurate diagnosis of the presentations is essential. Ultrasonic confirmation of presentation is used when needed

2. Adequate pain control is important to gain maternal cooperation and facilitate assisted delivery if required. Sedatives and analgesics are administered with care because small babies are susceptible to drugs that depress the vital centers. Epidural anaesthesia is preferred to limit fetal drug effects while permitting rapid surgical intervention as necessary and limit the risks of general anesthesia

3. The higher incidence of postpartum hemorrhage calls for precautionary measures even to the extent of having cross-matched blood available, especially if the mother is anemic

4. Watchful expectancy is the procedure of choice during labor. The best results are obtained when the least interference is used

5. All women labouring with twins should have direct IV access for infusion of crystalloid. This precautionary measure has two uses:
   a. If uterine atony occurs either before or after the birth of one or both twins, oxytocin can be added to the solution to stimulate the myometrium
   b. If postpartum hemorrhage takes place, the route for the administration of fluids or blood is available immediately

6. The first baby is delivered in the usual way as if it were a single pregnancy

7. Care should be taken to avoid delayed cord clamping in monochorionic twins. This is to prevent the second baby from bleeding through the cord of the first in uniovular twins, in whom the placental circulations communicate

8. Intravenous uterotonic agents should not be given before birth of the second twin is complete. The strong contraction that results may result in compromise to the second twin still in utero, especially if he or she is malpositioned

9. Careful examination is made to determine the position and station of the second baby. If the vertex or breech is in or over the inlet and the uterus is contracting, the membranes should be ruptured artificially, care being taken that the cord does not prolapse. If uterine inertia has set in, an oxytocin drip may be commenced to reestablish uterine contractions; when this has been achieved, amniotomy is performed. The presenting part is guided into the pelvis by the vaginal hand. If necessary, pressure is made on the fundus with the other hand. Because the first baby has already dilated the birth canal, the second one descends rapidly to the pelvic floor

10. Once the presenting part is on the perineum, it is delivered spontaneously or by simple operative measures

11. If the presentation is abnormal, fetal or maternal distress supervenes, or spontaneous delivery of the second twin has not taken place within 30 minutes, operative intervention is considered because the risk to the second baby increases with time. Options include breech extraction or external cephalic version (ECV) if the second twin is

in breech presentation. The choice of the approach varies with the training and experience of the operator. Generally, breech extraction can be accomplished in a shorter time frame than ECV and before the cervix begins to clamp down. Internal podalic version and extraction is accomplished if the fetus is a cephalic presentation or transverse lie. Routine version and extraction is not advised for normal positions

12. The sudden reduction of the intrauterine contents by delivery of the first twin may lead to premature separation of the placenta, endangering the second baby. Accurate monitoring and documentation of the fetal heart rate and differentiation from the maternal heart rate is imperative for early detection of potential fetal compromise, which would expedite delivery

13. The placentas are delivered after both twins have been born

14. Cesarean section is not indicted for a sole indication of twins but is reserved for twins with comorbidity such as severe preeclampsia, placenta previa and abruption placentae, transverse lie, or prolapse of the umbilical cord. Twin pregnancy does not impose a special threat to the integrity of a preexisting low transverse cesarean scar. It is not necessary to schedule a repeat cesarean section any earlier for a twin pregnancy than for a singleton

15. Cesarean section for second twin: In approximately 7 percent of twins, vaginal delivery of the first twin is followed by emergency cesarean delivery of the second twin. These situations usually arise when acute fetal distress is encountered and vaginal delivery of the second twin cannot be effected promptly. Included here are separation of the placenta, contracted cervix, prolapse of the umbilical cord, and so on

Delayed Interval Delivery of Twins

In 1880, the first published report of a prolonged delivery interval between premature birth of co-twins at 27 and 32 weeks of gestation appeared in the medical literature with survival of the second twin. Since the late 1970s, there has been renewed interest in this management strategy, with several reports of cases of successful delayed interval deliveries of multiples reported in both twins and triplets. Interval delays in delivery have been reported from 1 day to 153 days in attempted cases.

COMPLICATED LABOR

The relative statistical rarity of this approach has precluded attempts at prospective trials addressing outcome. Much of the published work in this area originates from case reports and small retrospective case series. Lack of published experience utilizing a structured, standardized approach to management, coupled with concerns over potential reporting bias in the literature makes informed patient counseling challenging.

Recently, experience from a single tertiary care center using a standard protocol for delayed interval delivery has been reported in a series of 93 twins and 34 triplets. Survival rates of first twins born beyond 25 weeks was 65 percent compared with 95 percent in corresponding second twins, with mean delays between delivery of twins of 19 days (range, 1-107 days). Overall, only 41 percent of twins and 35 percent of triplets were considered candidates for attempted interval delivery. Asynchronous delivery was not considered in the remaining 60 percent of multiples because of immediate delivery of the remaining fetuses or medical contraindications to prolonging the pregnancy. The elements of a standardized approach to intervention in these successful cases have included a four-step approach:

1. Preparation
   - Early identification of potential candidates at risk of extreme preterm delivery
   - Parent counseling and informed consent regarding procedural details, indications and contraindications, and risks and benefits
   - Administration of tocolytics (e.g., nifedipine, indomethacin)
   - Vaginal and urinary cultures
   - Administration of broad-spectrum antibiotics
   - Administration of maternal betamethasone to accelerate lung maturity beyond 24 weeks
2. Delivery of the first twin
   - Intrapartum use of tocolytics and antibiotics
   - Avoidance of episiotomy
   - Culture cervix and cord of the first baby
   - Avoidance of attempts at delivery of the placenta
   - Vaginal and cervical washing with chlorhexidine
   - High ligation of umbilical cord of the first twin with nonabsorbable ligatures
   - Avoidance of cerclage
   - Administration of anti-D prophylaxis as required
3. Interval delay between birth of the first and second twins
   - Avoidance of vaginal examination to assess the cervix
   - Transperineal ultrasound to assess cervical length and condition

- Daily temperature monitoring for signs of chorioamnionitis
- Serial cervical cultures and antibiotics as indicated
- Serial assessment of fetal well-being (ultrasound and cardiotocography)
4. Delivery of remaining multiples
   - Careful examination of the placenta to rule out retained products
   - Histologic examination of the placenta

Traditionally, delayed interval delivery has been thought to be contra-indicated in monochorionic twins because of concerns regarding higher infection rates limiting success. The standardized approach outlined above has been used with short-term success in four cases of monochorionic twins with a mean delay in delivery between twins of 9 days (range, 3-16 days).

Similar attempts at delayed delivery in triplet pregnancies have shown some success with an average delay in delivery between first and third fetuses of 18 days (range 1-118 days), but a small sample size prohibits conclusions regarding significant outcome differences between fetuses.

Informed consent for this intervention requires parental counseling regarding maternal complications of this approach, which may include chorioamnionitis (24%), abruption placentae (5%), postpartum hemorrhage greater than 1 L (11%), and manual removal of the placenta (11%).

The use of cervical cerclage after delivery of the first twin is controversial in the literature. Similarly, published case series have suggested an improved success rate when the first fetus has delivered at a previable stage, i.e. less than 24 weeks.

TRIPLET AND QUADRUPLET PREGNANCY

In the past, multiple pregnancy involving more than two infants was rare, but the widespread use of ovulation induction agents, such as clomiphene citrate and gonadotropins, as well as other ART, have increased the incidence of higher order plural births significantly. Between the years 1980 and 1997 in the United States, a 400 percent rise in triplet births was noted. Since that time, from 1998 to 2005, a substantive drop (16%) in the birth of these higher order multiples has been witnessed. This dramatic change may be multifactorial in nature, resulting from better control of the reproductive cycle, enhanced vigilance regarding the number of embryo transfers per cycle, and/or increased access to MFPR of triplets to twins or singletons.

COMPLICATED LABOR

Irrespective of the cause of this decline, reduction in the number of higher order multiples is welcome news because of the inherent risks of these plural births, as outlined in Table 29-1.

TABLE 29-1: RISKS FOR TWINS AND HOM VERSUS SINGLETONS

	Singletons	Twins	HOM
Mortality rate		5-7 times higher	10-12 times higher
Gestational age at delivery	39-40 weeks	35.8-36 weeks	32.5-34 weeks
RDS	60%	70%	15% higher (75%)
Cerebral palsy	1.6%	7.4%	28%

RDS, respiratory distress syndrome; HOM, higher order multiples.

This list does not address the other confounder, chorionicity, which is an additional independent risk factor that influences morbidity and mortality for higher order multiples just as it does in twin pregnancy.

In general, all of the special issues and complications of twin pregnancy for mothers and fetuses are augmented in higher order multiples. Fetal outcomes tend to decline with increasing plurality, with perinatal mortality rates about 10 to 12 times higher than those found in singletons.

The prime cause of high fetal loss is preterm labor, often preceded by spontaneous rupture of the membranes. The mean gestational age at delivery is 32.5 to 34 weeks. Of particular concern is the cerebral palsy rate in higher order multiples, which is more than 15 times greater than in singleton pregnancies. Spastic diplegia and bilateral cerebral palsy are more common in this group.

Management

As in twins, modern clinical management includes (1) early diagnosis, (2) enhanced fetal surveillance, (3) serial assessment of fetal growth and well-being, (4) close observations for signs of impending preterm birth, with frequent cervical assessment (by digital evaluation) or ultrasound assessment of cervical length, (5) prophylactic steroids (betamethasone 12 mg intramuscularly every 24 hours for two doses) to accelerate fetal lung maturity if early preterm birth (<34 weeks) is anticipated.

Mode of Delivery in Triplets

Routine use of cesarean section for delivery of these higher order multiples is recommended when fetal viability is reached. The liberal use of operative delivery avoids intrauterine instrumentation and manipulation in an overdistended uterus and minimizes maternal trauma. Careful planning with neonatal staff is imperative because the sudden unheralded arrival of three premature infants with special needs can overwhelm any intensive care nursery. Delayed interval delivery of triplets has been successfully implemented when at least one fetus delivers at a previable gestational age.

SELECTED READING

Aaronson D, Harlev A, Sheiner E, Levy A: Trial of labor after cesarean section in twin pregnancies: maternal and neonatal safety. J Matern Fetal Neonatal Med 23:550, 2010

Arabin B, van Eyck J: Delayed-interval delivery in twin and triplet pregnancies: 17 years of experience in 1 perinatal center. Am J Obstet Gynecol 200:154.e1-8, 2009

Arabin B, van Eyck J: The role of ultrasound in multiple pregnancy. Twin Res 4:141, 2001

Barigye O, Pasquini L, Galea P, Chambers H, Chappell L, Fisk NM: High risk of unexpected late fetal death in monochorionic twins despite intensive ultrasound surveillance: A cohort study. PLoS Med 2:e172, 2005

Chalouhi GE, Stirnemann JJ, Salomon LJ, Essaoui M, Quibel T, Ville Y: Specific complications of monochorionic twin pregnancies: Twin-twin transfusion syndrome and twin reversed arterial perfusion sequence. Semin Fetal Neonatal Med 15:349, 2010

Chauhan SP, Scardo JA, Hayes E, Abuhamad, AZ, Berghella V: Twins: prevalence, problems, and preterm births. Am J Obstet Gynecol 203:305, 2010

Fisk NM, Duncombe GJ, Sullivan MHF: The basic and clinical science of twin-twin transfusion syndrome. Placenta 30:379, 2009

Ford AA, Bateman BT, Simpson LL: Vaginal birth after cesarean delivery in twin gestations: A large, nationwide sample of deliveries. Am J Obstet Gynecol 195:1138, 2006

Glinianaia SV, Obeysekera MA, Sturgiss S, Bell R: Stillbirth and neonatal mortality in monochorionic and dichorionic twins: A population-based study. Hum Reprod 26:2549, 2011

Hubinont C, Santolaya-Forgas J: A systematic approach to first-trimester ultrasound assessment of twins. Am J Perinatol 27:595, 2010

Ishii K, Murakoshi T, Hayashi S, Saito M, Sago H, Takahashi Y, Sumie M, et al: Ultrasound predictors of mortality in monochorionic twins with selective intrauterine growth restriction. Ultrasound Obstet Gynecol 37:22, 2011

Karageyim Karsidag AY, Kars B, Dansuk R, Api O, Unal O, Turan MC, Goynumer G: Brain damage to the survivor within 30 min of co-twin demise in monochorionic twins. Fetal Diagn Ther 20:91, 2005

Lee KA, Oh KJ, Lee SM, Kim A, Jun JK: The frequency and clinical significance of twin gestations according to zygosity and chorionicity. Twin Res Hum Genet 13:609, 2010

Lewi L, Valencia C, Gonzalez E, Deprest J, Nicolaides KH: The outcome of twin reversed arterial perfusion sequence diagnosed in the first trimester. Am J Obstet Gynecol 203:213.e1-4, 2010

Oyelese Y, Ananth CV, Smulian JC, Vintzileos AM: Delayed interval delivery in twin pregnancies in the United States: Impact on perinatal mortality and morbidity. Am J Obstet Gynecol 192:439, 2005

Roman AS, Fishman S, Fox N, Klauser C, Saltzman D, Rebarber A: Maternal and neonatal outcomes after delayed-interval delivery of multifetal pregnancies. Am J Perinatol 28:91, 2011

Rossi AC, D'Addario V: Laser therapy and serial amnioreduction as treatment for twin-twin transfusion syndrome: A metaanalysis and review of literature. Am J Obstet Gynecol 198:147, 2008

Rossi AC, Mullin PM, Chmait RH: Neonatal outcomes of twins according to birth order, presentation and mode of delivery: A systematic review and meta-analysis. BJOG 118:523, 2011

Sabourin J, DeDoming E, Chandra S, Jain V: Twin reversed arterial perfusion syndrome. J Obstet Gynaecol Can 33:315, 2011

Shinwell ES, Haklai T, Eventov-Friedman S: Outcomes of multiplets. Neonatology 95:6, 2009

Smith NA, Wilkins-Haug L, Santolaya-Forgas J, Acker D, Economy KE, Benson CB, Robinson JN: Contemporary management of monochorionic diamniotic twins: Outcomes and delivery recommendations revisited. Am J Obstet Gynecol 203:133.e1-6, 2010

Stock S, Norman J: Preterm and term labor in multiple pregnancies. Semin Fetal Neonatal Med 15:336, 2010

Valsky DV, Eixarch E, Martinez JM, Crispi F, Gratacós E: Selective intrauterine growth restriction in monochorionic twins: Pathophysiology, diagnostic approach and management dilemmas. Semin Fetal Neonatal Med 15:342, 2010

Vayssière C, Benoist G, Blondel B, Deruelle P, Favre R, Gallot D, Jabert P, et al: Twin pregnancies: Guidelines for clinical practice from the French College of Gynaecologists and Obstetricians (CNGOF). Eur J Obstet Gynecol Reprod Biol 156:12, 2011

Wan JJ, Schrimmer D, Taché V, Quinn K, Lacoursiere DY, James G, Benirschke K, et al: (2011). Current practices in determining amnionicity and chorionicity in multiple gestations. Prenat Diagn 31:125, 2011

Zhang J, Hamilton B, Martin J, Trumble A: Delayed interval delivery and infant survival: a population-based study. Am J Obstet Gynecol 191:470, 2004

PART VI

Other Issues

CHAPTER 30

Preterm Labor

Griffith D. Jones

DEFINITION

In pregnancy, *term* refers to the gestational period from 37^{+0} to 41^{+6} weeks. Preterm births occur between 24^{+0} and 36^{+6} weeks. Although births earlier than this are referred to as miscarriages, occasional survivors are seen after delivery at 23 weeks, which has become the "gray zone" for viability.

Early births occur either because delivery is believed to be in the best interests of the mother or baby (indicated deliveries) or because the mother develops spontaneous contractions or membrane rupture earlier than normal (spontaneous deliveries). The latter group has two subdivisions: spontaneous preterm labor (PTL) and preterm prelabor rupture of membranes (PPROM). Indicated deliveries, PTL, and PPROM each account for approximately one-third of early births.

PREVALENCE

From 2005 to 2009, 647,088 women delivered between 24 and 42 weeks of gestation in Ontario (BORN Ontario, Niday Perinatal Database). A total of 7.5 percent of these births were preterm, occurring before 37 weeks, but the percentage of very early births is much smaller (Fig. 30-1). Although almost identical to 2005 data from the United Kingdom, significantly higher rates of preterm birth of up to 12 percent are reported from the United States. Conversely, many Nordic countries with very reliable data collection quote rates around 5 percent. This must reflect, at least in part, differing socioeconomic and cultural factors. There is

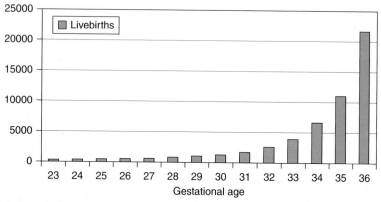

FIGURE 30-1. Ontario preterm live births, 2005–2009. (Data supplied by: BORN Ontario, Niday Perinatal Database.)

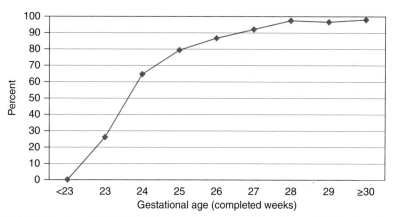

FIGURE 30-2. Survival to NICU discharge versus gestational age at birth. (From the 2010 Canadian Neonatal Network Report, published with permission.)

no evidence that the incidence of preterm birth is declining. In fact, the rate appears to be slowly increasing, partly because of an increasing incidence of multiple pregnancy. The 2008 Canadian Perinatal Health Report by the Public Health Agency of Canada reports that the preterm birth rate has increased from 6.4 percent in 1985 to 8.2 percent in 2004. Although just under 1 percent of singletons delivered before 32 weeks, this complicated 8.3 percent of twins and nearly 21 percent of higher multiples.

Preterm births contribute significantly to perinatal mortality, half of which results from babies born before 32 weeks. The survival to discharge for very preterm infants admitted to Canadian neonatal intensive care units (NICUs) in 2010 is shown in Figure 30-2. Predicted survival can be modified if accurate information concerning fetal sex, weight, and well-being is available. Parents are particularly anxious about the risks of later disability and handicap. These risks are especially significant before 26 weeks' gestation. When assessed at 6 years of age, nearly half the survivors at 23 to 25 weeks' gestation have a moderate or severe disability. Furthermore, many of these disabilities only become apparent after 2 to 3 years of age. Survival with no disability is only seen in 1, 3, and 8 percent of live births at less than 24, 24, and 25 weeks, respectively. There are other long-term worries after very preterm births, including subsequent growth, educational needs, and social behavior. There may also be influences on later adult health. Fortunately, both morbidity and mortality fall dramatically with increasing gestation.

It is important to recognize the effect of denominator differences in survival figures, especially at the earliest gestations. If the figures are based

OTHER ISSUES

on fetuses alive at the start of labor, the survival rates will be lower because there is an inherent risk of intrapartum death. If the figures are based on NICU admissions, the figures will be higher because some live births will succumb during initial resuscitation in the maternity unit. At 25 weeks or less, such statistical manipulations may lead to a significant change in the quoted survival figures. Of note, not all centers in the Canadian Neonatal Network included delivery room deaths; therefore, the above survival data may be overestimated at the lowest gestations.

CLASSIFICATION

For reasons related to etiology, outcome, and recurrence risk, preterm births should be divided into three gestational periods: mildly preterm births at 32^{+0} to 36^{+6} weeks (incidence, 6.4%), very preterm births at 28^{+0} to 31^{+6} weeks (incidence, 0.7%), and extremely preterm births at 24^{+0} to 27^{+6} weeks (incidence, 0.4%).

ETIOLOGY

Labor at term and before term share a common pathway involving uterine contractility, cervical effacement and dilatation, and membrane rupture. At term, the activation of this pathway is physiologic. However, a variety of pathologies underlie labor remote from term. It has been suggested by some authors that preterm labor be considered a syndrome in order to emphasize its multifactorial nature.

Infection

Subclinical intrauterine infection of the choriodecidual space and amniotic fluid is the most widely studied etiologic factor underlying spontaneous preterm births. The uterine cavity is normally sterile, but the vagina contains commensal bacteria. Depending on the bacterial load and cervical resistance, the bacteria may ascend through the cervix and reach the fetal membranes. This may activate the decidua, increase prostaglandin release, and trigger contractions. Alternatively, it may weaken the membranes, leading to rupture. Early-onset neonatal sepsis, maternal postpartum endometritis, and histologic chorioamnionitis are all significantly more common after preterm birth, particularly very early deliveries before 32 weeks.

Overdistension

The most common cause of uterine overdistension is multiple gestation. Polyhydramnios has a similar effect. Overstretching of the myometrium (and possibly the membranes) leads to increased contractile activity and premature shortening and opening of the cervix.

Vascular

Disturbance at the uteroplacental interface may lead to intrauterine bleeding. The blood can track down behind the membranes to the cervix and be revealed. Alternatively, it may track away from the cervix and be concealed. Either way, the blood irritates the uterus, leading to contractions, and damages the membranes, leading to early rupture.

Surgical Procedures and Intercurrent Illness

Serious maternal infective illnesses such as pyelonephritis, appendicitis, and pneumonia are associated with preterm labor. In these cases, preterm labor is presumed to be caused by either direct bloodborne spread of infection to the uterine cavity or indirectly to chemical triggers, such as endotoxins or cytokines. Many other illnesses, such as cholestasis of pregnancy, and non-obstetric surgical procedures, are associated with preterm labor, although the mechanisms for this remain obscure.

Amniocentesis is a pregnancy-specific procedure associated with an increased risk of late miscarriage and early birth. It is most commonly performed at 15 to 18 weeks' gestation. It is associated with a 0.5 percent chance of subsequent pregnancy loss before viability. This may happen in the days after the procedure, but many losses occur several weeks later, and a small increased risk of preterm delivery persists after reaching viability.

Abnormal Uterine Cavity

A uterine cavity that is distorted by congenital malformation may be less able to accommodate a developing pregnancy. Associated abnormal placentation and cervical weakness may also contribute. Fibroids in a submucosal position may also lead to complications. However, fibroids are common, and most pregnancies are successful despite their presence.

OTHER ISSUES

Cervical Weakness

Because of previous surgical damage or a congenital defect, the cervix may shorten and open prematurely. The membranes then prolapse and may be damaged by stretching or by direct contact with vaginal pathogens. These same pathogens may ascend and trigger contractions. Often referred to as *cervical incompetence*, *weakness* may be a better term. The evidence suggests that gradations of deficiency exist, rather than an "all-or-nothing" phenomenon. It may also vary from one pregnancy to the next.

This remains a notoriously difficult diagnosis to make, as dilatation of the cervix remains the final common pathway for all late miscarriages and early births. Reliably distinguishing between such dilatation being the primary event or secondary to other pathologies is challenging.

Idiopathic

In many cases, especially late preterm births between 34 and 36 weeks of gestation, no cause will be found. In these cases, the physiologic pathways to parturition may simply have been turned on too early.

RISK FACTORS

Nonmodifiable, Major

Last birth preterm: 20 percent risk
Last two births preterm: 40 percent risk
Twin pregnancy: 50 percent risk
Uterine abnormalities
Cervical anomalies:
• Cervical damage (cone biopsy, repeated dilatation)
• Fibroids (cervical)
Factors in current pregnancy:
• Recurrent antepartum hemorrhage
• Intercurrent illness (e.g., sepsis)
• Any invasive procedure or surgery

Nonmodifiable, Minor

Teenagers having second or subsequent babies
Parity (0 or ≥5)
Ethnicity (black women)

Poor socioeconomic status
Education (not beyond secondary)

Modifiable

Smoking: twofold increase of PPROM
Drugs of abuse: especially cocaine
Body mass index (BMI) <20: underweight women
Interpregnancy interval <1 year

When assessing symptomatic patients, the recognition of major risk factors in particular can help to modify an individual's actual risk of preterm delivery, especially in the absence of definitive signs.

CLINICAL FEATURES

History

Always check the dating of the pregnancy by reviewing the menstrual history and, if possible, any prior ultrasound examinations. This is critical at gestations near viability.

Fewer than 50 percent of all women presenting with symptoms suggesting a risk of early delivery will deliver within 7 days. Too much emphasis is often placed on the contraction frequency. In isolation, it correlates poorly with the risk of preterm birth. Markers of intensity, such as analgesic requirements or simple bedside clinical impression, may add refinement. Vague complaints such as increased discharge, pelvic pressure, or low backache are sometimes reported, with the latter two often showing a cyclical pattern. Nonetheless, the diagnosis of preterm labor remains notoriously difficult unless contractions are accompanied by advanced dilatation (>3 cm), ruptured membranes, or significant vaginal bleeding.

Examination

A brief general examination is important to assess overall health. This should include pulse, blood pressure, temperature, and state of hydration.

Abdominal examination may reveal the presence of uterine tenderness, suggesting abruption or chorioamnionitis. A careful speculum examination by an experienced clinician may yield valuable information; pooling of amniotic fluid, blood, and/or abnormal discharge may be

OTHER ISSUES

observed. A visual assessment of cervical dilatation is usually possible and has been shown to be as accurate as digital examination findings. Digital examinations should be limited because they are known to stimulate prostaglandin production and may introduce organisms into the cervical canal.

Differential Diagnosis

- Urinary tract infection (UTI)
- Red degeneration of fibroid
- Constipation
- Gastroenteritis

Investigations

Bedside Fibronectin

Fetal fibronectin (fFN) is a "gluelike" protein binding the choriodecidual membranes. It is rarely present in vaginal secretions between 23 and 34 weeks of gestation. Any disruption at the choriodecidual interface results in fFN release and possible detection in the cervicovaginal secretions. Its use is confined to symptomatic women who do not meet the major diagnostic criteria for preterm labor, namely advanced dilatation, PPROM, or significant bleeding.

Bedside fFN testing offers a rapid assessment of risk in symptomatic women with minimal cervical dilatation. If performed correctly, the test has a greater predictive value than digital examination. In one study, 30 percent of women with a positive fibronectin test result delivered within 7 days compared with only 10 percent of women who were 2 to 3 cm dilated. Only 1 percent of women who test negative for fFN deliver within 1 week. Aggressive intervention can be avoided in these women.

Cervical Length

Cervical length measurement by transvaginal ultrasound has also been shown to improve diagnostic accuracy. A normal cervix measures approximately 35 mm in length (Fig. 30-3A). Significant cervical shortening is often accompanied by dilatation and funneling of the membranes down the cervical canal (Fig. 30-3B). Although measurements can be repeated frequently, skilled ultrasonographers and suitable machines with transvaginal probes are required.

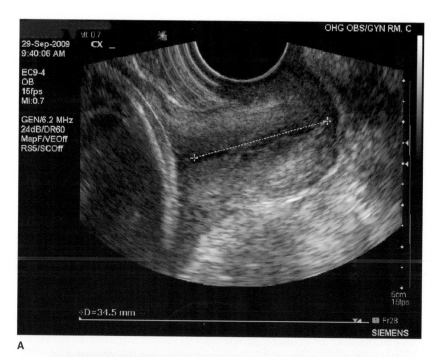

A

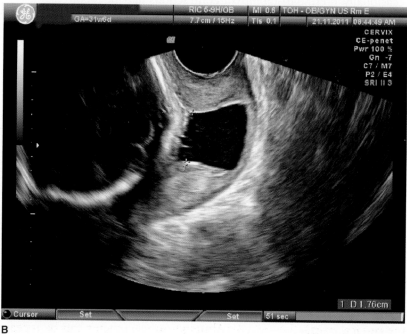

B

FIGURE 30-3. A, Normal cervical appearance on transvaginal scan. **B,** A shortened cervix with membrane funneling on transvaginal scan.

Repeat Vaginal Examination

Repeat vaginal examination in 1 to 4 hours should be considered essential in the absence of specialized tests. The interval between assessments should be guided by the severity of the symptoms.

CLINICAL FEATURES: PRETERM PRELABOR RUPTURE OF THE MEMBRANES

History

The most reliable diagnostic feature of PPROM from the history is the report of a "gush of fluid" vaginally, usually followed by a more or less continuous dribble. This "history" is as powerful as commonly relied upon tests, such as nitrazine swabs and ferning. This must be distinguished from leaking urine because incontinence or a UTI may present in a similar way. The presence of any vaginal discharge should be ascertained. Fetal movements may be reduced in strength or frequency after PPROM, and occasionally, uterine irritability or contractions may be reported.

Examination

Infection may lead to an increased pulse and temperature and a flushed appearance. Abdominal examination may reveal a clinical suspicion of oligohydramnios or uterine tenderness if chorioamnionitis is present. The definitive diagnosis of PPROM can only be made by performing a sterile speculum examination, preferably after the patient has been resting supine for 20 to 30 minutes. A pool of amniotic fluid in the posterior vagina is diagnostic. It is also important at this point to visualize the cervix. Fluid may be seen trickling through the external os, and dilatation can be visually assessed. Digital vaginal examinations should be avoided if possible in PPROM because they are associated with a significant reduction in the latent interval before labor. This reduction is most dramatic at the earliest gestations.

Differential Diagnosis

- Urine loss: Incontinence and UTIs are both more common in pregnancy
- Vaginal infection
- Leukorrhea: The cervical glands often become overactive during pregnancy

Investigations

Nitrazine Testing
Amniotic fluid is alkaline, whereas the vaginal secretions are usually acidic. An elevated pH turns a nitrazine stick black. Some units use nitrazine sticks to define the presence of amniotic fluid. Unfortunately, false–positives occur in 17%, with blood, semen, and even urine limiting its usefulness. However, the predictive value of a negative test result is very high.

Fern Testing
A drop of vaginal fluid from the posterior fornix is placed on a slide, allowed to dry, and examined under the high power of a microscope. Sodium chloride and proteins from the amniotic fluid, when allowed to dry on a clean slide, will crystallize and will show a characteristic fern pattern. Again, a sensitivity of 90% is achieved with a 6% false-positive rate.

Highly Specific Swab Tests
Highly specific markers for amniotic fluid can be detected using rapid bedside tests. These include immunoassays for insulin-like growth factor-binding protein-1 and of placental alpha-microglobulin-1 (Amni-Sure). The latter has a reported sensitivity of 98.9 percent for ruptured membranes, with 100 percent specificity. As always, cost is an issue.

Genital Tract Swabs
A high vaginal swab (HVS) may help to guide antibiotic therapy if subsequently required. Screening for group B streptococcus (GBS) can also be performed because there is a substantial risk of labor in the next few days.

Ultrasound
Ultrasound can give valuable information about the amniotic fluid volume. The presence or absence of oligohydramnios provides further diagnostic support. In established PPROM, there is a direct correlation between the amount of amniotic fluid remaining and the latency period. Unlike preterm labor, cervical length measurements have limited predictive ability in PPROM.

Amniocentesis
A sample of amniotic fluid can be sent for Gram stain, microscopy, and culture to establish whether an intrauterine infection (chorioamnionitis) is present. However, there is a risk of stimulating preterm labor by performing

OTHER ISSUES

an invasive test, and amniocentesis can be technically very difficult when there is little amniotic fluid.

Follow-up Monitoring

Maternal Well-Being. This should include regular assessment of the mother's blood pressure, pulse, and temperature. Some advise serial white blood cell (WBC) counts and C-reactive protein (CRP) as early markers of infection, although this has not been shown to improve management.

Fetal Well-Being. Serial antepartum cardiotocography is important after PPROM because a gradually increasing baseline heart rate or fetal tachycardia can be the first sign of intrauterine infection.

MANAGEMENT OF SYMPTOMATIC WOMEN

Communication and Support

A holistic approach to the situation is essential. Sympathy, explanations, and reassurance are mandatory. There are two vital areas of communication in the management of threatened preterm labor or PPROM. Communication with the woman and her family ensures that they have a full understanding of the risks involved and enables a clear management plan to be discussed. Communication with the neonatal unit staff ensures that adequate and appropriate resources are available at the time of delivery. Parents often also appreciate the opportunity to have discussed the care of their baby with the neonatology staff in advance of delivery.

Maternal Steroids

Current evidence shows that a single course of maternal steroids (two injections 12-24 hours apart) given between 24 and 34 weeks' gestation and received within 7 days of delivery results in markedly improved neonatal outcomes. This is primarily because of a reduction in neonatal respiratory distress syndrome (RDS). Maximum benefit from the injection is seen after 48 hours. Courses received less than 48 hours or more than 7 days before delivery still lead to benefit. They are not usually indicated before 24 weeks. The steroids most commonly used are 12 mg of either betamethasone or dexamethasone.

There is considerable reassuring evidence about the long-term safety of single courses of maternal steroids, with pediatric follow-up into the teenage years. However, there is growing concern about adverse consequences of multiple dosing. Similar to antibiotics, steroids have the potential for harm in pregnancy and should be used carefully.

Tocolytics

The Canadian Preterm Labor Trial remains the most influential tocolytic trial to date. It concluded that ritodrine, a beta-agonist that relaxes smooth muscle, had no significant benefit on perinatal mortality or the prolongation of pregnancy to term. However, it was able to reduce the number of women delivering within 2 days by 40 percent. This 48-hour window of opportunity is the sole reason for using tocolytics. Beta-agonists have significant maternal side effects, and maternal deaths from acute cardiopulmonary compromise are described. Other smooth muscle relaxants used to treat preterm labor include nifedipine and glyceryl trinitrate. The former has become popular because it is inexpensive, is given orally, and has a low side effect profile. A common nifedipine dosing regime is 20 mg orally followed by 10 to 20 mg every 6 to 8 hours to a maximum daily dose of 60 mg. The oxytocin antagonist atosiban has a product license in some countries but not in North America. Although side effects are seen less frequently than with ritodrine, the cost is much higher. Because prostaglandins appear to be one of the pivotal chemicals involved in parturition, nonsteroidal anti-inflammatory drugs such as indomethacin have attracted considerable interest as tocolytics. They have been associated with significant fetal cardiovascular side effects, although these can be mitigated by limiting them to short-term use (<72 hours) and only at gestational ages less than 30 weeks.

Unfortunately, despite a multitude of pharmacologic approaches, no tocolytic medication has yet been conclusively shown to improve neonatal outcomes. At the time of writing, the role for tocolysis is to allow a course of steroids for fetal lung maturation to be completed and to facilitate transfer of the undelivered mother to a unit able to provide appropriate neonatal care if delivery occurs. They should be used with caution in the presence of ruptured membranes.

Neuroprotection

Magnesium sulphate has been shown to lead to a reduction in cerebral palsy after very preterm birth. Not surprisingly, it has the greatest benefit

OTHER ISSUES

at the earliest gestations. However, the upper gestational age limit for use remains unclear and lies somewhere between 30 and 33 weeks. It is suggested that units use the same dosage regimen as they currently use for eclampsia prevention, with both a loading dose and maintenance therapy for up to 24 hours. Treatment should only be initiated in patients at imminent risk of preterm birth, and there is currently no evidence to support repeat courses.

Antibiotics

Broad-spectrum antibiotics offering aerobic and anaerobic coverage are necessary in the presence of overt clinical infection, such as chorioamnionitis. The role of antibiotics in the absence of clinical signs of infection is much less clear.

The MRC Oracle Study initially concluded that the use of prophylactic antibiotics in uncomplicated preterm labor before 37 weeks with intact membranes did not confer any short-term neonatal benefit. Worryingly, subsequent long-term follow-up of survivors actually showed a significant increase in neurodevelopmental disability in those who received either erythromycin or co-amoxiclav.

In PPROM, the same study concluded that a 10-day course of erythromycin led to improved short-term neonatal outcomes. A much smaller U.S. study that only enrolled women below 32 weeks with PPROM also confirmed the benefit of antibiotics in the short term.

Most North American centers continue to give intrapartum antibiotics to women in preterm labor unless GBS status is known to be negative. For reasons that are unclear, the risk of early-onset neonatal disease appears much less in other countries, such as the United Kingdom.

Fetal Assessment

After 24 weeks, maternal steroid therapy can suppress both fetal activity and heart rate variability, although Doppler studies are not influenced. Whenever possible, the presentation in preterm labor should be confirmed by ultrasound, because clinical palpation is notoriously unreliable. An estimated fetal weight, particularly before 28 weeks, can be helpful. Preterm infants have less reserve to tolerate the stress of labor, particularly in the presence of oligohydramnios. Therefore, continuous fetal monitoring may be required, although there may be considerable difficulties interpreting the fetal heart rate pattern in extremely preterm infants. At the extremes of viability, parents may decline intervention for suspected fetal compromise or aggressive resuscitation of the newborn. In these cases, continuous monitoring would be inappropriate.

In Utero Transfer

If local resources are unable to care for a viable neonate, in utero transfer to a unit with adequate neonatal facilities is recommended. It is generally accepted that this will improve the outcome for babies, particularly before 30 weeks of gestation. However, one must be careful not to convert a hospital delivery into a roadside one. A repeat assessment immediately before transfer is mandatory.

Modification of Activity

Randomized trials of social support in the United Kingdom failed to improve pregnancy outcomes, and in some studies, hospitalization for bed rest led to an increase in preterm birth. Roles for sexual abstinence and/or psychological support are no clearer. Patients should be informed that there is no evidence that their activity level influences outcome. This should be tempered by the realization that there is a natural tendency to analyze the days leading up to a preterm birth, looking for triggers. Patients should be somewhat cautious and avoid overexertion or extreme stress, if only to minimize subsequent feelings of guilt, however misplaced.

Emergency Cervical Cerclage

When a patient presents with an open cervical os and bulging membranes before viability, the idea of closing the cervix by passing a stitch around it seems logical. However, the results of emergency cervical cerclage are poor and are related to the cervical dilatation at insertion. The procedure itself can be technically challenging. A dilatation of more than 3 cm with an effaced cervix poses extreme difficulties even for the most experienced operator. Every effort should be made to detect and treat other causes of the uterine instability. If persistent placental bleeding is leading to secondary opening of the cervix, suturing the cervix clearly does not address the primary issue and is unlikely to be successful. Bleeding, contractions, and infection are all contraindications to cerclage. Depending on the initial dilatation of the cervix, the chance of the pregnancy proceeding beyond 26 weeks may be less than 50 percent.

OTHER ISSUES

Induction or Augmentation

In some cases, it may be judged appropriate to hasten delivery because the maternal or fetal risks of continuing the pregnancy are judged too high. After 24 weeks, if there is no evidence of acute maternal or fetal compromise, induction with milder prostaglandins, such as Cervidil, or conventional-dose oxytocin can considered as an alternative to a planned cesarean section. Great care must be exercised if there is already clinical evidence of chorioamnionitis. In these cases, delay in ending the pregnancy may lead to worsening infection and consequent morbidity for both the mother and baby. Augmenting labor may be the most appropriate management. After extremely or very preterm PPROM, an initial period of conservative management is commonly undertaken. Close observation for evidence of clinical chorioamnionitis, such as maternal fever, uterine tenderness, and fetal tachycardia, is necessary. There is no evidence that serial WBC counts or CRP levels add to clinical examination. There is evidence appearing that supports active management after 33 completed weeks, particularly after a course of steroids has been completed.

Analgesia

For intrapartum analgesia, an epidural is frequently advocated. Postulated benefits include avoiding expulsive efforts before full dilatation or a precipitous delivery, a relaxed pelvic floor and perineum, and the ability to proceed quickly to abdominal delivery.

Mode of Delivery

Many clinicians believe that the combination of high fetal morbidity and mortality; difficulty in diagnosing intrapartum hypoxia or acidosis; and maternal risk of complications, both intraoperatively and in subsequent pregnancies, do not justify cesarean section for fetal indications before 25 weeks. As gestation advances, both neonatal outcomes and the ability to diagnose fetal compromise improve, and intervention for fetal reasons becomes appropriate. It is often appropriate to leave the membranes intact even if oxytocin is required. There is little risk of dystocia, and an intact gestation sac cushions both the fetal head and umbilical cord. The safety of preterm breech vaginal delivery is often questioned and cesarean section commonly performed, although evidence to support this policy is weak.

Type of Cesarean Section

At the earliest gestations and in the presence of oligohydramnios, the lower segment is often poorly formed. Vertical uterine incisions may be necessary. This "classical" uterine incision carries an up to 5 percent risk of uterine rupture in subsequent pregnancies, some of which will occur before the onset of labor.

SELECTED READING

Royal College of Obstetricians and Gynaecologists: Antenatal Corticosteroids to Reduce Neonatal Morbidity and Mortality. Green-top Clinical Guideline No.7. 2010, *http://www.rcog.org.uk/guidelines*

Royal College of Obstetricians and Gynaecologists: Preterm Pre-labour Rupture of the Membranes. Green-top Clinical Guideline No.44. 2010, *http://www.rcog.org.uk/guidelines*

Royal College of Obstetricians and Gynaecologists: Tocolysis for Women in Preterm Labour. Green-top Clinical Guideline No. 1b. 2011, *http://www.rcog.org.uk/guidelines*

Society of Obstetricians and Gynaecologists of Canada: Clinical Guidelines – Magnesium Sulphate for Fetal Neuroprotection. J Obstet Gynaecol Can 33:516, 2011

OTHER ISSUES

Antepartum Hemorrhage

Griffith D. Jones

Hemorrhage in the second half of pregnancy can pose a serious threat to the health of both mother and child. In the majority of cases, the exact cause will remain unknown antenatally.

CAUSES

1. Placenta previa
2. Abruptio placentae
3. Vasa previa
4. Early labor
5. Local lesions (e.g., cervical ectropion or polyp)
6. Unknown or idiopathic: no discoverable cause

PLACENTA PREVIA

In this condition, the placenta is implanted in the lower uterine segment and lies over or near the internal os of the cervix. It is below the presenting part of the fetus. The incidence is 1:350 pregnancies. It is responsible for about 10 percent of antepartum hemorrhages. The late development of the lower uterine segment after 28 weeks leads to the phenomenon of placental migration, in which an apparent placenta previa in early pregnancy moves away from the internal os toward term.

Etiology

The etiology is unknown. Epidemiologic associations include a previous pregnancy with placenta previa, previous cesarean sections, and advanced maternal age. Weaker risk factors include multiparity, endometrial trauma such as curettage, and cigarette smoking.

Classification

The clinical classification of placenta previa is now based on the ultrasound findings (Fig. 31-1). Because of the possibility of placental migration, final decisions regarding mode of delivery in asymptomatic patients should only be based on the ultrasound appearance at 35+ weeks. Before then, its appearance should only guide decision making if the patient labors preterm, although a placenta that overlaps the internal os by more than 20 mm is associated with a low chance of migration.

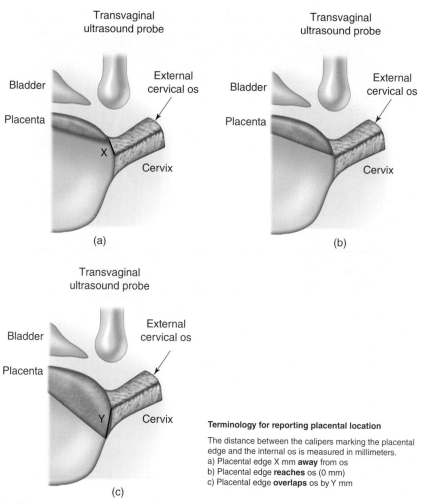

Terminology for reporting placental location

The distance between the calipers marking the placental edge and the internal os is measured in millimeters.
a) Placental edge X mm **away** from os
b) Placental edge **reaches** os (0 mm)
c) Placental edge **overlaps** os by Y mm

FIGURE 31-1. Modern approach to the ultrasonographic assessment of a low-lying placenta.

1. Lower edge of placenta >20 mm from internal os: The risk of significant intrapartum bleeding necessitating delivery by cesarean section is low, and vaginal delivery can be attempted
2. Lower edge of placenta within 20 mm of the internal os but does not overlap it: Studies have shown that some women will have successful vaginal births in this situation but that the incidence of emergency cesarean section is high (40%-90%). Intrapartum management should be dictated by individual clinical circumstances and local resources
3. The lower edge of placenta overlaps the internal os by any amount (Fig. 31-2): Delivery should be by cesarean section

OTHER ISSUES

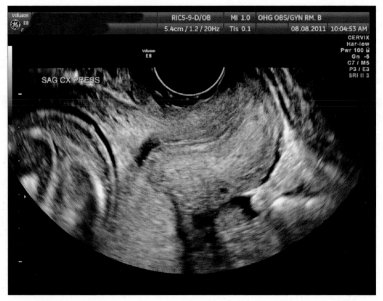

FIGURE 31-2. A posterior placenta with the lower edge just crossing the internal os on transvaginal ultrasound.

Clinical Manifestations

The classic symptom is painless vaginal bleeding. A feature of placenta previa is that the degree of anemia or shock is equivalent to the amount of blood lost. In most cases, the bleeding is unprovoked, but it may be preceded by trauma or coitus. For some patients, it remains an ultrasound diagnosis that never leads to any symptoms. Other patients have a single bleed that leads to the diagnosis and never recurs. A worrying group is those patients with recurrent episodes of bleeding (so-called warning bleeds) who have a higher risk of presenting with major hemorrhage.

Associated Findings

1. Failure of engagement of the presenting part
2. Abnormal presentations, such as breech and transverse lie, are more common
3. The uterus is soft and nontender
4. The fetal heart rate (FHR) pattern is often reassuring because the degree of placental separation is minimal, and there is little prior fetal compromise
5. Placenta accreta: The incidence is higher than when the placenta is implanted in the upper segment of the uterus. This is especially so

if the placenta is anterior and the patient has had previous cesarean deliveries. The risk increases in line with the number of previous cesareans. The diagnosis and management of placenta accreta is covered in more detail in Chapter 19, "Delivery of the Placenta, Retained Placenta, and Placenta Accreta"

Diagnosis

Ultrasound examination is the safest and most accurate method and is the procedure of choice. It is universally accepted that transvaginal scanning is the optimal method of assessment with the greatest precision. When transvaginal probes are not available, transperineal or translabial scanning (using the transabdominal probe) is a reasonable alternative. Transabdominal imaging can be challenging with a posterior placenta or in overweight patients and is associated with a higher incidence of false-positives.

ABRUPTIO PLACENTAE

This condition, known also as premature placental separation, involves the detachment of the placenta from the wall of the uterus. Abruptio placentae is initiated by hemorrhage, leading to a variable degree of separation of the placenta with a hematoma forming between the it and the uterus.

In most cases, the bleeding progresses to the edge of the placenta. At this point, it may break through the membranes and enter the amniotic cavity or, more often, the blood tracks down between the chorion and the uterine wall until it exits via the cervix. Occasionally, there is extensive extravasation of blood into the myometrium, a condition described as Couvelaire uterus. The incidence of abruptio placentae is around 1 percent.

Etiology

The cause of placental abruption is not known. The condition is associated with the following:

1. History of a previous pregnancy complicated by an abruption
2. Other manifestations of placental dysfunction in the current pregnancy, such as hypertensive disorders, intrauterine growth restriction and abnormal serum screening markers, especially a low pregnancy-associated plasma protein A (PAPP-A) result
3. PPROM: There is a strong interrelationship between these two clinical entities, perhaps linked by infection because PPROM is associated

OTHER ISSUES

with subclinical chorioamnionitis. A subchorionic collection of blood is an ideal culture medium for bacteria leading to secondary chorioamnionitis and membrane weakening. Alternatively, when subclinical chorioamnionitis is the primary event leading to membrane rupture, the associated vasculitis may trigger an abruption

4. Overdistention of the uterus (i.e., multiple pregnancy or polyhydramnios), especially if there is an acute volume reduction
5. Trauma: Most commonly motor vehicle accidents
6. Substance abuse: Most commonly cigarettes, but even higher risks are associated with the use of cocaine

Classification

1. Revealed or *external* (Fig. 31-3A): The blood may be bright red or dark and clotted. The pain is mild to moderate unless the patient is in labor. The degree of anemia and shock is equivalent to the apparent blood loss
2. Concealed or *internal* (Fig. 31-3B): There is little vaginal bleeding. The blood is trapped in the uterus. If it is a major abruption, the pain is severe, and the uterus is hard and tender. The degree of shock is greater than expected for the amount of visible bleeding. The FHR may suggest significant compromise or may be absent
3. *Mixed or combined:* A varying mixture of the above groups is seen

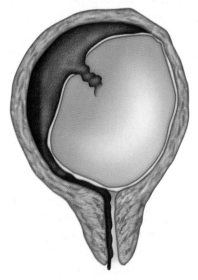 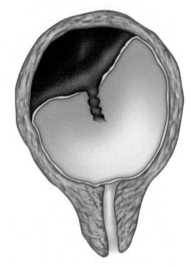

A. External or apparent.   B. Internal or concealed.

FIGURE 31-3. Revealed and concealed placental abruption.

Clinical Manifestations

This depends on the location of the blood (apparent or concealed) and the amount of blood lost. The latter may be relatively small or large enough to lead to hypovolemic shock and even maternal death. The clinical picture includes vaginal bleeding, abdominal pain, and uterine tenderness. Atypical back pain can be reported with a posterior placenta. The uterus may exhibit a woodlike rigidity and may enlarge as blood accumulates in the cavity. Often the patient is in labor.

Associated Findings

1. Labor, especially preterm labor, can be triggered by abruption. This is presumably caused by blood and coagulation products leading to myometrial contractility
2. Fetal distress is common, and a nonreassuring FHR tracing is often seen. With a major abruption involving more than 50 percent of the placenta, fetal demise may occur. The perinatal mortality rate ranges from 25 to 50 percent

Diagnosis

The diagnosis of abruptio placentae is made on clinical grounds. Ultrasonography has a low sensitivity for abruption, detecting only 15 percent of cases. It is used simply to rule out placenta previa. Kleihauer testing is of no diagnostic value but can guide WinRho or RhoGAM dosing in Rh-negative mothers. The diagnosis may only be confirmed at delivery when inspection of the placenta reveals an adherent retroplacental clot with disruption of the underlying tissue. However, subsequent pathologic examination of the placenta may be normal, especially in the setting of acute hemorrhage.

VASA PREVIA

Vasa previa is a condition in which the umbilical vessels, unsupported by either the umbilical cord or placental tissue, traverse the fetal membranes of the lower uterine segment and lie over the internal os of the cervix in front of the presenting part (Fig. 31-4). The branching vessels run between the amnion and the chorion and, unprotected by Wharton jelly, are vulnerable to compression or rupture. In either case, fetal death can occur.

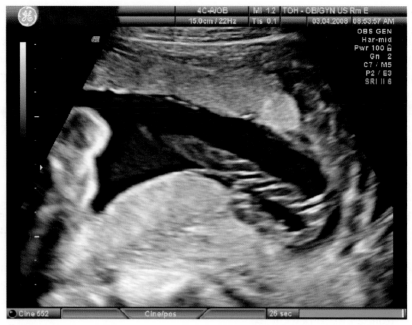

A

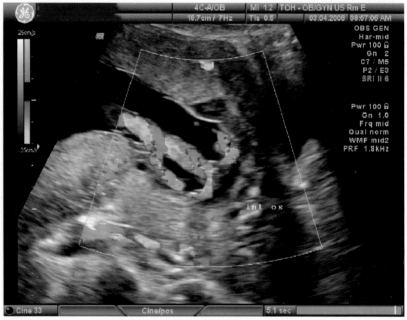

B

FIGURE 31-4. Transabdominal ultrasound images demonstrating a vasa previa.

In the vast majority of cases, the placenta is low lying, and one of two clinical situations exists: (a) There is a velamentous insertion of the cord, or (b) there is a separate accessory placental lobe. Some evidence indicates that the incidence is also increased in in vitro fertilization pregnancies and in multiple pregnancies.

The overall incidence of vasa previa is estimated at approximately 1 in 3000. However, in association with known velamentous insertion of the cord, the incidence of vasa previa rises to 1 in 50.

Clinical Picture

Antenatal diagnosis is possible using ultrasound, most often transvaginally. Targeted screening should be performed in women identified as having the major risk factors outlined above. Conventional management of women diagnosed with vasa previa prenatally includes hospital admission from 28 to 32 weeks and a planned cesarean delivery at 35 to 36 weeks. If labor or membrane rupture occurs spontaneously before then, prompt emergency cesarean section should be undertaken.

Intrapartum Diagnosis

In the absence of prenatal diagnosis, this includes:

1. *FHR:* Vasa previa may be suspected when a relatively minor episode of painless vaginal bleeding is followed by a nonreassuring FHR tracing
2. *Vaginal examination:* The vessels may be felt by the fingers. The condition may be confused with presentation of the umbilical cord
3. *Amnioscopy:* The blood vessels may be seen within the membranes
4. *Apt test:* This acid-elution procedure demonstrates the presence of fetal red blood cells and establishes that the bleeding is of fetal origin

The clinical reality is that the majority of undiagnosed cases will proceed to cesarean section for suspected fetal compromise, with the diagnosis made after delivery. The resources and skills to perform amnioscopy or a bedside Apt test are unlikely to be available.

EARLY LABOR

Some patients may present with a heavy "show" that is indistinguishable from an antepartum hemorrhage. However, most of these patients lack

OTHER ISSUES

features associated with pathologic diagnoses. They do not have pain between contractions, and the FHR tracing remains normal. Over time, the cervix effaces and dilates. Often the bleeding abates as the presenting part descends and compresses veins within the cervix and lower segment.

LOCAL LESIONS

Although usually only associated with relatively minor episodes of bleeding, cervical polyps or an ectropion are readily detected on speculum examination. Chlamydial cervicitis can be diagnosed by swab. Rare cases of cervical cancer are also diagnosed in these circumstances. Caution should be exercised in ascribing bleeding to any local lesion before all other obstetric causes have been assessed as unlikely.

IDIOPATHIC

Frequently, no cause or reason for the bleeding is ever found. The bleeding is usually small in quantity, and there is no effect on the mother, fetus, or pregnancy. Treatment involves the ruling out of serious conditions followed by expectant management. Most patients go to term.

GENERAL MANAGEMENT OF THIRD TRIMESTER BLEEDING

Preliminary Evaluation

1. Assess maternal hemodynamic status

   a. Check maternal vital signs and perform a clinical examination
   b. Estimate prior blood loss from history and visual inspection
   c. Determine ongoing blood loss, local lesions, and cervical dilatation by speculum examination

2. Assess fetal well-being (initially by fetal heart rate monitor)

3. Confirm precise gestational age

4. Placental localization: Determine from previous ultrasound reports or by a bedside scan whether a placenta previa exists

Management should always be guided by the risk to the mother and risk to the fetus. To be put into the correct context, the gestational age must be taken into account.

Preliminary Management

In all but the most minor episodes of bleeding, the following steps should be considered:

1. An intravenous infusion with a large-bore catheter is established
2. Blood is taken for a baseline blood count, creatinine, and type and screen. Cross-matching should be considered with more significant bleeds, especially in the presence of abnormal placentation. If the patient is rhesus negative, a Kleihauer test should be performed to ensure the correct dose of WinRho is given
3. The patient is admitted to the labor and delivery unit for observation. At preterm gestations, maternal steroids for fetal lung maturity should be considered

Maternal or Fetal Compromise Suspected

Initial steps should be directed at stabilizing or resuscitating the mother. All obstetric units should have a multidisciplinary protocol in place for the recognition and management of major obstetric hemorrhage. Of particular note, placental abruption can be deceiving. Not only can some or all of the bleeding be hidden, but a seemingly normotensive woman may be profoundly hypovolemic if preeclampsia was the aetiologic factor behind the abruption. In this circumstance, bladder catheterization will confirm significant proteinuria and document oliguria.

Either immediately after or simultaneous with maternal resuscitation, steps should be taken toward emptying the uterus. In the presence of a major abruption, the cervix may already be significantly dilated, and artificial rupture of the membranes (ARM) followed by vaginal delivery may be the best option. Fetal condition will influence decision making. If the FHR pattern is preterminal or there has been a prolonged severe bradycardia, the chance of fetal survival is slim, and the risks to the mother from surgery may be too high. Less severe degrees of suspected fetal compromise will push toward emergency cesarean delivery. In the presence of a

OTHER ISSUES

significant previa (placental or vasa), delivery should be by emergency cesarean section.

No Compromise Suspected

In the absence of any previa, if speculum examination reveals cervical dilatation and the gestation is suitably advanced, augmentation of labor may be appropriate. In other circumstances, expectant management will be undertaken. The duration of this depends on many factors, including the placental site, severity of blood loss, whether a recurrent problem is present, and the gestational age. Local resources should also be taken into account, particularly if specialized services such as interventional radiology may be required at delivery. In general, the threshold for delivery is inversely related to the severity and/or frequency of bleeding and the gestational age.

Double Setup Examination

This procedure is carried out when the diagnosis is uncertain and no ultrasound facilities exist locally. Although rarely, if ever, required in developed countries, it may still be necessary in underresourced areas. The patient is taken to the operating room, where all preparations have been made for immediate cesarean section. Under anesthesia, abdominal and vaginal examinations are performed to ascertain the fetal presentation, the condition of the cervix, and the location of the placenta. Vaginal examination begins in the fornices, assessing for any soft tissue mass between the presenting part and the examining fingers. Only after a major previa is excluded should a cervical assessment be performed, gently feeling for a placental edge. Treatment is based on these findings. However, vaginal examination may provoke heavy bleeding and is reserved for patients whose placenta previa is only suspected or whose vaginal bleeding is of unclear etiology.

SELECTED READING

Royal College of Obstetricians and Gynaecologists: Antepartum Haemorrhage. Green-top Clinical Guideline No. 63. 2011, *http://www.rcog.org.uk/guidelines*

Royal College of Obstetricians and Gynaecologists: Maternal Collapse in Pregnancy and the Puerperium. Green-top Clinical Guideline No. 56. 2011, *http://www.rcog.org.uk/guidelines*

Royal College of Obstetricians and Gynaecologists: Placenta praevia, placenta praevia accrete and vasa praevia: diagnosis and management. Green-top Clinical Guideline No. 27. 2011, *http://www.rcog.org.uk/guidelines*

Society of Obstetricians and Gynaecologists of Canada: Clinical Guideline No. 115: Hemorrhagic Shock. J Obstet Gynaecol Can 24:504, 2002

Society of Obstetricians and Gynaecologists of Canada: Clinical Guideline No. 189: Diagnosis and Management of Placenta Previa. J Obstet Gynaecol Can 29:261, 2007

Society of Obstetricians and Gynaecologists of Canada: Clinical Guideline No. 231: Guidelines for the Management of Vasa Previa. J Obstet Gynaecol Can 31:748, 2009

CHAPTER 32

Maternal Complications in Labor

Dan Boucher
Samantha Halman
Alan Karovitch
Erin Keely

PREGESTATIONAL DIABETES

Diabetes is the leading endocrine condition that complicates pregnancy, and the incidence is rising with the obesity epidemic and advancing maternal age. It is estimated that 5 percent of pregnancies are complicated by diabetes, with the vast majority caused by gestational diabetes mellitus (GDM) and the remainder caused by type 1 or type 2 diabetes mellitus (DM).

Physiologic Changes in Pregnancy

Pregnancy is associated with accelerated starvation, which results in increased ketogenesis and lower fasting plasma glucose levels, especially in the first trimester. The increased ketogenesis predisposes mothers to episodes of diabetic ketoacidosis. In early gestation, especially during weeks 7 to 12, there may be a 10 to 20 percent drop in insulin requirements before insulin-resistant placental hormones rise. This period is associated with an increased risk of hypoglycemic episodes without autonomic warnings. Maternal hypoglycemia unawareness is an important risk factor for the development of severe hypoglycemia.

In mid to late pregnancy, increased levels of human placental lactogen (hPL), human placental growth hormone (hPGH), cortisol, and prolactin lead to an insulin-resistant state. This leads to maternal insulin resistance at the level of skeletal muscle and adipose tissue to meet metabolic fetal demands that are 80 percent derived from glucose. It is important to note that if insulin requirements decrease significantly late in gestation, it may be a sign of placental failure. Changes in therapeutic requirements in patients with diabetes should be anticipated during this time by health care providers.

Important Comorbidities

Diabetes during pregnancy is associated with an increased risk of preeclampsia (15%-30%), polyhydramnios (15%-20%), and cesarean section or instrumental delivery (25%-40%).

Patients with diabetes also have important comorbidities that may need to be addressed during pregnancy, such as hypertension and obesity. There is evidence of an increased risk of progression of retinopathy and nephropathy.

Ominous Signs

- Maternal hypoglycemia and unawareness
- Maternal acidosis
- Uncontrolled maternal hyperglycemia
- Severe fetal macrosomia
- Polyhydramios and progressive growth restriction

Diabetic Ketoacidosis

Women with type 1 diabetes are at increased risk of diabetic ketoacidosis (DKA) during pregnancy because of increased ketogenesis, chronic compensated respiratory alkalosis and thus lower buffering capacity, increased rates of infection, and use of corticosteroids for fetal lung maturation. DKA most commonly occurs in the second or third trimesters. Although the presentation is similar to that in nonpregnant patients, glucose levels may be much lower, and the acidosis more pronounced. Ketones readily cross the placenta, and DKA is associated with high fetal mortality. Treatment is the same as in nonpregnant patients and requires prompt recognition, intravenous (IV) rehydration, electrolyte replacement, and IV insulin therapy. Identification of the triggering condition is crucial. Concise guidelines on the treatment of DKA in pregnancy are available.

Intrapartum Management of Diabetes

Timing and Mode of Delivery
Diabetes in itself is not an indication for cesarean section, and the route of delivery in women whose diabetes is well controlled should be based on the same criteria that apply to nondiabetic patients. Timing of delivery varies but is generally believed to be best between the 38th and 40th weeks of gestation. The American College of Obstetricians and Gynecologists guidelines does not advocate for routine delivery before 40 weeks, but the American Diabetes Association states that prolongation of gestation past 38 weeks increases the risk of fetal macrosomia without reducing cesarean section rates and that delivery during the 38th week is recommended unless obstetric considerations dictate otherwise.

Glycemic Control During Labor and Delivery
Because of decreased production of epinephrine and norepinephrine in pregnancy, patients are at increased risk of hypoglycemia unawareness. It is important to avoid hypoglycemia for maternal safety.

OTHER ISSUES

In early labor, while the patient is still eating, subcutaneous insulin should be continued, and doses may require adjustments to account for oral intake. When the patient is in active labor and no longer eating, IV dextrose and insulin should be used. Target glycemic values are between 4 and 7 mmol/L (72-126 mg/dL).

In general, women with type 1 DM require 1 to 1.5 U/h, whereas women with type 2 DM or GDM, who are more insulin resistant, may require more. Patients who are using an insulin pump may continue their basal infusion during labor, although the rate may need to be reduced. Once the patient has delivered and is eating, IV insulin should be discontinued two hours after subcutaneous insulin resumed. Patients previously controlled on diet and/or oral agents can often resume oral therapy, but their control needs to be closely monitored.

Many local health centers have standardized orders that can be applied (Fig. 32-1).

Neonatal Considerations

Neonates should have frequent capillary glucose monitoring. If the glucose level is below 2 mmol/L (36 mg/dL), oral feeding or IV dextrose needs to be initiated. Institutions should have protocols for neonatal hypoglycemia. Early breastfeeding has been shown to reduce the incidence of neonatal hypoglycemia.

Postpartum

Immediately postpartum, insulin requirements decrease. In women with type 1 DM, there may be a "honeymoon" period 24 to 48 hours postpartum during which they do not require insulin therapy to maintain glycemic values at 6 to 10 mmol/L (108-180 mg/dL). It is recommended that one-half to two-thirds of the prepregnancy insulin requirements is an appropriate starting dose in the postpartum period.

Insulin, second-generation oral sulfonylureas, and metformin are deemed safe for breastfeeding. No safety data are available for other oral agents. Angiotensin-converting enzyme (ACE) inhibitors can be reintroduced and are safe during breastfeeding.

HYPERTENSION

Hypertension is the most common chronic medical condition in pregnancy, and its incidence is likely to rise with increasing rates of obesity and advanced maternal age. It is estimated that up to 8 percent of all pregnancies are complicated by a hypertensive disorder. Generally, arterial blood pressure (BP) decreases by 10 to 15 mm Hg during pregnancy, with a greater decrease in diastolic blood pressure. This decrease begins in the

The Ottawa Hospital ☐ Civ ☐ Gen / **L'Hôpital d'Ottawa**	**PHYSICIAN'S ORDERS** **ORDONNANCES MÉDICALES** **Birthing/Mother Baby Units** **Unités des naissances/Maman-bébé**

Medication Allergies/Reactions

Substances or Food Allergies/Reactions

☐ None known-aucune connue ☐ None known-aucune connue

DIABETES MANAGEMENT - POSTPARTUM - GESTION DU DIABÈTE

☐ Type 1 DM   ☐ Type 2 DM

DIET: Regular maternity no added sugar.
BLOOD GLUCOSE MONITORING:
• Test blood glucose TID before meals, qhs using hospital meter.
• If on insulin postpartum, also test at 03:00 or when up to feed baby at night.

DIABETES MEDICATIONS:
☐ Discontinue all insulin and oral diabetes medications.
☐ Discontinue all insulin and start oral diabetes medications:_____
☐ Discontinue IV insulin infusion and start SC insulin when usual next does due (see order below). Transfer to Mother Baby Unit when obstetrically stable.
☐ Start SC insulin when usual next does due (see order below), continue intrapartum IV insulin protocol until 2 hours after first postpartum SC insulin injection or insulin pump restarted and patient tolerating food or fluids containing carbohydrates (at least 2 of these items: 175 mL of juice, 250 mL of milk, 1 slice of bread, ¾ cup of cereal, 6 crackers). Transfer to Mother Baby Unit when IV insulin is discontinued.

SUBCUTANEOUS INSULIN ORDERS:

☐ **PATIENT MANAGED**
- May self administer and adjust own insulin dose
- Nurse to monitor blood glucose using hospital meter and document.

☐ **PATIENT/FAMILY TO MANAGE with insulin pump**
- Nurse to monitor blood glucose using hospital meter and document.
• Recommended basal rate:_____
_____
• Recommended bolus:_____
_____

• **If patient unable to self-manage follow NURSE MANAGED ORDERS**

OR ☐ **NURSE MANAGED**

Basal Insulin (longer acting):   ☐ Novolin NPH ☐ Humulin N ☐ Other:_____
☐ 08:00 _____ units
☐ HS _____ units
☐ Other: _____ units

Mealtime Insulin (shorter acting):   ☐ Novorapid ☐ Humalog ☐ Other:_____
☐ With breakfast _____ units
☐ With lunch _____ units
☐ With supper _____ units • Hold meal time insulin if NPO

Supplemental scale: TID with meals only (once IV disconitnued)

Blood glucose (mmol/L)	Shorter acting insulin as above.	
<4	Give 175 mL juice po if unable to eat/NPO, give 25 mL D50W IV direct. Retest in 15 min and treat again if <4 mmol/L.	
4.1–8	Give usual mealtime dose.	
8.1–12	Add	units to mealtime dose.
12.1–16	Add	units to mealtime dose.
16.1–20	Add	units to mealtime dose.
≥20.1	Add	units to mealtime dose and call MD.

☐ Inform Dr _____ of patient's transfer to MBU during office hours at tel.: _____

☐ Social work consult

☐ Dietitian consult   ☐ Diabetes Nurse Specialist consult

☐ Other:

☐ Follow-up outpatient appointment with Dr _____ in _____ weeks

Date (yyaa/mm/dj):	Time-Heure:	Physician-Médecin (printed-imprimé):	Signature:
Date (noted-notée):	Time-Heure:	Processed by-Traitée par:	Signature: (Nurse-Infirmière):

OTHER ISSUES

FIGURE 32-1. Examples of peripartum insulin orders.

The Ottawa Hospital ☐ Civ ☐ Gen	L'Hôpital d'Ottawa	**PHYSICIAN'S ORDERS** **ORDONNANCES MÉDICALES** **Birthing Units-Unités des naissances**

Medication Allergies/Reactions	Substances or Food Allergies/Reactions
☐ None known-aucune connue	☐ None known-aucune connue

DIABETES MANAGEMENT - PRE DELIVERY-GESTION DU DIABÈTE - AVANT L'ACCOUCHEMENT

☐ Type 1 DM   ☐ Type 2 DM

DIET: Regular maternity no added sugar.   If NPO initiate IV insulin protocol
BLOOD GLUCOSE MONITORING: Test blood glucose TID before meals, qhs and 03:00, using hospital meter.

SUBCUTANEOUS INSULIN ORDERS: While patient eating

☐ PATIENT MANAGED - May self administer and adjust own insulin dose - Nurse to monitor blood glucose using hospital meter and document. ☐ PATIENT/FAMILY TO MANAGE with insulin pump - Nurse to monitor blood glucose using hospital meter and document. • Recommended basal rate:_____ _____ • Recommended bolus:_____ _____ ☐ Discontinue insulin pump when patient NPO and start IV insulin ☐ Continue insulin pump throughout labour and delivery • **If patient unable to self-manage follow NURSE MANAGED ORDERS**	OR ☐ NURSE MANAGED

OR ☐ NURSE MANAGED

Basal Insulin (longer acting):	☐ Novolin NPH	☐ Humulin N	☐ Other:_____
☐ 08:00 _____ units			
☐ HS _____ units			
☐ Other: _____ units			

Mealtime Insulin (shorter acting):	☐ Novorapid	☐ Humalog	☐ Other:_____
☐ With breakfast _____ units			
☐ With lunch _____ units			
☐ With supper _____ units			

Supplemental scale: TID with meals only

Blood glucose (mmol/L)	Shorter acting insulin as above
<4	Give 175 mL juice, if unable to eat or drink give 25 mL D50W IV direct. Retest in 15 min and treat again if <4 mmol/L.
4.1–8	Give usual mealtime dose.
8.1–10	Add 2 units to usual mealtime dose, retest in 4 hrs. If blood glucose > 8 mmol/L at next test, initiate IV insulin protocol.
> 10	Initiate IV insulin protocol.

IV INSULIN PROTOCOL TO BE INITIATED IN ALL PATIENTS IF (except those remaining on insulin pump):
• **Planned C-section: start upon admission.**
• **Blood glucose remains > 8 mmol/L X2 consecutive readings or > 10 mmol/L x 1.**
• **Patient is NPO.**

• Discontinue subcutaneous insulin/insulin pump.
• IV D5W at 100 mL/hr.
• IV regular insulin 50 units/500 mL NS (flush IV tubing with 50 mL insulin infusion prior to starting drip and piggy back insulin into D5W).
• Test blood glucose q1h: if 4–8 mmol/L x 2 consecutive hours, monitor q2h. Resume q1h monitoring if any change to infusion rate.

Adjust IV insulin dose as follows:

Blood glucose (mmol/L)	insulin infusion rate mL/hr (units/hr). Concentration 1 unit insulin/10 mL NS.	
<4	5 mL/hr	(0.5 unit/hr) and give D50W 25 mL IV direct. Retest in 15 min and treat again if blood glucose remains <4 mmol/L, notify MD for new IV insulin orders.
4.1–6	10 mL/hr	(1 unit/hr) or 0.5 unit/hr if previous blood glucose was < 4 mmol/L.
6.1–8	15 mL/hr	(1.5 units/hr).
8.1–10	20 mL/hr	(2 units/hr).
10.1–12	25 mL/hr	(2.5 units/hr).
12.1–14	30 mL/hr	(3 units/hr): if 2 consecutive results ≥ 12.1 mmol/L, notify MD for new IV insulin orders.
> 14	40 mL/hr	(4 units/hr): if 2 consecutive results ≥ 14.1 mmol/L, notify MD for new IV insulin orders.

Date (yyaa/mm/dj):	Time-Heure:	Physician-Médecin (printed-imprimé):	Signature:
Date (noted-notée):	Time-Heure:	Processed by-Traitée par:	Signature: (Nurse-Infirmière):

FIGURE 32-1. *(Continued)*

first trimester and reaches a nadir towards the end of the second trimester, with a return to baseline during the third trimester. New onset hypertension after 20 weeks should prompt evaluation for preeclampsia. See Table 32-1 for the differential diagnosis of hypertension in pregnancy.

TABLE 32-1: DIFFERENTIAL DIAGNOSIS OF HYPERTENSION IN PREGNANCY

Condition	Definitions	Associated Conditions
Chronic hypertension	BP ≥140/90 mm Hg with particular focus on dBP ≥90 mm Hg before 20 weeks gestation or 12 weeks postpartum or patient already taking hypertensive medications at the onset of pregnancy	20% risk of developing preeclampsia; without preeclampsia, risk of IUGR or placental abruption likely <1%
Transient hypertension of pregnancy	Isolated BP >140/90 mm Hg toward term	Hypertension resolves quickly postpartum; no previous documentation of hypertension; may be predictor of developing chronic hypertension
Severe hypertension in pregnancy	sBP ≥160 or dBP ≥110 mm Hg	sBP ≥160 mm Hg is associated with an increased risk of stroke
Preeclampsia	Maternal hypertension and proteinuria presenting after 20 weeks of gestation	Neurologic, renal, hepatic, and hematologic complications (see section below)
Eclampsia	Development of seizures in pregnancy	May predate other manifestations of preeclampsia

BP, blood pressure; dBP, diastolic blood pressure; IUGR, intrauterine growth restriction; SBP, systolic blood pressure.

Preeclampsia

Preeclampsia affects up to 6 percent of all first pregnancies and is the most common cause of pregnancy-associated mortality worldwide. Predisposing factors include extremes of age (younger than 20 or older than 40 years), elevated body mass index, underlying chronic hypertension, history of insulin resistance, and previous preeclampsia. Generally accepted diagnostic criteria include demonstration of hypertension that occurs after 20 weeks of gestation in a woman with previously normal

OTHER ISSUES

blood pressure and presence of proteinuria, defined as urinary excretion of 0.3 g of protein or higher in a 24-hour specimen.

The pathophysiology of preeclampsia is thought to be secondary to an abnormal vascular response to placentation, specifically to the second wave of trophoblastic invasion. This ultimately leads to increased systemic vascular resistance, endothelial cell dysfunction, activation of the coagulation cascade, and enhanced platelet aggregation. It is associated with numerous maternal and fetal complications. Although there are many risk factors for the development of preeclampsia, the most common ones are chronic hypertension, obesity, and nulliparity. Symptoms include headache, visual disturbances, epigastric or right upper quadrant pain, and worsening edema. Signs on clinical examination include hypertension, abdominal tenderness, clonus, and hyperreflexia. Serious manifestations are listed in Table 32-2.

Laboratory Investigation

If a diagnosis of preeclampsia is considered, fetal monitoring studies and the following laboratory investigations should be undertaken to look for concerning features:

- Complete blood count (CBC): hemolysis or anemia, thrombocytopenia
- Blood film: red blood cell fragments
- Hemolysis screen: elevated lactate dehydrogenase (LDH) and bilirubin, low haptoglobin

TABLE 32-2: SERIOUS MANIFESTATIONS OF PREECLAMPSIA

Maternal	Fetal
Seizures (eclampsia)	Placental abruption
Stroke	Preterm delivery
Congestive heart failure	Fetal growth restriction
Acute renal impairment	Fetal hypoxia
HELLP syndrome	Perinatal death
DIC	
Hepatic infarction, hemorrhage, rupture	
Diabetes insipidus	

DIC, disseminated intravascular coagulation; HELLP, hemolysis, elevated liver enzymes, and low platelets.

- Coagulation studies: international normalized ratio (INR), partial thromboplastin time (PTT), D-dimer, fibrinogen, and fibrin degradation products (FDP) to assess for coagulopathy
- Urinalysis to screen for proteinuria
  - Formal assessment of proteinuria by protein: creatinine ratio or 24-hour urine collection for protein
  - Significant proteinuria can be diagnosed when protein excretion is greater than 0.3 g/24 hours or 30 mg/mmol urinary creatinine
  - More information is needed to determine the utility of the urinary albumin:creatinine ratio
- Creatinine and urea: assess volume status and renal function
- Uric acid: most sensitive test for preeclampsia and is elevated in 80 percent of cases
- Liver enzymes: aspartate aminotransferase (AST) and alanine aminotransferase (ALT) elevation above two to three times normal is concerning for significant liver damage. Alkaline phosphatase (ALP) is produced by the placenta and may be slightly elevated in pregnancy

Intrapartum Hypertension Management

Timing and Mode of Delivery
If there is clear evidence of preeclampsia after 37 weeks of gestation, delivery should be advocated. At earlier gestational ages, evidence of severe fetal compromise or maternal risk should lead to consideration of delivery. Severe manifestations that may warrant delivery before 37 weeks are seizures, acute onset of renal failure (Cr >88 umol or oliguria <500 mL/24 hr), severe hypertension, thrombocytopenia with platelet count below 100,000/μL, evidence of hemolysis, elevated liver enzymes greater than two to three times normal, symptoms suggestive of end-organ damage, retinal hemorrhage or papilledema, pulmonary edema, or evidence of significant fetal compromise. This should be balanced by the neonatal risks associated with delivery, which are gestationally dependent. Below 34 weeks' gestation, the mother should be given corticosteroids to promote fetal lung maturation. Unless there is an obstetric indication for cesarean section, vaginal delivery should be considered for women with any hypertensive disorder of pregnancy.

Seizure Prophylaxis
All women with a firm diagnosis of preeclampsia and a decision to deliver should have initiation of therapy with magnesium sulfate to prevent

progression to eclampsia. An IV bolus of 4 to 6 g followed by IV infusion of 1 to 4 g/hr is recommended, with caution in women with renal insufficiency. Signs of toxicity, such as hypotension, muscular weakness, and respiratory distress, can be reversed with administration of IV calcium. The management of eclampsia is described elsewhere.

Treatment of Hypertension

There is no specified targeted blood pressure in the setting of preeclampsia. BP above 180/110 mm Hg should be treated urgently, and it is recommended that BP be lowered to sBP below 160 mm Hg and dBP below 100 mm Hg. When urgent BP reduction is required, IV labetolol is recommended as the first-line agent. Other agents such as hydralazine or nifedipine can also be used.

- Labetolol: 10 to 20 mg IV pushes followed by infusion of 0.5 to 2.0 mg/min or 100 to 600 mg orally twice to three times a day (maximum oral dose, 2400 mg/day)
- Nifedipine: fast-acting capsules (bitten and swallowed) or intermediate-release (PA) tablets can be given 10 mg orally every 30 minutes to a maximum of 50 mg acutely, with maintenance doses of 10 to 20 mg orally three times a day of PA tablets or 30 to 120 mg once daily of extended-release tablets
- Hydralazine: 2.5 to 10 mg IV every 30-minutes boluses; maintenance doses of 10 to 50 mg orally four times a day

In cases of nonsevere hypertension with or without preeclampsia, it is recommended that in women without comorbid conditions, antihypertensive drugs be used to keep sBP at 130 to 155 mm Hg and dBP at 80 to 105 mm Hg. In women with premorbid conditions, target sBP at 130 to 139 mm Hg and dBP at 80 to 89 mm Hg. Methyldopa (250-500 mg orally twice to four times a day), labetolol (100-400 mg twice to three times a day), and nifedipine XL (20-60 mg orally OD; maximum, 120 mg/day) are the mostly commonly used medications. ACE inhibitors and angiotensin receptor blockers (ARBs) should not be used. Atenolol and prazosin are not recommended.

Management and Prevention of Complications

Judicious administration of fluids is recommended to avoid pulmonary edema. Acute treatment of pulmonary edema includes supplemental oxygen administration, diuretic use, and morphine if needed. In the setting of oliguria and rising creatinine, small IV boluses (250 cc) of saline can be used cautiously to try to improve urine output.

Postpartum Considerations

It is important to remember that both preeclampsia and eclampsia can present postpartum. Blood pressure from preeclampsia may remain elevated for 6 to 12 weeks postpartum even without underlying chronic hypertension. Platelets, liver function tests, and renal function must be closely monitored until results are normal. Antihypertensive agents acceptable for use in breastfeeding include nifedipine XL, labetalol, methyldopa, captopril, and enalapril.

ACUTE DYSPNEA IN PERIPARTUM PATIENTS

The degree and severity of dyspnea in pregnant patients can range from mild discomfort in keeping with the normal physiologic changes of pregnancy to severe, life-threatening respiratory distress and ultimately respiratory failure. Early recognition of ominous signs and symptoms is crucial in the successful management of critically ill patients. This chapter focuses on the identification, diagnosis, and management of severely ill patients in the peripartum period. The ominous signs are listed in Table 32-3.

Normal Respiratory Changes in Pregnancy

It is important for clinicians to have a fundamental understanding of the normal alterations in maternal respiratory physiology during pregnancy. Minute ventilation increases during pregnancy, which reduces alveolar and arterial pCO_2. Therefore, a normal arterial pCO_2 in pregnant patients is lower (28-30 mm Hg) than in their nonpregnant counterpart (35-40 mm Hg). Compensation occurs through the loss of bicarbonate ions in the kidney. Therefore, pregnancy is normally associated with a compensated respiratory alkalosis. This is important to keep in mind when interpreting arterial blood gas (ABG) values.

Pulmonary Function in Pregnancy

Pregnancy is associated with an increase is tidal volume (TV) and a decrease in residual volume (RV) and functional residual capacity (FRC).

TABLE 32-3: OMINOUS SIGNS OF ACUTELY DYSPNEIC PATIENTS

Asterixis	May be observed with severe hypercapnia
Myoclonus and seizures	May occur with severe hypoxemia
Accessory muscle use	Indicates diaphragmatic fatigue
Cyanosis	Indicative of severe hypoxemia or intracardiac shunt
Tachypnea	(RR >30-40 breaths/min)
Difficulty speaking	(i.e., three- or four-word dyspnea)
Somnolence or alteration of mental status	May occur as a result of severe hypoxemia or hypercapnia
Crackles upon auscultation	May suggest pulmonary edema
Severe hypoxia refractory to oxygen therapy	(PaO_2/FiO_2 <200)
Hypercapnia or respiratory acidosis	PaO_2 >35 mm Hg; pH <7.35

FiO_2, fraction of inspired oxygen; PaO_2, partial pressure of oxygen in arterial blood; RR, respiratory rate.

Forced vital capacity (FVC), forced expiratory volume in 1 second (FEV_1), and total lung capacity (TLC) remain unchanged.

General Management

Regardless of the etiology of dyspnea, the initial steps in management of the patient with respiratory distress will be similar. Transfer of the patient to a high-dependency setting including continuous cardiac monitoring and pulse oxymetry as well as appropriate monitoring for the fetus should be pursued immediately. Close attention to hemodynamic and respiratory changes should prompt more urgent intervention.

Supportive care including supplemental oxygen and IV access is also mandatory in this setting. The level of delivered oxygen depends largely on the extent of hypoxemia, and it is recommended that maternal oxyhemoglobin levels be kept above 95 percent, corresponding to a PaO_2 (partial pressure of oxygen in arterial blood) of approximately 70 mm Hg. If this level of oxygenation cannot be maintained, noninvasive or invasive positive-pressure ventilation should be considered.

General Investigations

Initial investigations must include a focused history and physical examination to narrow the differential diagnosis and to direct more specific testing. An ABG analysis, a chest radiograph, and an electrocardiogram should also be included in the initial workup. Further investigations will be case specific and will be addressed in detail in the discussion of each individual diagnosis.

PULMONARY EDEMA

Pulmonary edema occurs when there is a net movement of fluid from the pulmonary vasculature to the alveolar space and pulmonary interstitium. This process can occur in response to a variety of underlying conditions. However, for the purpose of this chapter, pulmonary edema can simply be classified into cardiogenic and noncardiogenic causes. In pregnancy, a number of normal physiologic changes predispose patients to the development of pulmonary edema. These include an increased effective circulating volume (ECV), a relatively low oncotic pressure, and a decreased FRC, which promotes atelectasis and alveolar collapse. During labor and delivery, additional hemodynamic factors must be considered, including a sudden increase in both cardiac output and blood pressure secondary to the pain of uterine contractions and an abrupt increase in ECV resulting from autotransfusion.

Diagnosis

The diagnosis can be made using a combination of clinical examination and radiographic investigations. The presence of new bilateral rales on pulmonary auscultation should suggest pulmonary edema. A chest radiograph demonstrating bilateral airspace and interstitial infiltrates would further support the diagnosis. An elevated jugular venous pressure and increased cardiac silhouette may point to a cardiac cause. A transthoracic echocardiogram, if available, would also assist in identifying a cardiogenic etiology.

Cardiogenic Pulmonary Edema

Cardiogenic pulmonary edema can occur when left-sided cardiac filling pressures rise sufficiently to cause high pulmonary capillary pressure, resulting in extravasation of fluid from the pulmonary vasculature. A variety of mechanisms can account for left-sided filling pressures; the most common are presented below.

Arrhythmia

Although rarely a cause of pulmonary edema, acute supraventricular arrhythmias can compromise left ventricular filling in a patient with underlying cardiac dysfunction. More ominous ventricular arrhythmias can lead to homodynamic instability and even death.

Valvular

Severe aortic stenosis and symptomatic aortic insufficiency and symptomatic mitral valve lesions (stenosis or regurgitation) represent the highest risk to pregnant patients.

Peripartum Cardiomyopathy

Peripartum cardiomyopathy (PPCM) is a condition that causes subacute dilatation of the myocardial tissue, resulting in left ventricular dysfunction and clinical heart failure. The prognosis for patients with peripartum cardiomyopathy is variable, with reported mortality rates ranging from 10 to 40 percent in some studies. To establish a diagnosis of PPCM, a patient must meet all of the following criteria:

1. An ejection fraction less than 45 percent by echocardiography or radionuclide ventriculography
2. Clinical symptoms of heart failure
3. Development of cardiac failure in the last month of pregnancy or within 5 months of delivery
4. Absence of identifiable cause of cardiac failure
5. Absence of recognizable heart disease before the last month of pregnancy

Ischemia and Infarction

Fortunately, acute myocardial infarction in pregnant patients is a relatively uncommon problem. However, as maternal age continues to increase, clinicians are faced with patients with preexisting cardiovascular disease. Electrocardiographic and cardiac biomarkers (creatine kinase, troponin I) may assist in diagnosis.

Noncardiogenic Pulmonary Edema

In contrast to cardiogenic pulmonary edema, noncardiogenic pulmonary edema occurs in the context of normal pulmonary capillary pressure.

In this situation, the net movement of fluid into the alveolar and interstitial space can be accounted for by increased permeability of the pulmonary capillaries or low oncotic pressure.

Acute Respiratory Distress Syndrome

Acute respiratory distress syndrome (ARDS) is the most common cause of noncardiogenic pulmonary edema and can be seen in conditions such as pneumonia, sepsis, disseminated intravascular coagulation (DIC), and inhalation injury. In addition, there are a number of pregnancy-associated causes of ARDS, such as tocolysis, preeclampsia or eclampsia, and amniotic fluid embolism. The most common pregnancy-associated etiologies are discussed below.

Tocolysis

The use of tocolytic beta-adrenergic receptor agonists (e.g., ritodrine and terbutaline) to suppress preterm labor is associated with the development of ARDS. Although the etiology remains unclear, it is postulated that prolonged exposure to beta-agonists may cause myocardial dysfunction. These drugs are also known to promote sodium and water retention.

Preeclampsia

Preeclampsia is also associated with the risk of developing ARDS. It is estimated that approximately 3 percent of patients with severe preeclampsia will develop pulmonary edema, with maternal mortality rates reported to be as high as 11 percent. As a result, judicious use of IV fluids is necessary in patients with preeclampsia.

Amniotic Fluid Embolism

Although amniotic fluid embolism (AFE) is a relatively rare condition, the diagnosis must be considered in any peripartum patient with acute dyspnea. Predisposing factors include prolonged labor, multiparity, advanced maternal age, and cesarean or instrumental delivery. Although AFE is a known cause of ARDS, the presentation is usually fulminant and is not limited to respiratory symptoms. Patients can present with profound hypotension and circulatory collapse, respiratory failure, and ultimately DIC. Treatment is largely supportive and is best managed in a critical care setting. Urgent cesarean delivery may be indicated if the patient is critically ill.

OTHER ISSUES

Medical Management

In a peripartum patient with pulmonary edema, management will not differ significantly from management of nonpregnant patients. Identification and treatment of the underlying cause is important and help in the definitive management and prevention of recurrence. However, treatment of symptoms and hypoxia is similar in most cases. In addition to the management discussed in the introduction, the following treatment is recommended to treat acute pulmonary edema.

Diuretics

Treatment with diuretics is indicated in patients with pulmonary edema. Loop diuretics are generally preferred over thiazide diuretics, but either may be used. Loop diuretics such as furosemide have been shown to decrease jugular venous pressure and pulmonary congestion as well as improve cardiac function. Monitoring of blood work should be considered because electrolyte abnormalities are common. Pregnant women usually have higher than normal glomerular filtration rates (GFRs), and often only low doses of diuretics are required to treat pulmonary edema and induce diuresis.

Nitrates

Nitrates are potent venodilators that are commonly used in acute decompensated heart failure. They rapidly decrease cardiac preload and have an effect on peripheral arterial tone. Nitrates can be safely used in pregnancy and can be administered sublingually, transdermally, or via the IV route.

Special Considerations

Although ACE inhibitors, ARBs, and spironolactone are standard therapy in heart failure, they should generally be avoided in pregnant patients.

ACUTE PULMONARY EMBOLISM

Pregnancy is associated with an increased incidence of pulmonary embolism (PE). It is estimated that the risk of venous thromboembolism (VTE) in pregnant women is approximately 5 to 10 times higher than in their nonpregnant counterparts. This is because of a number of hematologic and hemodynamic factors that lead to a relatively hypercoagulable state.

Despite advances in the diagnosis and treatment of acute thrombo-embolic events, untreated PE remains the commonest cause of maternal mortality in the developed world (as high as 30%). With early recognition and appropriate treatment, PE-associated mortality decreases to less than 10 percent. It is therefore imperative that diagnosis be made promptly and appropriate treatment be instituted without delay.

Diagnosis

Establishing the diagnosis of PE in pregnant patients is of particular importance given the high mortality rate in untreated patients. It is equally important to disprove the presence of a PE because erroneous diagnosis may delay treatment for other important conditions and would also expose a patient to unnecessary treatment with potentially harmful anti-coagulant medications.

There are multiple strategies and algorithms to assist clinicians managing patients with suspected PE. A combination of history and physical examination are used to first develop a pretest probability of VTE. A number of imaging modalities are available to subsequently establish a diagnosis.

History and Physical Examination

In addition to dyspnea, clinical features that may suggest PE may include signs and symptoms of peripheral deep vein thrombosis (i.e., lower extremity tenderness, edema and/or erythema), pleuritic chest pain, tachycardia, or hemoptysis. A personal or family history of VTE or history of active malignancy would also increase the pretest probability.

Imaging

Many imaging modalities exist to diagnose PE, each with its potential strengths and weaknesses. The most common approaches are ventilation-perfusion scintigraphy and contrast-enhanced helical computed tomography (CT).

Ventilation–perfusion scintigraphy is a reasonable first option in the diagnosis of suspected PE in patients with normal chest radiograph. A low probability test all but rules out the diagnosis, and a high-risk result confirms it. However, an indeterminate or moderate probability test would likely lead to further imaging, exposing the mother and fetus to further ionizing radiation.

Contrast-enhanced helical CT (CT pulmonary angiography) is another commonly used imaging modality to diagnose PE. Although this modality is often favored in the nonpregnant population, its use in pregnancy is

OTHER ISSUES

also a reasonable option. With respect to radiation exposure, CT pulmonary angiography exposes the fetus to similar amounts of ionizing radiation as ventilation–perfusion scintigraphy. Both tests fall well within acceptable levels of fetal exposure to ionizing radiation and are considered safe in pregnancy. However, the amount of radiation delivered to a woman's breasts through CT angiography is orders of magnitude higher than through ventilation–perfusion scintigraphy. The potential risks of any imaging test must be weighed against the benefits and may be patient and center specific.

Treatment

Once a baseline CBC, PTT, and INR are obtained, treatment with IV unfractionated heparin (UFH) or low-molecular-weight heparin (LMWH) should be initiated immediately. The decision to treat with UFH versus LMWH will depend largely on the clinical context and the time to expected delivery.

There are limited data to support the use of one agent over another, and guidelines are dated or based on anecdotal evidence. LMWH is often selected as the treatment of choice because of its ease of administration and lower incidence of heparin-induced thrombocytopenia (HIT).

One of the greatest challenges in treating pregnant women with acute PE is what to do at the time of labor and delivery. In the authors' center, if the VTE is remote from term, then LMWH is continued until a date of induction of labor or cesarean section. Postpartum, a smaller dose of LMWH is used starting on PP day 1 until hemostasis is achieved. Then the usual dose of LMWH is restarted.

If the VTE occurs within 4 weeks of delivery, then consideration of using IV UFH during labor and delivery is reasonable. This will allow for a potentially shorter duration whereby anticoagulation needs to be interrupted.

In the authors' center, placement of an inferior vena cava (IVC) filter is considered if the diagnosis of PE is made at or near term (greater than 38 weeks' gestation). Again, IV UFH would be used if the event is close to term.

Thrombolytic therapy is associated with severe bleeding and should be reserved for patients with severe hemodynamic instability in the context of confirmed PE. If thrombolysis is indicated, tissue plasminogen activator (tPA) at a dose of 200 mg administered IV over 2 hours is the recommended treatment.

PNEUMONIA

Community-acquired pneumonia (CAP) is a common cause of respiratory distress in both in pregnant and nonpregnant patients. However,

CAP seems to be more common in the pregnant population and can have a more severe course. This may be because of a high prevalence of gastroesophageal reflux disease and alterations in cell-mediated immunity.

Diagnosis

Clinical features that may be useful in differentiating an infectious cause of dyspnea from other causes may include general malaise fever; chills or rigors; a productive cough; and less frequently, pleuritic chest pain.

A chest radiograph is a safe imaging modality in pregnancy (especially with proper shielding) and may assist in diagnosis if there is evidence of airspace disease or consolidation. Concomitant peripheral leukocytosis would further support an infectious cause. Blood cultures may assist in selecting to more specific antibiotic treatment.

Treatment

Treatment with antibiotics is indicated in any patient suspected to have pneumonia. In general, broad-spectrum empiric treatment is initiated to include coverage for typical and atypical bacterial infections. Initial treatment is empiric treatment and may include macrolide monotherapy (e.g., azithromycin, clarithromycin) in otherwise healthy patients who are not acutely unwell. In critically ill patients, a second- or third-generation cephalosporin in combination with a macrolide should be considered.

Special consideration should also be given to viral pathogens, particularly influenza. Data from the 2009 H1N1 pandemic support the notion that pregnant women are more likely to have a severe course of illness with a higher risk of intensive care unit admission and death. Prompt recognition and treatment with an appropriate antiviral medication such as neuraminidase inhibitors (i.e., oseltamivir and zanamivir) should be considered. Early treatment with osteltamivir may diminish the severity of illness and decrease mortality in pregnant patients with influenza.

ACUTE EXACERBATION OF ASTHMA

Asthma is a common chronic illness in women and as such is an important consideration when assessing the peripartum patient with dyspnea.

OTHER ISSUES

The rate of acute exacerbations among pregnant women with asthma is higher than in the nonpregnant population and may be associated with poor outcomes for the mother and fetus.

Treatment

The treatment of acute asthma exacerbations in pregnancy is similar to the management in the nonpregnant patient. In addition to usual supportive care, the cornerstone of treatment in the acute setting is bronchodilator therapy. Concomitant treatment with both inhaled short-acting beta-adrenergic agonists (SABAs) and inhaled anticholinergic medication is warranted. Both agents can be delivered by metered-dose inhalers (MDIs) with aero-chambers or by nebulization and facemask.

Guidelines suggest that three treatments be administered every 20 to 30 minutes for initial therapy. The frequency of further treatment will vary depending on response (i.e., improvement in airflow obstruction and associated symptoms). In patients who do not respond to this initial regimen or who have severe airflow limitation (i.e., <40% of predicted value for either FEV_1 or peak expiratory flow), continuous administration of inhaled beta-agonists may be more effective than intermittent administration.

In addition, the use of systemic corticosteroids may also be warranted to decrease airway inflammation in severe cases. Steroids are generally recommended in all patients with moderate to severe airflow obstruction as well as patients who do not respond to initial bronchodilator therapy. The dose of systemic corticosteroids in pregnancy is the same as those recommended for nonpregnant patients.

Serial measurements of peak flow may help to monitor response to therapy and alert the clinician to worsening symptoms. If signs of impending respiratory failure are present (see Table 32-3), prompt recognition and consultation with critical care specialists is recommended. Early intubation and mechanical ventilation are crucial, as respiratory failure can progress rapidly and can be difficult to reverse.

CARDIAC ARREST

Owing to the younger population with less comorbidities, cardiac arrest is rare in pregnancy, with an incidence estimated at 1 in 30,000. The most common causes are listed in Table 32-4.

TABLE 32-4: MOST COMMON CAUSES OF CARDIAC ARREST IN PREGNANCY

VTE	Amniotic fluid embolus
Hypertensive disorders of pregnancy	Obstetric hemorrhage
Sepsis	Trauma
Preexisting heart disease	Iatrogenic (medication allergies, anesthesia complications)

VTE, venous thromboembolism.

There are little changes to established protocols for cardiopulmonary resuscitation (CPR) and advanced cardiac lifesaving (ACLS). The following should be taken into consideration:

- Placing a wedge or a rescuer's knee under the patient's right hip to relieve vena cava obstruction will improve venous return and may increase cardiac output by 25 to 30 percent
- Intubate as soon as possible to prevent aspiration
- Remove fetal monitoring devices when considering cardioversion/defibrillation to prevent cardiac arcing
- No drug should be withheld because of pregnancy, if believed to be lifesaving compared with an alternate choice
- Avoid vasopressin as an alternative to epinephrine in scenarios of pulseless ventricular tachycardia or ventricular fibrillation because the placenta produces vasopressinase, which may degrade the drug

The key in maternal cardiac arrest is rapid performance of a cesarean section. It is well described that performing a cesarean section within 4 to 5 minutes of an arrest in a patient who has reached a viable gestational age (>24 weeks) will not only improve fetal outcomes but also hasten maternal recovery. In fact, 70 percent of infants who survive a perimortem cesarean section were delivered within 5 minutes and 95 percent within 15 minutes. It is important that CPR be continued through the delivery process.

In the rare and unfortunate instances in which maternal brain death occurs, there have been reported cases of somatic support until delivery. The longest reported duration of such support is 107 days. This issue raises a number of ethical and medical challenges and warrants in-depth discussion with the patient's family, the health care team, and possibly ethics committees.

OTHER ISSUES

THROMBOCYTOPENIA IN PREGNANCY

Thrombocytopenia occurs in 6 to 10 percent of all pregnancies and is second only to anemia in terms of common hematologic disorders in pregnancy. Normal pregnancy is associated with a physiologic fall in the platelet count that is characterized by a leftward shift in the platelet count distribution. Platelet counts usually remain within the normal range, but a 10 percent drop is deemed acceptable. The differential diagnosis of thrombocytopenia in pregnancy includes conditions that are specific to pregnancy and those that can also been seen in the general population (Table 32-5).

Ominous Signs

- Diffuse petechia, ecchymoses, or purpura
- Spontaneous bleeding
- Platelet counts of less than 20,000/μL
- Postpartum hemorrhage
- Coagulopathy
- Association with hypertension, renal dysfunction, or liver dysfunction

Investigations

The diagnosis is made based on platelet count on a CBC. When platelets are low, other investigations should include a CBC, blood film, coagulation studies including INR/PT, PTT, fibrinogen, D-dimer, liver function testing, electrolytes, creatinine, and urinalysis for proteinuria (Table 32-6).

General Guidelines for Management of Thrombocytopenia in Labor and Delivery

Maternal bleeding is uncommon unless the platelet count is below 20,000/μL. Maternal hemorrhage most commonly occurs at the time of delivery. Generally, treatment is recommended in asymptomatic patients with platelet counts of less than 20,000/μL. Expert recommendations suggest that in anticipation of delivery, third-trimester counts below 40,000 to 50,000/μL should be treated. Patients who are actively bleeding should always be treated, and a hematologic consultation is required. Although platelet transfusions are generally the primary mean of treatment, certain disease conditions require specific treatment. These are discussed in detail below. Guidelines recommend a platelet count of at least 75,000/μL for safe placement of an epidural catheter.

TABLE 32-5: DIFFERENTIAL DIAGNOSIS OF THROMBOCYTOPENIA IN PREGNANCY

Gestational thrombocytopenia
AFLP
HELLP syndrome
Preeclampsia or eclampsia
	Decreased production
	  Myelodysplasia
	  Bone marrow infiltration
	  Hematologic malignancy
	  Chronic alcoholism
	  Megaloblastic anemia (e.g., vitamin B_{12}, folate deficiency)
	  Aplastic anemia
	  Alcohol
	  Chemotherapy

	Increased destruction:
	  Primary immune-mediated
	    ITP
	  Secondary immune-mediated
	    Infectious (viral: HIV, EBV, CMV, HCV)
	    Drug induced (e.g., heparin)
	    Autoimmune disorders (e.g., SLE)
	    Antiphospholipid antibodies
	    Posttransfusion purpura
	  Thrombotic microangiopathies
	    TTP
	    HUS
	  DIC
	  Sepsis
	  Liver failure
	  Drugs (e.g., antimicrobials, NSAIDs, antiepileptics)
	  Inherited thrombocytopenias

	Splenic sequestration or hypersplenism

AFLP, acute fatty liver of pregnancy; CMV, cytomegalovirus; DIC, disseminated intravascular coagulation; EBV, Epstein-Barr virus; HCV, hepatitis C virus; HELLP, hemolysis, elevated liver enzymes, and low platelets; HUS, hemolytic uremic syndrome; ITP, immune thrombocytopenia; NSAID, nonsteroidal anti-inflammatory drug; SLE, systemic lupus erythematosus; TTP, thrombotic thrombocytopenic purpura.

Specific Etiologies of Thrombocytopenia in Pregnancy

Gestational

This accounts for 75 percent of the causes of thrombocytopenia in pregnancy. It is a diagnosis of exclusion and is generally reserved for cases of mild thrombocytopenia in the third trimester (usually counts >70,000/μL) when there has been no prior diagnosis and there is spontaneous resolution

TABLE 32-6: LABORATORY INVESTIGATIONS TO DIFFERENTIATE CAUSES OF THROMBOCYTOPENIA

Condition	Hgb	Blood Film	Platelets	INR/PT	PTT	Fibrinogen	D-Dimer/FDP	Liver
Gestational	N	N	↓	N	N	N or ↑	N	N
ITP	N	Giant platelets	↓	N	N	N or ↑	N	N
TTP or HUS	↓	Fragments	↓	N	N	N or ↑	N or ↑	N
Preeclampsia	↓ or N	N or Fragments	↓	N	N	N or ↑	N or ↑	N
HELLP	↓	Fragments	↓	N	N	N or ↑	↑	↑
DIC	↓	Fragments	↓	↑	↑	N or ↓	↑	N

DIC, disseminated intravascular coagulation; FDP, fibrin degradation products; HELLP, hemolysis, elevated liver enzymes, low platelet syndrome; Hgb, hemoglobin; HUS, hemolytic uremic syndrome; INR, international normalized ratio; ITP, immune thrombocytopenia; N, normal; PT, prothrombin time; PTT, partial thromboplastin time; TTP, thrombotic thrombocytopenic purpura postpartum with no associated fetal thrombocytopenia or adverse outcomes. No treatment is required.

Preeclampsia

Preeclampsia is the leading cause of pregnancy-associated mortality worldwide. It is defined as hypertension diagnosed after 20 weeks of gestation with evidence of proteinuria.

The details regarding the diagnosis, presentation, and management of preeclampsia is described in the section pertaining to hypertension. Thrombocytopenia occurs in up to 50 percent of women with preeclampsia and may precede other manifestations of the disorder. The definitive treatment of preeclampsia is delivery.

HELLP Syndrome

HELLP syndrome is a syndrome of hemolysis, elevated liver enzymes, and low platelets. It affects 0.5 to 0.9 percent of all pregnancies, is most common in multiparous women, and develops in 10 percent of patients with preeclampsia. Up to 70 percent of cases occur before term, and the remainder usually occur within 48 hours of delivery, although thrombocytopenia and elevated LDH can last as long as several weeks postpartum.

Diagnosis rests on demonstrated evidence of microangiopathic hemolytic anemia, increased LDH, increased AST (usually no more than 400 IU/L), and thrombocytopenia. There are many associated features and overlap with preeclampsia. Up to 75 percent of patients have proteinuria, and 50 to 60 percent have hypertension. Symptoms include malaise, right upper quadrant pain (obstructed blood flow to hepatic sinusoids), nausea, and vomiting. Hypotension or rapidly dropping hemoglobin should prompt consideration of a liver capsule hematoma or hepatic rupture, especially in the setting of transaminases above 500 IU/L.

There is a consensus that delivery is indicated beyond 34 weeks of gestation or earlier if there is evidence of multiorgan dysfunction, DIC, liver infarction or hemorrhage, renal failure, suspected abruptio placentae, or nonreassuring fetal status. Recovery may be hastened by administration of corticosteroids. Evidence suggests that administration of dexamethasone 10 mg IV every 12 hours for 2 doses followed by 5 mg every 12 hours for 2 doses may improve liver enzymes and platelet count and reduce blood pressure. Patients with suspected liver rupture should undergo a CT scan or magnetic resonance imaging (MRI). Management of hepatic rupture requires surgical intervention, although hepatic artery embolization appears to be most effective.

OTHER ISSUES

Immune Thrombocytopenia

The incidence of immune thrombocytopenia (ITP) is between 1 in 1000 and 1 in 10,000 pregnant women. Unlike other causes of thrombocytopenia, it may precede pregnancy or manifest at any time during pregnancy. Clinical features are easy bruising, mucosal bleeding, and petechiae. Only 30 percent of cases require therapy during pregnancy.

First-line therapy for treatment is IV immunoglobulin (IVIG), and/or corticosteroids. IVIG works rapidly (within 2-3 days) and lasts 2 to 3 weeks. There is no consensus on optimal dosing, but most centers recommend 1 g/kg/day for 2 days. Side effects include fever, headaches, chills, and chest pain. Corticosteroids are equally efficacious in pregnant women. The usual dose recommended is prednisone 1 mg/kg or high-dose pulse steroids (methylprednisolone 1g/day for 2 days). The maximal effect is reached after 2 to 4 weeks. Corticosteroid use may be associated with premature rupture of membranes and placental abruption along with an increased risk of gestational diabetes and hypertension when used longer term. It is recommended to use them sparingly and at the lowest efficacious dose. Women treated with long-term corticosteroids may have underlying adrenal suppression and should be considered for stress steroids dosing at the time of delivery.

Alternative treatments in patient actively bleeding include tranexamic acid and recombinant factor VIIa. Rarely, splenectomy can be performed during cesarean section in selected patients.

Of note, antiplatelet antibodies cross the placenta and may cause fetal thrombocytopenia, the degree of which does not correlate with maternal thrombocytopenia. About 15 percent of the offspring of mothers with ITP will have platelet counts below 100,000/μL, 10 percent below 50,000/μL, and only 4 percent will have severe thrombocytopenia with counts below 20,000/μL. Studies have shown that there is no increased risk of intracranial hemorrhage with vaginal delivery even when fetal thrombocytopenia is documented by cordocentesis.

Neonatal platelet counts should be determined in cord blood immediately on delivery and for the next five days as it may take several days to reach the nadir neonatal platelet count. Some centers recommend routine transcranial ultrasound, even in asymptomatic neonates, when the platelet count is below 50,000/μL.

Thrombotic Thrombocytopenic Purpura and Hemolytic Uremic Syndrome

These two conditions are collectively referred to as thrombotic microangiopathies. Although they are not pregnancy specific, there is a slightly increased incidence of thrombotic thrombocytopenic purpura (TTP) in pregnancy. TTP is caused by a deficiency in ADAMTS-13, a metalloprotease that cleaves von Willebrand factor (vWF). This deficiency leads to ultra-larger vWF multimers that promote platelet agglutination and microthrombotic events. It can be difficult to distinguish from other disorders such as preeclampsia, HELLP syndrome, and acute fatty liver, which are commonly associated with microangiopathic hemolytic anemia (MAHA) and thrombocytopenia. TTP is classically associated with the pentad of MAHA, thrombocytopenia, fever, renal dysfunction, and neurologic impairment (confusion, headaches, seizures, coma). Of the nonhematologic manifestations of TTP, the neurologic changes are most common. Hemolytic uremic syndrome (HUS) is seen predominantly in children, and the renal impairment is typically the most important feature.

The management is the same as in the nonpregnant population, with plasma exchange yielding an 80 percent response rate. Although there are no randomized trials to support the use of corticosteroids in TTP, some authors recommend their use given the immune nature of the disorder. Importantly, unlike preeclampsia and the HELLP syndrome, termination of pregnancy does not induce remission of TTP.

Disseminated Intravascular Coagulation

Disseminated intravascular coagulation (DIC) is the final common pathways resulting in overactivation of coagulation and/or fibrinolytic system that leads to unopposed production of thrombin, resulting in microvascular thrombotic obstruction and bleeding from a consumptive coagulopathy. Obstetric causes include placental abruption, amniotic fluid embolism, retained fetal products, massive obstetrical hemorrhage, preeclampsia or eclampsia, and uterine rupture. Non–pregnancy-related causes include trauma, hemolytic reactions, tissue damage, cancer, leukemia, and sepsis. The laboratory diagnosis rests on evidence of anemia and presence of red blood cell fragments (schistocytes), thrombocytopenia, increased PT or PTT, and increased fibrin degradation products or D-Dimer. The fibrinogen level is normally elevated in pregnancy and may remain normal or decreased in severe cases.

The primary treatment is reversal of the cause. Prompt evacuation of the uterus followed by hemodynamic and hemostatic support usually leads to complete reversal of the coagulopathy. Vaginal delivery is possible in the majority of cases, but local measures to reduce bleeding are crucial. With adequate fluid resuscitation, uterotonic medications, and hemostatic management, most patients have a spontaneous resolution of bleeding.

OTHER ISSUES

Transfusions are indicated for ongoing bleeding. The American Society of Anesthesiologists suggests the following transfusion parameters:

- Platelet transfusion to maintain counts more than 50,000/μL
- Fibrinogen (10 units of cryoprecipitate) should be given to patients with levels less than 1.0 g/L. If cryoprecipitate is not available, fresh-frozen plasma (FFP) can be used, although is not as rich in fibrinogen
- FFP if INR greater than 1.5

In rare cases when severe bleeding persists, potential pharmacologic options include antithrombin, tissue factor pathway inhibitors, and activated protein C, although recent trials have shown no proven benefits. Recombinant factor VIIa may be potentially useful. Aminocaproic acid, a fibrinolysis inhibitor used in postoperative bleeding, should not be used because it may predispose to thrombotic events. Surgical interventions include selective pelvic arterial embolization.

ACUTE FATTY LIVER OF PREGNANCY

Acute fatty liver of pregnancy (AFLP) occurs in the third trimester and is thought to be part of a spectrum of diseases related to impaired fatty acid transport. It is characterized by accumulation of microvascular fat within the liver parenchyma. The differential includes HELLP syndrome, hepatic hemorrhage, and rupture, all of which can be seen with preeclampsia and intrahepatic cholestasis of pregnancy (Table 32-7).

Clinical Presentation

There is a wide spectrum of presentation for AFLP. Patients may range from being asymptomatic to having nonspecific malaise, including nausea, vomiting, and lethargy. This may be followed by jaundice and hepatic failure. Early recognition is important as it may lead to coma and maternal or fetal demise. Diagnosis rests on the clinical history, and laboratory investigations should include a coagulation panel, ammonia level, CBC and film, liver and renal panel, and glucose levels. Acetaminophen toxicity should be ruled out.

Ominous Signs

- Encephalopathy
- Hyperammonemia

TABLE 32-7: DIFFERENTIAL DIAGNOSIS OF LIVER PATHOLOGY IN PREGNANCY

Variable	Intrahepatic Cholestasis	HELLP Syndrome	Rupture	Infarction	AFLP
Timing	Late second or third trimester	≥20 weeks	≥20 weeks	≥20 weeks	Third trimester
Clinical signs	Pruritus	Abdominal pain, preeclampsia	Abdominal swelling or tenderness, shock	Fever, abdominal pain	Asymptomatic nausea, vomiting, jaundice, preeclampsia
Laboratory values	Elevated bile salts +/- transaminases	Hemolysis, thrombocytopenia, elevated AST	Anemia, second-degree bleeding	Anemia, very high AST (>1000 IU/L)	Elevated transaminases but <1000 IU/L, increased PTT, decreased fibrinogen, hypoglycemia, increased INR
Management	Ursodeoxycholic acid, rapid resolution after delivery	Delivery, treatment of preeclampsia, potentially steroids	Surgical, hepatic artery embolization	Surgical, hepatic artery embolization; may require transplantation	Supportive, prompt delivery; may require transplant

AST, aspartate aminotransferase; INR, international normalized ratio; PTT, partial thromboplastin time.

- Hypoglycemia
- Coagulopathy (hallmark features are increased PTT and decreased fibrinogen)
- Sepsis

Intrapartum Management

The treatment of ALFP is delivery and supportive care. Continuous fetal monitoring should be undertaken. It is recommended that broad-spectrum antibiotics be administered because of the high risk of sepsis. Proton pump inhibitors or H2 antagonists are commonly used for gastric mucosal protection. An IV glucose drip should be considered. Depending on presentation, lactulose or neomycin may be required to treat encephalopathy. If the patient is not in labor, induction should be planned as soon as possible. ALFP is not an absolute contraindication to vaginal delivery, but coagulation should be optimized. The same general principles as in DIC apply. Frozen plasma is indicated if the INR is greater than 1.5. Cryoprecipitate should be given if the fibrinogen level falls below 1.0 g/L.

Postpartum Considerations

In mild cases, resolution is prompt after delivery and is reflected by improvement in the prothrombin time. In severe cases, patients require ongoing support because a variety of complications may ensue. These include gastrointestinal hemorrhage, respiratory distress, acute pancreatitis, and nephrogenic diabetes insipidus. Patient should be monitored in the hospital until all signs of liver function and coagulation have returned to normal.

SEIZURES IN PREGNANCY

Epilepsy

The most common cause of seizures in pregnancy is preexisting epilepsy. The prevalence of epilepsy among women of childbearing age is higher than in the general population given that epilepsy is more common in young people. Plasma volume expansion, induction of hepatic microsomal enzymes, increased renal clearance, and decreased volume of plasma proteins lead to reductions in therapeutic levels of all antiepileptic drugs (AEDs) during pregnancy. In addition, estrogen has been shown to

TABLE 32-8: CAUSES OF SEIZURES IN PREGNANCY

Preexisting epilepsy	Cerebral arterial or venous thrombosis
Eclampsia	Metabolic anomalies
Encephalitis or meningitis	Hypoglycemia
Intracranial lesion	Porphyria
Hydrocephalus	Vitamin B_6 deficiency
Postpartum pituitary hemorrhage	Epidural anesthesia
Cavernous angioma	Postepidural blood patch

decrease the seizure threshold through interactions with GABA (gamma-aminobutyric acid) receptors. AEDs in themselves have the potential for significant impact on fetuses, including teratogenicity, the details of which are beyond the scope of this section. Table 32-8 details a differential diagnosis of seizures in pregnancy.

Fetal monitoring of seizures during labor and delivery has demonstrated late decelerations and reduced variability. It is reported that a single brief generalized tonic-clonic seizure can be associated with fetal heart rate depression lasting more than 20 minutes.

Eclampsia

Eclampsia is the most common cause of reactive seizure in pregnancy. The presence of seizures defines eclampsia. It is important to note, however, that classic preeclamptic signs may be absent in a fair proportion of patients at the onset of seizures. Preeclampsia is detailed in a previous section. Many neurologic symptoms may be experienced in preeclampsia and include headache, blurred vision, diplopia, hyperreflexia, agitation, or coma. In upwards of 15 percent of patients, eclamptic seizures occur in the postpartum period, with reports of seizures occurring as late as 26 days. Although the incidence of eclampsia has decreased with recognition and treatment of preeclampsia, when it does occur, it is associated with 5 percent rate of maternal mortality and perinatal mortality rates up to 30 percent.

The physiology behind eclamptic seizures is thought to depend on a number of factors. Accelerated or profound hypertension can exceed the realms of cerebral autoregulation and result in cerebral vasospasm and/or ischemia, particularly in watershed areas. This is particularly important

OTHER ISSUES

in the posterior areas owing to visual changes. Cerebral edema, metabolic encephalopathy, and cerebral microhemorrhages are also thought to play a role.

Diagnosis and Investigations

Once the diagnosis has been made and management initiated, the etiology of the seizure should be investigated if not apparent by history and physical examination. Initial tests should include a basic chemistry panel to rule out a metabolic anomaly (electrolytes, magnesium, calcium, liver enzymes, thyroid-stimulating hormone), CBC to rule out infection, AED levels in patients on chronic therapy, coagulation studies in suspected eclampsia, and toxicology panel for potential abuse or withdrawal. When imaging is required, MRI is preferred to CT. An electroencephalogram may be required to determine the type of seizure or to rule out nonconvulsive status epilepticus in patients whose level of consciousness remains altered for extended periods of time. Finally, a lumbar puncture may be needed to rule out a central nervous system infection.

Management of Acute Seizures

The first steps involve basic resuscitation. The ABCs (airway, breathing, and circulation) should be constantly monitored. It is important to relieve IVC obstruction by putting the patient in the left lateral decubitus position and applying and supplemental oxygen. First-line therapy to terminate a seizure is the use of IV benzodiazepines. Lorazepam (1-2 mg IV bolus) and diazepam (5-10 mg IV bolus) are most commonly used.

The drug of choice for definite management in eclamptic seizures is magnesium sulphate ($MgSO_4$). A landmark trial revealed that magnesium sulphate is better than phenytoin or benzodiazepines for preventing eclamptic seizures and markedly decreased the risk of recurrence. The recommended initial bolus is 4 to 6 g IV over 20 minutes followed by an infusion at 2 g/hr. A repeat dose of 2 to 4 g IV over 5 to 10 minutes can be given for seizure recurrence. Therapy should be continued for 24 hours postpartum. Patients taking $MgSO_4$ need to be monitored for signs of toxicity, which include loss of deep tendon reflexes, decreased urine output, hypotension, and respiratory depression. The routine monitoring of magnesium levels is not recommended.

Up to 10 percent of patients with eclampsia are resistant to $MgSO_4$ and require phenytoin. Phenobarbital, valproic acid, and phenytoin can all be given IV. It is important to note that other components of preeclampsia and eclampsia, such as hypertension, also need to be addressed to prevent recurrence.

Route of Delivery

Vaginal delivery is not contraindicated when seizures are resolved during labor. Cesarean section should be performed when the mother experiences frequent, uncontrolled generalized tonic-clonic seizures during labor or if she is unable to cooperate with labor because of altered level of consciousness or absence or complex partial seizures.

Postpartum Considerations

Although breast milk has been found to have small levels of AEDs, the American Academy of Neurology guidelines suggest that breastfeeding is safe for patients on AEDs. Of note, barbiturates, clonazepam, and ethosuximide can cause excessive drowsiness in infants and should be reserved for refractory cases only.

SELECTED READING

American College of Obstetricians and Gynecologists: ACOG Practice Bulletin: Diagnosis and management of preeclampsia in pregnancy. Obstet Gynecol 99:159, 2002

American College of Obstetricians and Gynecologists: ACOG Practice Bulletin: Gestational Diabetes: Clinical management guidelines for obstetrician-gynecologists. Obstet Gynecol 98:525, 2001

American Diabetes Association: Gestational diabetes mellitus. Diabetes Care 27(Suppl):S88, 2004

Bandi VD, Munnur U, Matthay MA: Acute lung injury and acute respiratory distress syndrome in pregnancy. Crit Care Clin 20:577, 2004

Bonow R, Carabello B, Chatterjee K, et al: ACC/AHA 2006 Guidelines for the Management of Patients With Valvular Heart Disease. Circulation 114:e84, 2006

Bourjeily G, Paidas M, Khalil H, Rosene-Montella K, Rodger M: Pulmonary embolism in pregnancy. Lancet 375:500, 2010

Camargo C, Rachelefsky G, Schatz M: Managing asthma exacerbations in the emergency department. Summary of the National Asthma Education and Prevention Program Expert Panel Report 3 Guidelines for the Management of Asthma Exacerbations. Proc Am Thorac Soc 6:357, 2009

Elkayam U: Pregnancy and cardiovascular disease. In: Zipes DP, Libby P, Bonow RO, Braunwald E, editors. Braunwald's Heart Disease: A Textbook of Cardiovascular Medicine, 7th ed. Philadelphia: Elsevier, 2005

Magee LA, Helewa M, Moutquin J-M, et al: Diagnosis, evaluation, and management of the hypertensive disorders of pregnancy. J Obstet Gynaecol Canada 30:S1, 2008

OTHER ISSUES

Mallampalli A, Powner DJ, Gardner MO: Cardiopulmonary resuscitation and somatic support of the pregnant patient. Crit Care Clin 20:747, 2004

Marik PE, Plante LA: Venous thromboembolic disease and pregnancy. N Engl J Med 6;359:2025, 2008

McCrae KR: Thrombocytopenia in pregnancy. Hematol Am Soc Hematol Educ Program 397-402, 2010

Murphy VE, Gibson P, Talbot PI, Clifton VL: Severe asthma exacerbations during pregnancy. Obstet Gynecol 106:1046, 2005

National Heart, Lung and Blood Institute: Clinical practice guidelines: Managing exacerbations of asthma. http://www.nhlbi.nih.gov/guidelines/asthma/11_sec5_exacerb.pdf

National Heart, Lung and Blood Institute: Guidelines for the diagnosis and management of asthma. http://www.nhlbi.nih.gov/guidelines/asthma/asthgdln.htm

National Institute for Health and Clinical Excellence: NICE guidelines: Diabetes in pregnancy management of diabetes and its complications from preconception to the postnatal period. [CG 63], London: National Institute for Health and Clinical Excellence, 2008. http://www.nice.org.uk/nicemedia/pdf/CG063Guidance.pdf

Parker JA, Conway DL: Diabetic ketoacidosis in pregnancy. Obstet Gynecol Clin North Am 34:533, 2007

Provan D, Stasi R, Newland AC, et al: International consensus report on the investigation and management of primary immune thrombocytopenia. Blood 115:168, 2010

Sheffield JS, Cunningham FG: Community-acquired pneumonia in pregnancy. Obstet Gynecol 114:915, 2009

Sliwa K, Fett J, Elkayam U: Peripartum cardiomyopathy. Lancet 368:687, 2006

CHAPTER 33

Labor in the Presence of Fetal Complications

Laura M. Gaudet

INTRAUTERINE GROWTH RESTRICTION

Background

Prenatal care seeks to diagnose pathologically small fetuses carrying an increased risk of perinatal morbidity and mortality. Intrauterine growth restriction (IUGR) occurs when fetuses are unable to achieve their genetic potential for in utero growth. To exclude healthy but constitutionally small fetuses, many clinicians define IUGR as estimated fetal weight (EFW) less than the third percentile. Others prefer to use a broader definition, often referred to as *small for gestational age* (SGA), which identifies fetuses with an EFW below the 10th percentile. Ultrasound-derived EFW's should be plotted against gestational age-specific growth charts. Some institutions use customized growth charts that account for local population differences and maternal factors, including height, weight, past obstetric history, and ethnicity.

IUGR can be described as symmetrical or asymmetrical. Symmetrical IUGR has traditionally been thought to reflect reduced fetal growth potential, as seen with genetic conditions, congenital anomalies, or intrauterine infection. Approximately one-third of infants with IUGR display this pattern of growth in which all biometric parameters are smaller than expected. It usually has an early onset, before 32 weeks of gestation. Asymmetrical IUGR reflects reduced fetal growth support and impaired placental transfer of nutrients. This leads to a decrease in soft tissue mass and, in particular, a decreased deposition of glycogen in the fetal liver. Because the liver is the predominant intraabdominal organ, the abdominal circumference is reduced. The fetus compensates with cerebral redistribution of blood flow to protect growth of the brain and head. This results in the typical head-sparing asymmetry in which the abdominal circumference and femur length lag behind expected. Often, asymmetric growth is not recognized until after 32 weeks' gestation. There is considerable overlap between the two forms of IUGR, and with increased duration and severity, either may attain a symmetric profile of growth restriction.

Of all fetuses with an estimated fetal weight under the 10th percentile, approximately 80 to 85 percent are constitutionally small but healthy; 10 to 15 percent have true IUGR caused by placental insufficiency; and 5 to 10 percent are affected by a pathologic condition, including aneuploidy, structural anomalies, or intrauterine infection (Fig. 33-1). Although the proportion of constitutionally small babies in a given population remains relatively stable, the prevalence of pathologic growth restriction is less predictable.

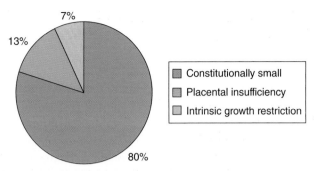

FIGURE 33-1. Causes of fetal growth restriction.

IUGR may be detected fortuitously after an ultrasound performed for another indication or deliberately after serial assessments of a high-risk patient. Some advocate routine third-trimester growth ultrasound for all women. The benefits of this have not been substantiated and would be impossible in resource-challenged settings. Clinical palpation of the abdomen and measurement of the symphyseal-fundal height (SFH) may raise the suspicion of growth restriction but is not sufficiently sensitive or specific; both techniques identify, at best, 30 percent of fetuses with IUGR. Diagnosis should rely on basic ultrasound biometric measurements as a minimum. When available, Doppler studies can lead to some refinement and assessment of acute fetal compromise and reserve.

As soon as the diagnosis of IUGR is considered, pregnancy dating must be reviewed for accuracy. Gestational dating based on first-trimester ultrasound measurements is the most accurate and is now the recommended standard of care in the United Kingdom. Although menstrual dating is notoriously unreliable, it remains the primary method in many countries. When ultrasound data are available, pregnancy redating should be undertaken if there is a significant difference between menstrual and ultrasound dating (≥5 days before 12 weeks, ≥10 days from 16 to 21 weeks). If no ultrasound was done before the third trimester and pregnancy redating is considered, follow-up ultrasonography is indicated in 2 weeks to ensure adequate interval growth.

For fetuses with true IUGR caused by placental insufficiency, labor presents the ultimate challenge. Fetuses who are barely able to compensate when the uterus is quiescent and umbilical artery blood flow is relatively stable are often unable to tolerate the increased demands of labor. This is especially prominent in IUGR fetuses with concomitant oligohydramnios. Labor attendants must make individual decisions about the timing and mode of delivery based on gestational age, presentation, estimated fetal weight, and an assessment of acute fetal well-being.

OTHER ISSUES

Labor with Prenatally Diagnosed Intrauterine Growth Restriction

Preterm Intrauterine Growth Restriction

Fetuses with preterm IUGR present a notable challenge to intrapartum care providers. The important benefits of gaining gestational age in utero must be carefully balanced with the risk of imminent intrauterine demise. Several studies have consistently shown that gestational age, rather than birthweight, is the dominant predictor of neonatal outcome. For this reason, at very early gestational ages, delivery should be delayed until necessary for survival.

Once the limits of viability are reached, fetuses with IUGR are generally followed carefully with serial assessments of well-being and growth and Doppler studies if resources allow. Maternal corticosteroid administration for fetal lung maturity should be considered. Many clinicians opt for prelabor cesarean section in preterm IUGR fetuses who require delivery. Fetal reserve may be inadequate to tolerate the reduction in uterine blood flow seen with contractions, and noncephalic presentations are very common. In the earliest gestations, the lower segment may be poorly formed, and a classical or vertical uterine incision becomes necessary.

The possibility of a trial of labor may be considered if continuous fetal monitoring is available and there is a cephalic presentation, particularly if favorable circumstances (e.g., multiparity) are present. The patient should be well-informed of the potential for fetal compromise resulting in need for cesarean section. Consideration should be given to epidural analgesia because its use may decrease the "decision to delivery time" if cesarean section is required.

With induction, cervical ripening is essential to minimize the intrauterine pressures required. Mechanical methods, such as an intracervical Foley catheter or Laminaria tents, result in less uterine activity than prostaglandins. If oxytocin use is necessary, caution should be exercised. A "gentle" protocol starting at low dose (1 milliunits/min) and increasing slowly by 1 milliunits/min every 30 minutes may be appropriate to allow increased control over the frequency and intensity of uterine contractions. If the fetal heart rate (FHR) becomes abnormal, oxytocin should be discontinued and consideration given to operative delivery. Once the cervix is fully dilated and pushing is initiated, the second stage is usually accomplished quickly thanks to the smallness of the passenger.

True IUGR from placental insufficiency sometimes manifests as severe growth restriction in the late second trimester. In the absence of maternal complications, delivery should generally be delayed until two criteria are met—gestational age must be greater than 24 weeks *and* estimated fetal weight must be greater than 500 g. Patients with severe IUGR (especially in the presence of abnormal Doppler study results) who are identified before these thresholds should be warned of the potential for prelabor intrauterine demise. If significant maternal complications develop (e.g., preeclampsia) and the fetus is judged to be previable, induction of labor and vaginal delivery are preferred when possible. Intrapartum or neonatal demise is expected, and fetal monitoring in labor is usually foregone.

Term Intrauterine Growth Restriction

Many fetuses with IUGR that reach term with a normal umbilical artery Doppler result usually represent either constitutional smallness or intrinsic growth restriction (aneuploidy, chronic infection, or congenital anomaly). These fetuses should have ongoing surveillance with delivery if there is any question of acute compromise.

Fetuses with growth restriction and abnormal Doppler studies are more likely because of placental insufficiency. The degree of Doppler abnormality is considered in determining when to intervene and deliver the fetus.

Studies suggest that it is reasonable to offer most patients with IUGR at term a trial of labor, especially if there is adequate amniotic fluid. Timing of delivery remains debatable, with either induction of labor at 37 weeks or expectant surveillance being acceptable. Continuous intrapartum fetal monitoring is recommended for all pregnancies with suspected IUGR. In a term trial of labor, many of the precautions recommended for fetuses with preterm IUGR are also advised. Unlike preterm fetuses, operative vaginal delivery can be considered for abnormal FHR or failure to descend in the second stage.

Labor with Unanticipated Intrauterine Growth Restriction

Given that clinical assessment by abdominal palpation and symphyseal fundal height fails to detect 70 percent of fetuses with IUGR and that many clinicians work in limited-resource settings, many fetuses with IUGR are undiagnosed prenatally. In this scenario, the labor attendant may be the first to suspect IUGR, usually because of abnormalities in fetal heart monitoring.

Postnatal Investigations

Newborns with IUGR often require additional medical attention after delivery. All infants should have their birthweight plotted on a standardized growth curve. Most newborn care centers have clinical protocols to be followed when the birthweight is under the 10th percentile. Infants with IUGR, particularly if marked, should undergo a thorough physical examination to rule out evidence of congenital problems, including anomaly, infection, aneuploidy, and other genetic conditions. If resources allow, the placenta may also be sent for pathologic examination.

CONGENITAL ANOMALIES

Background

A congenital anomaly can be defined as any unusual variation or abnormality in the shape, structure, and/or function of a tissue, organ, or body part that is present at birth. Congenital anomalies can be classified in several ways: internal versus external, single (isolated) or multiple, and major or minor. They develop through four major pathways (Table 33-1).

A European population-based registry of congenital anomalies, covering 1.5 million births annually, recorded a total prevalence of major congenital anomalies of 23.9 in 1000 between 2003 and 2009. Of infants with congenital anomalies, 80 percent were live born, and 2.5 percent were stillborn (after 20 weeks' gestation); a further 17.6 percent of infants with congenital anomalies underwent termination of pregnancy after prenatal diagnosis. Of these therapeutic abortions, nearly half had associated aneuploidy.

TABLE 33-1: PATHOGENESIS OF CONGENITAL ANOMALIES

	Mechanism	Example
Malformation	Intrinsically dysfunctional developmental process	Anencephaly
Deformation	Mechanical forces on the embryo or fetus	Potter's sequence secondary to prolonged, early oligohydramnios
Disruption	Extrinsic factor that disrupts normal development	Limb amputation from amniotic bands
Dysplasia	Abnormal organization of cells in a particular tissue	Abnormal cartilage formation in achondroplasia

The most common congenital anomalies among chromosomally normal fetuses were congenital heart disease (6.5 in 1000 births), limb defects (3.8 in 1000 births), anomalies of the urinary system (3.1 in 1000 births), and nervous system defects (2.3 in 1000 births).

Labor with Prenatally Diagnosed Congenital Anomalies

Several issues should be considered when contemplating a trial of labor for a fetus with a prenatally diagnosed congenital anomaly. Ideally, discussion with the parents occurs before the onset of labor so that all options can be fully explored. The content of that discussion must be individualized to reflect the best interests of both the fetus and the mother. In some circumstances, with the family's informed consent, intervention on behalf of the fetus may be desired, indicated, and necessary. In others, comfort measures and palliative care may be appropriate. In either case, consideration should be given to ensuring that delivery occurs in a facility that can best accommodate the infant's condition while allowing for close family involvement. This may require delivery in a center with an advanced neonatal intensive care unit, medical subspecialists (e.g., pediatric surgeons, otolaryngologists, cardiac surgeons), and paramedical support (e.g., lactation consultants or prosthetists). Ideally, delivery is accomplished at as late a gestational age as is safely possible; prematurity increases the morbidity and mortality of infants with congenital anomalies, particularly if early surgical correction is required.

The Role of Prelabor Cesarean Section

For several reasons, operative delivery in the form of cesarean section before the onset of labor may be entertained, including:

1. *Malpresentation:* Noncephalic presentation is more common in fetuses with congenital anomalies, particularly in those with polyhydramnios. If the family's aim is to have a live-born infant, cesarean section may be indicated for transverse or breech presentations
2. *Protection of the mother:* Occasionally, fetal congenital anomalies (e.g., macrocephaly, conjoined twins) place the mother at risk for complications during labor by preventing vaginal delivery, particularly as pregnancy advances. In this scenario, delivery by cesarean section may be indicated
3. *Protection of the anomalous area:* Some external congenital anomalies (e.g., omphalocele involving the liver, vascular sacrococcygeal teratoma)

OTHER ISSUES

may be at risk for damage because of the process of labor and delivery. If the goal is to have a live-born infant and correct the anomaly postnatally, cesarean section may be beneficial. As always, care should be taken to avoid inadvertent laceration of the fetus and undue manipulation of the affected area. If the fetus has a congenital anomaly that may obstruct the upper airway, an ex utero intrapartum treatment (EXIT) procedure may be considered, for which cesarean delivery is performed

4. *Minimizing fetal distress:* In the presence of certain congenital anomalies (e.g., osteogenesis imperfecta and related fractures), the fetus may experience unnecessary or detrimental distress. Delivery by cesarean section could be considered if the process of vaginal delivery is believed likely to cause significant pain to the fetus and the goal is a live birth. This should be balanced by the recognition that cesarean delivery is not entirely atraumatic

The Role of Fetal Monitoring in Labor

The wishes of the family are important in planning fetal monitoring. For major anomalies or aneuploidy in which intervention for fetal indications is not being entertained, it is appropriate to forego fetal monitoring to minimize anxiety of the parents and maternity care providers. It is important that the patient also accepts the risk of intrapartum demise. For less severe anomalies (or if the family has a strong desire to have monitoring despite major anomalies or aneuploidy), intrapartum monitoring may be considered.

The potential impact of the congenital anomaly on fetal monitoring must be taken into account. External fetal monitoring is the preferred route. If this is unsatisfactory, internal fetal monitoring in the form of a scalp electrode may be useful, providing there are no concerns that the congenital anomaly could interfere with placement. Expectations regarding the tracing should be appropriate to the anomaly. For example, cardiac anomalies may be accompanied by intermittent or sustained arrhythmias despite adequate fetal oxygenation. Similarly, fetuses with anomalies of the central nervous system may not display the usual variability and accelerations that are characteristic of a normal tracing. When monitoring is used, there should be clear parameters for intervention.

Impact of the Congenital Anomaly on Progress of Labor

It has been recognized that some congenital anomalies have the potential to interfere with the progress of labor. The classic example of this situation are fetuses with anencephaly. Although it is uncommon in the current obstetric era to encounter postdate pregnancy complicated by anencephaly, it is recognized that the natural history of the condition includes postdate pregnancy in a significant proportion of fetuses. As such, induction of labor may be necessary. Furthermore, the active phase of labor may not progress as expected because of the irregularity of the presenting part.

Impact of the Congenital Anomaly on Vaginal Delivery

Special considerations may arise during planned vaginal delivery of fetuses with known congenital anomalies. In some situations, intervention is required to facilitate vaginal delivery of the infant. For example, a fetus with megacystis may require vesicocentesis to allow the abdomen to be delivered through the maternal pelvis. Some additional information on destructive procedures is found at the end of this chapter. It is taken directly from the fifth edition of this textbook and retained as a reference for those working in underdeveloped countries.

Role of the Neonatal Team

The role of the neonatal team also depends on the ultimate goal of treatment. If the family wishes full or limited resuscitation, an appropriate neonatal team should be present for delivery and assume care of the infant as soon as possible after delivery. If the plan is for palliation with comfort care, routine newborn care measures such as swaddling and use of a warmer should be provided. Regardless of the neonatal care plan, the obstetric team should be involved in providing information and comfort to the parents in a timely and sensitive manner.

Fetuses with Unanticipated Congenital Anomalies

Because prenatal ultrasound has become routine in most countries, it is relatively uncommon to deliver a fetus with an unanticipated major congenital anomaly. Sonographic detection rates for anomalies such as neural tube defects and gastroschisis approach 100%. Detection rates are considerably lower for some conditions, however, including cleft palate. Furthermore, a small number of patients who have not had an ultrasound (perhaps by choice or because they were unable to access prenatal care) present in labor. It should be remembered that there may be no hint of an abnormality before delivery. Therefore, all maternity care providers should be prepared for the possibility of an unanticipated congenital anomaly in every patient. Upon recognition of an abnormality, the most responsible person should inform the parents of the finding. This may be the attending obstetrician, midwife, or pediatrician, depending on the setting. In general, as much available information as possible should be provided as soon as it is reasonable to do so. The impact of the abnormality on the health of the infant should be explained clearly and further treatment and investigation offered if appropriate (including karyotype, diagnostic imaging, and genetic examination). Several congenital anomalies have the potential to be life threatening; it is crucial that emergent conditions be excluded (as with ambiguous genitalia secondary to congenital adrenal hyperplasia and electrolyte abnormalities). At a later date, once the diagnosis is confirmed, the family should be provided with as much information as possible regarding recurrence risk.

Neglected Labor and Fetal Anomalies: Destructive Operations on the Fetus

The following paragraphs are taken from the fifth edition of the textbook. Although there is little role for them in advanced countries, they may occasionally be required in the developing world.

Indications

The purpose of destructive operations on an unborn child is to reduce his or her size (head, shoulder girdle, or body) to enable the vaginal delivery of a baby that is too large to pass intact through the birth canal. This procedure is tolerable only on a fetus who is dead or so deformed that survival is impossible. The risk of abdominal delivery to the mother has decreased to the point where embryotomy on a living normal child is never justified. Indeed, the operation is so unpleasant and the dangers to the mother are such that destructive procedures are rarely performed today. After delivery, the birth canal must be examined thoroughly to be certain that no injury has been caused by the instruments or the sharp edges of the skull bones.

Contraindications

1. Living normal fetus
2. Markedly contracted pelvis
3. Cervix less than three-fourths dilated (full dilatation preferable)
4. Neoplasms obstructing the pelvis

Dangers

1. Lacerations of the vagina, cervix, and uterus, as well as fistulas in the bladder or rectum

2. Uterine rupture, especially through the thinned-out lower segment, when labor has been obstructed
3. Hemorrhage from lacerations and uterine atony
4. Infection
5. Risks attendant on prolonged deep anesthesia

Types of Destructive Operation

Encephalocentesis
The purpose of encephalocentesis is to reduce the bulk of the head. The only indication acceptable today is hydrocephalus. The excess cerebrospinal fluid can be removed, even in a live infant, by inserting a large-bore needle (16-18 gauge) through the scalp. The size of the head is reduced and its delivery made possible.

The most direct approach to encephalocentesis is vaginal. The needle is inserted through the cervical os and into the cranial cavity through a fontanel or suture. The sagittal sinus should be avoided. If necessary, the needle can be pushed through one of the cranial bones. When the presentation is breech, drainage of the cerebrospinal fluid can be achieved by spondylectomy or, if the head is reachable, by direct entry into the ventricles beneath the occipital plate or behind the ear.

When the head cannot be reached through the vagina, an alternative route is the transabdominal one. The needle is passed through the abdominal and uterine walls and through the fetal cranial bones into the interior of the skull.

Decapitation
Severing the head from the body may be done for neglected transverse presentations when the child is dead and version and extraction or cesarean section is contraindicated. It may be done also when twins have become interlocked chin to chin. A blunt hook is placed over the neck to steady the fetus, and decapitation is performed with scissors. The fingers of the other hand are used to protect the mother's soft tissues. After decapitation, the body is extracted by pulling on an arm or a lower limb. The head is delivered either by forceps or by inserting a finger in the mouth and exerting traction on the jaw. This must be done slowly.

Cleidotomy
Cleidotomy is indicated when there is shoulder dystocia and a dead fetus. One or both clavicles are cut with scissors. The shoulder girdle then collapses, and delivery is accomplished.

SELECTED READING

Dolk H, Loane M, Garne E: The presence of congenital anomalies in Europe. Adv Expl Med Biol 686:349, 2010

Royal College of Obstetricians and Gynaecologists: The investigation and management of the small-for-gestational-age fetus. Green-top Clinical Guideline No. 31, 2002. *http://www.rcog.org.uk/guidelines*

Smale LE: Destructive operations on the fetus. Am J Obstet Gynecol 119:369, 1974

Thornton JG, The GRIT Study Group: A randomized trial of timed delivery for the compromised preterm fetus: short term outcomes and Bayesian interpretation. BJOG 110:27, 2003

CHAPTER 34

Intrapartum Infections

Andrée Gruslin

Infections are increasingly recognized as important contributors of maternal, fetal, and neonatal complications. Although the exact incidence of infections complicating labor is difficult to ascertain, available data suggest that it varies from 1 to 4 percent of all births and up to 60 percent of preterm births. These can generally be divided into two major categories, ascending genital tract infections and hematogenously spread infections from the mother. The symptoms associated with infections during labor can vary significantly, and it is not infrequent for some of these entities to be subclinical. As such, a high index of suspicion is required, along with appropriate knowledge of preventive and therapeutic approaches. Diagnostic tools include serologic testing; culture of blood, amniotic fluid, placenta, and membranes; pathologic examination of the placenta; and umbilical cord and molecular approaches.

ASCENDING INFECTIONS

Ascending genital tract infections are usually bacterial and almost always polymicrobial. These can occur in the context of intact or ruptured membranes and can be either subclinical or present as full-blown chorioamnionitis with maternal and fetal symptoms.

Chorioamnionitis

Chorioamnionitis is an infection of the chorion and amnion, which can progress to involve the umbilical cord, placenta, and fetus itself. It is characterized by the infiltration of these membranes by neutrophil polymorphs, which starts at the interface between the decidua and chorion at the level of the os. The most common microorganisms involved include *Ureaplasma* spp., *Mycoplasma* spp., enterococci, streptococci, coliforms, and staphylococci.

Intrapartum risk factors for the development of chorioamnionitis include multiple examinations during labor, prolonged labor, nulliparity, bacterial vaginosis or group B streptococcal (GBS) colonization, meconium, use of internal monitoring, and epidural anesthesia. Finally, alcohol use and cigarette smoking are predisposing factors.

Frequently associated with preterm prelabor rupture of the membranes (PPROM) and preterm labor (PTL), chorioamnionitis is often suspected as playing a causative role in these pathologies. Ascension of microorganisms via the genital tract to the membranes results in the production and release of proinflammatory cytokines and chemokines, which in turn may weaken the membranes and lead to PPROM. In addition, the release of prostaglandins associated with the process of inflammation may induce cervical changes and result in preterm delivery. The incidence of microbial invasion of amniotic cavity (MIAC) is as high as 30 percent in women with PPROM. Up to 34 percent of women with term PROM and 13 percent of women with an episode of PTL have been shown to have MIAC. The role of inflammation in the cascade of intraamniotic infection is extremely important. A recent study of 224 women with PPROM who underwent amniocentesis revealed a proven intraamniotic infection in 23 percent and a rate of intraamniotic inflammation of 42 percent. Infectious agents most commonly isolated included *Ureaplasma urealyticum* (38 samples), *Candida* spp. (five samples), and *Escherichia coli* (two samples). These data clearly demonstrated that inflammation of the amniotic cavity, independent of the presence of positive cultures, is associated with a higher risk of preterm delivery, chorioamnionitis, low APGAR scores, admission to the neonatal intensive care unit, and low birth weight.

In addition, exposure of a fetus to such a proinflammatory environment in the context of an invasion by polymicrobes can lead to the development of an intense inflammatory reaction in the fetal compartment itself. This is referred to as fetal inflammatory response syndrome (FIRS), which is characterized by elevated levels of interleukin-6 (IL-6) in the fetal blood and by the possibility of multiorgan damage, including effects on the hematopoietic system, lungs, brain, heart, kidneys, and adrenal glands. Long-term sequelae for these newborns include bronchopulmonary dysplasia and cerebral palsy. A recent meta-analysis examining the association between chorioamnionitis and cerebral palsy reported a 140 percent increased risk for fetuses exposed to clinical chorioamnionitis and an 80 percent increased risk for a histologic but asymptomatic chorioamnionitis.

Clinical Presentation

Chorioamnionitis can present with maternal and fetal signs or be subclinical. Maternal fever is often associated with general malaise and may present with uterine contractions. In addition, the presence of a tender uterus and a foul-smelling discharge help strengthen the diagnosis. Associated with this are maternal and fetal tachycardia (>100 and >160 beats/min, respectively) and a nonreassuring tracing. Although these symptoms and signs can raise the possibility of chorioamnionitis, they are neither sensitive nor specific, and as such, an overall evaluation of the risk factors present and the clinical presentation are both important.

OTHER ISSUES

Diagnostic Criteria

Laboratory investigations in cases of suspected chorioamnionitis are based on the presence of a maternal response and the presence of inflammation and of an invading microorganism. As such, an evaluation of maternal leukocytosis or a left shift may help the clinician but remain nonspecific, particularly in the context of labor, which may be associated with increases in maternal leukocyte counts because of dehydration or the administration of steroids.

In an attempt to achieve an earlier diagnosis, C-reactive protein (CRP), an acute phase reactant, has been evaluated in multiple studies. A recent meta-analysis examined results from four studies aiming to evaluate the predictive value of CRP for chorioamnionitis in women with PPROM. A total of 330 women were included, but unfortunately, the heterogeneity of the results precluded their pooling. The authors concluded that CRP only moderately predicted histologic chorioamnionitis but that the current literature did not support the use of CRP in this context at the present time. In the presence of maternal fever and tachycardia, a maternal blood culture, although not useful in diagnosing chorioamnionitis itself, may be helpful in certain complex cases for selection of antibiotics.

Finally, the evaluation of amniotic fluid has been the scope of much research in the hope to uncover a specific and sensitive diagnostic strategy. Various testing methodologies have been evaluated, including Gram stain; glucose levels; IL-6, matrix metalloproteinase-8 (MMP-8), and MMP-9 concentrations; and obviously cultures and molecular methods such as polymerase chain reaction (PCR) for the search of specific organisms.

Although levels of cytokines (especially IL-6) and MMPs (especially MMP-8) were consistently found to be higher in the amniotic fluid of women with a chorioamnionitis and their sensitivities and specificities were acceptable, the need for an amniocentesis has severely limited their use clinically. Similarly, although Gram stains have been found to be very specific (98%) and glucose levels relatively specific (73.5%), the same limitations regarding the need for invasive testing applies.

Finally, whereas cultures have been recognized as the "gold standard," they also require obtaining amniotic fluid. Furthermore, the time required for testing is often too long in a clinical setting, where rapid decisions regarding delivery must be made. In addition, recent data are now revealing the presence of unsuspected microorganisms, which would not necessarily be identified on culture. Innovative technologies such as proteomics may assist the clinician in this context in the future.

For now, the search for specific organisms via the use of PCR has been shown to be reliable in its sensitivity and specificity. However, this applies to clinical scenarios in which a specific and particular microorganism is suspected and therefore cannot be used in the overall evaluation of clinical chorioamnionitis, which is polymicrobial.

Management

Supportive Care. Upon diagnosis of chorioamnionitis, supportive measures for both the mother and fetus must be put in place and a plan for delivery initiated. Given the possible maternal risks of sepsis, attention to intravenous (IV) fluids is essential. A Foley catheter may be useful to assess fluid balance. Monitoring of vital signs is crucial, with prompt attention paid to hypotension and tachycardia. Oxygen saturation should be evaluated regularly and maintained at 95 percent and above. Antipyretics should be administered to normalize maternal temperature given the association between maternal fever and adverse neonatal outcomes, including encephalopathy. Electronic fetal monitoring should be implemented.

The mode of delivery in these cases should be dictated by obstetrical determinants because cesarean delivery has not been shown to improve outcomes for either the mother or the fetus upon initiation of appropriate antibiotic use.

Antibiotics

Parenteral antibiotics must be administered promptly and their choice based on the most commonly found microorganisms. In that context, it is suggested to treat with a combination of ampicillin 2 g IV every 6 hours (or vancomycin 1 g IV every 12 hours for those with allergy to penicillins) and gentamicin 1.5 mg/kg every 8 hours. Although this particular administration of gentamicin is widely used, a once-daily dosage approach (one dose of 5 mg/kg) has been found to be as efficacious in treating the infection.

Finally, if better anaerobic coverage is desired (e.g., if a cesarean section is planned), the addition of clindamycin (900 mg IV every 8 hours) or metronidazole (500 mg IV every 8 hours) may be wise.

The duration of treatment generally is limited. In the case of a vaginal delivery, antibiotics can usually be discontinued at delivery or after one postpartum dose has been administered. However, in the context of a cesarean delivery, most clinicians continue antibiotics until the patient has been afebrile for a period of 24 hours.

OTHER ISSUES

Group B Streptococcus

Group B streptococcus is a gram-positive organism responsible for infections mostly in infants and pregnant women. Maternal colonization of the lower gastrointestinal (GI) and urinary tracts with GBS occurs in 15 to 30 percent of women. As such, this organism is considered to be part of the "normal" flora of the vagina. However, GBS also represents one of the most important causes of neonatal mortality and morbidity, with a case fatality rate that can be as high as 50 percent. Two types of neonatal infection can occur: early onset or late onset. Early-onset disease (EOD) manifests itself in the first 7days of life and is the result of transmission from mother to fetus. The incidence of this serious disease is reported as 0.3 per 1000 infants.

Risk Factors for Early-Onset Disease

1. Maternal colonization: The most important risk factors for EOD is maternal colonization. A pregnant woman with positive GBS vaginal or rectal culture near term has 25-fold increased risk of having an infant with EOD. The GI tract serves as the reservoir for GBS, and it is noteworthy that colonization during pregnancy can be transient or persistent. In addition, the extent of colonization also plays a role in disease transmission, with heavy colonization representing an even higher risk to the infant. Finally, the presence of GBS in the urine at any time during pregnancy also carries a much higher risk of EOD
2. Gestational age less than 37 completed weeks
3. Prolonged duration of membrane rupture (12-18 hours)
4. Intrapartum temperature more than 37.5°C
5. Intraamniotic infection
6. Previous delivery of an infant with invasive GBS disease
7. Young maternal age, black race, and low maternal levels of GBS-specific anticapsular antibody

Prevention

Since the 1970s, multiple approaches toward prevention of EOD have been examined, including treatment of women with risk factors only and universal screening for GBS with intrapartum treatment of those who are culture positive. A multicenter study conducted by the American Centre for Disease Control involving 626,912 infants revealed that universal screening of all pregnant women with appropriate treatment in labor was superior to a risk-based approach. This is the basis for the Society of Obstetricians and Gynaecologists of Canada (SOGC) and American

TABLE 34-1: ANTIBIOTIC DOSAGES FOR THE PREVENTION OF EARLY-ONSET DISEASE DUE TO GROUP B STREPTOCOCCUS

Penicillin G 5 million units IV; then 2.5 million every 4 hours
Penicillin-allergic, no risk of anaphylaxis: cefazolin 2 g IV; then 1 g every 8 hours
Penicillin allergic and at risk of anaphylaxis: clindamycin 900 mg IV every 8 hours or erythromycin 500 mg IV every 6 hours
In rare cases, GBS resistance may occur; vancomycin is then the antibiotic of choice

GBS, group B streptococcus; IV, intravenous.

College of Obstetricians and Gynecologists (ACOG) recommendations, and as such, all pregnant women should be offered screening with a rectovaginal swab at 35 to 36 weeks gestation. The negative predictive value of GBS cultures performed 5 weeks or less before delivery is 95 to 98 percent. However, because of a decrease in negative predictive value, the clinical utility decreases when a prenatal culture is performed more than 5 weeks before delivery.

Treatment of all women with a positive GBS culture at 35 to 37 weeks or unscreened women with risk factors as described in Table 34-1 should be initiated at the onset of labor or rupture of membranes.

Recommended antibiotics are listed in Table 34-1. Although both ampicillin and penicillin are efficacious against GBS, penicillin has a narrower spectrum. Because it is less likely to result in resistant organisms, it is the antibiotic of choice. In the case of penicillin allergy but no anaphylaxis, cephazolins are considered appropriate. Otherwise, clindamycin or erythromycin is recommended for those with anaphylaxis to penicillins.

Because several other important risk factors have also been shown to be associated with a significant risk of EOD GBS, recommendations for treatment in labor applies to all women in the categories listed in Table 34-2.

Human Immunodeficiency Virus

The World Health Organization estimates that 1.4 million pregnant women are infected with human immunodeficiency virus (HIV). Mother-to-child transmission (MTCT) can occur antenatally, intrapartum, or postpartum through breastfeeding. Most commonly, the infant acquires the infection intrapartum. Without maternal screening and antiretroviral (ARV) therapy,

TABLE 34-2: RISK FACTORS REQUIRING ANTIBIOTIC TREATMENT INTRAPARTUM OR AT THE ONSET OF MEMBRANE RUPTURE FOR THE PREVENTION OF GROUP B STREPTOCOCCUS EARLY-ONSET DISEASE

Women with a positive rectovaginal culture at 35 to 37 weeks[a]

Women with a previously affected infant

Women with GBS bacteriuria at any time during pregnancy (regardless of the amount of colony-forming units present)

Women at less than 37 weeks gestation unless a negative swab has been obtained in the 5 weeks before presentation

Women with intrapartum fever (>38°C)

Women with an unknown GBS status and with ruptured membranes at term for greater than 18 hours

Women with GBS (rectovaginal or urine) and prelabor rupture of membranes at term (should also initiate induction of labor)

[a]A recent publication by the Centers for Disease Control and Prevention and endorsed by the American College of Obstetricians and Gynecologists has also added to this list "intrapartum nucleic acid amplification test," a form of rapid testing available in the United States.

GBS, group B streptococcus.

the risk of transmission to the fetus or infant is as high as 25 percent but can decrease to below 2 percent with appropriate management, including ARV therapy and careful selection of the mode of delivery.

Screening in Pregnancy

Given that the most common risk factor for HIV acquisition in women of childbearing age is heterosexual contact, it is essential to offer universal screening to all pregnant women. After being identified as HIV positive, the pregnant woman must be followed closely by a team with expertise in infectious disease and obstetrics. Of importance is the need for maximum viral suppression to minimize the risk of transmission to the infant. This is accomplished by the use of ARV therapy, which must be administered antenatally and during labor to the mother and to the infant after birth. In women who are receiving a cytochrome P (CYP) 3A4 enzyme inhibitor such as a protease inhibitor or non-nucleoside reverse transcriptase inhibitor, methergine (ergot) is to be avoided because these drugs depend on the enzyme CYP3A for their metabolism, and their concomitant use may lead to increased plasma levels, which can result in life-threatening side effects. Other drugs in this category include amiodarone, cisapride,

TABLE 34-3: RISK FACTORS FOR MOTHER-TO-CHILD TRANSMISSION OF HIV

High maternal viral load (the amount of HIV RNA in the plasma)

Breastfeeding

Sexually transmitted infections

Chorioamnionitis

Prolonged rupture of membranes

Young maternal age

History of stillbirth

Vaginal mode of delivery (in the context of high viral load)

Low CD4 count

Advanced maternal HIV disease

Bleeding during labor (episiotomy, perineal laceration, and intrapartum hemorrhage)

flecainide, midazolam, propafenone, quinidine, rifampin, pimozide, and triazolam.

In addition to drug therapy, labor must be managed in a way to minimize the potential exposure of the fetus to maternal blood. Careful selection of mode of delivery also contributes to reducing the risk of transmission. Significant risk factors for mother-to-child transmission are listed in Table 34-3.

Intrapartum Care

Antiretroviral Therapy

- Intrapartum IV zidovudine is recommended for all HIV-infected pregnant women, regardless of their antepartum regimen, to reduce perinatal transmission of HIV
- Women who are receiving an antepartum combination ARV drug regimen should continue this regimen on schedule as much as possible during labor and before scheduled cesarean delivery
- Women receiving combination regimens that include zidovudine should receive IV zidovudine during labor while other oral ARV components are continued

OTHER ISSUES

Cesarean Delivery

- For women who have either an unknown or a significant viral load (i.e., HIV RNA >50 copies/mL at 34 to 36 weeks) in late pregnancy, delivery by scheduled cesarean delivery is recommended in Canada. This is regardless of the use of antepartum ARV drugs
- It is not clear whether cesarean delivery after ruptured membranes or onset of labor provides benefit in preventing perinatal transmission. Management of women originally scheduled for cesarean delivery who present with ruptured membranes or in labor must be individualized based on duration of rupture, progress of labor, plasma viral load, current ARV regimen, and other clinical factors

Trial of Labor. Women with maximally suppressed viral loads (<50 copies/mL) can be offered a vaginal delivery. However, it is essential to minimize the contact with maternal blood or body fluids and secretions during that time. As such, the following is recommended:

- Avoid routine use of fetal scalp electrodes for fetal monitoring
- Avoid artificial rupture of membranes unless clear obstetric indications are present
- Operative delivery with forceps or a vacuum extractor and/or episiotomy should be performed only if there are clear obstetric indications

Postpartum

- The infant should be carefully washed before any injections are administered
- Breastfeeding is contraindicated
- Contraceptive counseling is recommended

Herpes Simplex Virus

In Canada, the incidence of type 2 herpes simplex virus (HSV-2) seropositivity in pregnant women varies from 7.1 to 28.1 percent, and the incidence of neonatal HSV is of one in 17,000 births. Neonatal HSV (as opposed to congenital, which is acquired antenatally) is acquired intrapartum as a result of exposure to genital tract lesions. It is diagnosed based on clinical presentation and cultures of the infant 48 hours after birth. The infant can develop a variety of complications, which have been categorized according to their potential morbidity and mortality. These are listed in Table 34-4.

TABLE 34-4: CATEGORIES OF NEONATAL HERPES SIMPLEX VIRUS COMPLICATIONS

1. Skin, eye, and mouth infection (rarely fatal; however, 38% may develop neurologic disease)

2. Central nervous system disease (encephalitis with or without skin, eye, and mouth infection)

3. Disseminated disease (the most serious form of infection, which has a 90% mortality rate if untreated)

It is imperative to recognize and treat maternal infections with HSV for the adequate prevention of neonatal disease. Maternal HSV can be categorized in primary (no antibodies to HSV-1 or -2) or recurrent infections (has antibodies to HSV-1 or -2). The greatest risk of neonatal infection occurs in the context of a primary infection in the third trimester because this does not confer sufficient time for transplacental passage of maternal antibodies to the newborn for his or her protection.

Primary Infection
Because primary infection in the third trimester carries a neonatal risk of HSV of 30 to 50 percent, most authorities, including the SOGC, recommend that these women be delivered by cesarean section. Neonatal cultures should then be performed and the infant observed closely.

Recurrent Disease
In these circumstances, maternal antibodies are present, and as such, the risk of neonatal disease is much reduced, given the protection provided by the transplacental passage of these antibodies. In this context, women presenting in labor with a genital lesion carry a risk of neonatal disease of 2 to 5 percent. The absence of such lesions at delivery carries a small risk of asymptomatic shedding of 1 percent, with a calculated risk of neonatal disease of 0.02 to 0.05 percent. Unfortunately, cultures are not predictive of neonatal disease in these instances.

Therefore, women with recurrent infection presenting at delivery should be examined carefully for the presence of HSV lesions. If lesions are seen in the genital area or even as far as over the thighs or buttocks or if prodromal symptoms are present, cesarean delivery is recommended. Table 34-5 summarizes these recommendations regarding mode of delivery. Because this infection is ascending, the cesarean section should be performed within 4 hours of ruptured membranes. In addition, scalp sampling and scalp electrodes should be avoided in women with a history of recurrent HSV.

OTHER ISSUES

TABLE 34-5: SUMMARY OF RECOMMENDATIONS FOR MODE OF DELIVERY WITH HERPES SIMPLEX VIRUS

1. Primary infection any time in the third trimester

↓

Caesarean delivery

2. Recurrent infection without lesions or prodrome

↓

Acyclovir prevention during pregnancy, may consider vaginal delivery

3. Recurrent infection with lesion or prodrome

↓

Cesarean delivery

HEMATOGENOUS INFECTIONS

The risk of fetal infection hematogenously spread from the mother is much less common during labor. This is partly related to the physiologic, mechanical, and immunologic barriers provided by the placenta. However, rarely, organisms such as staphylococci, streptococci, or pneumococci may infect the pregnant woman, resulting in a significant degree of maternal bacteremia. This then reaches the placenta and occasionally crosses to the fetus. These patients may present with classical symptoms of maternal fever, tachycardia, malaise, and uterine tenderness. The fetus may show evidence of tachycardia. Prompt treatment with antibiotics should be initiated, and delivery should be planned accordingly, as suggested in cases of chorioamnionitis earlier.

A more common group of organisms involved in hematogenous infections are viruses. These include cytomegalovirus (CMV), rubella, enteroviruses, and parvovirus. However, these infections usually present antenatally and are not very significant contributors to intrapartum infections.

Listeriosis

Perhaps the most relevant hematogenous infection that may affect the women is listeriosis. Although rare (12 per 100,000 in pregnancy), this gram-positive bacillus has severe consequences for the fetus and newborn. Maternal listeriosis is associated with increased risks of fetal demise, preterm delivery, neonatal sepsis, meningitis, pneumonia, and death. The perinatal mortality rate varies between 27 and 33 percent.

Listeria monocytogenes has a particular predilection for pregnant women, who are 20 times more likely to become infected compared with the general population. The organism is acquired by the mother through contaminated water and food such as milk, cheese, chicken, coleslaw, undercooked meat, fruits, and vegetables. It can then spread transplacentally to the fetus. Mothers infected with *Listeria* are often asymptomatic or present with nonspecific flu-like symptoms. A high index of suspicion is thus necessary.

The predilection for pregnant women is well illustrated by a 1981 Canadian outbreak, which affected 100 individuals, of whom 34 were pregnant. In this group were nine stillbirths, 23 neonatal infections, and only two live healthy births.

Diagnosis

Confirmation of diagnosis can be done reliably by cultures of amniotic fluid, meconium, membranes, placenta, blood, or spinal fluid. Placental pathologic examination may reveal the presence of acute villitis and of multiple microabscesses.

Because *Listeria* is an intracellular organism and can resemble diphtheroids, pneumococci, or hemophilus, Gram stains are helpful clinically only one-third of the time. Cultures of the vagina or stools are not recommended because women can be normal carriers without being infected. Serologic test of listeriosis are also not recommended. Therefore, if a pregnant woman presents with a clinical scenario suggestive of listeriosis, blood cultures are recommended.

Treatment

The antibiotics recommended for the treatment of listeriosis must be given in high dose to cross the placenta and to penetrate intracellularly. These include ampicillin as a first line and erythromycin as a second line. In women allergic to penicillins, trimethoprim–sulfamethoxazole has been effective. Therapy should continue for 7 to 14 days (Table 34-6).

PREVENTION OF MATERNAL INFECTIONS

Infections are among the five most important causes of maternal mortality and morbidity. In this context, the most important risk factor is delivery by

OTHER ISSUES

TABLE 34-6: RECOMMENDED TREATMENT APPROACHES MATERNAL LISTERIOSIS

First line:
- Ampicillin 2 g every 6-8 hours

Second line:
- Erythromycin 4 g/day
- Penicillin-allergic women: trimethoprim–sulfamethoxazole 1-2 tablets every 6 hours

cesarean section. Women delivered by cesarean section are 20 times more likely to suffer a postpartum infection compared with those delivered vaginally. These infections include endomyometritis, wound infection and infection of the urinary tract, pelvic abscess, septic pelvic thrombophlebitis, pneumonia, and sepsis.

To reduce this risk, a significant number of studies have investigated the use of prophylactic antibiotics before performing a cesarean section. A recent Cochrane review reported on 81 randomized controlled trials and found a significantly decreased risk of endometritis and wound infections when prophylactic antibiotics are administered to women undergoing emergency or elective cesarean sections. These data with others have led to recommendations by SOGC and ACOG that all women delivered by cesarean section should be offered prophylactic antibiotics (Table 34-7). Administration of antibiotics does not reduce the risk of subsequent infections in operative vaginal deliveries, and there are insufficient data to recommend for or against antibiotic prophylaxis in cases of manual removal of the placenta and postpartum dilatation and curettage. However, a randomized control trial involving 107 women with a third- or fourth-degree perineal laceration found a significant decrease in perineal wound complications in the treatment group.

TABLE 34-7: SUMMARY OF RECOMMENDATIONS FOR PROPHYLACTIC ANTIBIOTICS

- Women undergoing either an elective or emergency cesarean section should receive antibiotic prophylaxis

- Women with third- or fourth-degree laceration may benefit from antibiotic prophylaxis

- There is no benefit of prophylaxis with antibiotics in cases of manual removal of the placenta and dilatation and curettage or operative vaginal delivery

TABLE 34-8: ANTIBIOTIC PROPHYLAXIS: RECOMMENDATIONS FROM THE SOCIETY OF OBSTETRICIANS AND GYNAECOLOGISTS OF CANADA

1. Emergency or elective cesarean section
- Cefazolin 1-2 g IV 15-60 minutes before skin incision
- Penicillin-allergic women: clindamycin 600 mg IV or erythromycin 500 mg IV

2. Third- or fourth-degree lacerations
- Cefotetan 1 g IV or cefoxitin 1 g IV

IV, intravenous.

Choice of Antibiotics

Most studies have examined the use of cephalosporins in the context of prophylaxis at cesarean section. With adequate coverage of gram-positive and modest coverage of gram-negative organisms, this class of agents carries a spectrum that is narrow enough to minimize the risk of developing resistance. In women with penicillin allergy, clindamycin or erythromycin has been suggested.

Finally, cefotetan or cefoxitin is recommended for women with third- or fourth-degree perineal tears. Table 34-8 summarizes the SOGC recommendations regarding antibiotic prophylaxis and obstetric procedures.

CONCLUSION

Infections represent a major complication associated with preterm rupture of membranes, preterm delivery, and maternal and perinatal morbidity and mortality. Evidence is now accumulating to suggest that microorganisms are responsible for an increasing amount of perinatal complications, many of which present in labor. However, often the diagnosis requires a high index of suspicion and remains based on the clinical presentation. The development of new approaches to assist in the diagnosis of both ascending and hematogenous infections during pregnancy will help further unravel the implications of infectious agents in obstetric complications and will assist the clinician in establishing a rapid diagnosis, which is often crucial in cases of intrapartum infections.

OTHER ISSUES

SELECTED READING

Money D. Dobson S, Boucher M, et al: The prevention of early-onset neonatal group B streptococcal Disease. J Obstet Gynaecol Can 26:826, 2004

Money D, Steben M, Wong T, et al: Guidelines for the management of herpes simplex virus in pregnancy. J Obstet Gynaecol Can 30:514, 2008

Panel on Treatment of HIV-Infected Pregnant Women and Prevention of Perinatal Transmission: Recommendations for use of antiretroviral drugs in pregnant HIV-1-infected women for maternal health and interventions to reduce perinatal HIV transmission in the United states,, 1-207, 2011. http://aidsinfo.nih.gov/contentfiles/PerinatalGL.pdf

Shatrov JG, Birch SC, Lam LT, Quinlivan JA, McIntyre S, Mendz GL: Chorioamnionitis and cerebral palsy: A meta-analysis. Obstet Gynecol 116(2 Pt 1):387, 2010

Smaill F, Hofmeyr GJ: Antibiotic prophylaxis for caesarean section. Cochrane Database Syst Rev (3):CD000933, 2002

Van Schalkwyk J, Van Eyk N, Yudin M et al: Antibiotic prophylaxis in obstetric procedures. J Obstet Gynaecol Can 32:878, 2010

Verani JR, McGee L, Schrag SJ; Division of Bacterial Diseases, National Center for Immunization and Respiratory Diseases, Centers for Disease Control and Prevention (CDC). Prevention of perinatal group B streptococcal disease—revised guidelines from CDC, 2010. MMWR Recomm Rep 59(RR-10):1-36, 2010.

CHAPTER 35

Postterm Pregnancy

Laura M. Gaudet

INTRODUCTION

Definition

Postterm refers to a pregnancy that has reached or exceeded 42 weeks of gestation or 294 days from the first day of the last menstrual period (LMP). Confusion often arises when patients are referred to as "postterm" at 41 weeks of gestation. This appears to have evolved as a result of current recommendations for postterm surveillance, which generally begin at 41 weeks' gestation. Maternity care providers should be clear about gestational age when using the phrase "postterm," which in this chapter refers to pregnancies at or beyond 42 weeks unless otherwise specified.

Prevalence

In general, postterm pregnancy occurs in approximately 7 percent of gestations, with up to 1.4 percent of pregnancies reaching at least 301 days (43 weeks). When first- or second-trimester ultrasound is used for pregnancy dating, rates of postterm pregnancy are decreased. In one study, the incidence fell from 12.1 percent using LMP data to 3.4 percent using an ultrasound estimate. Over time, the number of deliveries occurring at 42 weeks has decreased (from 7.1% in 1980 to 2.9% in 1995).[3] This pattern reflects the decision of many women to undergo delivery at 41 weeks of gestation based on recommendations from national organizations.

Risk Factors

There are several recognized risk factors for postterm pregnancy, including primiparity and history of previous postterm pregnancy. Genetic predisposition appears to also play a role, as do excess maternal weight and male fetal sex. Rare associations include fetal anencephaly and placental sulfatase deficiency. In the absence of ultrasound dating, postterm pregnancy correlates with predictors of inaccurate recall of LMP, including young mothers, those of non-optimal prepregnancy weight, and smokers.

Complications of Postterm Pregnancy

The potential for complications in the postterm pregnancy has long been recognized. Much effort has been put into identifying and quantifying

TABLE 35-1: RISKS ASSOCIATED WITH POSTTERM PREGNANCY

Maternal Risks	Fetal and Neonatal Risks
Increased rate of labor induction	Perinatal death
Dysfunctional labor	Meconium aspiration syndrome
Macrosomia-related birth trauma	Macrosomia and related birth trauma
Postpartum hemorrhage	

these risks. Table 35-1 highlights the generally accepted maternal and fetal and neonatal risks associated with postterm pregnancy.

The Cochrane review and meta-analysis of induction to improve birth outcomes found the data concerning cesarean section difficult to interpret because of heterogeneity of trial methodology. They also identified significant sources of confounding, including cervical ripeness at the time of induction. However, they recently concluded that a policy of induction of labour is associated with a significant reduction in abdominal delivery.

In contrast, data on postterm pregnancies between 2000 and 2003 from the British Columbia Perinatal Database Registry showed consistently higher rates of cesarean section among nulliparous women who were induced compared with women who entered labor spontaneously at 41, 42, and greater than 42 completed weeks' gestation. These pragmatic data include all deliveries and partially addresses concerns that data arising from trials may be different than population-level statistics because the trial setting is often more rigorous.

Other maternal risks are largely related to the fetal overgrowth that frequently accompanies postterm pregnancy. For example, dysfunctional labor, shoulder dystocia, perineal trauma, and postpartum hemorrhage are all more common in prolonged pregnancies.

For the neonate, there may be a gradual increase in perinatal morbidity and mortality in the postterm period, although epidemiologic studies reported inconsistent findings. A U.K. study classified the risk of perinatal death as a function of ongoing pregnancies (as opposed to all births) and found the risk rose steadily from 0.7 per 1000 at 37 weeks to 5.8 per 1000 at 43 weeks (Fig. 35-1).

The Cochrane review on induction of labor for improving birth outcomes identified fewer perinatal deaths in women who had labor induced than in those who were followed expectantly. When women at 41 and 42 completed weeks are combined, the relative risk of perinatal death

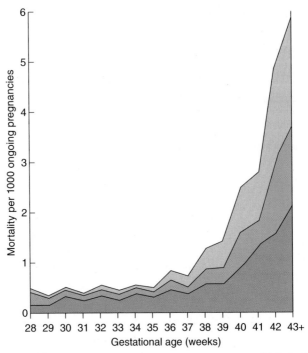

FIGURE 35-1. Perinatal mortality per 1000 ongoing pregnancies. (Hilder L, Costeloe K, Thilaganathan B: Prolonged pregnancy: evaluating gestation-specific risks of fetal and infant mortality. B J Obstet Gynecol 105:169, 1998.)

was 0.30 (95% confidence interval [CI], 0.09-0.99) for women who were induced. If deaths caused by congenital anomalies are excluded, there were no deaths in the labor induction group and nine deaths in the expectant management group.

The presence of meconium in the amniotic fluid is often a normal physiologic finding in postterm pregnancy. In the absence of in utero hypoxia, risks to the fetus related to meconium are minimal. Meconium aspiration syndrome (MAS) is thought to result from fetal gasping of meconium-stained amniotic fluid secondary to hypoxia, resulting in a chemical pneumonitis. The Cochrane database reports a significant decrease in the risk of MAS among fetuses in the induction group compared with the expectant management group (0.29; 95% CI, 0.12-0.68). Labor induction was also associated with a reduction in the prevalence of fetal macrosomia (birthweight greater than 4000 g) in three of the four trials that reported this outcome. Other investigators have reported increased rates of macrosomia-related birth trauma among postterm women who are managed expectantly, including clavicle fracture and Erb's palsy.

PREVENTION

Accurate Pregnancy Dating

Ensuring accurate pregnancy dating is the most important factor in reducing the incidence of postterm pregnancy. Traditionally, pregnancies are dated by using menstrual history and Naegele's rule. Based on the assumption of a 28-day menstrual cycle with day 14 ovulation, the estimated date of confinement (EDC) is then determined using the following formula: EDC = date of LMP + 1 year − 3 months + 7 days. Most commonly, this is done using handheld pregnancy "wheels" or computer software. In limited-resource settings, this may be the only option. However, maternity care providers must be aware of the limitations of using LMP to determine gestational age. When questioned, many women are uncertain of the first day of their LMP, particularly in the roughly 50 percent of pregnancies that are unplanned. Even when a woman is certain of her menstrual dating, there is marked variation in the follicular phase of the menstrual cycle, making exact timing of ovulation difficult to determine. Furthermore, it has been demonstrated that there is a pattern of "digit preference" in reporting of the date of the LMP.

Research suggests that ultrasound, performed as early as possible, represents a safe and acceptable means of reducing the prevalence of postterm pregnancy by up to two-thirds. In the United Kingdom, the National Institute for Clinical Excellence issued guidelines for antenatal care in 2010 recommending that all pregnancies have their gestation assigned on the basis of an ultrasound scan, ideally using a crown–rump length between 10 and 14 weeks or the head circumference at later gestations. Menstrual history is only used to time the scan appointment.

Membrane Sweeping

Sweeping the membranes is a procedure in which a digital cervical assessment is completed with the examining finger advanced between the membranes and the lower uterine segment as far as possible and rotated 360°, thus separating the membranes from the lower uterine segment. It is thought that this elicits endogenous release of prostaglandins that subsequently soften the cervix and potentially augment uterine activity. Some clinicians also advocate stretching of the cervix at the same time.

A Cochrane review assessed the effectiveness of membrane sweeping after 38 weeks for the prevention of postterm pregnancy and concluded that it significantly reduced the frequency of postterm birth at 41 weeks or

OTHER ISSUES

later (relative risk [RR], 0.59; 95% CI, 0.46-0.74) and at 42 weeks or later (RR, 0.28; 95% CI, 0.15-0.50). Some evidence suggests that the benefits of membrane sweeping are most marked in the population of nulliparous women with an unfavorable cervix.

MANAGEMENT

Identifying Complicated Pregnancies at Term

At every stage of pregnancy, care providers must make decisions about whether it is safer to continue the pregnancy or to deliver the infant. Before term, the well-being of the premature infant generally precludes delivery unless there is significant risk to the mother or fetus of continuing the pregnancy. Once term is reached, the threshold for delivery in the presence of any maternal or fetal complication falls precipitously because the risks to continuing the pregnancy usually outweigh the risks associated with delivery.

Among postterm pregnancies, the option to manage the pregnancy expectantly may be chosen when complications have been excluded. For this purpose, an ultrasound for fetal growth and well-being along with an assessment of amniotic fluid volume is recommended when the pregnancy reaches 41 weeks. If the ultrasound findings are reassuring and the mother is in good health and prefers nonintervention, expectant management may be offered with full discussion of its risks and benefits.

Induction of Labor Versus Expectant Management

Despite much investigation and discussion of the ideal management of uncomplicated postterm pregnancies, controversy continues to exist. After excluding contraindications to labor, the American College of Obstetricians and Gynecologists recommends a discussion of risks, benefits, and alternatives to induction of labor versus expectant management with appropriate surveillance. Gestational age, results of antepartum testing, condition of the cervix, and maternal preference should then be taken into consideration and a plan formulated (Fig. 35-2).

Surveillance During Expectant Management

If an informed patient declines induction, expectant management should be provided with appropriate surveillance. There is no consensus on the

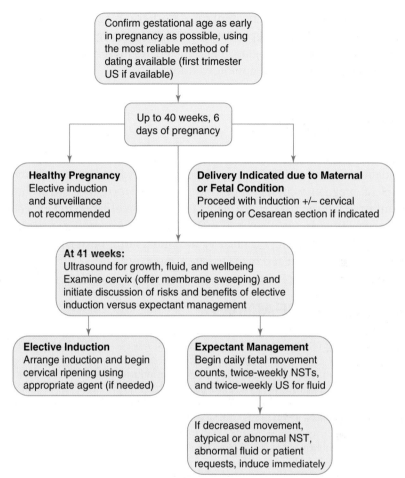

FIGURE 35-2. Algorithm for management of postterm pregnancy. NST, nonstress test; US, ultrasonography.

optimum time to initiate postterm surveillance, nor is there agreement on the frequency of monitoring. It is reasonable to instruct the mother to perform daily fetal movement counts. Women should perceive six fetal movements in an interval of 2 hours. Failure to meet these criteria should prompt women to contact their maternity care provider or hospital as soon as possible for further antenatal testing. After 41 weeks' gestation, formal surveillance should be offered, such as follow-up ultrasound assessments of amniotic fluid volume and nonstress tests, both performed twice weekly until delivery. Throughout this period, the woman and her care provider should be in close contact and have a low threshold to proceed with induction. Nonetheless, expectant management with appropriate surveillance is a reasonable care plan for uncomplicated postterm pregnancies. The small increase in absolute risk of perinatal mortality and maternal and newborn complications of continuing pregnancy postdates must be weighed against the patient's preference for nonintervention.

CONCLUSIONS

Postterm pregnancy occurs in 2 to 10 percent of pregnancies, depending on definition and determination of postterm pregnancy. Once maternal and fetal pregnancy complications have been excluded, the patient should be informed of the risks and benefits to induction of labor and expectant management with surveillance. If induction is chosen, cervical ripening is essential for maximizing the chances of vaginal birth. Birth complications should be anticipated and managed appropriately.

SELECTED READING

American College of Obstetricians and Gynecologists: Practice Bulletin No.55. Management of Postterm Pregnancy. Obstet Gynecol 104:639, 2004.

Boulvain M, Stan C, Irion O: Membrane sweeping for induction of labour. The Cochrane Database of Systematic Reviews (1):CD000451, 2005

British Columbia Reproductive Care Program: Obstetric Guideline 7: Postterm Pregnancy, 2005. http://www.perinatalservicesbc.ca/Guidelines.htm

Gülmezoglu AM, Crowther CA, Middleton P: Induction of labour for improving birth outcomes for women at or beyond term. The Cochrane Database of Systematic Reviews (4):CD004945, 2012

Hannah ME, Hannah WJ, Hellmann J, et al: Induction of labor compared with serial antenatal monitoring in post-term pregnancy. N Eng J Med 326:1587, 1992

Hilder L, Costeloe K, Thilaganathan B: Prolonged pregnancy: Evaluating gestation-specific risks of fetal and infant mortality. B J Obstet Gynecol 105:196, 1998

Mandruzzato G, Alfirevic Z, Chervenak F, et al: Guidelines for the management of postterm pregnancy. J Perinatal Med 38: 111, 2010

Society of Obstetricians and Gynaecologists of Canada: Guidelines for the Management of Pregnancy at 41+0 to 42+0 Weeks. J Obstet Gynaecol Can 30:800, 2008

CHAPTER 36

Obstetric Anesthesia and Analgesia

Catherine Gallant

The practice of obstetric anesthesia began in 1847 when Sir James Young Simpson introduced ether, or "twilight sleep," into obstetric practice for the final stages of labor and delivery. Today obstetric anesthesia has evolved into a complex subspecialty. Although the majority of deliveries are uncomplicated, parturients are presenting with increasingly complex comorbidities such as cystic fibrosis and corrected congenital heart disease because of medical and surgical advances in the treatment of their underlying conditions. Modern regional anesthetic techniques have contributed to maternal and neonatal safety.

This chapter provides an overview of the physiologic changes seen with pregnancy, describes commonly used methods of labor analgesia, and provides an overview of anesthetics administered during pregnancy for cesarean section and non-obstetric surgery.

PREPARATION FOR PAIN DURING LABOR

The majority of parturients experience moderate to severe pain during labor and delivery, which they describe as being more intense than any other previous pain experience. Women who deliver for the first time describe the pain as more intense than that of subsequent labors. It is reported that the pain is exceeded only by traumatic amputation or causalgia.

The American Society of Anesthesiologists (ASA) states:

> There is no other circumstance where it is considered acceptable for an individual to experience untreated severe pain, amenable to safe intervention, while under a physician's care. In the absence of a medical contraindication, maternal request is a sufficient medical indication for pain relief during labor.

Lack of proper psychological preparation can contribute to the pain experienced during labor and delivery. Prenatal classes may dissipate fear about the birthing process and give details about what to expect. Considerable evidence exists that preparation for childbirth can significantly modify the amount of pain experienced.

Psychoprophylaxis, of which Lamaze is the most well-known method, postulates that the pain arising from uterine contractions and perineal distension can be replaced with conditioned "positive" reflexes. This technique promotes a natural delivery and avoids routine medical interventions. A partner who functions as a coach helps the parturient concentrate on breathing techniques and on releasing muscle tension. Education about labor and delivery is believed to give the parturient a sense of control over the birthing process. It may reduce the request for analgesia and anesthesia. However, two-thirds of mothers following this technique still require some kind of analgesic. Following this technique does not guarantee painless labor and may contribute to a sense of failure and lowered self-esteem in those who do request analgesics.

Excessive pain may result in more harm to the fetus than the judicious use of analgesics and anesthetics. The pain and stress of labor contribute to elevated levels of circulating catecholamines, especially epinephrine. Epinephrine has beta-adrenergic tocolytic effects on the myometrium. Adequate labor analgesia reduces plasma epinephrine levels and may shift a dysfunctional to a normal labor pattern.

Elevated plasma catecholamine levels observed during labor may lead to increases in maternal cardiac output and peripheral vascular resistance, as well as decreased uteroplacental perfusion.

Hyperventilation consistently accompanies labor pain. It leads to maternal hypocarbia, which can inhibit ventilatory drive between contractions and result in maternal hypoxemia. Maternal alkalosis shifts the oxygen–hemoglobin curve to the left, thus reducing the offloading of oxygen to the fetus. Maternal alkalosis can cause uteroplacental vasoconstriction and impair oxygen transfer to the fetus. Epidural analgesia has been shown to reduce plasma levels of maternal epinephrine, beta-endorphin and cortisol, likely by reduced pain and anxiety.

CAUSES OF PAIN DURING LABOR

In the first stage of labor, pain is caused by uterine contractions and dilatation of the cervix. It is visceral or cramplike in nature. Pain impulses are carried by the visceral afferent type C fibers (sympathetic) entering the spinal cord from T10 to L1. Pain can be referred to the abdominal wall, lower back, and thighs.

In the second stage, pain caused by distension of the vaginal vault and perineal stretching is carried by the sacral nerves S2 to S4. Pain is more severe. The parturient experiences rectal pressure and the urge to bear down as the presenting part descends into the pelvic outlet.

Various factors may influence the degree and intensity of the pain that is experienced with labor and delivery. Some of these are listed in Table 36-1.

OTHER ISSUES

TABLE 36-1: FACTORS THAT MAY INFLUENCE THE PAIN OF LABOR AND DELIVERY

The parturients psychological state

Mental preparation

Family support

Presence of trained support person such as doula

Medical support

Cultural background

Parity

Previous childbirth experiences

Size and presentation of fetus

Size and anatomy of pelvis

Use of medications to augment labor

Duration of labor

MATERNAL PHYSIOLOGY

Profound physiologic changes affecting most maternal organ systems occur during pregnancy, which may affect anesthetic management. A summary of these changes is given in Table 36-2.

SUPINE HYPOTENSIVE SYNDROME

In up to 15 percent of parturients, the gravid uterus may compress the inferior vena cava (IVC) when the parturient lies supine. This may be seen as early as week 20 and increases in frequency in the third trimester. There is an increased risk in parturients with polyhydramnios and in multiple pregnancy because of the increased size of the uterus.

With IVC compression, there is reduced venous return to the heart. This may lead to signs of shock in the parturient such as maternal hypotension, diaphoresis, nausea, vomiting, and altered mentation. Venous pressure in the lower limbs and uterus increases. Uterine blood flow is not autoregulated but depends on the difference between arterial and venous pressures. There may be a reduction in uterine blood flow, resulting in fetal distress or asphyxia.

TABLE 36-2: THE PHYSIOLOGIC CHANGES OF PREGNANCY

Nervous System			
Variable	Change	Cause	Importance
General Anesthesia	MAC requirements decrease by 25% to 40%	CNS effect of progesterone and (or) beta-endorphin	General anesthesia drug requirements are decreased.
Regional anesthesia	LA dose requirements decrease by ~40%	Decrease in size of epidural space caused by engorged epidural veins and (or) hormonal changes	Increased epidural spread of LA may occur, especially if aortocaval compression is not prevented.
Cardiovascular System			
Blood volume (BV)	Total BV ↑ by 35% Plasma BV ↑ by 45% RBCs' BV ↑ by 20%	Hormonal effect	An ↑ of ~1000 mL compensates for the 400-600 mL of blood loss with delivery.
Cardiac output (CO)	↑ by 40% at 10 weeks' gestation Labor↑ CO 45% above prelabor values After delivery, CO ↑ 60% above prelabor values	Increases in CO are in response to increased metabolic demands (stroke volume increases more than heart rate)	Patients with preexisting heart disease may decompensate (e.g., pulmonary edema may occur during labor or after delivery in the patient with significant mitral stenosis).
Peripheral circulation	BP normal or ↓ SVR ↓ by 15% Venous return from legs decreases	SVR decreases to compensate for ↑ in CO, leaving BP normal or ↓	Supine hypotensive syndrome (see text)

(Continued)

OTHER ISSUES

TABLE 36-2: THE PHYSIOLOGIC CHANGES OF PREGNANCY (*Continued*)

Cardiovascular System			
Variable	**Change**	**Cause**	**Importance**
Regional blood flow	Uterus increases blood flow by 500 mL/min	Blood flow in the placenta depends on blood pressure	Placental blood flow cannot ↑ but can ↓ with maternal ↓ BP because of blood loss, aortocaval compression, or catecholamines.

Respiratory System			
Upper airway	Mucosal edema makes the parturient prone to bleeding	Capillary engorgement	Trauma may occur with suctioning and placing nasal or oral airways. Choose a smaller ETT.
Ventilation	Minute ventilation increases by 50% Tidal volume ↑ 40% Respiratory rate ↑ 10%.	Increases in O_2 consumption begin in the first trimester Labor may increase O_2 consumption more than 100%	Normal resting maternal $PaCO_2$ ↓ to ~30 mm Hg in the first trimester. Pain from labor and delivery result in further hyperventilation.
Lung volumes	FRC ↓ 20% No change in VC	By the fifth month, the rising uterus begins to force the diaphragm up	Uptake of inhaled anesthesia occurs faster because of increased minute ventilation with a smaller FRC.
Arterial oxygenation PaO_2	Increased by 10 mm Hg	Caused by hyperventilation	Decreased FRC with increased O_2 consumption results in very rapid decreases in PaO_2 during apnea (e.g., induction of general anesthesia). Pulse oximetry is important.

(*Continued*)

TABLE 36-2: THE PHYSIOLOGIC CHANGES OF PREGNANCY (*Continued*)

Respiratory System			
Variable	**Change**	**Cause**	**Importance**
Gastrointestinal System			
Gastric fluid volume	Increased	Enlarged uterus displaces pylorus Gastric emptying delayed	All parturients are considered to have a "full stomach." Pain, anxiety, and drugs (especially narcotics) all slow gastric emptying. Metoclopramide may be useful in reducing volume.
Gastric fluid acidity	Increased	Gastrin secreted by placenta Stimulates H+ secretion	Use of H2-receptor antagonists (ranitidine) and (or) a nonparticulate antacid (Na citrate) is recommended to increase gastric pH.
Gastroesophageal junction	Decreased competence	Enlarging uterus distorts the angle of the junction	Pulmonary aspiration of gastric contents is the major risk of general anesthesia. Placement of an ETT is mandatory in every parturient rendered unconscious by anesthesia.

BP, blood pressure; CNS, central nervous system; ETT, endotracheal tube; FRC, functional residual capacity; LA, local anesthesia; MAC, minimum alveolar concentration; RBC, red blood cell; SVR, systemic vascular resistance; VC, vital capacity.

OTHER ISSUES

However, it is important to appreciate that a lack of maternal symptoms does not exclude decreased placental perfusion.

Displacing the uterus to the left during labor with the placement of a right hip wedge helps prevent this phenomenon from occurring. A minimum left lateral tilt of 15° should be used. In women who remain symptomatic, increasing the tilt may be beneficial because individual susceptibility to this syndrome varies.

PAIN MANAGEMENT OPTIONS DURING LABOR AND DELIVERY

The wide range of options available for pain relief during labor are summarized in Table 36-3.

Opioid Analgesia

Opioid analgesia includes intravenous (IV) and intramuscular (IM) techniques. Advantages include ease of use and patient acceptance. It is useful for those who prefer less invasive techniques and when regional anesthetics are contraindicated or unavailable.

TABLE 36-3: OPTIONS FOR PAIN MANAGEMENT

Nothing
Psychological support (birthing coach, partner, other family members)
Behavioral modification (Lamaze)
Hypnotherapy (relaxation exercises practiced before presentation to birthing unit)
Education (prenatal classes)
Massage, walking, various birthing positions
Nitrous oxide (Entonox)
Opioid analgesics
Epidural analgesia
Spinal anesthesia
Combined spinal and epidural anesthesia
Local infiltration
Pudendal block
Paracervical block

Although sedatives and tranquilizers have been used in the past, the increasing availability of regional anesthesia has largely replaced their use. However, opioids are still used in many cases either as the sole agent for labor analgesia or in early labor as a temporizing measure until regional anesthesia is available. There is a risk of maternal and neonatal depression with their use. All parenteral opioids readily cross the placenta and cause central nervous system (CNS) depression. The choice of drug, timing of administration, and method of administration must be carefully considered.

Side effects common to all opioids include respiratory depression, orthostatic hypotension, delayed gastric emptying, nausea, and vomiting.

1. *Morphine:* The dose used is approximately 0.1 mg/kg maternal body weight every 3 to 4 hours. Peak effect is seen 1 to 2 hours after IM injection and 20 minutes after an IV injection, with a duration of action of 4 to 6 hours. The effect on the fetus depends on the time relationship of administration to delivery. If given within 3 hours of delivery, the risk of fetal narcosis is high

2. *Meperidine:* The dose is 1 mg/kg every 3 to 4 hours. Peak effect is 40 to 50 minutes after an IM injection and 5 to 10 minutes after an IV injection. The duration of action is 3 to 4 hours. Maternal effect is similar to morphine. It is quickly transferred across the placenta, but peak levels are reached in the fetus 2 to 3 hours after administration. Infants born 2 to 3 hours after administration are most susceptible to opioid-induced respiratory depression. Elimination may take 2 to 3 days, and this manifests as lower APGAR scores and impaired neurobehavioural scores for the first 3 days of life. Normeperidine, an active metabolite, may be responsible for these changes

3. *Nalbuphine,* a mixed agonist antagonist, provides good pain relief without respiratory depression and may be a better choice. Doses of 10 to 20 mg IM every 4 to 6 hours usually provide adequate analgesia

4. *Fentanyl* is a synthetic opioid. It has been used to provide pain relief in labor, but because of its short duration of action, it must be administered IV, usually through a patient-controlled analgesia (PCA) pump. Remifentanil is an ultra-short-acting synthetic opioid that has been used as an alternative to fentanyl in PCA pumps. Remifentanil has a half-life of 2 minutes and is rapidly metabolized by fetuses, so there should be minimal neonatal depression. Use of remifentanil PCA requires one-to-one nursing because of the risk of maternal hypoventilation Narcotic effects in the newborn are best antagonized with naloxone, 5 to 10 mcg/kg

OTHER ISSUES

Nitrous Oxide

Nitrous oxide is a weak analgesic and amnesic. It is relatively insoluble in blood, so induction and recovery are both rapid. For labor analgesia, it is offered in a 50:50 mixture in oxygen (Entonox) to decrease the chances of maternal hypoxemia. Advantages are ease of use, the safety profile for the mother and infant, rapidity of onset of effect (50 seconds), and widespread availability. It is relatively simple to use because the patient self-administers it using a handheld face mask. To be effective, there must be adequate analgesic concentrations of nitrous oxide present in the blood and the brain at the peak of uterine contractions. This requires maternal cooperation. Some patients may become drowsy. However, this effect is short lived after discontinuation of the agent.

Accumulation is negligible, and neonatal depression is rare.

Disadvantages are that if it is not administered correctly, peak analgesic effect may be delayed until after the contraction. The patient must begin using the Entonox at the beginning of each contraction and continue until the end. Studies on its effectiveness have shown mixed results. It may be ineffective in up to half of parturients. Specialized equipment is required for its administration. Efficient scavenging is difficult, resulting in environmental pollution. It is unclear what, if any, the effects of long-term exposure to subanesthetic concentrations of nitrous oxide are.

Epidural Analgesia

This is the gold standard of labor analgesia. It is the most effective way to block the pain of labor. It involves the injection of a dilute local anesthetic, usually combined with an opioid analgesic, into the lumbar epidural space. The drugs diffuse across the dura into the subarachnoid space, where they act on the spinal nerve roots to provide analgesia. Various combinations of drugs have been used as either intermittent nurse-controlled boluses or more commonly by continuous infusion.

Placement of an epidural catheter allows analgesia to be maintained until after delivery. If a cesarean delivery is deemed necessary, conversion to epidural anesthesia can be completed rapidly, avoiding the need for general anesthesia in most cases.

Epidural analgesia produces a segmental and sensory nerve block with the onset of pain relief. Blood pressure may normalize because of vasodilatation and may lower in some instances. This may be beneficial in patients with pregnancy-induced hypertension (PIH). There may be a significant improvement in uteroplacental blood flow, both in healthy patients and those with PIH. This is because of a reduction in vascular resistance as long as blood pressure is maintained.

More recently, patient-controlled epidural analgesia (PCEA) has become increasingly popular. A low baseline infusion is given and the patient has the ability to "top up" with bolus doses of the same mixture. Alternatively, there is no background infusion, and the patient gives herself bolus doses on demand only. There is high satisfaction with this method and overall less medication is given than by the conventional infusion technique.

Contraindications to Epidurals

Absolute contraindications include patient refusal or inability to cooperate, uncorrected coagulopathy, sepsis or infection at the puncture site, uncorrected hypovolemia, and raised intracranial pressure. Any preexisting neurologic disease should be carefully documented before initiation of the epidural.

Technique of Epidural Analgesia

Before the initiation of the epidural, several steps must be taken. The anesthetist must review the patient's obstetric history; review her medical and anesthetic history; and perform a focused physical examination, including the vital signs, airway, heart, lungs, and back. Emergency resuscitation equipment must be readily available. An IV catheter should be placed. Most anesthesia providers administer a 500-mL bolus of crystalloid, although the ASA Taskforce on Obstetric Anesthesia has stated that a fixed volume of IV fluid is not required before placement of a labor epidural. With the use of more dilute local anesthetics for epidural analgesia, severe hypotension is rarely seen. However, one study did show a deterioration in fetal heart rate (FHR) patterns when the fluid preload was omitted.

After obtaining informed consent, the patient is either seated or placed in the lateral decubitus position. The lumbar area is prepped with an antiseptic solution. In the authors' institution, 2 percent chlorhexidine in 70 percent isopropyl alcohol is the agent of choice. A sterile drape is placed over the prepped area. In the second or third lumbar interspace, the skin is infiltrated with 1 or 2 percent lidocaine. Either a paramedian or midline technique with a 16- or 17-gauge Tuohy needle is used, using loss of resistance to saline or air. The epidural space is identified, and a 20-gauge polyurethane multi orifice catheter is threaded 3 to 5 cm into the epidural space through the Tuohy needle, which is then withdrawn. The catheter is secured to the mothers' back with an adhesive dressing and tape.

There is increasing support in the literature for the use of saline rather than air to identify the epidural space using the loss of resistance technique. Incomplete analgesia may be more likely with loss of resistance to air. Studies comparing air versus saline have shown a statistically significant increase in the incidence of postdural puncture headache (PDPH) with air. Numerous case reports of immediate-onset headache caused by pneumocephalus after loss of resistance to air have been published. One study from 1998 involving almost 4000 patients found no difference in dural puncture rates with air versus saline. However, when dural puncture was documented, 66.7 percent of the patients in the loss of resistance to air group developed headache versus 9.8 percent in the loss of resistance to saline group.

In the past, a test dose of 3 mL of lidocaine 1.5 percent with epinephrine 1:200,000 was injected at this point to rule out intrathecal or intravascular catheter placement. If the dose was injected intravascularly, the patient would experience tinnitus, a metallic taste, and dizziness. Tachycardia would be seen because of the beta-adrenergic effects of the epinephrine. However, because of the wide variations in heart rate that occur with contractions, this effect may be masked. It is recommended that the traditional test dose should be given immediately after a contraction to maximize sensitivity.

The use of a traditional test dose is controversial. Epinephrine may reduce placental blood flow by producing uterine artery constriction. It is relatively contraindicated in cases such as diabetes mellitus or preeclampsia, where there may be decreased uteroplacental blood flow. An undesirable side effect of the traditional test dose is that it produces motor block. There may be maternal hypotension caused by block of sympathetic nerves.

Today the anesthetist may elect to "test" the epidural with a more dilute solution that will be used for infusion. The epidural is loaded with 3- to 5-mL increments of the epidural solution. Examples are 0.0625 to 0.1 percent bupivacaine with fentanyl 2 mcg/mL or 0.08 to 0.125 percent ropivacaine with fentanyl 2 mcg/mL. A total of 15 to 20 mL of these solutions can be used to incrementally load the epidural while watching the vital signs.

Effects on Labor and Delivery

Many studies have attempted to identify factors associated with cesarean delivery. Observational studies have suggested that epidural analgesia, particularly when administered in early labor, is associated with an increased risk of cesarean delivery. Studies are difficult to perform because it is not ethical to assign women to a placebo group with no analgesia. Most studies compare epidural analgesia with systemic opioids, mostly IM or IV meperidine. Meta-analyses of these have concluded that epidural analgesia does not increase the risk of cesarean delivery. Impact studies comparing cesarean delivery rates at an institution before and after the introduction of an epidural service show similar results.

Epidural anesthesia may increase the rate of instrumented vaginal deliveries. There may be a dose-response effect in that this rate is increased with the use of traditional or higher dose anesthetics for labor analgesia (bupivacaine 0.25%). Results of studies have been inconsistent in this area. High concentrations of epidural local anesthetic may cause maternal motor block with pelvic floor relaxation. This may interfere with rotation of the fetus during descent and reduce the effectiveness of maternal expulsive efforts.

Multiple observational studies have found that early initiation of epidural analgesia (cervical dilatation 3-5 cm) is associated with a higher risk of cesarean delivery. Randomized controlled trials have not shown this to be true. In 2006, the American College of Obstetricians and Gynecologists (ACOG) stated that it had "previously recommended that practitioners delay initiation of epidural analgesia in nulliparous women until cervical dilation reached 4 to 5 cm. However, more recent studies have shown that epidural analgesia does not increase the risks of cesarean delivery. ... The fear of unnecessary cesarean delivery should not influence the method of pain relief that women can choose during labor."

Studies have attempted to address whether or not neuraxial analgesia prolongs the duration of the first and second stages of labor. Studies are conflicting regarding the effect on the first stage of labor. If it does prolong it, it is to a minor degree. The bulk of evidence suggests that neuraxial analgesia does prolong the second stage of labor. However, neonatal outcomes do not appear to be affected.

Risks of Epidural Analgesia

Risks of epidural analgesia and anesthesia should be disclosed to the patient. Studies looking at informed consent have shown that patients want to be informed of significant material risks even if the incidence is low.

In the past, hypotension and motor block were commonly seen with the use of more concentrated local anesthetic solutions. It was believed that these agents contributed to pelvic wall muscle relaxation and an inability to push, which may have contributed to an increase in instrumented deliveries. This led to changes in practice and the introduction of less concentrated agents along with PCEA regimens.

Common side effects include pruritus and nausea. There is a failure rate of up to 12 percent in labor epidurals. The risk of PDPH is quoted at 1 percent, but this incidence is increased with new trainees and is reduced with experience. It is common to have backache at the site of skin entry, especially if there are multiple passes with the Tuohy needle. This may last for up to several weeks.

Infection at the site of insertion is rare, as is meningitis. It has been reported in the literature. Meticulous sterile technique during insertion and during top ups of the epidural must be observed.

Traumatic injury to a vessel in the epidural space leading to an epidural hematoma is rare. If a patient has back pain or a worrisome neurologic examination, then imaging should be obtained urgently. Surgical decompression should be performed urgently or paralysis may result.

Systemic toxicity is related to high plasma levels of local anesthetics and is extremely rare. Most commonly, it is caused by accidental IV injection. Initial signs and symptoms include tinnitus and disorientation and ultimately seizures and cardiovascular collapse. It is more likely to be seen after epidural than after spinal because the doses are higher for epidurals, especially when dosing epidurals for cesarean sections. The risk of toxicity is reduced by dosing incrementally and by aspirating the catheter before injecting.

If signs of CNS toxicity occur, the injection should be stopped. Seizures should be treated with benzodiazepines (midazolam 2-5 mg) or barbiturates (thiopental 50-100 mg). The airway should be secured and supplemental oxygen provided.

If cardiovascular toxicity develops, advanced cardiac life support protocols should be followed. The airway should be secured. When performing chest compressions, the uterus must be displaced leftward after 20 weeks' gestational age so that the major vessels are not compressed by the enlarged uterus. If spontaneous circulation has not returned, the current recommendation is to deliver the baby within 5 minutes after cardiac arrest.

Early administration of lipid emulsion (20% intralipid) is recommended for local anesthetic toxicity. After the airway has been secured, a bolus of 1.5 mL/kg is administered IV over 1 minute followed by an infusion of 0.25 mL/kg/min for at least 10 minutes after return of spontaneous circulation. The bolus may be repeated. Total dose should not exceed 10 mg/kg over 30 minutes.

Failed Blocks

There is a failure rate of up to 12 percent in labor epidurals. The definition of a failed block is inadequate analgesia or anesthesia after an epidural. Failed blocks may be caused by inadequate dosing of drugs, patient factors, or technical issues related to the placement of the epidural. If inadequate amounts of drugs are injected, then the required spinal segments will not be blocked and analgesia will not be achieved. Scar tissue or other anatomical features in patients may rarely cause epidural failure. Another factor to consider is that the Tuohy needle or the catheter may not be sited within the epidural space. The catheter may migrate after being positioned, either out through an intervertebral foramen or back out through the skin. With multiorifice catheters, one or more of the orifices may not be in the epidural space. The catheter may be positioned more to one side, causing a unilateral block. Ideally, the catheter should be placed 3 to 5 cm within the epidural space to avoid migration of the catheter.

Spinal Anaesthesia and Combined Spinal Epidural

Spinal anesthesia is not often used alone for labor analgesia because of the finite duration of action of the agents used. However, it may be combined with epidural analgesia for rapid onset of pain relief. This can be done either with a needle through needle technique or a specifically designed combined spinal epidural (CSE) kit.

Small doses of local anesthetic combined with opioids, such as bupivacaine 2 mg and fentanyl 10 to 15 mcg, may be combined with epidural anesthesia to give rapid onset of analgesia. The duration of analgesia is about 90 minutes. If the patient has not delivered within that time period, the epidural catheter can be activated. The author starts the epidural infusion immediately rather than waiting for patient request so that there is uninterrupted analgesia. In this situation, the epidural test dose is omitted.

The CSE technique does result in a greater incidence of fetal bradycardia compared with epidural techniques. The mechanism is believed to be attributable to a transient imbalance in epinephrine compared with norepinephrine levels. This results in a relative increase in uterine tone and may lead to a prolonged tetanic contraction. This is usually short lived and does not result in increased cesarean delivery rates.

With the use of pencil point or atraumatic spinal needles for this technique, the risk of PDPH is not significantly increased.

Postdural Puncture Headache

Headache is one of the most common symptoms seen in the postpartum period. When the dura is breached by a 16-gauge Tuohy needle, a PDPH will develop in up to 88 percent of parturients. The headache is believed

OTHER ISSUES

to be caused by leakage of cerebrospinal fluid through the rent in the dura, which causes intracranial hypotension. When standing, there is traction on pain-sensitive structures. Cerebral vasodilatation is also believed to play a role. This headache has a strong postural component with relief of symptoms when supine. The International Headache Society has defined PDPH as a bilateral headache that develops within 7 days after lumbar puncture and disappears within 14 days after the lumbar puncture. The headache worsens within 15 minutes of assuming the upright position and disappears or improves within 30 minutes of resuming the recumbent position.

The headache is usually described as occurring in the frontal and/or occipital areas, but may also involve the neck and upper shoulders. The usual onset of symptoms is within 48 hours of the dural puncture, but in 25 percent of cases, it presents later than 3 days. Nausea, vomiting, nuchal rigidity, hearing loss, and diplopia may be seen.

This headache can be debilitating and may significantly impair the mother's ability to care for herself and her infant. The natural history is that symptoms will resolve over 10 days, but there have been case reports of persistent headaches for weeks to months. The duration is headache is usually related to the gauge of the needle that breached the dura.

Management of the second stage may affect the incidence of headache after accidental dural puncture. One study of 33 patients who had accidental dural puncture showed that the incidence of headache was 10 percent (1 in 10) in those who went on to have cesarean section compared to 74 percent (17 of 23) in those who pushed.

Epidural blood patch is the definitive treatment for severe headache. However, treatment of PDPH usually begins with conservative measures such as bed rest and analgesics. This delay increases the success rate of the blood patch, which has a failure rate of up to 71 percent if performed within the first 24 hours of dural puncture versus a failure rate of 4 percent if performed later than 24 hours after dural puncture. The optimal volume of autologous blood to be injected is believed to be 20 mL. Success rates vary from 75 to 93 percent.

Paracervical Block

This method is now rarely used in North America for labor analgesia because there has been a high incidence of complications with its use, specifically fetal asphyxia and poor neonatal outcome, especially with the use of bupivacaine. However, it is an easily performed method of achieving pain relief during the first stage of labor. It is ineffective for the second stage of labor. Its main advantage is that the block can be performed by the obstetrician, and the attendance of an anesthetist is not required. It is more commonly used to provide analgesia for other gynecologic procedures.

The injection is made transvaginally into the posterolateral fornices, thus blocking the sensory pathways at the junction of the uterosacral ligaments with the cervix. The procedure can be carried out in the patient's bed or the delivery table. The block is instituted during the active phase of labor with the cervix at least 3 to 4 cm dilated.

Equipment consists of a 20-gauge needle, 13 to 18 cm long, with a sheath or needle guide of such length that 1.5 cm of the tip of the needle protrudes when it is inserted up to its hub. The needle sheath is guided by the fingers into the vagina and placed in the fornix just lateral to the cervix at a tangent to the presenting part. The needle (with the attached syringe) is introduced through the guide until the point rests against the mucosa. With quick, slight pressure, the needle is pushed through the mucosa to a depth of 6 to 12 mm. Aspiration is performed to guard against direct intravascular injection. If no blood returns, the desired amount of anesthetic agent is used. It is advisable to wait for a few minutes after the injection of one side. Fetal heart auscultation is performed, and if it is normal, the other side is injected. If fetal bradycardia occurs, the procedure should be discontinued. Mepivacaine, lidocaine, and procaine in 1 percent concentrations are effective. Bupivacaine is not recommended because of a high incidence of fetal bradycardia.

Sites of injection vary. Some inject at 3 and 9 o'clock, but others give several injections at 3, 4, 8, and 9 o'clock. In any case, 10 mL is given on each side in single or multiple doses.

Most parturients experience complete or partial relief from pain almost immediately with a duration of about 1 hour. If the cervix is not yet fully dilated, a second block may be required. Other forms of anesthesia are required for the actual delivery.

Transient numbness and paresthesias of one or both lower extremities occur commonly as a result of spread of the local anesthetic to the sciatic nerve or part of the lumbosacral plexus.

Rapid absorption or intravascular injection may cause symptoms of local anesthetic toxicity, including dizziness, anxiety, shaking, and occasional seizures and loss of consciousness. Occasionally, transient hypotension may occur. There is a risk of hematoma formation at the site of injection. There have been case reports of parametritis.

The main concern of paracervical block is the effect on the fetus. Changes in FHR can be seen in up to 30 percent of cases with the majority

OTHER ISSUES

being fetal bradycardia. In up to 20 percent of the cases when bradycardia is seen, it is sufficient to impair tissue perfusion, with acidosis and neonatal depression the ultimate result.

The etiology of the bradycardia is complex and likely occurs by several pathways:

1. Uterine artery vasoconstriction because of the proximity of the injection, leading to placental hypoperfusion and fetal asphyxia
2. Direct uterine artery injection
3. Direct intramyometrial injection
4. Diffusion of local anesthetic through the uterine arteries and deposition into the intervillous spaces with subsequent fetal uptake and direct fetal cardiotoxicity
5. Direct fetal injection

Changes in FHR are seen more frequently in primigravidas, in those with previous nonreassuring FHR patterns, and in very low birthweight infants (less than 2500 g). Onset is usually within 2 to 10 minutes after injection and may last 3 to 30 minutes. With prolonged bradycardia, fetal acidosis and neonatal depression may be seen, especially if delivery is within 30 minutes of injection.

Due to the high risk of complications, this technique should be avoided if the fetus is compromised, as in cases of placental insufficiency, prior fetal distress, and prematurity. Use only small doses of dilute local anesthetics. Avoid vasoconstrictors such as epinephrine. Do not perform this block if delivery is anticipated within 30 minutes. If the cervix is dilating rapidly, the chance of aberrant injection is increased, and the block should not be performed. The FHR should be monitored continuously during and after the block.

Do not use this block if there is a known sensitivity to local anesthetics or if there is vaginal bleeding or infection.

Direct Infiltration Anesthesia

The main purpose of perineal infiltration is to permit incision and repair of episiotomy, as well as suturing of lacerations

1. Xylocaine 1 percent provides a rapid onset of action and profound anesthesia. Total volume of 30 to 50 mL is sufficient for most cases
2. Either the needle is inserted at the posterior fourchette and the injections are made lateral *or* the needle is inserted at a point halfway

between the anus and the ischial tuberosity and the injections are made toward the midline

3. Using a 25- to 27-gauge needle, a wheal is made by injecting a small amount of the local anesthetic solution into the skin where the needle is to be inserted

4. The needle is then changed to a 22 or 20 gauge, which is inserted through the wheal. Multiple injections are made into the subcutaneous tissue, muscles, and fascia after aspiration to ensure that the needle is not intravascular

5. Adequate analgesia is achieved within 5 minutes

The technique is simple to perform, with no special anatomic knowledge necessary. The success rate is almost 100 percent. However, complete perineal anesthesia is not achieved because only the infiltrated areas are anesthetized.

Pudendal Nerve Block

The pudendal nerve originates from S2, S3, and S4. It exits the pelvis through the lower part of the greater sciatic foramen, curves around the ischial spine, crosses the sacrospinous ligament close to the attachment to the ischial spine and then reenters the pelvis alongside the internal pudendal artery at the lesser sciatic foramen. At this point, the pudendal nerve breaks up into the inferior hemorrhoidal (rectal) nerve, the perineal nerve, and the dorsal nerve of the clitoris. These nerves are best blocked at the ischial tuberosity. Additional innervation is received from the pudendal branch of the posterior femoral cutaneous nerve, which supplies the posterior labial portion of the perineum. A secondary innervation is provided by the ilioinguinal and genitofemoral nerves. These nerves must be blocked by supplemental infiltration to achieve thorough anesthesia of the anterior portions of the labia majora and mons pubis.

The timing of administration of this block is important to its success. In primigravidas, it is done when the cervix is fully dilated and the presenting part is at station +2. In multiparas, the block is administered at 7- to 8-cm dilatation. Pudendal anesthesia is sufficient for spontaneous delivery or low forceps extractions, breech delivery, and repair of episiotomy and lacerations. It may be combined with local infiltration. Before the widespread availability of epidurals, it was the preferred analgesic technique for delivery. It can be used when contraindications to neuraxial anesthesia exist or when low forceps delivery is required.

Either a transvaginal or transperineal approach may be used. The transvaginal approach is most commonly used.

Transperineal Approach

The local anesthetic is injected around the pudendal nerve through a 5-inch, 20-gauge needle. A commonly chosen agent is 1 percent lidocaine. Effective analgesia is achieved within 15 minutes. After an intradermal wheal has been raised, the needle is inserted through the skin midway between the anus and the ischial tuberosity. As the needle is advanced, small amounts of local anesthetic are injected. The index finger of the left hand is inserted into the vagina or rectum to palpate the tuberosity of the ischium. The needle is then directed toward the ischial spine. A number of injections are made:

1. Five to 10 mL is injected at the anterolateral aspect of the spine, as well as under the tuberosity, to block the inferior pudendal branch of the posterior cutaneous nerve. At this point, the syringe can be detached from the needle and refilled
2. The needle is then advanced to the medial aspect of the ischial spine, where another 5 to 10 mL is injected to block the branches of the pudendal nerve. Because the pudendal artery and vein run parallel to the nerve, intermittent aspiration to ensure the needle is not intravascular should be performed
3. Another 5 to 10 mL of the solution is injected as the needle is advanced 2.5 cm past the ischial tuberosity into the ischial fossa. This blocks the pudendal nerve in Alcock's canal
4. The point of the needle is advanced posteriorly to the ischial spine. The finger can palpate the sacrospinous ligament, and it guides the needle in this direction until a "popping" sensation indicates that the needle has pierced the ligament. The needle is advanced another 0.5 cm, and 5 to 10 mL of solution is injected at this point to block the pudendal needle before it divided. The needle is withdrawn, and the other side is blocked
5. The final step is to infiltrate the area that lies 1.5 cm lateral and parallel to the labia majorum from the middle of the labium to the mons pubis. This effectively blocks the secondary innervation from the iliohypogastric, ilioinguinal, and genitofemoral nerves. This must be done bilaterally

Transvaginal Approach

A 10- or 20-mL syringe is attached to a 5-inch, 20-gauge needle. The left pudendal nerve is blocked first. The index and middle fingers of the left hand are inserted into the vagina, and the ischial spine and sacrospinous ligament are palpated.

Holding the syringe in the right hand, the needle is placed in a specialized pudendal needle sheath, such as an Iowa trumpet with the sharp tip retracted into the sheath. Using the groove formed by the apposition of the index and middle fingers, the needle is inserted into the wall of the vagina toward the tip of the ischial spine. The needle is advanced 1.5 cm into the sacrospinous ligament, and 5 to 10 mL of local anesthetic solution is injected. The needle is then advanced until it "pops" through the sacrospinous ligament, and 5 to 10 mL of local anesthetic is injected with intermittent aspiration to ensure the needle is not intravascular. Supplementary infiltration of the area lateral to the labia majora is carried out as described in the section on transperineal technique. The procedure is then repeated on the other side.

CESAREAN SECTION

Cesarean delivery now accounts for approximately one-third of all deliveries in North America. The updated Practice Guidelines for Obstetric Anesthesia from the ASA Task Force on Obstetrical Anesthesia observe that neuraxial techniques (spinal, epidural, and CSE) are associated with improved outcomes for both mother and baby when compared with general anesthesia, especially in the presence of a high body mass index and airway issues. However, the choice of anesthetic should be made in each instance after a careful assessment of patient, medical, anesthetic, and obstetric issues.

Complications related to anesthesia are the sixth leading cause of peripartum maternal mortality in the United States. Most commonly, these deaths result from failures in oxygenation and ventilation and may be seen at extubation as well as induction of anesthesia.

At the authors' institution, most cesarean sections are performed under regional anesthesia. For elective cesarean sections with no contraindication to regional anesthesia, spinal anesthesia is preferred. After establishing IV access with a 16- or 18-gauge IV and with standard monitors in place, the back is prepped with a 2 percent chlorhexidine in 70 percent isopropyl alcohol solution. Using sterile technique, the intrathecal space is identified with an atraumatic 25- to 27-gauge spinal needle. Bupivacaine 9 to 12 mg with 15 mcg of fentanyl and 100 mcg of preservative-free morphine are then injected.

The patient is then placed supine with left uterine displacement. If hypotension and nausea occur, small boluses of phenylephrine 50 to 100 mcg are

OTHER ISSUES

given, or alternatively an infusion of phenylephrine is started at 50 mcg/min and titrated to effect.

If an epidural is in situ and functioning well, then the catheter is topped up with a combination of 2 percent lidocaine, fentanyl, and bicarbonate 8.4 percent. One mL of bicarbonate is added for each 10 mL of 2 percent lidocaine. Twenty mL of this combination, with 50 to 100 mcg of fentanyl, is given in 3- to 5-mL increments through the epidural catheter. Preservative-free morphine given in doses of 2.5 to 3.75 mg provides analgesia for about 18 hours.

When the surgery may be prolonged, a CSE technique is used. General anesthesia is reserved for the emergencies when there is no time to establish a regional block.

After the baby is delivered, an infusion of oxytocin is started with 10 units added to 1 L of crystalloid. If there is uterine atony, additional oxytocin may be added to the infusion. Alternatively, 100 mcg of carbetocin may be injected IV over 1 minute. If atony persists, prostaglandin F2 (PGF2) alpha or Hemabate 250 mcg should be given intramuscularly or intramyometrially. Ergonovine is reserved for resistant uterine atony.

Postoperative analgesia routines include 500 mg of acetaminophen and 400 mg of ibuprofen every 4 hours. This provides excellent analgesia in the majority of patients. Tramadol and hydromorphone may be added if necessary.

Currently, the author administers prophylactic antibiotics before skin incision in all cesarean sections. Cefazolin is the agent of choice, with clindamycin or vancomycin being the alternate drugs in case of allergy.

NON-OBSTETRIC SURGERY DURING PREGNANCY

Elective non-obstetric surgery is avoided during pregnancy because of increased risk to the mother and child. However, incidental surgery is sometimes necessary. Anesthetic considerations in these patients must include any underlying medical conditions, the reason for the surgery, the physiologic effects of the pregnancy, and any potential effects on the fetus.

Surgical diagnosis of an acute abdomen may be made more difficult because of the presence of the gravid uterus. The white blood cell count is normally elevated during pregnancy. Surgical technique and patient positioning must take into account the gravid uterus.

Because surgery is normally avoided during pregnancy, patients who do present are usually more seriously affected. Surgery is generally delayed until the second trimester if at all possible because of the risks of teratogenicity.

Anesthetic management should include a careful assessment of the airway. The supine position should be avoided, especially after 18 to 20 weeks of gestation. The choice of general versus regional anesthesia should be carefully weighed for each case. However, most women require an urgent laparotomy for exploratory surgery and require general anesthesia.

General anesthesia usually consists of rapid-sequence induction with standard agents, tracheal intubation, and maintenance with a volatile agent. Minimum alveolar concentration (MAC) is decreased by up to 40 percent. Drugs with an established safety record in pregnancy should be used rather than newer drugs.

Maternal arterial CO_2 levels should be kept in the normal pregnant range during ventilation (32-34 mm Hg); otherwise, fetal acidosis may result in fetal myocardial depression. Maternal alkalosis may lead to decreased uterine blood flow. Maternal hypotension must be treated aggressively with fluids and vasopressors. Data suggest that phenylephrine is the vasopressor of choice.

As pregnancy is a hypercoagulable state, there is an increased risk of thromboembolic events postoperatively. The need for anticoagulants should be determined on a case-by-case basis.

SELECTED READING

American College of Obstetricians and Gynecologists: Analgesia and Cesarean Delivery Rates. ACOG Committee Opinion Number 339, June 2006. Obstet Gynecol 107:1487, 2006, reaffirmed 2010

Chestnut DH, Polley LS, Tsen LC, Wong CA: Chestnut's Obstetric Anesthesia: Principles and Practice, 4th ed. Philadelphia: Mosby Elsevier, 2009

Eisenach JC, Pan PH, Smiley R, et al: Severity of acute pain after childbirth, but not type of delivery, predicts persistent pain and postpartum depression. Pain 140:87, 2008.

Shenouda PE, Cunningham BJ: Assessing the superiority of saline versus air for use in the epidural loss of resistance technique: A literature review. Reg Anesth Pain Med 28:48, 2003

OTHER ISSUES

Intrapartum Imaging

Griffith D. Jones

CHAPTER 37

ULTRASOUND

In the diagnosis of obstetric and fetal conditions, ultrasound is a valuable and frequently used tool. Traditionally, labor and delivery units have managed with "hand-me-down" scanners, retired from the hospitals' main ultrasound department. More recently, numerous feature-packed and extremely portable ultrasound machines have appeared that are designed for bedside imaging in the acute setting. This has allowed advances in prenatal ultrasound to be transferred to the intrapartum setting and enabled novel approaches to age-old assessments. Changing patient demographics, including increasing maternal obesity, are further drivers for change.

The chapter focuses on imaging techniques directly applicable to the process of labor and birth, the focus of the book. Labor units often function as an out-of-hours walk-in clinic or emergency room, triaging a variety of obstetric complaints, such as reduced fetal movement or nonspecific pain. Imaging undertaken in these situations is more related to the operational hours of the obstetric ultrasound unit and is not covered. Some other diagnostic uses of ultrasound, including preterm labor and antepartum hemorrhage, are covered in other chapters.

Safety of Ultrasonography

The American Institute of Ultrasound in Medicine Bioeffects Committee has noted in its "2008 Statement on Mammalian In Vivo Ultrasonic Biological Effects" that "information from experiments using laboratory mammals has contributed significantly to our understanding of ultrasonically induced biological effects and the mechanisms that are most likely responsible. The following statement summarizes observations relative to specific diagnostic ultrasound parameters and indices.

In the low-megahertz frequency range there have been no independently confirmed adverse biological effects in mammalian tissues exposed in vivo under experimental ultrasound conditions, as follows:

1. Thermal Mechanisms

   a. No effects have been observed for an unfocused beam having free-field spatial-peak temporal-average (SPTA) intensities below 100 mW/cm^2, or a focused beam having intensities below 1 W/cm^2, or thermal index values of less than 2

   b. For fetal exposures, no effects have been reported for a temperature increase above the normal physiologic temperature, ΔT, when $\Delta T < 4.5 - (\log_{10} t/0.6)$, where t is exposure time ranging from 1 to 250 minutes, including off time for pulsed exposure"

Basic Intrapartum Imaging

The following ultrasound assessments should be within the skill set of most obstetricians practicing on labor and delivery. A key practical point is to always ensure the probe orientation matches the screen orientation. This ensures "left" and "cranial" are always depicted correctly on the screen. Gently moving your finger on one corner of the probe and observing the screen will confirm this before you start scanning.

Because ultrasound is transmitted poorly through air, the face of the transducer must be coupled to the patient's skin by a fluid medium, such as gel, so that the sound waves may penetrate the skin surface–air interface. Higher ultrasound frequencies are used on vaginal probes, giving finer, more detailed resolution of structures. However, the higher frequency beam can only penetrate a short distance, and therefore the field depth is limited. Lower frequency probes are used transabdominally, giving greater depth and penetration.

Fetal Viability

Using real-time ultrasound, fetal cardiac motion can be readily appreciated within the fetal chest. By applying color or power Doppler, the movement of blood within the cardiac chambers and the great vessels can also be appreciated. An approximate heart rate can be estimated visually. Alternatively, this can be more precisely defined using pulse-wave Doppler and either counting manually or using the machine's integrated software.

Fetal Presentation

Probably one of the commonest uses of portable ultrasound in birthing units has been to assess presentation. The position of the head and orientation of the longitudinal axis of the spine should be used (Fig. 37-1A, B).

Amniotic Fluid Volume

It is widely accepted that a significant reduction in amniotic fluid volume is associated with an increased incidence of nonreassuring fetal heart rate (FHR) patterns and subsequent emergency cesarean section. Evidence also suggests that the knowledge that the amniotic fluid volume is low alters obstetric decision making and results in increased cesarean sections. What is much less clear is whether it is associated with any significant reduction in neonatal morbidity.

Amnioinfusion continues to be used to relieve variable decelerations in the presence of oligohydramnios. In this situation, amniotic fluid volume assessments can guide therapy.

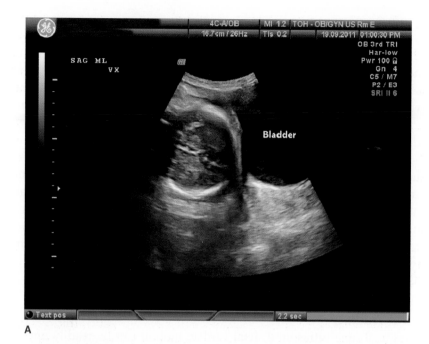

A

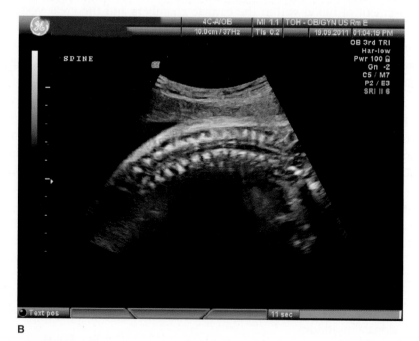

B

FIGURE 37-1. A, Cephalic presentation. **B,** Fetal lie assessment using a longitudinal image of the spine.

On occasion, a patient may be seen for whom no previous scan results are available. This may be because the patient has not had any prenatal care or did not even recognize she was pregnant. Although uncommon in developed countries with socialized medicine, this remains a familiar situation in areas of socioeconomic deprivation. In other cases, the patient will have moved, be traveling away from home, or her own doctor may not have transferred information to the hospital. In many European countries, patients carry their obstetric notes and this presents little difficulty. However, most North American centers have been reluctant to adopt this standard and the issue arises frequently. Additional indications for scanning would then include:

Fetal Number
Before the routine use of prenatal ultrasound, up to 50 percent of twin gestations were only diagnosed after delivery of the leading twin.

Placental Localization
Transabdominal ultrasound can usually exclude previa, but a transvaginal or transperineal approach is required to diagnose it (see Chap. 31). Clinicians should avoid the temptation to search for abruption because the diagnostic sensitivity of ultrasound is poor.

Biometry
Routine measurements (biparietal diameter, head circumference, abdominal circumference, and femur length) can give a reasonably accurate composite estimate of gestational age and fetal weight; the latter usually within 15 percent. When the operator does not feel confident in his or her measurement technique, the unique shape of the cerebellum is readily recognized and its length easily measured (Fig. 37-2). This can provide an approximate estimate of gestation when other options are limited.

Advanced Intrapartum Imaging

Head Position
Occipitoposterior (OP) positions remain a prominent cause of dystocia in labor and operative delivery. Transabdominal ultrasound can reliably assess head position using the position of the fetal eyes and the spine in cross-section through the chest (Fig. 37-3A, B). It has shown that transient OP positions are seen in up to one-third of labors but that the majority rotate

OTHER ISSUES

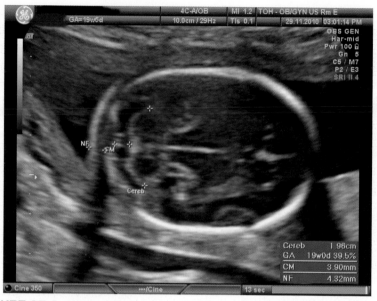

FIGURE 37-2. Fetal cerebellum. Its unique shape and simple measurement allow for an approximate assessment of preterm gestational age.

to occipitoanterior (OA) even after full dilatation. Epidural anaesthesia has been shown to reduce this rotation, leading to a higher persistence of posterior positions. Most importantly, ultrasound has shown how inaccurate digital vaginal examination is at assessing head position, with some studies reporting error rates as high as 75 percent. The accuracy of digital assessment was poorest when the head was in a non-OA position or when the station was not below the ischial spines. These are the exact clinical situations that can be associated with difficult instrumental deliveries. Correct placement of the ventouse cup or forcep blades is predicated by an accurate assessment of fetal position.

Type of Breech

There has been renewed interest in vaginal breech delivery. Most guidelines recommend knowledge of the type of breech presentation to identify the footling breech at risk of cord complications. The longitudinal orientation of the cervical spine should be visualized to exclude the hyperextended "star-gazing" position associated with an increased risk of neurologic complications. Finally, attempts at vaginal birth are often tied to certain birth-weight ranges. If the breech was previously undiagnosed, some attempt at assessing this using biometry will be necessary.

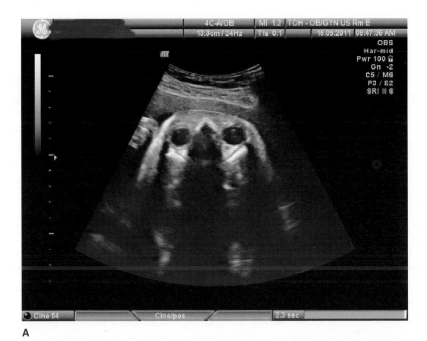

A

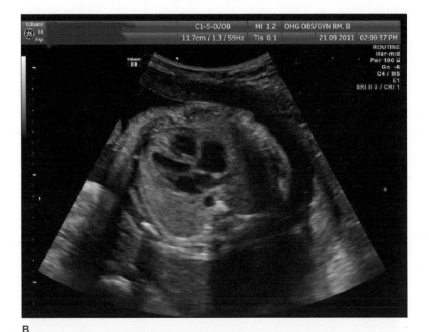

B

FIGURE 37-3. A, Fetal eyes looking straight upward in a direct occipitoposterior position. **B,** Transverse section of the fetal chest shows the spine and vertebra to be left posterior.

Management of Twin Delivery

After delivery of the first twin, the lie of the remaining twin needs to be assessed along with the FHR. These can both be accomplished quickly and efficiently by real-time scanning. Knowing the fetal cardiac position allows prompt and accurate placement of the external monitors' Doppler probe. Alternatively, the heart rate can be monitored by ultrasound, because the relatively rapid descent that will occur will require frequent readjustments of the Doppler probe. If either a breech extraction or internal podalic version is required, the position of the fetal feet can be identified before the procedure is started. Real-time guidance can be provided to the accoucheur during intrauterine manipulation.

Cord Presentation

On occasion, the suspicion of a cord presentation will arise either from a vaginal examination or from marked decelerations related to contractions. Transperineal or transvaginal ultrasound, aided by color Doppler, can assist diagnosis (Fig. 37-4). Abdominal delivery is the only option for an abnormal heart rate. If there is no suspicion of fetal compromise, expectant management can be undertaken provided there is rapid access to emergency cesarean section because there is an ever-present risk of acute cord prolapse. Cases with intrapartum resolution of the cord presentation

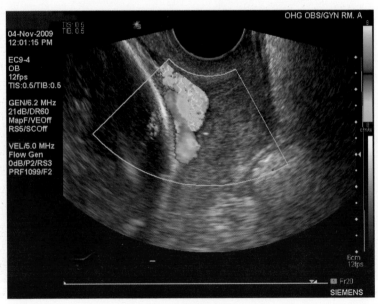

FIGURE 37-4. Color Doppler TV scan highlights a cord presentation just above the internal os.

as labor progresses have been reported. It is also important to distinguish cord presentation from vasa previa. The latter may be associated with an accessory placental lobe and will usually only have two vessels. Alternatively, there may be a membranous cord insertion into the lateral margin of a low placenta.

Preoperative Mapping

When cesarean section is being undertaken for a placenta previa with an anterior component, for vasa previa, or for obstructive or lower segment fibroids, mapping can be performed immediately before surgery to help guide the optimal uterine incision site.

Third Stage Complications

The placental bed vessels vasoconstrict after delivery of the fetus, and this precedes placental expulsion. Abnormal placental adherence can be identified if flow persists. If retained products are suspected, guidance can be given to aid the manual removal or curettage of retained tissue. On one occasion, the author has imaged acute uterine inversion after vaginal delivery, providing guidance during manual replacement and confirming correct repositioning.

Invasive Procedures

Amnioreduction

In the presence of marked polyhydramnios, a gradual reduction in fluid volume can play a part in a stabilizing induction and minimize the risk of acute abruption sometimes seen with a sudden reduction in uterine volume.

Drainage of Abnormal Fetal Fluid Collections

Excessive fluid collections within the fetal head or abdomen can lead to dystocia. After appropriate counseling as to risk, ultrasound-guided drainage can be performed. Bilateral pleural effusions can seriously compromise neonatal respiratory function during delivery. Even a partial drainage in utero can significantly lower the ventilation pressures needed after intubation.

Non-obstetric Imaging

Bladder Residual Volumes

Bladder dysfunction with retention is common in the immediate postnatal period. It can be related to a transient pelvic nerve apraxia or an epidural

OTHER ISSUES

effect. The concern is that large-volume retention, if unrecognized, can lead to prolonged difficulties with bladder emptying. Bladder volume can be measured noninvasively using ultrasound. Indeed, there are now portable ultrasound machines whose sole purpose is to assess bladder volume using built-in software.

Catheter Insertion

Using probes that allow imaging of the superficial structures, ultrasound guidance can be used to guide epidural or central line placement. This improves the accuracy of needle placement and reduces the risk of complications.

Imaging Techniques of Limited Use on Labor and Delivery

Nuchal Cord

The positive predictive value for identifying a nuchal cord on ultrasound before delivery is only 30 percent. Furthermore, it cannot differentiate between cords found to be tight at delivery and those found to be loose.

Biophysical Profile

Although a low biophysical profile (BPP) score has been associated with a higher risk of delivery by cesarean section, it has little routine role in routine intrapartum care. Fetal heart monitoring remains the mainstay supplemented by ST analysis, oxygen saturation, or scalp blood sampling, as necessary.

Advanced Cervical Dilatation and Head Descent

Monitoring advanced cervical dilatation by ultrasound has proven problematic. Although techniques for assessing head descent have been devised, they rely on artificially created reference points and are not yet easily applicable on labor and delivery units.

Fetal Doppler

No intrapartum role has yet been found for these tests.

Placental Maturity

A "mature" placenta, as reflected by a Grannum grade III appearance, was originally thought to identify a fetus with lung maturity. This is no longer considered true. It remains contentious as to whether this test has any role in fetal assessment. Certainly, there is considerable interobserver variability in assessing grade, with a significant tendency to overcall the more advanced grades.

RADIOGRAPHY

As a diagnostic aid, x-ray has a limited range of uses in modern obstetrics. The use of diagnostic ultrasound has almost eliminated the need for x-ray examination of developing fetuses.

Multiple Pregnancy

With an advanced pregnancy at term, particularly in the presence of a pendulous abdomen, it can occasionally be challenging to confidently exclude an undiagnosed twin gestation in patients presenting for the first time. Higher multiples can be even more difficult when there is no scan before the third trimester. In these cases, a plain abdominal x-ray may be diagnostic.

Pelvimetry

In general, radiological pelvimetry is not recommended as a routine test to predict the likelihood or safety of vaginal birth. Clinical pelvimetry along with a serial assessment of progress in labor is believed to be adequate. There may be specific clinical circumstances, such as a congenital pelvic anomaly or a history of an unstable or displaced pelvic fracture, in which individual clinicians may request this test. However, in most of these situations, testing will have been organized prenatally.

Although radiological pelvimetry can be undertaken by conventional x-ray, computed tomography, or magnetic resonance imaging, in the acute intrapartum setting, a limited plain x-ray pelvimetry using the standing lateral view will be the most likely imaging mode. Details of this assessment taken from the fifth edition of this textbook are included below for reference.

Standing Lateral View

A lateral view of the pelvis is taken with the patient erect. A metal ruler with notches or perforations 1 cm apart is placed in the gluteal folds between the buttocks. The ruler has the same degree of distortion as the pelvis, and the desired diameters can be measured.

OTHER ISSUES

Information Obtained

1. Inclination, curve, and length of the sacrum
2. Depth of the pelvis
3. Relationship of the promontory of the sacrum to the inlet
4. Sacrosciatic notch—whether it is wide or narrow
5. Anteroposterior diameters of the inlet, the obstetric conjugate; midpelvis, the plane of least dimensions; and the outlet
6. Posterior sagittal diameter of the midpelvis and the outlet
7. Size and shape of the ischial spines. Are they small or large? Are they prominent and posterior? Do they shorten the posterior sagittal diameter and narrow the sacrosciatic notch?
8. Length and inclination of the symphysis
9. Station of the fetal presenting part
10. In cephalic presentations, the presence of synclitism or asynclitism
11. Attitude of the fetus: flexion or extension
12. Relationship or fit of the head to the pelvis

In 1986, this chapter's author wisely concluded that:
"X-ray pelvimetry is needed rarely in modern times because:

1. In most cases the decision can be made on clinical examination and a trial of labor
2. Often the reason for failure of progress is not demonstrated by x-ray
3. In cases of disproportion the cause is a large baby more often than a contracted pelvis
4. Inefficient labor is a frequent factor when progress ceases, and this is not shown by x-ray
5. Most cesarean sections are performed in women with normal pelves"

SELECTED READING

Maharaj D: Assessing cephalopelvic disproportion: back to the basics. Obstet Gynecol Surv 65:387, 2010

Molina FS, Nicolaides KH: Ultrasound in labor and delivery. Fetal Diagn Ther 27:261, 2010

Sherer DM: Intrapartum ultrasound. Ultrasound Obstet Gynecol 30:123, 2007

Society of Obstetricians and Gynaecologists of Canada: Guidelines for ultrasound in labor and delivery. J Soc Obstet Gynaecol Can 23:431, 2001

Vintzileos AM, Chavez MR, Kinzler WL: Use of ultrasound in labor and delivery. J Maternal-Fetal Neo Med 23:469, 2010

The Puerperium

Felipe Moretti

CHAPTER 38

NORMAL CHANGES

The puerperium is the period that begins after the delivery of the placenta and lasts until the reproductive organs have returned to approximately their prepregnant condition. The puerperium is usually considered to last 6 weeks.

Anatomic and Physiologic Changes

Shivering

Postpartum shivering is observed in 25 to 50 percent of women after normal delivery. The pathogenesis of postpartum chills is not clear. No treatment is necessary other than supportive care. When shivering is anaesthesia related, it can be treated pharmacologically.

Uterine Involution

After the delivery of the placenta and membranes, contractions reduce the size of the uterus so that it can be felt as a hard globular mass lying just below the umbilicus. Contraction of interlacing myometrial muscle bundles constricts the intramyometrial vessels, impeding blood flow and preventing postpartum hemorrhage. Moreover, large vessels at the placental site thrombose, a secondary hemostatic mechanism for preventing blood loss at this site.

The uterus weighs 1000 to 1200 g immediately after delivery. It rapidly falls to 500 g by 7 days, disappears into the pelvis by 2 weeks, and is back to its nonpregnant weight of 50 to 70 g by 6 weeks. This reduction is the result mainly of a decrease in the size of the myometrial cells rather than of their number.

Involution of the placental site also takes up to 6 weeks. Immediately after delivery, the placental site is elevated, irregular, and friable and is composed of thrombosed vascular sinusoids. These undergo gradual hyalinization. Most of the decidua basalis is shed over a period of weeks and is replaced by regenerating endometrium. Failure of normal involution of the placental site may lead to late postpartum hemorrhage.

Lochia

The basal portion of the decidua remains after delivery of the placenta. The decidua divides in two layers: the superficial layer and the deep layer. The deep layer, which contains some endometrial glands, regenerates new endometrium. Restoration of the endometrial cavity is rapid and is complete in 16 to 21 days. The superficial layer of decidua surrounding the placental site becomes necrotic and is sloughed off during the first 5 to 6 days. This postpartum vaginal discharge, made up of a mixture of blood and necrotic decidua, is called "lochia." It is red for 2 to 3 days (lochia rubra), becomes paler as the bleeding is reduced (lochia serosa), and by 7 days is yellowish-white (lochia alba). The total volume of postpartum lochial secretion is 200 to 500 mL and lasts from 3 to 6 weeks.

Regeneration of the Endometrium
The deeper part of the decidua that contains some endometrial glands remains intact and is a source of a new lining of the uterine cavity. Restoration of the endometrium is rapid; by the seventh day, it resembles the nonpregnant state and is complete by 16 to 21 days.

Cervix
Immediately after delivery, the cervix is floppy and ragged with several small tears and bleeding points that are insignificant. The cervical os closes gradually. It admits two to three fingers for the first 4 to 7 days and by the end of 10 to 14 days is barely dilated.

The glandular hypertrophy and hyperplasia of pregnancy regresses gradually, and this process is complete by about 6 weeks. The squamous epithelium that was lacerated during delivery heals and undergoes rapid re-epithelialization, but not all cervices regain their prepregnant appearance. Persistence of glandular epithelium on the exocervix is described as a cervical ectropion.

Vagina
After delivery, the vagina is a spacious, smooth-walled cavity with poor tone. Gradually, the vascularity and edema decrease, and by 4 weeks, the rugae reappear, although they are less prominent than in nulliparas. The vaginal epithelium appears atrophic for some time (longer in lactating women) but looks normal by 6 to 10 weeks.

Lacerations of the lower vagina and perineum heal gradually. Perineal care is a matter of hygiene. Showers and washing with soap and water are sufficient for most patients. Hot sitz baths reduce perineal tenderness and promote healing of episiotomy and lacerations. The suggestion has been put forward that ice baths, by causing vasoconstriction, reducing edema, inflammation, and bleeding. It may also decrease the excitability of nerve endings, relieving muscular irritability and spasm. This may relieve pain more effectively and for a longer period than hot baths. The drawback to

OTHER ISSUES

this treatment is that the patient has to endure the sensation of cold, burning, and aching until the numbness and analgesia supervene.

Fallopian Tubes

The cells decrease in size and number. Two weeks after delivery, the tubal epithelium is similar to that seen in menopause, with atrophy and deciliation. After 6 to 8 weeks, the normal structure has been regained.

Ovaries and Ovulation

The puerperal period is one of relative infertility, especially for women who are lactating. In nonlactating mothers, initial postpartum ovulation can occur within 6 weeks. In women who exclusively breastfeed without supplementation, ovulation is usually reliably delayed by at least 6 months. The incidence of conception in this situation is only 2 percent, but additional contraception should be considered, depending on individual circumstances.

The occurrence of the first menstruation varies, but most nonlactating women have menstruated by 12 weeks after delivery. The return of menstruation is usually delayed in lactating women. Menses within the first 6 weeks are rarely ovulatory.

Breasts

In the early puerperium, the breasts undergo marked changes. Between the second and fourth day, the breasts become engorged with increased vascularity and areolar pigmentation. There is enlargement of the lobules resulting from an increase in the number and size of the alveoli. At this time, lactation begins, controlled by various hormones. The production of milk occurs spontaneously but is enhanced by suckling. Once lactation is established, the most important stimulus for the continuation of the production of milk is suckling. A message is sent via the nervous system to the hypothalamus, and there is an increase in the production and release of oxytocin. Oxytocin stimulates the myoepithelial cells of the alveoli of the breasts to contract, causing milk to be transported to, and sometimes through, the nipple. This is the "letdown" reflex.

Some mothers are unable to breastfeed their infants for a variety of reasons, including insufficient milk, inverted nipples, diseases of the breast, or the need to take drugs that may be excreted in the milk and effect the baby. Others simply choose not to.

In 60 to 70 percent of women who do not wish to breastfeed, lactation can be suppressed by the use of a tight bra and the avoidance of stimulation of the nipple. Pharmacologic suppression is no longer advised because of a high incidence of rebound phenomenon.

Cardiovascular System
The cardiac output increases during the first and second stages of labor. It rises even higher immediately after the birth as the reduction in uterine size squeezes an additional amount of fluid into the circulation. After a short interval, the cardiac output decreases to about 40 percent above the prelabor levels and returns to normal after 2 to 3 weeks. The decrease in heart rate is partly responsible for the reduced cardiac output. Changes in blood volume result from loss of blood at delivery and from the mobilization and excretion of extravascular fluid.

Urinary Tract
The dilatation that takes place in the urinary collecting system during pregnancy does not return to normal for more than 6 weeks. The combination of loss of tone, trauma to the bladder during delivery, and anesthesia (especially of the conduction variety) may lead to retention of urine, necessitating catheterization.

Gastrointestinal Tract
Mobility of the intestines, which is decreased during pregnancy, gradually returns to normal. The use of excessive analgesia may delay this process. Laxatives or an enema may be required.

BREASTFEEDING

Advantages

Breastfeeding is convenient, economical, and emotionally satisfying to most women. It also helps to contract the uterus, decreasing maternal blood loss.

Breast milk is digestible, has the ideal temperature and nutrient composition, and has no bacterial contamination. Colostrum and milk contain immunologic components such as immunoglobulin A (IgA), complement, macrophages, lymphocytes, lactoferrin, lactoperoxidase and lysozymes.

Breastfed infants have decreased incidences of diarrhea, respiratory infections, otitis media, urinary tract infections (UTIs), necrotizing enterocolitis, invasive bacterial infection, and sudden death. Additionally, cognitive development and intelligence may be improved.

OTHER ISSUES

Breastfeeding should always be encouraged by care-givers. Mothers and infants who are able to start breast feeding within one to two hours after delivery are more successful than those whose initial interactions are delayed for several hours.

Contraindications

Breastfeeding is contraindicated in women who abuse drugs or alcohol, have human immunodeficiency virus (HIV) or untreated tuberculosis, are undergoing treatment for breast cancer, take certain medications (Table 38-1), or who have infants with galactosemia.

TABLE 38-1: DRUGS THAT HAVE BEEN ASSOCIATED WITH SIGNIFICANT EFFECTS ON SOME NURSING INFANTS

Drug	Reported Effect[a]
Acebutolol	Hypotension, bradycardia, tachypnea
5-Aminosalilcylic acid	Diarrhea (one case)
Atenolol	Cyanosis, bradycardia
Bromocriptine	Suppresses lactation; may be hazardous to the mother
Aspirin (salicylates)	Metabolic acidosis (one case)
Clemastine	Drowsiness, irritability, refusal to feed, high-pitched cry, neck stiffness (one case)
Ergotamine	Vomiting, diarrhea, convulsions; doses used in migraine medications
Lithium	One-third to half therapeutic blood concentration in infants
Phenindione	Anticoagulant: increased PT and PTT in one infant; not used in United States
Phenobarbital	Sedation; infantile spasms after weaning from milk containing phenobarbital; methemoglobinemia (one case)
Primidone	Sedation, feeding problems
Sulfasalazine	Bloody diarrhea (one case)

PT, prothrombin time; PTT, partial thromboplastin time.

[a]Blood concentration in the infant may be of clinical importance.

From the American Academy of Pediatrics, American College of Obstetricians and Gynecologists. Guidelines for Perinatal Care, 6th ed. Elk Grove Village, IL: Author, 2007.

Breast Fever

Puerperal fever from breast engorgement is common and may occur in 13 percent of all women postpartum. Fever can range from 37.8° to 39°C. Treatment of engorgement consists of firm breast support, analgesics, and applying ice bags. Pumping of the breast or manual expression is recommended.

Mastitis

Infection of the mammary glands is often caused by coagulase-positive *Staphylococcus aureus*. Most frequently, symptoms of a painful erythematous lobule in one quadrant of the breast are noted during the second or third week of the puerperium.

Infection may be limited to the subareolar region but more frequently involves an obstructed lactiferous duct and the surrounding breast parenchyma. If cellulitis is not properly treated, a breast abscess may develop. If the infected breast is too tender to allow suckling, gently pumping until nursing can be resumed is recommended. Apply local heat and provide good support. Penicillins or cephalosporins are the antibiotics of choice. Erythromycin is given to women who are penicillin sensitive. Treatment should be continued for 10 to 14 days.

Breast Abscess

Clinical suspicion occurs when a mass is palpable or a fever fails to subside after 48 to 72 hours. Pitting edema over the inflamed area and some degree of fluctuation are indicative of abscess formation. If an abscess occurs, it is usually necessary to undertake drainage. Ultrasound-guided needle aspiration followed by antibiotics has an 80 to 90 percent success rate.

ENDOMETRITIS

Postpartum endometritis is essentially an infection of the decidua. It may also extend to the myometrium (called endomyometritis) or involve the parametrium (called parametritis). The route of delivery is the most important single risk factor for puerperium infection. The French Confidential Enquiry on Maternal Deaths cited a nearly 25-fold increased infection-related mortality rate with cesarean section versus vaginal

OTHER ISSUES

delivery. The incidence of cesarean section has increased rapidly in Europe and in the rest of the world, with some places in Latin America reporting rates of 50%.

Antibiotic prophylaxis is widely used to reduce the incidence of puerperium infection after cesarean section, resulting in a two-thirds reduction in endometritis and a decrease in wound infection. In contrast, endometritis is relatively uncommon after vaginal delivery.

Risk Factors for Endometritis

1. Antepartum

  a. Low socioeconomic status
  b. Lack of prenatal care
  c. Anemia
  d. Maternal diabetes mellitus
  e. Obesity
  f. Bacterial colonization of the lower genital tract (e.g., group B streptococcus)
  g. HIV infection

2. Intrapartum

  a. Prolonged membrane rupture
  b. Prolonged labor
  c. Multiple cervical examinations
  d. Intrapartum chorioamnionitis
  e. Intrauterine fetal monitoring

3. During delivery

  a. Cesarean section
  b. Manual removal of the placenta
  c. Operative vaginal delivery
  d. Hemorrhage
  e. Devitalization of tissue from episiotomy and lacerations

Pathogenesis of Endometritis

The cervicovaginal flora may have access to uterine cavity during labor and delivery. It can be facilitated by the risk factors mentioned earlier. The colonization of the decidua may lead to invasive infection of the myometrium and parametrium. The potential for invasive infection is enhanced in cesarean births because of the presence of foreign bodies such as suture material, myometrial necrosis at the suture line, and formation of hematomas or seromas. A wide range of bacteria may be involved, including both aerobes and anaerobes. Broad-spectrum coverage is necessary for treatment.

Clinical Manifestations

The most common symptom is pyrexia. It is considered postpartum fever when the temperature is 38°C or more. After the first 24 hours, two episodes of fever within 10 days postpartum is suggestive of infection. Other symptoms include uterine tenderness, foul lochia, chills, and lower abdominal pain. The uterus may be soft and subinvoluted, which can lead to excessive uterine bleeding.

Other common causes of fever are:

- Surgical site infection (cesarean delivery incision, episiotomy incision, perineal laceration)
- Mastitis or breast abscess
- UTI
- Aspiration pneumonia
- Deep vein thrombosis (DVT) and pulmonary embolism (PE)

Laboratory Studies

Leukocytosis is a normal finding during labor and early puerperium. However, white blood cell counts as high as 20,000/mL can be expected with an infection. Urinalysis should be routinely performed to rule out a UTI. Lochia cultures should be obtained using speculum to allow direct visualization of the cervix. Accurate cultures can be achieved only if specimens obtained transcervically are free from vaginal contamination.

Imaging

Postpartum imaging is often used to rule out any other cause of fever such as pneumonia, DVT, or pulmonary embolus if there is persistent postpartum fever. Patients refractory to 48 to 72 hours of adequate antimicrobial therapy should be imaged, searching for abscesses, retained products of conception, hematomas, and septic pelvic thrombophlebitis. Imaging can be also be used to guide therapy, such as abscess drainage.

OTHER ISSUES

Treatment

Treatment of mild metritis after vaginal delivery with outpatient oral antibiotics is usually sufficient. For moderate to severe infections, intravenous broad-spectrum antibiotic therapy is recommended. The response of therapy should be monitored clinically and by laboratory testing as needed. Improvement follows in 48 to 72 hours in nearly 90 percent of women treated with one of the several standard regimens. Deterioration or failure of treatment requires a complete reevaluation.

Antimicrobial Regimens

In mild endometritis, outpatient treatment with ampicillin (1 g every 6 hours) has been shown to be effective and should be given up to 2 to 3 days after remission of fever and clinical improvement.

In moderate or severe cases or after cesarean section, intravenous therapy with a broad-spectrum antimicrobial agent regimen, such as clindamycin 900 mg + gentamicin 1.5 mg/kg every 8 hours, should be administered. If sepsis or enterococcal infection is suspected, ampicillin (1 g intravenously every 6 hours) should be added to the regimen.

Alternative Regimens

- Clindamycin + aztreonam (gentamicin substitute with renal insufficiency)
- Cefoxitin + clindamycin or metronidazole
- Ceftriaxone
- Imipenem + cilastatin

WOUND INFECTION

Cesarean Section Incision

When prophylactic antibiotics are given, the incidence of wound infection is usually less than 2%. Fever that persists to the fourth or fifth postoperative day suggests a wound infection. Wound infection is characterized by local erythema and tenderness. Spontaneous drainage may occur and is often accompanied by reduction of symptoms and signs.

Treatment

The incision should be opened, encouraging drainage of infected material. Mechanical cleansing of the wound is the mainstay of therapy. The wound can be packed with saline-soaked gauze two to three times per day, which will remove necrotic debris each time the wound is unpacked. The wound can be left open to heal or it can be closed secondarily when granulation tissue has begun to form.

Episiotomy Infection

The incidence is 0.5 to 3 percent, and clinical findings are characterized by local pain. Spontaneous drainage is frequent, and inspection of the episiotomy site shows disruption of the wound and a gaping incision. A necrotic membrane may cover the wound and should be debrided if possible.

Treatment
By opening and cleaning the episiotomy wound, the formation of granulation tissue is promoted. Warm sitz baths may help the debridement process.

URINARY TRACT INFECTION

The incidence of postpartum UTI is approximately 2 to 4 percent. The anatomical proximity of the lower gastrointestinal tract and genital tract exposes the urinary tract to bacteria present in the vicinity. Asymptomatic bacteriuria is found in 2 to 7 percent of women during pregnancy and up to 13 percent postpartum. Catheterization significantly increases the rate of bacteriuria. Operative delivery, epidural anesthesia, and frequent pelvic examinations are also associated with increased risk for a UTI. Moreover, after delivery, the bladder and lower urinary tract remain somewhat hypotonic, and residual urine and reflux result, which provides an excellent environment for infection.

Cystitis

Most UTIs are limited to the bladder. The presenting symptoms are frequency and dysuria. Rarely is there fever or malaise.

Escherichia coli is the most common organism isolated from infected urine postpartum. In women with persistent or repeated infections, bacteria such as *Proteus*, *Pseudomonas*, *Enterobacter*, and *Klebsiella* spp. are often cultured. Treatment consists of antibiotics with specific activity against the causative organism. These drugs include sulfonamides, nitrofurantoin, trimethoprim–sulfamethoxazole, oral cephalosporins, and ampicillin.

OTHER ISSUES

Pyelonephritis

Patients who develop pyelonephritis appear unwell. They develop fever, shaking chills with fever spikes, pain in the back and flank, and tenderness in the costovertebral angle. In contrast with cystitis, pyelonephritis requires initial therapy with high doses of intravenous antibiotics such as ampicillin 8 to 12 g/day or a first-generation cephalosporin such as cefazolin 3 to 8 g/day. When the patient has clinical signs of sepsis or a resistant organism, aminoglycoside can be added. The response to therapy may be fast and after resolution of fever, antibiotics should be continued intravenously or orally for a total of 10 days. Urine cultures should be obtained to guide any necessary modification in drugs.

DEEP VENOUS THROMBOSIS AND PULMONARY EMBOLISM

Venous thromboembolism (VTE) complicates between one in 500 and one in 2000 pregnancies and is more common postpartum than antepartum. PE is the leading direct cause of maternal death in the United Kingdom (1.56 of 100,000 maternities) and is the second most cause of maternal death overall (11% of maternal deaths).

The highest incidence of VTE, PE in particular, is during the postpartum period. Cesarean section is a significant risk factor, but women having vaginal deliveries are also at risk, and 55 percent of the postpartum maternal deaths from VTE in the United Kingdom between 1997 and 2005 occurred in women who had delivered vaginally. DVT is more common in the left than the right leg. The risk of VTE is twice as high after cesarean section than vaginal delivery.

Pathogenesis

Pregnancy itself puts all women at higher risk of VTE, with a four- to 10-fold increase compared with an age-matched nonpregnant female population. Venous stasis, endothelial injury, and a hypercoagulable state (Virchow's triad) are marked in pregnancy and the postpartum period, increasing the risk of thromboembolic events. Major additional risk factors are a previous VTE and/or a documented thrombophilia. A history of thrombosis increases the risk of pregnancy-related VTE to up to 12 percent.

Clinical Manifestations

Clinical diagnosis of DVT and PE is unreliable and is even more inaccurate during pregnancy. DVT can present with leg discomfort, leg swelling, pitting edema, discoloration, and warmth. PE is the most difficult diagnosis. Dyspnea, the most common symptom of PE, occurs in up to 70 percent of normal pregnancies, often stabilizing near term. Usually PE is considered in the differential diagnosis of many clinical presentations, including chest pain, dyspnea, hemoptysis, and unexplained tachycardia.

Thromboprophylaxis

The management strategy for postpartum thromboprophylaxis should be based on assessment of prepregnancy and antenatal risk factors for VTE, modified by intrapartum events, including mode of delivery and any obstetric complications (Table 38-2).

Postpartum Thromboprophylaxis

Thromboprophylaxis involves both nonpharmacologic and pharmacologic measures. Early mobilization after delivery and hydration should be encouraged. Graduated compression stockings and pneumatic compression boots may also be used to achieve improved blood flow and reduce stasis in the femoral and popliteal vessels. Women with known thrombophilia should be considered for heparin prophylaxis for at least 7 days postpartum even if they did not receive antenatal thromboprophylaxis. It can be extended to 6 weeks if there is a family history or other risk factors present. Patients who have an emergency cesarean section should be considered for thromboprophylaxis with heparin for 7 days after delivery. For patients who have an elective cesarean section and have one or more risk factors such as body mass index greater than 30 should also receive thromboprophylaxis for 7 days after delivery. Where resources allow it, low-molecular-weight heparin (LMWH) is appropriate for postpartum thromboprophylaxis (Table 38-3). If women are receiving long-term anticoagulation with warfarin, this can be started when the risk of hemorrhage is low, usually 5 to 7 days after delivery. Heparin and warfarin are safe when breastfeeding.

Contraindications to Anticoagulation

- Active antenatal or postpartum bleeding
- Increase risk of major hemorrhage such as placenta previa

OTHER ISSUES

TABLE 38-2: RISK FACTORS FOR VENOUS THROMBOEMBOLISM IN PREGNANCY

Preexisting		
Previous Venous Thromboembolism		
Thrombophilia	Inherited	Antithrombin deficiency
		Protein C deficiency
		Protein S deficiency
		Factor V Leiden
		Prothrombin gene G20210A
	Acquired (antiphospholipid syndrome)	Persistent lupus anticoagulant
		Persistent moderate or high-titer anticardiolipin antibodies
		Persistent moderate or high-titer β2 glycoprotein 1 antibodies
Medical comorbidities	(e.g., inflammatory diseases, nephrotic syndrome, sickle cell disease,[a] IV drug user)	
Age >35 years or parity ≥3		
Obesity (BMI >30 km/m²)		
Smoking		
Gross varicose veins	Symptomatic or above knee or with associated phlebitis, edema, or skin changes)	
Obstetric		
Multiple pregnancy		
Assisted reproductive therapy		
Preeclampsia		
Prolonged labor, midcavity rotational operative delivery		
Cesarean section		
PPH (>1 L) requiring transfusion		

(Continued)

TABLE 38-2: RISK FACTORS FOR VENOUS THROMBOEMBOLISM IN PREGNANCY (Continued)

New Onset or Transient

Surgical procedure in pregnancy or puerperium

Hyperemesis, dehydration

Ovarian hyperstimulation syndrome

Admission or immobility (≥3 days bed rest)

Systemic infection (requiring antibiotics or admission to hospital)

Long-distance travel (>4 hours)

[a]Villers MS, Jamison, MG, De Castro LM, James AH. Morbidity associated with sickle cell disease in pregnancy. *American Journal of Obstetrics and Gynecology* 199:125 e1-125, 2008

BMI, body mass index; IV, intravenous; PPH, postpartum hemorrhage.

From Royal College of Obstetricians and Gynaecologists. Reducing the risk of thrombosis and embolism during pregnancy and the puerperium. Green-top Guideline No. 37a. November 2009, with permission.

TABLE 38-3: THROMBOPROPHYLACTIC DOSE FOR ANTENATAL AND POSTNATAL LOW-MOLECULAR-WEIGHT HEPARIN

Weight (kg)	Enoxaparin	Dalteparin	Tinzaparin (75 U/kg/day)
<50	20 mg/day	2500 units/day	3500 units/day
50-90	40 mg/day	5000 units/day	4500 units/day
91-130	60 mg/day[a]	7500 units/day[a]	7000 units/day[a]
131-170	80 mg/day[a]	10000 units/day[a]	9000 units/day[a]
>170	0.6 mg/kg/day[a]	75 units/kg/day[a]	75u/Kg/day[a]
High prophylactic dose	40 mg 12-hourly	5000 units 12 hourly	4500 units 12 hourly for women weighing 50-90 kg

[a]May given in two divided doses.

From the Royal College of Obstetricians and Gynaecologists. Reducing the risk of thrombosis and embolism during pregnancy and the puerperium. Green-top Guideline No. 37a. November 2009 with permission.

OTHER ISSUES

- Bleeding diathesis, such as von Willebrand's disease, hemophilia, or acquired coagulopathy
- Thrombocytopenia
- Acute stroke in the past 4 weeks (ischemic or hemorrhagic)
- Severe renal disease
- Severe liver disease
- Uncontrolled hypertension (systolic blood pressure greater than 200 mm Hg and diastolic blood pressure greater than 120 mm Hg)

SEPTIC PELVIC THROMBOPHLEBITIS

The incidence of septic pelvic thrombophlebitis (SPT) is approximately 1 in 3000 deliveries (1 in 9000 vaginal deliveries and 1 in 800 cesarean sections). There are two types of SPT, ovarian vein thrombophlebitis (OVT) and deep septic thrombophlebitis (DSPT). The pathogenesis is similar to that of VTE.

Clinical Manifestation

Ovarian vein thrombophlebitis usually presents within 1 week of delivery. Patients appear clinically ill and develop fever and abdominal pain localized to the flank, the back, or the side of the affected vein. Pelvic tenderness may be present.

Patients with DSPT usually present with fever in the early postpartum or postoperative period. They are not usually clinically ill. Fever or chills may be the only symptoms, and patients appear clinically well between spikes. DSPT is frequently diagnosis of exclusion and should be suspected in persistent postpartum fever despite antibiotic therapy.

Diagnosis

SPT is often a diagnosis of exclusion. It should be suspected in the setting of unexplained fever during the week after delivery or persistent postpartum fever despite antibiotic therapy for metritis. Imaging should be obtained to evaluate SPT. CT or MRI can be useful for diagnosis of OVT but not for DSPT.

Treatment

Antibiotic therapy combined with anticoagulation is the most common treatment for this condition. Most patients have already been receiving

TABLE 38-4: EMPIRIC ANTIBIOTIC THERAPY FOR SEPTIC PELVIC THROMBOPHLEBITIS

Options for empiric gram-negative and anaerobic coverage include:

Monotherapy with a beta-lactam/beta-lactamase inhibitor, such as one of the following:

Ampicillin–sulbactam (3 g every 6 hours)

Piperacillin–tazobactam (4.5 g every 8 hours)

Ticarcillin–clavulanate (3.1 g every 4 hours)

A third-generation cephalosporin such as ceftriaxone (1 g IV every 24 hours) plus metronidazole (500 mg IV every 8 hours)

For patients with beta-lactam intolerance, alternative empiric regimens include:

A fluoroquinolone (e.g., ciprofloxacin 400 mg IV every 12 hours or levofloxacin 500 mg/day IV daily) plus metronidazole (500 mg IV every 8 hours)

Monotherapy with a carbapenem, such as one of the following:

Imipenem (500 mg every 6 hours)

Meropenem (1 g every 8 hours)

Ertapenem (1 g/day)

parenteral antibiotics for endometritis. Options for appropriate antibiotic regimens are shown in Table 38-4.

Anticoagulation is recommended, and unfractionated heparin in an initial bolus of 5000 units followed by continuous infusion of 16 to 18 U/Kg can be used. Therapeutic doses of LMWH are also used by many clinicians.

SELECTED READING

Benson MD, Haney E, Dinsmoor M, Beaumont JL: Shaking rigors in parturients. J Reprod Med 53:685, 2008

Confidential Enquiry into Maternal and Child Health: Saving Mothers' Lives: Reviewing Maternal Deaths to Make Motherhood Safer, 2003-2005. The Seventh Report of the Confidential Enquiries into Maternal Deaths in the United Kingdom. London: CEMACH; 2007

Deneux-Tharaux C, Carmona E, Bouvier-Colle MN, Bréart G: Postpartum maternal mortality and cesarean delivery. Obstet Gynecol 108:541, 2006

OTHER ISSUES

Liu S, Liston RM, Joseph KS, et al: Maternal mortality and severe morbidity associated with low-risk planned Caesarean delivery versus planned vaginal delivery at term. CMAJ 176:455, 2007

Marik PE, Plante LA: Venous thromboembolic disease and pregnancy. N Engl J Med 359:2025, 2008

Negishi H, Kishida T, Yamada H, Hirayama E, Mikuni M, Fujimoto S: Changes in uterine size after vaginal delivery and cesarean section determined by vaginal sonography in the puerperium. Arch Gynecol Obstet 263:13, 1999

Royal College of Obstetricians and Gynaecologists: Reducing the risk of thrombosis and embolism during pregnancy and the puerperium. Green-top Guideline No. 37a, 2009. http://www.rcog.org.uk/guidelines

Smaill FM, Gyte GM: Antibiotic prophylaxis versus no prophylaxis for preventing infection after cesarean section. Cochrane Pregnancy and Childbirth Group Cochrane Database Syst Rev (1):CD007482 2010

Villar J, Valladares E, Wojdyla D, et al: Caesarean delivery rates and pregnancy outcomes: the 2005 WHO global survey on maternal and perinatal health in Latin America. Lancet 367:1819, 2006

Witlin AG, Mercer BM, Sibai BM: Septic pelvic thrombophlebitis or refractory postpartum fever of undetermined etiology. J Matern Fetal Med 5:355, 1996

CHAPTER 39

The Newborn Infant

Nadya Ben Fadel
Samira Samiee

ADAPTATION TO EXTRAUTERINE LIFE

After delivery, the newborn child must undergo major physiologic changes to adapt to a new environment and way of life. The most vital of these are:

1. The establishment of regular breathing and exchange of gases
2. Circulatory alterations

Respiration

In utero, the fetal lung produces fluid that passes through the tracheo-bronchial tree until it reaches the oropharynx. There it is swallowed or mixes with the pool in the amniotic cavity. In animals, catecholamines secreted by fetuses during labor decrease lung fluid production. During vaginal delivery, the thorax is compressed as it traverses the birth canal. This expresses some fluid from the upper airways. Most of what remains is absorbed by the pulmonary capillaries and lymphatics.

The mechanical expansion of the lungs at first breath and the rise in alveolar Po_2 lead to a rapid decrease in pulmonary vascular resistance and an increase in pulmonary blood flow. A number of factors are involved in the initial stimulus to respiration. Perhaps the most important is the fall in Po_2 and the rise in Pco_2 that follow the cessation of umbilical circulation. Tactile, thermal, and proprioceptive inputs also play significant roles.

Circulation

The changes in the circulation include:

1. Absolute and relative pressure changes
2. Closure of fetal channels

Changes in Pressure

Fetal circulation is characterized by relatively high right ventricular and pulmonary artery pressures. These are maintained by elevated pulmonary arteriolar resistance and by the presence of a large ductus arteriosus. The ductus equalizes pressures between the pulmonary artery and aorta and directs most of the right ventricular output into the systemic circulation. Systemic pressures are decreased by the presence of the umbilical circulation, which acts as a low-pressure shunt.

As outlined earlier, with the first breath, there is a drop in pulmonary vascular resistance and consequently in right ventricular pressure. Clamping of the umbilical cord leads to a sudden rise in systemic vascular resistance. Left ventricular pressure is now elevated above that of the right ventricle.

Closure of Fetal Vascular Channels

1. *Foramen ovale:* The increase in pulmonary venous return leads to a rise in left atrial pressure. This compresses the valve of the foramen ovale and produces functional closure of the interatrial septum. Anatomic closure takes place over a period of months or years
2. *Ductus arteriosus:* The ductus arteriosus closes functionally over the first 24 to 72 hours of life. This process is related to the rise in arterial oxygen saturation and is mediated by prostaglandins

IMMEDIATE CARE OF THE INFANT IN THE DELIVERY ROOM

Of all newborn infants, 10 percent will need some assistance to initiate and establish breathing, and around 1 percent will need more extensive resuscitation. Before the actual delivery, it is important to identify infants who may need support for their initial transitioning to extrauterine life. This step helps to minimize any delay in resuscitative measures, thereby improving prognosis and outcome.

Some examples of infant groups that may warrant the presence of a neonatal resuscitation team at time of their birth include:

1. Newborns with intrauterine growth restriction (IUGR)
2. Preterm newborns
3. Nonreassuring intrapartum fetal monitoring
4. Assisted deliveries (forceps or vacuum)
5. Presence of meconium
6. Shoulder dystocia
7. Newborns with significant congenital abnormalities

To rapidly and efficiently identify newborns needing support during early neonatal transition, physicians should consider the American Academy of Pediatrics (AAP) guidelines, the most recent version of which was published in 2010.

OTHER ISSUES

Upon the birth of any newborn, the following four questions should be asked:

1. Is this a term newborn?
2. Is the newborn crying?
3. Does the newborn have good muscle tone?
4. Is there any meconium present?

If, after considering the above four questions, no concerns are identified, then the newborn should be dried, immediately placed skin to skin on the mother, and covered by a dry blanket to avoid heat loss. Such newborns simply need to be monitored for their respiratory pattern and their color.

If concerns are identified, then the newborn needs extra support and should be transferred to a bed equipped with a warmer, oxygen source, appropriate size bag and mask, and suction. During the first 30 seconds, resuscitation aims to dry and stimulate the newborn followed by clearing the airway. Suctioning the mouth is followed by the nose if necessary. The primary assessment of breathing pattern and heart rate via chest auscultation should follow immediately after the above primary supportive steps have been taken. If newborn does not respond to these measures by establishing a strong cry and a heart rate above 100 beats/min, the pediatrician should be paged and the following sequential steps in resuscitation should be undertaken:

1. A baby who has heart rate below 100 beats/min *or* is apneic *or* is gasping needs to be started on positive-pressure ventilation with room air immediately and have the preductal circulation assessed using an oxygen saturation monitor attached to the right hand. If an oxygen saturation monitor is not available, the assessment of the color should take place every 30 seconds. The most sensitive indication of successful resuscitation is an increase in heart rate
2. If prompt increase in heart rate does not happen, the adequacy of the positive-pressure ventilation needs to be assessed. The correct position of the bag and appropriate seal of the mask, the resulting chest wall movement, and the adequacy of the inflation pressure should be confirmed. One hundred percent supplemental oxygen should also be started. Assisted ventilation should be delivered at a rate of 40 to 60 breaths/min to promptly achieve or maintain a heart rate above 100 beats/min. Endotracheal intubation should be considered if adequate ventilation is not being achieved by bag and mask ventilation. At

any point during the resuscitation, if newborn initiates strong breathing efforts and maintains a heart rate above 100 beats/min, positive-pressure ventilation should be stopped

3. Chest compressions are indicated if there is no response to 30 seconds of adequate ventilation with supplemental oxygen. Compressions should be delivered to the lower third of the sternum using a depth of approximately one-third of anteroposterior diameter of the chest. Compressions and ventilation should be coordinated with a 3:1 ratio of compressions to ventilation. Coordinated chest compressions and ventilations should continue until the spontaneous heart rate is 60 beats/min or above

4. If heart rate remains below 60 beats/min despite adequate ventilation with 100 percent oxygen and chest compressions, administration of epinephrine, volume expansion, or both is indicated, and 0.01 to 0.03 mg/kg per dose of epinephrine should be administered intravenously. If intravenous access has not yet been established, a higher dose of epinephrine can be administered via an endotracheal tube (0.05-0.1 mg/kg/dose)

5. Newborns who required resuscitation are at increased risk of deterioration after their vital signs returned to normal. These newborns should be transferred to an environment where close monitoring can be provided

6. In any newborn with an undetectable heart rate after 10 minutes of effective resuscitation, consideration should be given to discontinuing resuscitation.

For detailed information on this topic refer to the 2010 American Heart Association Guidelines for Cardiopulmonary Resuscitation and Emergency Cardiovascular Care

PERINATAL ASPHYXIA

Asphyxia results from impairment of fetal blood supply and/or impairment of fetal gas exchange before or during delivery. In mild asphyxia, apnea is the principal clinical manifestation. In severe cases, the neonate is flaccid and pale with hypotension and bradycardia.

When fetal blood supply and oxygenation are adequate, energy requirements during labor and delivery are met by aerobic glycolysis. Uterine contractions reduce placental blood flow and may compress the umbilical cord. There is a transient decrease in oxygen supply and buildup of carbon dioxide, for which normal fetuses can readily compensate.

OTHER ISSUES

If, however, the supply of blood or oxygen falls below a critical level, the production of energy changes to less efficient anaerobic glycolysis. During this process, lactic and pyruvic acids accumulate with the development of increasingly severe metabolic acidosis, leading to multiorgan failure.

Epidemiology

According to the World Health Organization, perinatal asphyxia is one of the top 20 leading causes of burden of disease in all age groups (in terms of disability life-adjusted years) and is the fifth largest cause of death of children younger than 5 years. In the United States and in most technologically advanced countries, the incidence of hypoxic-ischemic encephalopathy (HIE) ranges between one and eight cases per 1000 births. The incidence is reportedly higher in countries with limited resources.

The incidence of long-term complications depends on the severity of HIE. As many as 80 percent of infants who survive severe HIE develop serious complications, 10 to 20 percent develop moderate disabilities, and up to 10 percent are healthy. Among the infants who survive moderately severe HIE, 30 to 50 percent may have serious long-term complications, and 10 to 20 percent have minor neurologic morbidities. Infants with mild HIE tend to be free from serious central nervous system (CNS) complications.

Diagnostic Criteria for Perinatal Asphyxia

Guidelines from the AAP and the American College of Obstetricians and Gynecologists (ACOG) for HIE indicate that all of the following must be present for the designation of perinatal asphyxia severe enough to result in acute neurologic injury:

1. "Sentinel" obstetric event (e.g., uterine rupture, placental abruption) occurring immediately before or during labor
2. A previously normal fetal heart rate (FHR) pattern that becomes grossly abnormal after the sentinel event
3. Need for significant resuscitation after birth (APGAR scores of 0-3 beyond 5 minutes)
4. Profound metabolic acidosis (pH <7, base excess [BE] ≥12) in an umbilical artery blood sample
5. Neonatal encephalopathy (e.g., seizures, coma, hypotonia)
6. Evidence of multiorgan dysfunction (e.g., kidney, lungs, liver, heart, intestines)

7. Exclusion of other causes of neonatal encephalopathy. (e.g., congenital anomalies of the CNS)

Infants may have experienced asphyxia or brain hypoxia remote from the time of delivery and therefore may not meet all the criteria set forth by the AAP and ACOG for intrapartum causation.

Risk Factors for Perinatal Asphyxia

A wide range of risk factors contribute to neonatal encephalopathy secondary to perinatal asphyxia.

1. Maternal causes (e.g., preeclampsia)
2. Placental causes (e.g., abruptio placentae)
3. Umbilical cord causes (e.g., cord prolapse)
4. Fetal causes (e.g., IUGR)

APGAR Score

The APGAR score is a method of grading newborns; 0, 1, or 2 points are awarded for each of five signs, depending on their presence or absence (Table 39-1). The grading is done at 1 minute after birth and may be repeated at 5 minutes. Most children are normal and fall in the 7- to 10-point range. A score of 3 to 6 indicates mild to moderate depression. When the APGAR score is 2 or less, the infant is severely depressed.

TABLE 39-1: APGAR SCORING OF NEWBORNS

Sign	0 Points	1 Point	2 Points
Heart rate	Absent	Under 100	Over 100
Respiratory effort	Absent	Slow, irregular	Good, crying
Muscle tone	Limp	Flexion of extremities	Active motion
Reflex irritability: response to catheter in nostril	No response	Grimace	Cough or sneeze
Color	Blue-white	Body pink; extremities blue	Completely pink

OTHER ISSUES

The APGAR scoring system has become established as the method by which the condition of babies is assessed immediately after birth. Recent investigations have shown that the APGAR score by itself is not a totally accurate index of the health of the neonate and that the predictive value of the system is limited. Analyses of blood from the umbilical cords of infants from mothers in the high-risk category revealed that many acidotic babies were born in a vigorous condition with high APGAR scores and that numerous infants with low APGAR scores did not have acidosis at birth. The conclusion is that although scoring the infant's condition by the APGAR criteria is important, other tests and examinations are necessary for full assessment.

Management of Perinatal Asphyxia

Preventive Management

The initial step in management is an intrapartum fetal monitoring plan based on a prenatal risk assessment that identifies fetuses at high risk of perinatal asphyxia. The plan must be modified based on new risk factors identified during the course of labor, such as significant meconium staining of the amniotic fluid. If perinatal asphyxia is suspected based on a screening test (e.g., the FHR pattern), it must be either resolved by intrauterine resuscitation or reassessed by a diagnostic test. If the suspected condition cannot be resolved or refuted, delivery should be expedited to minimize fetal exposure.

Supportive Management

The management of depressed infants is mostly supportive intensive care. Intervention strategies aiming to avoid any further brain injury in these infants include:

1. Immediate resuscitation of any infant with apnea following standard Neonatal Resuscitation Program (NRP) guidelines
2. Maintain adequate ventilation; avoid hypercarbia (which increases cerebral acidosis and impairs cerebrovascular autoregulation) and hypocarbia (which increases the of risk of periventricular leukomalacia in preterm and sensorineural hearing loss in full-term infants)
3. Maintain adequate oxygenation, avoiding hyperoxemia that may lead to additional brain injury. Keep in mind that most term asphyxiated infants, if adequately ventilated, even using room air, will recover
4. Maintain adequate perfusion and normal blood pressure using volume expanders and inotropic support, avoiding either hypotension or hypertension

5. Avoid hypoglycemia and hyperglycemia
6. Treat seizures
7. Fluid restriction is typically recommended for these infants until renal function and urine output can be evaluated. This is because of concern about acute tubular necrosis (ATN) and the syndrome of inappropriate antidiuretic hormone (SIADH) secretion

Neuroprotection
Extensive experimental data suggest that mild hypothermia (3-4°C below baseline temperature) initiated within the first 6 hours of birth is neuroprotective. The neuroprotective mechanisms are not completely understood.

Consequences of Perinatal Asphyxia

Severe perinatal asphyxia has profound effects on almost every organ system. Some of the most important of these are:

1. *CNS:* HIE results in extensive neural damage or destruction. The neonatal period may be complicated by altered state of consciousness, seizures, disturbances of tone and activity, and signs of damage to the brain stem (e.g., apnea, instability of temperature). The rate of mortality is significant, and morbidity occurs in the form of mental retardation, deafness, cortical blindness, and cerebral palsy (CP). However, only 10 percent of CP cases are believed to have an intrapartum origin
2. *Respiratory system:* Asphyxia increases the incidence of respiratory distress syndrome (RDS), probably because of damage to the surfactant producing type 2 alveolar cells and the persistent pulmonary hypertension. Pulmonary hemorrhage may also complicate asphyxia
3. *Cardiovascular system:* Profound hypoxia can cause acute myocardial failure and sever hypotension. In such cases, the electrocardiogram will show changes consistent with myocardial ischemia
4. *Urinary system:* Renal function is commonly impaired after severe perinatal asphyxia. Anuria or oliguria result from ATN. Cortical necrosis may also occur. In most cases, the changes are reversible, but occasionally, chronic renal disease results

BIRTH INJURY

Birth injuries are sustained during birth process and solely include injuries during labor and delivery. Some fetal-, maternal-, or delivery-related factors have

OTHER ISSUES

been shown to increase the risk of birth injuries. With changes in obstetric practice, the incidence of birth injuries has significantly decreased. However, they are still considered a major cause of neonatal morbidity.

Fracture of the Skull

Neonatal skull fractures, although uncommon, can happen secondary to a forceful vaginal delivery or a forceps-assisted delivery. The two common types of skull fractures in neonates are linear and depressed fractures. Linear skull fractures can be completely asymptomatic except if associated with internal bleeding or injury. Linear skull fractures at the base of skull can be particularly dangerous, with severe hemorrhage from the underlying venous system. This type of linear fracture is more common in breech deliveries. Uncomplicated linear fractures do not need any intervention. However, in case of hemorrhage or cerebrospinal fluid leak in basal skull fracture, appropriate supportive treatment, including transfusions and antibiotic therapy, should be considered.

Depressed fractures of the newborn skull are usually secondary to forceps delivery. Depressed fractures smaller than 2 cm can be observed without surgical intervention.

Intracranial Hemorrhage

Intracranial hemorrhage can be divided in to four main categories: subarachnoid hemorrhage, subdural hemorrhage, intraventricular hemorrhage, and intracerebellar hemorrhage.

Subarachnoid Hemorrhage
Bleeding occurs into the subarachnoid space, the interval between the arachnoid membrane and pia mater. Small subarachnoid hemorrhages can happen in preterm infants without causing any symptoms. Infants with larger subarachnoid hemorrhage may develop nonspecific neurologic signs and symptoms such as irritability or seizures, usually after the second day of life. It may also present with catastrophic deterioration after massive intracranial bleeding. MRI is the diagnostic modality of choice because ultrasound is not sensitive enough.

Subdural Hemorrhage
Small subdural hemorrhages are a common incidental finding on brain MRI of newborns, and their occurrence is not necessarily associated with birth trauma. In contrast, the presence of significant subdural hemorrhage

usually relates to birth trauma. Newborns maybe asymptomatic or present with signs of increased intracranial pressure, warranting emergency neurosurgical consult. Similar to subarachnoid hemorrhages, this type of bleed may not be detected on ultrasound, and MRI is the diagnostic test of choice.

Intracerebellar Hemorrhage

Intracerebellar hemorrhage mainly happens in preterm infants. It has been reported in up to 2.5 percent of preterm infants and even higher on autopsy results. The prognosis is guarded.

Intraventricular Hemorrhage

Intraventricular hemorrhage (IVH) is the most concerning of all intracranial hemorrhages. The overall incidence of IVH is estimated at 10 to 20 percent, which has shown a decline during the recent decades. This type of hemorrhage is caused by the prominence of germinal matrix vessels, which regress by term. Therefore, most IVHs happen in infants between 24 and 32 weeks' gestational age. Screening ultrasound is necessary for diagnosis in preterm infants younger than 32 weeks' gestational age. There are four types of intraventricular hemorrhage, previously named as grades I to IV:

1. Subependymal germinal matrix hemorrhage
2. IVH with no ventricular dilatation
3. IVH with ventricular dilatation
4. IVH associated with intraparenchymal hemorrhage

Infants with IVH accompanied by ventricular dilatation (grade III) or intraparenchymal bleeding (grade IV) are at risk of developing hydrocephalus and have poor long-term neurodevelopment outcomes.

Acute intraventricular bleed in a neonate may present with signs and symptoms of anemia with or without increased intracranial pressure and may require emergency resuscitation.

Management

1. *Prevention:* Minimize trauma at delivery or preterm births
2. *Early detection:* Newborns with signs or symptoms suspected of intracranial hemorrhage should be transferred to a center equipped with neonatal intensive care unit (NICU) as soon as possible after initial stabilization

3. *Supportive management:* Newborns with intracranial hemorrhage should be under close monitoring until they are transferred to a NICU. The initial supportive management may include securing the airway, supporting oxygenation and ventilation, blood transfusion, and seizure control.

Extracranial Hemorrhage

Caput Secundum

This type of scalp swelling is very commonly seen in newborns of vaginal birth. On examination, soft edema with or without overlying skin trauma will be noticed. It is predominantly tissue edema, but there may be a serosanguineous component. The differentiating sign of caput secundum is that the superficial edema may pass the suture line and fontanels. Except for rare, very severe cases, the newborn is usually asymptomatic, and no special intervention is necessary.

Subgaleal Hemorrhage

Subgaleal hemorrhage can be considered the most important type of extracranial bleeding. The potential for a large amount of blood to accumulate in the loose connective tissue of the subgaleal space can lead to hemorrhagic shock and death. Operative vaginal deliveries, especially the more difficult forceps and vacuum deliveries, are known risk factors. Fetal risk factors such as coagulopathies, prematurity, or macrosomia can also play a role. On the initial examination, there is a fluctuating edema crossing the suture line and fontanel, which spreads over to the neck and back of the ears as bleeding progresses. Newborns present with pallor, irritability, and eventually shock. A newborn physical examination should take place after all attempted vacuum deliveries. These infants should be observed closely for signs of extracranial bleeding, including an increase in head circumference, irritability, pallor, tachycardia, and shock. If bleeding is suspected, initial stabilization of newborn should take place, and prompt expert consult should be sought.

Cephalohematoma

This is an uncommon type of extracranial bleeding beneath the periosteum. The parietal region is most commonly affected. Prolonged vaginal deliveries and use of forceps are risk factors. During the examination, the swelling usually has demarcated, sharp borders and does not cross the suture lines. Up to 5 percent of affected newborns may have an underlying skull fracture.

This type of bleeding is usually uncomplicated and does not need any intervention. Infants are at higher risk for development of hyperbilirubinemia after the resorption of the hematoma. On rare occasions, excessive bleeding may happen.

Injury to the Spinal Cord

Spinal cord injuries in neonates are most commonly secondary to difficult deliveries, especially breech deliveries or those associated with extensive traction during labor. Upper cervical injuries are the most common type.

Ligamentous laxity and the lack of muscular support are the main causes of neonates' vulnerability to spinal cord damage without obvious vertebral fractures. However, in any neonate with suspicion of spinal cord injury, vertebral fractures should be ruled out. Bone scan or MRI is the modality of choice.

Clinical Outcome

The clinical outcome may be divided into four groups:

1. Stillbirth or early neonatal death because of lower brain stem injury
2. Respiratory failure leading to death or permanent ventilator dependence
3. Long-term survival with paralysis or weakness of the limbs
4. Survival with minimal neurologic damage. Most of these develop spasticity later and may be erroneously diagnosed as having CP

Management

Management is essentially supportive. It is important to rule out other possible conditions that might lead to a similar picture (e.g., an occult dysrhaphic lesion or a neuromuscular disorder). There is little evidence that there is a place for neurosurgical intervention in spinal cord injury. Supportive care, including mechanical ventilation and physiotherapy, minimizes disability in less severely affected infants.

Injury to Peripheral Nerves

Brachial Plexus

Paralysis of the arm from injury during birth was described by Smellie in 1764. It was Wilhelm Erb who, in 1872, localized the most common lesion to the fifth and sixth cervical roots that supply the upper trunk of the brachial plexus. In 1885, Klumpke described injury to the C8 to T1

OTHER ISSUES

nerve roots. The reported incidence of this injury is around 0.42 to 5.1 infants per 1000 live births.

The network of nerves is fragile and can be damaged by stretching, which can occur when the head and neck are forced away from the shoulder; such injury might happen during breech delivery when there is difficulty with the arms and in cephalic presentations with shoulder dystocia.

Types of Brachial Plexus Injury

1. **Erb palsy**, involving C5 and C6. The arm hangs limply by the side and is rotated internally. The elbow is extended, but flexion of the wrist and fingers is preserved, giving rise to the so-called "waiter's tip" position. The possibility of phrenic nerve injury (C3, C4, and C5) should be considered and diaphragmatic paralysis excluded
2. **Klumpke paralysis**, involving C8 and Tl. There is weakness of the wrist and finger flexors and of the small muscles of the hand. A true isolated Klumpke palsy is extremely rare. The term is sometimes loosely applied when there is total brachial plexus palsy. This pattern of injury is much less common than Erb's palsy. The prognosis is also poorer than in Erb's palsy
3. **Total plexus injury**, involving all brachial nerves, C5 to T1. Newborn will have a flaccid arm with absent reflexes throughout

Management. Daily physical therapy is the main treatment method. When an injury is judged unlikely to improve further, several surgical techniques can be used to aid the recovery. Nerve surgery is most effective when it is done between the ages of 5 and 12 months.

Prognosis. Some brachial plexus injuries are minor and completely recover in several weeks. Other injuries are severe enough that some permanent disability involving the arm can be expected.

The upper brachial injuries (e.g., Erb's palsy [C5, C6]) have the best prognosis of all brachial plexus injuries. Onset of recovery within 2 to 4 weeks is a favorable sign. Lower plexus and total plexus injuries (often signified by flaccid paralysis of an entire arm, or diaphragmatic injury, or Horner's syndrome) have worse prognoses. Recent evidence suggests that 20 to 30 percent of these infants will have residual deficit.

In general, if physical examination shows incomplete recovery by 3 to 4 weeks, full recovery is unlikely. If there are no signs of improvement by 3 to 6 months, spontaneous recovery is unlikely, and surgical exploration (nerve transfer) can be considered. Otherwise, the damage will most likely be permanent.

Facial Nerve

Injury to the seventh cranial (facial) nerve usually occurs distal to its emergence from the stylomastoid foramen of the skull. The result is weakness of the muscles on the affected side of the face. The characteristic signs are the failure of one side of the mouth to move and the eyelid to close. An oblique application of obstetric forceps may compress the nerve. However, this may occur after spontaneous vaginal delivery. It has been suggested that the lesion might result from pressure on the face from the sacral promontory. Clinical presentation depends on the site of injury. In central paralysis, forehead muscle function remains intact. In peripheral paralysis, the entire one side of the face will be affected, and the newborn will have difficulty closing the eye on the affected side.

Management. Treatment is limited to the protection of the eye when it is involved. Methylcellulose eye drops are applied, and the eye should be taped shut to avoid corneal injury.

The prognosis for affected infants is good. In most cases there is some return of function in 2 to 3 weeks and complete recovery by 2 to 3 months.

Bony Injuries

1. *Fracture of the clavicle:* This is the most common bony injury and usually occurs in association with shoulder dystocia. Most fractures are of the greenstick type, but complete fractures also occur. The diagnosis may be suspected by noting decreased or absent movements of the arm on the affected side. Tenderness, deformity, and crepitus may be elicited at the site of the injury. Usually no treatment is required other than care in handling the infant. In case of complete fracture, immobilization is required, and consultation with orthopaedic services should be considered. Humeral fracture or brachial plexus injury may be associated with clavicular fracture, which should be ruled out
2. *Fractures of the humerus or femur:* These occur rarely, and result from traumatic delivery. Newborns with these type of fractures need assessment and follow-up by pediatric orthopedic surgery team

Sternomastoid Muscle

A firm, painless swelling may be palpated in the midportion of the sternomastoid muscle at birth or within the first 1 to 2 weeks. It was postulated that this was fibrosis related to a hemorrhage into the muscle after birth trauma. Pathologic examination of such a tumor may show mature fibrous tissue, suggesting that the lesion originated earlier during intra-uterine life.

In the absence of treatment, shortening of the muscle can occur with the production of torticollis (wry neck) and eventual deformation of the skull. A regular program of passive stretching of the involved muscle should avoid this outcome and obviate the need for surgical intervention.

Abdominal Injury

Abdominal trauma is uncommon but can have serious consequences, and early diagnosis can prevent major morbidity and mortality. In infants presenting with shock, pallor, and abdominal distention, intraperitoneal bleeding must be considered. There may be bluish discoloration of the overlying skin.

1. *Hepatic rupture:* The liver is the organ most often injured or lacerated. A subcapsular hematoma may develop, increasing in size until it ruptures into the peritoneal cavity. Infants are at increased risk if:

   a. They have hepatomegaly (e.g., infants of diabetic mothers)
   b. They have a coagulation disorder
   c. They are asphyxiated at birth
   d. They are preterm or postterm
   e. They are delivered as breeches

2. *Splenic rupture:* This accident is less common than injury to the liver. Splenomegaly increases the danger of its occurrence, but in most cases, the damaged organ is of normal size

   Infants with either of the above injuries need urgent resuscitation and transfer to a tertiary care center for further management.

RESPIRATORY DISTRESS SYNDROME

RDS (hyaline membrane disease) or surfactant deficiency syndrome results from inadequate production or early inactivation of surfactant. Surfactant molecules form a layer over the interior of the alveoli, effectively reducing surface tension during expiration and preventing collapse. It mainly affects preterm infants, but it can certainly happen at term, especially after a nonlabor cesarean section.

The infant's first breath requires the production of negative pressure much greater than that needed for subsequent inspirations. The first expiration is accompanied by positive intrathoracic pressure, but some air remains trapped in the alveoli, so a functional residual capacity is built up over the first few breaths.

In the immature lung, where surfactant is deficient, progressive alveolar collapse tends to occur with each expiration. It is almost as if the first inspiration is repeated with each breath. Worsening lung compliance increases the work of breathing. Areas of atelectatic alveoli cause intrapulmonary shunting. The result of these changes is increasing respiratory failure and hypoxia.

Untreated, either recovery may occur in time as surfactant production increases or the baby may die in the absence of treatment of exhaustion or hypoxia. At autopsy, the lungs are collapsed and airless. Histologically, the bronchioles and alveoli are lined with hyaline membranes composed of fibrin and cellular debris.

Clinical and Laboratory Findings

Evidence of respiratory difficulty immediately or within the first few hours of life is the classical clinical syndrome. There is indrawing of the sternum and lower ribs on inspiration, flaring of the alae nasi, and an audible expiratory grunt. The baby can be cyanotic in room air, but his or her color improves with the administration of oxygen.

The condition may stabilize. More typically, however, there is deterioration over the first 24 to 48 hours. The baby's oxygen requirements increase. As the infant tires, he or she becomes increasingly hypercarbic and begins to have apneic spells. Hypoxia and acidosis may cause a reversion to the fetal circulatory pattern with pulmonary vasoconstriction, a rise in pulmonary artery pressure, and right-to-left shunting through the still patent ductus arteriosus.

Because the signs of respiratory distress are nonspecific, chest x-ray is important for diagnosis. This will show small, poorly aerated lungs with a granular appearance, the result of areas of microatelectasis. The airways stand out against the opaque lung fields as air bronchograms.

Treatment

1. Positive-pressure ventilation: Administering positive pressure to maintain the functional residual capacity and open the areas of microatelectasis is the mainstay of treatment. This can be done

OTHER ISSUES

using continuous positive airway pressure (CPAP) machines without needing to intubate the newborn or by use of invasive mechanical ventilation

2. Surfactant therapy was introduced in 1990 and had a significant impact on survival of newborns suffering from RDS. Different centers follow varying protocols regarding when to intubate and administer surfactant. However, in majority of centers, newborns who are on significant support from CPAP and still on considerable amount of oxygen are intubated to receive surfactant

Therapy is otherwise essentially supportive. Oxygen is given as necessary. A neutral thermal environment is provided to minimize oxygen consumption. Hypotension or hypovolemia are treated by blood volume expansion with plasma or albumin. Anemia is corrected by transfusion with packed red blood cells. Blood gases, glucose, calcium, and electrolytes are monitored carefully.

Prevention

Administering betamethasone to pregnant women at risk of preterm delivery less than 34 weeks of gestational age has been the main preventive measure. Obstetric decision making can be influential in births that are either late preterm (between 34 and 36 weeks) or nonlabor cesarean sections before 39 weeks, both scenarios now recognized as at increased risk of RDS. Either the timing of planned delivery can be changed or maternal steroids considered.

MECONIUM ASPIRATION SYNDROME

Unlike RDS, which is mostly a disease of preterm infants, this condition is usually seen in term or postterm babies. Intrauterine stress may cause in utero passage of meconium into the amniotic fluid. Meconium staining of the amniotic fluid can probably be regarded as a physiologic finding that does not, in itself, indicate the presence of asphyxia. The great majority of infants who are born with meconium staining are well at birth and have no respiratory problems.

If asphyxia occurs before delivery, the fetus may be stimulated to make gasping respiratory movements and thereby draw meconium into the upper airways. After delivery, further gasping draws this material deep into the respiratory tract.

Meconium aspiration syndrome (MAS) is defined as a respiratory distress in an infant born through meconium-stained amniotic fluid (MSAF) whose symptoms cannot be otherwise explained. Hallmarks of this syndrome include an early onset of respiratory distress in a meconium-stained infant, hypoxia and characteristic radiologic lung appearances caused by chemical irritation, and physical partial or complete obstruction of small airways.

Clinical and Laboratory Findings

The infant shows signs of respiratory distress, with grunting, indrawing, and cyanosis in room air. Severe refractory hypoxia may result from the persistence pulmonary hypertension. Chest x-ray shows the presence of areas of pulmonary collapse as well as areas of hyperinflation. Air leak with pneumothorax or pneumomediastinum is a common complication. The picture is frequently complicated by other signs of perinatal asphyxia such as seizures and anuria.

Management

Prevention
The most important form of management is prevention. This approach begins with recognition of high-risk pregnancies and maternal factors that may cause uteroplacental insufficiency and subsequent fetal hypoxia during delivery.

In the presence of meconium staining, the fetus should be carefully monitored to detect early evidence of suspected fetal compromise. In the presence of confirmed compromise, delivery should be accomplished promptly by cesarean section if necessary.

There is no evidence that elective suctioning of babies' airways as they are being born, cricoid pressure to prevent aspiration, or thorax compression to prevent spontaneous breathing has any beneficial effect. In fact, these maneuvers may be potentially harmful, causing trauma, vagal stimulation, or induction of deep inspiration.

After birth, the appropriate management of infants born through MSAF depends on whether the infant is vigorous with spontaneous regular breathing or is nonvigorous and apneic. For vigorous infants, routine care only should be provided regardless of the meconium consistency. Infants who are depressed at birth should be intubated immediately and the trachea suctioned.

OTHER ISSUES

Treatment

Infants with meconium below the vocal cords are at risk of pulmonary hypertension, air leak, and chemical pneumonitis and must be observed closely for signs of respiratory distress.

Treatment of established MAS is mainly supportive and follows the general principles described above for RDS.

If mechanical ventilation is required, a gentle strategy with minimal pressures should be used to reduce the risk of pneumothorax. Infants with persistent pulmonary hypertension may have to be treated with high-frequency ventilation and inhaled nitric oxide.

The role of antibiotics in meconium aspiration is still controversial. There is some evidence that the presence of meconium facilitates bacterial growth. Because it is difficult to differentiate meconium aspiration from pneumonia radiographically, infants with infiltrate on chest radiographs should be started on broad-spectrum antibiotics after appropriate cultures have been obtained.

PERINATAL MORTALITY

The accurate and timely reporting of live birth and fetal and infant death is the cornerstone of perinatal mortality data. Because reducing fetal and infant mortality is among any nation's health goals, accurate definitions of these events are essential for understanding causes and researching potential solutions.

Perinatal mortality is defined as the sum of intrauterine deaths plus deaths in the first 7 days of life of infants, expressed per 1000 total births. The most recent data for Ontario, Canada, showed a perinatal mortality of 7 per 1000 total births in 2007. This is roughly split equally between stillbirths (fetal deaths) and neonatal mortality.

Etiology

Stillbirth

Deaths before or during delivery (stillbirths) are most commonly caused by anoxia. These may be associated with:

1. Placental insufficiency in which the placenta is small or its function impaired by infarcts or disease. There is usually evidence of decreased fetal growth, and some of these deaths may be avoidable by careful monitoring and early delivery when indicated

2. Antepartum hemorrhage, especially abruptio placentae. This accident can occur as an unexpected emergency 1 to 2 months before term and may result in immediate fetal death caused by extensive placental separation

3. Umbilical cord problems: Prolapse of the cord carries a high risk of fetal death. Knots or loops in the cord are considered causes of fetal death only when they are very tight and no other cause can be found

4. Maternal disease, especially diabetes. The risk of sudden unexpected fetal death has been much reduced by improved medical care of pregnant women with diabetes

5. Abnormalities of labor and delivery such as breech presentation and prolonged labor, particularly in underresourced settings

Neonatal Death

Early neonatal deaths are most commonly related to:

1. *Preterm delivery* with its attendant complications, especially RDS and intraventricular hemorrhage. Some infants born at 25 weeks' gestation or less show inadequate lung development to allow for gas exchange

2. *Congenital malformations:* Abnormalities causing early death include extensive lesions of the CNS and severe forms of congenital heart disease, especially the hypoplastic left heart syndrome. Pulmonary hypoplasia, incompatible with life, accompanies Potter syndrome and many cases of diaphragmatic hernia

3. *Infection:* Bacterial infections remain a serious problem in the neonatal period. The organism most frequently associated with overwhelming infection in term newborn is group B, beta-hemolytic streptococcus, while in preterm infants, *E coli* was recently found to be the most common cause of sepsis. Pneumonia or generalized sepsis may result, which, especially in preterm infants, have a very high mortality rate

4. *Intrapartum asphyxia or trauma:* Deaths from these causes have been reduced because of better fetal monitoring and the more judicious use of cesarean section. However, unexpected complications continue to cause occasional neonatal deaths

SELECTED READING

American Academy of Pediatrics Committee on Fetus and Newborn: Standard terminology for fetal, infant, and perinatal deaths. Pediatrics 128:177, 2011

OTHER ISSUES

Badawi N, Kurinczuk JJ, Keogh JM, et al: Antepartum risk factors for newborn encephalopathy: the Western Australian case-control study. BMJ 317:1549, 1998

Canadian Pediatric Society Fetus and Newborn Committee: Perinatal brachial plexus palsy. Paediatr Child Health 11:111, 2006

Kattwinkle J, Perlman J, Aziz K, et al: Neonatal Resuscitation: 2010 American Heart Association Guidelines for Cardiopulmonary Resuscitation and Emergency Cardiovascular Care, Pediatrics 126: e1400, 2010

Kliegman RM, Bonita MD, St. Geme J, et al. Nelson Textbook of Pediatrics. St. Louis: Elsevier, 2011

Martin R, Fanaroff A, Walsh M: Fanaroff & Martin's Neonatal-Perinatal Medicine. Diseases of the fetus and infants. St. Louis: Saunders Elsevier; 2011

Perlman JM: Brain injury in the term infant. Semin Perinatol 28:415, 2004

Note: Page numbers followed by f and t refer to figures and tables respectively.

A

Abdomen
  examination, 214, 220, 234, 240, 246, 252,
        255, 257
  injury, 740
  inspection, 90-93
Abdominal wall incisions, 467-469
  closure, 468-469
  pfannenstiel (transverse), 467
  postoperative complications, 469
  vertical, 468
Abruptio placentae, 591-593
  associated findings, 593
  classification, 592
  clinical manifestations, 593
  diagnosis of, 593
  etiology, 591-592
Acardiac twin, 545
Active phase of labor, 200-201
  first stage, 132-133, 133t
  primary dysfunctional labor, 201
  primigravidas, 200t
  prolonged, multipara, 200, 200t
  secondary arrest of dilatation,
        201
  second stage, 267, 269
Activity of uterus, recording, 151-152
Acute fatty liver of pregnancy, 628-630
  clinical presentation, 628
  differential diagnosis, 629t
  intrapartum management, 630
  ominous signs, 628-630
  postpartum considerations, 630
ALARMER, risk management, 347
Amniocentesis
  mortality, fetal, 453
  for preterm pre-labor rupture of membranes,
        579-580
Amnion nodosum, 354-355
Amnioscopy, 595
Amniotic fluid embolism, 615
Amniotic membranes, 133-136, 134f
  delivery, 357-358

Amniotomy, 135-136, 205-206
  advantages, 139
  conditions, 136
  disadvantages, 139
  indications, 136
  in labor management, 138-139
AmniSure test, 135
Analgesia and anesthesia, 672-693
  in breech presentation, 495
  cesarean section, 466, 691-692
    in obese patients, 466
      in emergency, 467
      in nonemergency, 467
      respiratory function, 467
  direct infiltration, 688-689
  epidural block, 680-684
    contraindications, 681
    effects, 682-683
    failure, 684-685
    risks, 683-684
    technique, 681-682
  fentanyl, 679
  labor
    first stage, 137, 139, 673
    second stage, 267, 673
  meperidine, 679
  morphine, 679
  nalbuphine, 679
  nitrous oxide, 680
  non-obstetric surgery, 692-693
  opioid, 678-679
  pain of labor, 672-673, 674t
    management, 678-691
  paracervical block, 686-688
  physiologic changes, 674, 675t-677t
  pudendal nerve block, 689-691
    transperineal approach, 690
    transvaginal approach, 690-691
  spinal block, 685-686
  supine hypotensive syndrome,
    674, 678
Anal triangle, 19
  anococcygeal body in, 19
  sphincter ani externus in, 19
Android pelvis, 47, 47f, 48f, 49t-52t
Aneurysm, umbilical vessel,
    531-532

Angiographic uterine artery
    embolization (UAE),
    364-365
Anococcygeal body, 19
Antepartum fetal health surveillance,
    145-150
Antepartum hemorrhage, 174,
    588-598
  abruptio placentae, 591-593
    associated finding, 593
    classification, 592
    clinical manifestations, 593
    diagnosis, 593
    etiology, 591-592
  causes, 588
  in early labor, 595-596
  idiopathic, 596
  local lesions, 596
  management, 596-598
    double setup examination,
      598
    fetal compromise, 597-598
    maternal compromise,
      597-598
    preliminary, 596-597
  placenta previa, 588-591
    associated findings,
      590-591
    classification, 588-589
    clinical manifestations, 590
    diagnosis, 591
    etiology, 588
  vasa previa, 593-595
    clinical picture, 595
    intrapartum diagnosis, 595
Anterior asynclitism, 83-85, 84f
Anterior shoulder delivery, 343f
Anthropoid pelvis, 47, 47f, 48f,
    49t-52t
Antibiotics
  for chorioamnionitis, 651
  group B streptococcus, 653t
  prevention of intrapartum infection,
    661, 661t
  prophylaxis, 466
Antiretroviral therapy, in intrapartum
    care, 655

Aortic compression
in postpartum hemorrhage, 381
in uterine rupture, 420
Apt test, intrapartum diagnosis, 595
Arborization test, 135
Arcuate uterus, 26*f*, 31
Artificial rupture of membranes.
See also Amniotomy
induction of labor, 183-184
contraindications to, 184
technique of, 183-184
in labor management, 138-139
Asphyxia, perinatal, 729-733. *See also*
Perinatal asphyxia
Assisted breech, 494-495
Asthma, acute exacerbation,
619-620
Asynclitism, 81-85
anterior, 83-85, 84*f*
posterior, 81-83, 83*f*
Atony uterus, 369-370, 374-384
Attitude, 66, 68*f*
military, 67, 240-242, 241*f*
Auscultation fetal heart, 93-95,
150-151
Axis of the birth canal, 39, 39*f*
Axis-traction forceps, 290

B
Bakri SOS tamponade balloon
catheter, 379-380,
379*f*
Barnes-Neville forceps, 290
Bearing down by patient
first stage, 137
management, 277
second stage, 272
Bicornuate uterus, 32, 33*f*, 212
Biochemical analysis, fetal blood,
168-171
Biometry, 699-700, 700*f*
Birth asphyxia, 338-339
Birth injury, 733-740
abdominal injury, 740
bone injury, 739
extracranial hemorrhage,
736-737

fracture
clavicle, 739
femur, 739
humerus, 739
skull, 734
intracranial hemorrhage,
734-736
meconium aspiration syndrome,
742-744
perinatal mortality, 744-745
peripheral nerves, 737-739
brachial plexus, 737-738
Erb palsy, 738
Klumpke paralysis, 738
management, 738
prognosis, 738
total plexus, 738
facial, 739
respiratory distress syndrome,
740-742
spinal cord, 737
clinical outcome, 737
management of, 737
sternomastoid muscle, 739-740
Bishop score, induction of labor,
178-179, 178*f*
Blood dyscrasias, 371
Blood transfusion, 373
B-lynch technique, 380, 380*f*
Body mass index (BMI), 464, 464*t*
Bones, pelvic, 4-5, 6*f*
coccyx, 5
ilium, 4
innominate, 4-5
ischium, 4
pubis, 4-5
sacrum, 5
Brachial plexus injury, 338-339,
737-738
Braxton Hicks contractions, 127
Breast
abscess, 713
fever, 713
postpartum, 710-711
Breastfeeding, 711-713
advantages, 711-712
contraindications, 712

Breech presentation, 68-69, 69*f*,
   472-512
abdominal examination, 476
anesthesia, 495
anterior, 476
arrest of progress
   arms, 505-508
   fracture, 507-508
   head, 499-501, 500*f*
      Mauriceau-Smellie-Veit
         maneuver, 500*f*, 501
      piper forceps, 500*f*, 501
      Wigand-Martin maneuver,
         499, 500*f*, 501
   neck, 505
   prophylaxis, 505
   rotation of body, 506
   shoulders, 505-508
   simple extraction, 505-506
cephalic version, 488-490
cesarean section, 491-492
classification
   complete, 475
   footling, 475
   frank, 475
   kneeling, 476
definition, 472
diagnosis, 476-478
etiology, 473
extraction
   head, 502-505
      airway, 502
      chin-to-pubis rotation, 503,
         505
      embryotomy, 505
   prerequisites, 510
   procedure, 510
failure of descent, 508-509,
   509*f*
   decomposition, 508
   disproportion, 508
   etiology, 508
fetal heart rate examination, 476
forceps, 502
incidence, 472
investigation at term, 488
Kristellar maneuver, 499

labor, mechanism of, 478-485,
   479*f*
   arms, 480-482
   footling, 485
   head, 482, 483*f*
   hips, 478-480, 480*f*
   kneeling, 485
   lower limbs, 478-480
   sacrum anterior, 482-483
   sacrum posterior, 484-485
   shoulders, 480-482, 481*f*
management
   in delivery, 490-499
      arms, 496, 497*f*
      body, 495-496
      cesarean section, 491-492
      classification, 490-493
         cesarean section, 491
         elective cesarean section,
            491-492
         trial of labor, 492-493
         vaginal, 490-491
      head, 497, 498*f*, 499
      shoulders, 496, 497*f*
      umbilical cord, 496, 496*f*
   in labor, 493-499
      first stage, 493
      second stage, 494-495
      trial, 492-493
   in late pregnancy, 488-490
morbidity, fetal, 486-487
mortality, fetal, 486-487
orientation, 501-502
positions, 472*f*
prognosis, 485-487
   fetal, 485-487
   maternal, 485
prolapse, 524
rotation of body, 506
sacrum anterior, 476-478, 477*f*,
   482-483
ultrasonography, 478, 488, 700
vaginal examination, 476
version, external, 488-490
Broad ligament hematomas,
   411
Brow presentation, 68, 233-240

definition, 233
diagnosis, 234
etiology, 233-234
incidence, 233
management, 239-240
mechanism of labor, 235-238,
    236f-239f
    descent, 236
    extension, 236, 237
    flexion, 236
    molding, 237
    restitution, 237
    rotation
        external, 237
        internal, 236
    persistent, 240
    prognosis, 239
Bulbocavernosus muscle, 18
Bulbospongiosus, 18

C
Caldwell-Moloy classification of pelvis,
    47, 47f, 48f, 49t-52t
Candida spp., 649
Caput secundum, 736-737
Caput succedaneum, 60-62, 61f
Carbetocin, in postpartum
        hemorrhage, 375
Cardiac arrest, pregnancy,
        620-621
Cardiovascular system, in puerperium,
        711
Catherization, bladder
    in labor management, 139-140
Cavity of pelvis, 38, 39f
Cephalic presentation, 67-68, 68f
    abnormal
        brow presentation, 233-240
        face presentation, 243-261
        malpresentation, 212-214
        median vertex presentation, 240-
            242
    passage of meconium, 136
    prolapse, 524
Cephalic prominence, 72-74, 73f
Cephalic version
    in breech presentation, 488-490

contraindications, 489
prerequisites, 489
procedure, 489-490
risk, 490
timing, 488-489
Cephalohematoma, 61f, 62-63, 736-
    737
Cephalopelvic disproportion, 195.
        See also Disproportion
Cervical dystocia, 207
Cervix, 23, 23f, 27, 204
    annular detachment, 414-416
        clinical picture, 415
        etiology, 415
        mechanism, 415
        prevention, 416
        prognosis, 416
        treatment, 415-416
    dilatation, 126, 131f
    Dührssen incisions, 413-414
        indication, 413
        technique, 413-414, 414f
    incompetent, 574
    lacerations, 408f, 412-414
        deep, 412
        diagnosis, 412
        etiology, 412
        repair, 412-413
    palpation, 95-96
    postpartum, 709
    ripeness, 177
        evaluation, 178-179
        pre-induction, 178-182
    ripening, 130-131
Cesarean section, 434-454, 527
    analgesia and anesthesia,
        691-692
    in breech presentation,
        491-492
    conjoined twin, 549
    frequency, 434
    HIV and, 656
    hysterectomy, 453-454
        complications, 454
        indications, 454
    incision infection, 716-717
    indications, 434-441

Cesarean section, indications (*Cont.*):
  dystocia, 436-437
  failure to progress, 437
  fetal, 439-440
    abnormal heart rate, 439
    herpes virus infection of the
      genital tract, 440
    HIV infection, 440
    placental insufficiency, 439
    postmortem, 440
    previous damage, 439
    previous death, 439
    rhesus incompatibility, 439
    umbilical cord prolapse, 439
  fetopelvic disproportion, 436
  hemorrhage, 438
    abruptio placentae, 438
    placenta previa, 438
  malposition, 436
  malpresentation, 436
  miscellaneous, 441
  neoplasm blocking passage,
    437
  pelvic contraction, 436-437
  previous uterine surgery,
    437-438
    cervical cerclage, 438
    cesarean section, 437
    hysterotomy, 437
    myomectomy, 438
  toxemia of pregnancy, 438
  uterine dysfunction, 436
  on maternal request, 441
  morbidity, maternal, 449-452
    antibiotics, 452
    complications, 449-451
    prevention, 451-452
  mortality
    fetal, 452-453
    maternal, 448-449
      causes of death, 448-449
      decline in rate, 449
      factors, risk to, 448
  in multiple pregnancy, 558, 561
  in obese women, 466-469
    abdominal wall incisions,
      467-469

  anesthesia, 466
    prophylactic antibiotics, 466
    skin care, 466
    thromboprophylaxis, 466
  in postterm pregnancy, 665
  role in congenital anomalies,
    641-642
  trial labor, previous cesarean
    section, 458-461
    considerations, 461
    contraindications, 458-459
    management guidelines, 459-460
    prerequisites, 458
    safety and results, 460-461
    signs of uterine rupture, 460
  types, 442-448
    position of the patient on the
      operating table, 442
    skin incisions, 442
      transverse, 442
      vertical, 442
    uterine incisions, 443-448,
      443*f*-444*f*
      advantages of, 445-446
      classical, upper segment, 444*f*,
        447-448
      disadvantages of, 446, 448
      indications for, 447
      J incision, 444*f*
      T incision, 444*f*
      transverse, 443-446
      vertical, 444*f*, 446-447
    uterine rupture, 418
Chorioamnionitis, 175, 648-651
  clinical presentation, 649
  diagnostic criteria, 650-651
  management, 651
  risk factors, 648-649
Cho technique, 380-381, 381*f*
Circumference
  fetal shoulders, 59
  fetal skull, 59
Circumvallate placenta, 354
Clamping, umbilical cord,
  281
Clavicle fracture, fetus, 346
Cleidotomy, 645

Coccyx, 5
Complete breech, 68, 475, 475*f*
Compound presentation
  classification, 524
  definition, 524
  diagnosis, 525-526
  etiology, 524-526
  incidence, 524
  management, 526-527
    arrest of progress, 526-527
      cesarean section, 527
      internal podalic version and
        extraction, 527
      reposition, 526
      progressing case, 526
    mechanism of labor, 526
    prognosis, 526
    prolapse
      cord, 527
      hand and arm, 524-526, 525*f*
      leg and foot, 524-526
Confinement, expected date, 120
Congenital anomalies
  classification, 640
  definition, 640
  fetal distress and, 642
  incidence, 640
  labor with prenatal diagnosis,
    641-643
  pathogenesis, 640*t*
  progress of labor, impact of,
    642-643
  role of prelabor cesarean section,
    641-642
  vaginal delivery, impact of,
    643
Congenital uterine anomaly, 441
Conjoined twin
  classification, 546-547
  diagnosis, 547-549
    fetal echocardiography,
      548
    MRI, 548
    ultrasonography, 547-548
    X-ray, 548-549
  etiology, 546
  incidence, 546

management, 549
  method of delivery, 549-550
  monoamniotic, 550-551
  multifetal reduction, 551
  selective intrauterine growth
    restriction, 550
  structural or chromosomal anomaly,
    552-553
  in utero death of co-twin, 551-552
Contraction of uterus, 204-205
  activity, 123
  coordination, 125-126
  definition, 122
  frequency, 123
  intensity, 123
  Montevideo units, 123
  normal labor, 122-127
  pacemakers, 126
  in pregnancy, 126-127
  propagation, 126
  strength, 129*t*
  triple descending gradient, 126
Contractions of pelvis, 212
  inlet, 195
  midpelvic, 195-196
  outlet, 196
Cord, umbilical. *See* Umbilical cord
Coronal suture, 56
Corpus of uterus, 23
Counting methods, in movement
    assessment, 146-147
Cranial vault, 55-56
C-reactive protein (CRP), 650
Crowning of fetus, 276
CRP (C-reactive protein), 650
Cyst, umbilical, 531
Cystitis, 717

D
Death, fetal
  neonatal, 745
    congenital malformations, 745
    infection, 745
    intrapartum asphyxia, 745
    preterm delivery, 745
    trauma, 745
  previous, 439

Decapitation, 645
Deep perineal pouch, 18
Deep transverse perineal muscles, 18
Deep venous thrombosis (DVT),
        616-618, 718-722
    clinical manifestation, 719
    diagnosis, 617-618
        history and physical examination,
            617
        imaging, 617-618
    pathogenesis, 718
    risk factors, 720t-721t
    thromboprophylaxis, 719-722, 721t
    treatment, 618
        heparin, 618
        thrombolytic therapy, 618
Deformation, as congenital anomaly, 640
DeLee forceps, 289
Delivery
    amniotic membranes, 357-358,
        358f
    in breech presentations, 490-499
    cesarean, 491-492
    delayed interval in twins, 561-563
    epidural block, 682-683
    fetus, 275-281
    in multiple pregnancy, 556-563
    operative, 208, 370
    pain management, 678-691
    placenta
        active management, 355
        delayed separation, 358-359
        examination, 358
        expulsion, 356
        manual removal, 359, 360f
        separation, 356
    positions, 272-274
        back elevated: semisitting,
            272, 273f
        dorsal, 272, 273f
        in epidural block, 274
        lithotomy, 272, 273f
        posterior arm and shoulder,
            342, 344f
    vaginal, 284-330
        breech, 490-491, 493-499
        conjoined twin, 550

failed instrumental assisted, 441
impact of congenital anomaly, 643
Denominator, 66, 71-72
Descent, 215
    breech presentation, 478
    brow presentation, 236
    face presentation, 248, 255, 257,
        260
    failure, 204, 508-509, 509f
        decomposition, 508-509
        disproportion, 508
        etiology, 508
    fetal, 275-276
    LOA, 104, 105f, 111f
    of the presenting part, 201
Destructive operation, fetus
    contraindications, 644
    dangers, 644-645
    indications, 644
    types of, 645
        cleidotomy, 645
        decapitation, 645
        encephalocentesis, 645
De Wees forceps, 286, 290
Dexamethasone, in HELLP syndrome,
        625
Diabetes mellitus
    fetal, 175
    gestational, 623-625
    maternal, 337, 439
    pregestational, 602-604
Diameter
    fetal skull, 58-59, 58f
        biparietal, 58
        bitemporal, 58
        occipitofrontal, 59
        submentobregmatic, 59
        suboccipitobregmatic, 59
        verticomental, 59
    pelvis, 40-41
Diazepam, 632
Dichorionic diamniotic twin, 543
Didelphys, uterus, 33-34, 34f
Dilatation of cervix, 126, 131f
Dipping, 78, 79f
Discoloration, 355
Disproportion

cephalopelvic, 195
face presentation, 250, 260
Disruption, as congenital anomaly, 640
Disseminated intravascular coagulation, 371, 627-628
Dizygous twin, 540
Doppler, umbilical cord, 535-536
Double uterus, 33-34, 34*f*
Ductus arteriosus, 727
Dührssen cervical incisions, 413-414
  indication, 413
  technique, 413-414, 414*f*
Duncan method, placental expulsion, 114, 116
DVT. *See* Deep venous thrombosis
Dyscrasias, blood, 371
Dysplasia, as congenital anomaly, 640
Dyspnea, acute
  in peripartum patients, 611-613, 612*t*
    investigations, 613
    management, 612
    normal respiratory changes in pregnancy, 611
    pulmonary function in pregnancy, 611-612
Dystocia
  cervical, 207
  definition, 120
  labor, 194-208
    classification of prolonged labor, 199-203
      active phase, 200-201, 200*t*
      descent of the presenting part, 201
      latent phase, 199-200, 200*t*
      second stage, 202-203
    complications, 197-198
      maternal, 197
      neonatal, 197-198
    definition, 194
    etiology and risk factors, 194-197
    graphic analysis, 198-199, 198*f*
    management, 203-208
      arrest of labor in the second stage, 207

cervical dystocia, 207
first stage, 205-207
  amniotomy, 205-206
  FHR monitoring, 207
  oxytocin, 206
  tachysystole, 206-207
  therapeutic rest, 205
operative delivery, 208
prevention strategies, 203
second stage, 270-271
uterine contractions, 204-205
vaginal examination, 204
mechanical, 436-437
shoulder, 334-348, 335*f*
  clinical presentation, 334-336
  definition, 334
  diagnosis, 340
  differential diagnosis, 336
  incidence, 334
  management, 340-347
    fetal clavicle fracture, 346
    McRoberts maneuver, 341-342
    posterior arm and shoulder delivery, 342, 344*f*
    risk, 347
    rolling over to "all fours" position, 346-347
    suprapubic pressure, 341-342
    symphysiotomy, 347
    Woods' corkscrew maneuver, 342, 344-345, 345*f*-346*f*
    Zavanelli maneuver, 347
  mechanism, 334
  risk factors, 336-338
    fetal macrosomia, 337
    history of, 337
    maternal diabetes mellitus, 337
    maternal obesity, 337
  sequelae of, 338-340
    birth asphyxia, 338-339
    brachial plexus injury, 338-339
    bruises, 339
    fractures, 339
    maternal morbidity, 339-340
soft tissue, 436

E
Early labor, 595-596
Echocardiography, fetal, 548
EFW (estimated fetal weight), 636
Elderly primigravidity, 441
Elective induction, 175
Electronic monitoring fetal heart, 152-167
Embolization of pelvic arteries, postpartum hemorrhage, 381-382
Embryotomy, 505
Emergency cesarean section, 467
Encephalocentesis, 645
Endometritis, 713-716
  clinical manifestation, 715
  imaging, 715
  laboratory studies, 715
  pathogenesis, 714-715
  risk factors, 714
  treatment, 716
Endometrium, regeneration, 709
Endomyometritis, 713
End-stage bradycardia, 268
Engagement, 78
  breech, 480, 482
  process, 79f
  in synclitism, 81, 82f
Epidural analgesia, 680-684
  contraindications, 681
  in delivery of twins, 559
  effects, 682-683
  failure, 684-685
  fetal rotation and, 700
  positioning during delivery, 274
  risks, 683-684
  in second stage of labor, 267
  spinal, 685-686
  technique, 681-682
Episiotomy, 278-279
  disruption, 396-399
    clinical course, 398
    etiology, 396, 398
    management
      secondary repair, 399
      supportive, 398-399
    predisposing factors, 396, 398

fetal benefits, 390
indications, 390-391
maternal benefits, 390
mediolateral, 395-396
  repair, 396, 397f
  technique, 396
midline
  advantage, 391, 393
  aftercare, 395
  disadvantage, 393
  repair, 393-395, 394f
  technique, 391, 392f
third stage of labor, 390-399
timing, 391
types, 391-396
wound infection in, 717
Erb palsy, 738
Ergotamine, in postpartum hemorrhage, 375-376
Escherichia coli, 649
Estimated fetal weight (EFW), 636
Estrogen, in labor onset, 121
Examination of the patient
  abdomen, 90-93
  Leopold maneuver, 90-93
  rectal, 98-100
  vaginal, 95-98
    membranes, 96
    palpation of cervix, 95-96
    position of fetus, 96
    presentation of fetus, 96
Expected date of confinement, 120
Extension, 68, 217
  brow presentation, 236, 237
  face presentation, 245, 255, 257, 259
  LOA, 107, 108f, 112f
External rotation, LOA, 108-109, 110f, 112f
Extracranial hemorrhage, 736-737
Extraction, head, 309-310, 309f

F
Face presentation, 243-261
  anterior, 243-252
    diagnosis, 244-245

management, 250, 252
mechanism of labor, 245-249
prognosis, 250
arrest, 252
definition, 243
etiology, 243
forceps for, 320-321
incidence, 243
mechanism of labor
descent, 248, 255, 257, 260
extension, 245, 255, 257, 259
external rotation, 249, 255, 259
flexion, 249, 255, 259
internal rotation, 248-249, 255,
257, 260
molding, 249
restitution, 249, 255, 259
persistent, 260-261
posterior, 255-261
diagnosis, 255-257
long arc rotation, 257-259, 258f
management, 260-261
mechanism of labor, 257
prognosis, 260
short arc rotation, 259-260, 259f
Thorn maneuver, 260, 261f
transverse, 252-255
diagnosis, 252
management, 255
mechanism of labor, 252-255,
253f-254f
Facial nerve injury, 739
Fallopian tubes, in puerperium, 710
False labor, 128-129
False pelvis, 38, 39f
Fentanyl, 679
Fern test, ruptured membranes, 579
Fetal assessment
indications, 144-145
during labor, 144-145
during pregnancy, 144
Fetal cotyledon, 354
Fetal echocardiography
conjoined twins, 548
Fetal heart rate (FHR), 268
abnormal, 439
auscultation, 93-95, 150-151

bradycardia, 268
examination during intrapartum
diagnosis, 595
location of, 94f
monitoring, 152-167
electronic, 207
in labor, 642
second stage, 268
monitoring, second stage, 268
Fetal inflammatory response syndrome
(FIRS), 649
Fetal macrosomia, 666
Fetal malposition, 194
Fetopelvic disproportion, 436. See also
Disproportion
Fetus, 54-64
blood, biochemical analysis,
168-171
correlation between FHR
patterns, 169-171
indications, 169
management during labor, 171
technique, 169
bruises, 339
clavicle fracture, 346
congenital anomalies
classification, 640
definition, 640
incidence, 640
pathogenesis, 640t
prenatally diagnosed,
641-643
damage, previous, 439
death
intrauterine, 174
previous, 439
delivery, 275-281
destructive operations
contraindications, 644
dangers, 644-645
indications, 644
types, 645
cleidotomy, 645
decapitation, 645
encephalocentesis, 645
distress, 232, 642
estimated fetal weight, 636

Fetus (*Cont.*):
  fractures, 339
  growth, 465
  head, 54-64
    hyperextension, 510-512,
      511*f*
      danger, 511-512
      diagnosis, 511
      etiology, 510-511
      prognosis, 512
    health determination
      auscultation fetal heart, 93-95
      oligohydramnios, 176
    health surveillance, in labor,
      143-171
    antepartum, 145-150
    auscultation fetal heart, 150-151
    blood, biochemical analysis, 168-
      171
    counting method, 146-147
    electronic monitoring, 152-167
    intrapartum, 150-167
    movement, 146-147
    negative response, 168
    nonstress test, 147-150, 149*f*
    positive response, 168
    psychological response, 167-168
    uterine activity recording,
      151-152
  heart tones
    breech presentation, 476
    brow presentation, 234, 240
    face presentation, 245, 252, 257
    malpresentation, 214, 220, 222
  indications for assessment, 144-145
  intrauterine growth restriction,
    175, 636-640, 639
    preterm, 638-639
    term, 639
    unanticipated, 639
  macrosomia, 175, 337
  malpresentation, 212-214
    transverse lie, 515-521
  membranes, 96
  meningocele, 64
  mortality, 421-422
    in cesarean section, 452-453

  ovoids, 54
  position, 66, 67*t,* 70-72, 96, 97*f*
  presentation, 96
  skull, 55, 55*f*
    bosses, parietal, 57
    bregma, 57
    caput succedaneum, 60-62, 61*f*
    cephalohematoma, 61*f,* 62-63
    diameters, 58-59, 58*f*
      biparietal, 58
      bitemporal, 58
      occipitofrontal, 57, 59
      submentobregmatic, 59
      suboccipitobregmatic, 59
      verticomental, 59
    fontanelle, 56-57
      anterior, 57
      posterior, 57
    fracture, 734
    glabella, 57
    molding, 56, 59-60, 60*f*
    nasion, 57
    occiput, 57
    sinciput, 57
    sutures, 56
      coronal, 56
      frontal, 56
      lambdoidal, 56
      sagittal, 56
    vertex, 57
  ultrasonography, fetal presentation,
    697, 698*f*
  umbilical cord prolapse, 439
FHR. *See* Fetal heart rate
Fibronectin, fetal, 576
FIRS (fetal inflammatory response
    syndrome), 649
First maneuver, 90-92, 91*f*
Fistula
  rectovaginal, 409
  vesicovaginal, 406-409
    management, 408-409
    occurrence, 406, 408
Flexed breech, 508
Flexion, 67, 217
  breech presentation, 478-479, 482
  brow presentation, 236

face presentation, 249, 255, 259
LOA, 104-105, 105*f*, 111*f*
Floating, fetus, 78, 79*f*
Fontanelle, 56-57
Footling breech, 69, 475, 475*f*, 485
Foramen ovale, 727
Forceps
after-coming head, 314, 317-318,
320*f*
application, 297
cephalic, 297, 302*f*
pelvic, 297, 302*f*
perfect, 297
axis-traction, 290
Barnes-Neville, 290
blades, 287, 300*f*-302*f*
breech presentation, 500*f*, 501, 502
causes of catastrophy, 321, 323-324
cephalic, 298*f*
classification, 293, 294*f*
contraindications, 291-292
curve, 287
DeLee, 289
De Wees, 286, 290
diameter, 287
face presentation, 320-321, 321*f*
failed, 310, 324
function
rotation, 311-321
traction, 303
handles, 286
indications, 290-291
fetal, 291
maternal, 291
prolonged active second stage,
291
Kielland, 286, 288*f*, 290, 311-312
left, 287
lock, 286, 302*f*
English, 286
French, 285*f*, 286
sliding, 285*f*, 286
Luikart, 288*f*, 289
mentum anterior, 320-321, 321*f*, 322*f*
Milne-Murray, 290
morbidity and mortality associated
with, 292-293

fetal risks, 292-293
maternal risks, 292
obstetric, 284-290, 285*f*-286*f*
application, 306*f*, 307*f*-308*f*
parts, 286-287
types, 287-290
uses, 290-297, 299-303
pelvic, 298*f*
perfect, 298*f*
piper, 289*f*, 290, 320*f*
breech, 500*f*, 501
prerequisites, 293-297
removal of, 305*f*
right, 287
rotational, 311-321
shank, 287
Simpson, 285*f*, 286, 288*f*, 289
Tarnier, 286, 290
trial, 324
Tucker-McLane, 287, 289*f*, 290
Wrigley's, 287, 289
Fourth maneuver, 91*f*, 93
Fracture, breech presentation,
507-508
Frank breech, 68, 475, 475*f*,
508-509
Friedman's curve, 199
first stage of labor, 132*f*
Frontal suture, 56
Fundus of uterus, 23
Funic presentation, 533

G
Gastrointestinal tract, puerperium,
711
Gestational age, 177
Gestational dating, 637
Grandmultiparity, 369
Graphic analysis of labor, 198-199,
198*f*
Gravidity, 74
Group B streptococcus, 652-653
antibiotics, 653*t*
prevention, 652-653
risk factors, 652, 654*t*
GTPAL System, 75
Gynecoid pelvis, 47, 47*f*, 48*f*, 49*t*-52*t*

H
Haultain procedure, 428
Head, fetus, 54-64
  controlled birth, 277-279
    bearing down, 277
    episiotomy, 278-279
    manual pressure, 277
    Ritgen maneuver, 277-278
  crowning, 276
  descent, 275-276
  extraction
    airway, 502
    chin-to-pubis rotation, 503, 505
    embryotomy, 505
    post-delivery, 279
  relationship to the pelvis, 93
  spontaneous birth, 275-276
Headache, postdural puncture,
      685-686
Head descent, ultrasonography of, 704
HELLP syndrome, 625
Hematomas
  broad ligament
    diagnosis, 411
    treatment, 411
  cephalohematoma, 61*f*, 62-63
  concealed, 410
  subgaleal, 63-64
  supravaginal/subperitoneal, 410
  vulvar and vaginal, 409-411
    diagnosis, 410-411
    treatment, 411
  vulvovaginal, 410
Hemolytic uremic syndrome,
      626-627
Hemorrhage
  fetal
    extracranial, 736-737
      caput secundum, 736-737
    intracranial, 734-736
      intracerebellar, 735
      intraventricular, 735
      management of, 735-736
      subarachnoid, 734
      subdural, 734-735
  maternal
    after cesarean section, 449

antepartum, 174
postpartum, 368-387. *See also*
      Postpartum hemorrhage
Hepatic rupture, 740
Herpes, genital, 440
Herpes simplex virus, 656-658
  neonatal complications, 657*t*
  primary infection, 657
  recommendations for mode of
      delivery, 658*t*
  recurrent, 657
Higher order multiples *versus*
      singleton birth, 564*t*
Human immunodeficiency virus (HIV)
      infection, 653-656
  cesarean section, 440
  intrapartum care
    antiretroviral therapy, 655
    cesarean delivery, 656
    trial of labor, 656
  postpartum, 656
  risk factors, 655*t*
  screening in pregnancy, 654-655
Huntington procedure, 428
Hyaline membrane disease. *See*
      Respiratory distress
      syndrome
Hygroscopic dilators, 180
  complications, 180
  technique, 180
Hyperextension, fetal head, 510-512,
      511*f*
  danger, 511-512
  diagnosis, 511
  etiology, 510-511
  prognosis, 512
Hypertension
  differential diagnosis, in pregnancy,
      607*t*
  intrapartum management,
      609-610
    seizure prophylaxis, 609-610
    timing and mode of delivery, 609
  management and prevention, 610-
      611
  maternal complications in labor,
      604-611

postpartum, 611
preeclampsia, 607-609
treatment of, 610
hydralazine, 610
labetolol, 610
nifedipine, 610
Hypotension, postural supine, 274
Hypoxia, 145
Hysterectomy
cesarean section, 453-454
for placenta accreta, 364
postpartum hemorrhage, 383-384

I
Iatrogenic prematurity, 452
Iliococcygeus muscle, 12
Immune thrombocytopenia (ITP), 626
Incision, closure of
midline vertical incision, 468, 468*f*
Smead-Jones, 468, 468*f*
subcutaneous tissue, 469
transverse incision, 468
Inclination, pelvis, 38-39, 39*f*
Indomethacin, tocolysis, 581
Induction of labor, 174-190
Bishop score, 178-179, 178*f*
cervical priming
mechanical, 179-181
hygroscopic dilators, 180
intracervical balloon catheters,
180-181
pharmacologic, 181-182
oxytocin, 182
prostaglandin, 181-182
contraindications, 176
hygroscopic dilators, 180
indications
fetal, 175-176
maternal, 174-175
intracervical balloon catheters, 180-
181
Lange score, 179*f*
methods, 183-190
artificial rupture of membranes,
183-184
membrane stripping, 183
oxytocin, 184-190

prerequisites, 177
risks associated with, 176-177
Infant, newborn. *See* Newborn infant
Infarcts, placental, 355
Infections
intrapartum, 648-661
ascending, 648-658
chorioamnionitis, 648-651
group B streptococcus,
652-653
Herpes simplex virus, 656-658
HIV, 653-656
hematogenous
listeriosis, 658-659
diagnosis, 659
treatment, 659, 660*t*
prevention, 659-661
antibiotics, 661, 661*t*
post-cesarean section, 449
postpartum
cesarean section incision,
716-717
episiotomy, 717
urinary tract, 717-718
cystitis, 717
pyelonephritis, 718
Inlet contraction, 195
Inlet of pelvis, 38, 41-43
Innominate bone, 4-5
Intermittent auscultation fetal heart,
150-151
Internal rotation, LOA, 105-107, 106*f*,
111*f*
Internal uterine pressure catheter, 152
Intracerebellar hemorrhage, 735
Intracervical balloon catheters,
induction labor, 180-181
Intracranial hemorrhage, 734-736
Intrapartum
fetal health surveillance in, 150-167
imaging, 696-706
biophysical profile, 704
of placental maturity, 704-705
radiography, 705-706
lateral view, standing, 705-706
in multiple pregnancy, 705
pelvimetry and, 705

Intrapartum, imaging (*Cont.*):
  ultrasonography, 696-705
    advanced imaging, 699-703
    amniotic fluid volume, 697,
      699
    basic imaging, 697-699
    cervical dilatation and head
      descent, 704
    fetal number, 699
    fetal presentation, 697, 698*f*
    fetal viability, 697
    invasive procedures
      abnormal fetal fluid
        drainage, 703
      amnioreduction, 703
      non-obstetric imaging
        bladder residual volume,
          703-704
        catheter insertion, 704
        nuchal cord identification,
          704
      placental localization, 699
    safety, 696
  infections, 648-661
    ascending, 648-658
    chorioamnionitis, 648-651
    group B streptococcus,
      652-653
    Herpes simplex virus,
      656-658
    HIV, 653-656
    listeriosis, 658-659
      diagnosis, 659
      treatment, 659, 660*t*
      prevention, 659-661
      antibiotics, 661, 661*t*
Intrauterine fetal death, 174
Intrauterine growth restriction (IUGR),
    636-640
  causes, 637*t*
  diagnosis, 637
  fetal, 175
  labor with prenatal diagnosis, 638-
    639
  labor with unanticipated, 639
  placental insufficiency and,
    637-638

postnatal investigation, 639-640
  preterm, 638-639
  selective, in conjoined twin, 550
  term, 639
  ultrasonography, 637
  unanticipated, 639
Intraventricular hemorrhage, 735
Inversion of uterus, 364, 422-428
  acute, 423-426
  causes, 423
  chronic, 424, 426-427
  classification, 423-424
  clinical picture, 424-425
  diagnosis, 425
  etiology, 422-423
  pathology, 424
  predisposing factors, 423
  prognosis, 428
  prophylaxis, 425
  subacute, 424, 426
  treatment
    acute, 425-426, 427*f*
    chronic, 426, 428
      Haultain procedure, 428
      Huntington procedure, 428
      Spinelli procedure, 426
    subacute, 426
Ischiocavernosus muscle, 18
Ischiococcygeus muscle, 12
Ischium, 4
Isoimmunization, 175
Isthmus of uterus, 23, 24*f*, 25-26
ITP (immune thrombocytopenia), 626
IUGR. *See* Intrauterine growth
    restriction

J
Joints, 6-8, 6*f*
  sacrococcygeal, 7
  sacroiliac, 6
  symphysis pubis, 7-8

K
Kielland forceps, 286, 288*f*, 290,
    311-312
Klumpke paralysis, 738
Kneeling breech, 69, 475*f*, 476, 485

Knots, umbilical
  false, 533
  true, 532-533
Kristellar maneuver, 499

L
Labor, 570-585
  abdominal examination, 518
  analgesia and anesthesia, 672-673,
      674*t*
  arrest of progress
    compound presentation,
        526-527
    left occiput transverse, 217,
        219
    management of, 219
    right occiput posterior, 222-223,
        232
  brow presentation, 233-240
  causes, 120-121
  clinical course, 116-117
  complication
    fetal, 636-645
    maternal, 602-633
    multiple pregnancy, 538-565
    oblique lie, 517*f*
    transverse lie, 515-521, 516*f*
      definition, 516
      diagnosis, 517-518
      etiology, 517
      general considerations, 516
      incidence, 517
      management, 520-521
      prognosis, 520
  congenital anomalies
    impact of, 642-643
    prenatally diagnosed,
        641-643
    role of fetal monitoring,
        642
    role of prelabor cesarean section,
        641-642
  contractions
    inlet, 195
    midpelvic, 195-196
    outlet, 196
  crowning, 276

definition, 120
descent, 201, 275-276
dystocia. *See* Dystocia, labor
early, 595-596
epidural block, 682-683
face presentation, 243-261
fetal complications, 636-645
fetal health surveillance, 143-171
fetal heart monitoring, 518
first stage, 90-100, 129-140,
    133*t*, 200*t*
  abnormal cephalic presentation,
      212-261
  amniotomy, 135-136
  breech, 493
  causes of pain, 673
  cervix, 130-131
  fetal health surveillance,
      143-171
  Freidman curve, 132*f*
  management, 136-140
  passage of meconium, 136
  phase
    active, 132-133, 133*t*,
        200-201, 200*t*
    fetal descent, 133
    latent, 132, 133*t*, 199-200,
        200*t*
fourth stage, 130, 133*t*, 140
graphic analysis, 198-199, 198*f*
induction, 174-190
  contraindications, 176
  versus expectant management,
      668
  hygroscopic dilators, 180
  risks associated with, 176-177
infections, 648-661
IUGR and
  prenatally diagnosed, 638-639
  preterm, 638-639
  term, 639
  unanticipated, 639
malpresentation, 212-214. *See also*
    Malpresentation
management
  ambulation, 136-137
  amniotomy, 138-139

Labor, management (*Cont.*):
  bearing down by patient, 137
  bladder catherization, 139-140
  breathing and relaxation
      technique, 137
  crystalloid infusion, 138
  hygiene, 139
  nutrition, 137
  physical examination, 138
  supportive care, 137
  maternal complications, 602-633
    acute exacerbation of asthma,
        619-620
    acute fatty liver of pregnancy,
        628-630
    cardiac arrest, 620-621
    dyspnea, acute, 611-613
    hypertension, 604-611
    pneumonia, 618-619
    preeclampsia, 607-609
    pregestational diabetes, 602-604
    pulmonary edema, 613-616
    pulmonary embolism, 616-618
    seizures, 630-633
    thrombocytopenia, 622-628
  mechanism. *See* Mechanism of labor
  median vertex presentation,
      240-242
  normal clinical course, 120-140
  obesity and, 464-465
  occiput posterior, 219-232, 221*f*,
      224*f*-228*f*, 230*f*
  onset, 104, 111*f*, 120-122
  oxytocin, 184-190
  pain
    back pain, 127
    causes, 127-128, 673, 674*t*
    false labor pains, 128-129
    incoordinate uterus, 127-128
    lower abdominal pain, 127
    management, 678-691
    preparation for, 672-673
  prelabor spontaneous rupture of
      membranes, 174
  preliminary phenomena, 122
  preterm. *See* Preterm labor
  prolonged, 199-203. *See also*
      Prolonged labor
  second stage, 130, 133*t*, 140,
      202-203, 266-281
    management
      active phases, 267, 269
      breech, 494-495
      causes of pain, 673
      definition, 266
      duration, 266*t*
      dystocia in, 270-271
      with epidural analgesia, 267
      etiology, 202-203
      fetal malpositioning, 271
      fetal monitoring, 268
      management, 268-274
        dystocia, 270-271
        Ottawa Hospital protocol,
            269, 270*t*
        passive phases, 267
        positioning in, 272-274
        postural supine
            hypotension, 274
        principles of care, 269
        pushing, 271-272
        transition, 266
        without epidural analgesia,
            266-267
  third stage, 130, 133*t*, 140, 390-399
  trial
    breech, 492-493
    previous cesarean section, 458-461
      considerations, 461
      contraindications, 458-459
      management guidelines, 459-
          460
      prerequisites, 458
      safety and results, 460-461
      signs of uterine rupture, 460
  ultrasonography, 518
  vaginal examination, 518
Lacerations
  anterior paraurethral, 404, 405*f*
  cervix, 408*f*, 412-414
    diagnosis, 412
    etiology, 412

repair, 412-413
superficial, 412
perineum, 399-403
classification, 400-403
fetal factors, 399-400
first-degree tear, 400
maternal causes, 399
repair, 400, 402
second-degree tear, 400
third-degree tear, 400, 402
postpartum hemorrhage, 370, 374,
384
vagina
deep, 404
lower anterior wall, 404
superficial small, 404
upper, 405-406
predisposing factors, 405
repair technique, 406, 407*f*
vulva, anterior, 404
deep, 404
location, 404
repair, 404
superficial small, 404
Lamaze method, 672-673
Lambdoidal suture, 56
Lange score, induction labor, 179*f*
Laparotomy, in uterine rupture, 420
Last menstrual period (LMP), 664,
667
Latent phase of labor, 199-200, 200*t*
first stage, 132, 133*t*
Left frontum anterior (LFrA),
234-238, 235*f*
Left occiput anterior (LOA), 102-114,
102*f*, 116-117
clinical course, 116-117
diagnosis
abdominal examination, 103
fetal heart, 103
vaginal examination, 103
mechanism of labor, 103-110, 104*f*,
111*f*-112*f*
descent, 104, 105*f*, 111*f*
extension, 107, 108*f*, 112*f*
external rotation, 108-109,
110*f*, 112*f*

extremities, 113
flexion, 104-105, 105*f*, 111*f*
internal rotation, 105-107, 106*f*,
111*f*
moulding, 113, 114*f*
restitution, 108, 108*f*, 112*f*
shoulders, 110-111, 113*f*
trunk, 113
Left occiput transverse (LOT), 110*f*, 112*f*
malpresentation, 214-220, 215*f*, 218*f*
Leopold maneuvers, 90-93
Levator ani muscle, 11-12
Lie, fetus, 66-70
longitudinal, 66-69
oblique lie, 69-70
transverse lie, 69-70
Ligaments, pelvis, 7
Ligation, postpartum hemorrhage
internal iliac artery, 382-383, 383*f*
uterine artery, 382
Lightening, 74
Listeria monocytogenes, 659
Listeriosis, 658-659
diagnosis, 659
treatment, 659, 660*t*
LMP (last menstrual period), 664
LOA. *See* Left occiput anterior
Lochia, 708-709
Long arc rotation
face presentation, 257-259,
258*f*
malpresentation, 223, 224*f*-225*f*,
229*f*
Longitudinal lie, 66-69
Lorazepam, 632
LOT. *See* Left occiput transverse
Lower segment of uterus, 25-26
Luikart forceps, 288*f*, 289

M

Macrosomia, fetal, 175, 337, 666
Magnesium sulphate
for seizures, 632
tocolysis, 581
Magnetic resonance imaging (MRI),
365, 548
Male and female pelvis, 8

Malformation, as congenital anomaly, 640
Malposition, 436
Malpresentation, 194, 212-214, 436
  clinical course, 217-220
  effects, 213-214
  mechanism of labor, 215-217, 216*f*, 218*f*
    arrest of progress, 217, 219, 222-223, 232
    descent, 215
    extension, 217
    external rotation, 217
    flexion, 217
    internal rotation, 217
    restitution, 217
    right occiput posterior, 222-230
  occiput posterior, 219-232
    definition, 219
    diagnosis of position, 220-222
    etiology, 220
    incidence, 220
    indications for intervention, 232
    long arc rotation, 223, 224*f*-225*f*, 229*f*
    management, 231-232
    mechanism of labor, 222-230
    molding, 228, 228*f*
    short arc rotation, 224-225, 226*f*-227*f*, 228, 230*f*
  occiput transverse, 214-220, 215*f*, 218*f*
    diagnosis of position, 214-215
  predisposing factors, 212
    fetal, 212
    maternal and uterine, 212
    placenta and membranes, 212
  transverse lie, 515-521
Maneuver
  first, 90-92, 91*f*
  fourth, 91*f*, 93
  Leopold, 90-93
  McRoberts, 341-342
  Ritgen, 277-278
  Scanzoni, ROP, 312, 313*f*-318*f*
  second, 91*f*, 92
  third, 91*f*, 92
  two-forceps, 319*f*
  Valsalva, 268
  Woods' corkscrew, 342, 344-345, 345*f*-346*f*
  Zavanelli, 347
MAS. *See* Meconium aspiration syndrome
Mastitis, 713
Mauriceau-Smellie-Veit maneuver, 500*f*, 501
McRoberts maneuver, 341-342
Mechanism of labor
  breech
    arms, 480-482
    footling, 485
    head, 482, 483*f*
    hips, 478-480, 480*f*
    kneeling, 485
    lower limbs, 478-480
    sacrum anterior, 478-483, 479*f*, 480*f*-481*f*
    sacrum posterior, 484-485
    shoulders, 480-482, 481*f*
  brow presentation, 235-238, 236*f*-239*f*
  compound presentation, 526
  descent, 104, 105*f*, 111*f*
  extension, 107, 108*f*, 112*f*
  external rotation, 108-109, 110*f*, 112*f*
  extremities, 113
  face presentation
    anterior, 245-249, 246*f*-248*f*, 252*f*
    posterior, 257
    transverse, 252-255, 253*f*-254*f*
  flexion, 104-105, 105*f*, 111*f*
  internal rotation, 105-107, 106*f*, 111*f*
  LOA. *See* Left occipital anterior
  malpresentation, 215-217, 216*f*, 218*f*
  median vertex presentation, 242
  moulding, 113, 114*f*
  occiput posterior, 222-230
  placenta, 114-116, 115*f*
  restitution, 108, 109*f*, 112*f*
  right occiput posterior, 222-230
  ROA, 117
  shoulders, 110-111, 113*f*
  transverse lie, 518-520

complications, 519f, 520
  neglected, 519-520
  spontaneous version, 519
  trunk, 113
Meconium, passage in cephalic
    presentations, 136
Meconium aspiration syndrome
    (MAS), 666, 742-744
  clinical and laboratory findings, 743
  management, 743-744
  prevention, 743
  treatment, 744
Median vertex presentation, 67,
    240-242, 241f
  definition, 240
  diagnosis, 204-241
  management, 242
  mechanism of labor, 242
  prognosis, 242
Mediolateral episiotomy, 395-396
  repair, 396, 397f
  technique, 396
Membrane stripping, 183
Meningocele, 64
Mentum, 243. See also Face presentation
Meperidine, 679
Methotrexate, in placenta accreta, 364
MFPR (multifetal pregnancy
    reduction), 551
Microanalysis, fetal blood, 169
Midline episiotomy
  advantage, 391, 393
  aftercare, 395
  disadvantage, 393
  repair, 393-395, 394f
  technique, 391, 392f
Midpelvic contraction, 195-196
Military attitude, 67, 240-242, 241f.
    See also Median vertex
    presentation
Milne-Murray forceps, 290
Misoprostol, 182
Mobility, pelvis, 8
Molding, 56, 59-60, 60f, 228f
  brow presentation, 237
  face presentation, 249, 249f
  malpresentation, 228

Monoamniotic twin, 543, 550-551
Monochorionic twin
  complication
    TRAP, 545
    twin transfusion syndrome,
      544-545
  diamniotic, 543
  monoamniotic, 543
Monozygous twin, 540, 543
  placentation in, 543-544
    conjoined twins—monochorionic
      monoamniotic, 544
    dichorionic diamniotic, 543
    monochorionic diamniotic,
      543
    monochorionic monoamniotic,
      543
Montevideo unit (MU), 123
Morbidity, maternal, 339-340
Morphine, 679
Mortality, perinatal, 666f
Moulding, 113, 114f
MRI. See Magnetic resonance imaging
Müllerian anomalies, 29
Multifetal pregnancy reduction
    (MFPR), 551
Multigravida, 74
Multipara, 75
Multiple pregnancy, 538-566. See also
    Twins
  ART, 539
  conduct of delivery, 559-561
  delayed interval delivery,
    561-563
  diagnosis, 553
  effect on labor, 555-556
  fetal effects, 554-555
  incidence, 538-539
  management, 556
    intrapartum, 559
  maternal effects, 553-554
  mode of delivery, 556-558
  radiography in, 705
  timing of delivery, 558-559
  triplets, 563-565
    management, 565
    mode of delivery, 565

Murphy drip, 187-188
Muscles
  bulbocavernosus, 18
  deep transverse perineal, 18
  iliococcygeus, 12
  ischiocavernosus, 18
  ischiococcygeus, 12
  levator ani, 11-12
  pubococcygeus, 11-12
  pubococcygeus proper, 12
  puborectalis, 12
  pubovaginalis, 11-12
  superficial transverse perineal, 18
Myomas of the uterus, 370
Myometrium, growth, 22-23,
        25

N
Nalbuphine, 679
Nasion, 57
Neonatal outcome, 465
Neoplasm blocking passage,
        212, 437
Newborn infant, 726-745
  adaptation to extrauterine life,
        726-727
    circulation, 726-727
      changes in pressure, 726-727
      closure of fetal vascular
          channels, 727
    respiration, 726
  immediate care in the delivery
      room, 727-729
Nifedipine, tocolysis, 581
Nitrazine test, ruptured membranes,
        579
Nitrous oxide, 680
Nonemergency cesarean section, 467
Nonstress test, fetal health
        surveillance, 147-150,
        149f
  abnormal, 149, 150
  atypical, 148-150
  normal, 148-150
Non-uterine bleeding, 385
Nullipara, 75

O
Obesity
  cesarean section in, 466-469
    abdominal wall incisions, 467-469
      closure, 468-469
      pfannenstiel (transverse), 467
      postoperative complications, 469
      vertical, 468
    anesthesia, 466
      in emergency, 467
      in nonemergency, 467
      respiratory function, 467
    prophylactic antibiotics, 466
    skin care, 466
    thromboprophylaxis, 466
  maternal, 337
  in pregnancy, 464-469
    definition, 464
    fetal growth and neonatal
        outcome, 465
    labor abnormalities, 464-465
    weight gain, 464, 464t
Oblique lie, 69-70
Obstetric forceps, 284-290
Obstetric shock, 386-387
  direct conditions, 386-387
  nonobstetric conditions, 387
  related conditions, 387
Occiput anterior, 106f, 109f,
        111f-112f, 295f
  direct forceps, delivery, 299-303, 306f
  left. See Left occiput anterior
  right, 117
Occiput posterior, 295f
  direct, delivery, 304, 307-310,
        307f-308f
  extraction of head, 309f
  indications for intervention, 232
  malpresentation, 219-232
  persistent, management, 231-232
  right, 220-230
Occiput transverse, 214-220, 295f
  left, 110f, 112f, 214-220, 215f,
        218f. See also Left occiput
        transverse
  right, 219

Oligohydramnios, 176
Operative delivery, 208, 370
  vaginal, 284-330
    documentation, 330
    incidence, 284
    obstetric forceps, 284-297,
      285*f*-286*f*
      parts, 286-287
      types, 287-290
      uses, 290-297, 299-303
Opioid analgesia, 678-679
Ottawa Hospital protocol,
        second stage of labor,
        269, 270*t*
Outlet contraction, 196
Outlet of pelvis, 38, 45-46, 45*f*
Ovary, in puerperium, 710
Overdistention uterus, 369
Ovoids, fetal, 54
Oxytocin, 206
  administration, 186-188
    intravenous route, 186-187
    technique, 187-188
  cervical priming, 182
  contraindications, 188
  danger, 189-190
    fetal, 190
    maternal, 189
    water intoxication, 189-190
  effects, 185-186
    breast, 186
    cardiovascular system,
      185-186
    kidneys, 186
    uterus, 185
  induction of labor, 182,
    184-190
  in intrauterine growth restricted
    labor, 638
  in labor onset, 121
  post-delivery management,
    355-356
  postpartum hemorrhage, 375
  prerequisites to use of, 188
  in second stage of labor, 271
  water intoxication, 189-190

P
Pacemaker, uterus, 125
Pack uterus, 378-380, 378*f*, 379*f*
Pain of labor, 127-128
  back pain, 127
  causes, 127-128
  false labor pains, 128-129
  incoordinate uterus, 127-128
  lower abdominal pain, 127
  management of, 678-691
Palpation, 90-93, 91*f*
  cervix, 95-96
Paracervical block, 686-688
Parametritis, 713
Parietal bosses, fetal skull, 57
Parity, 75, 177
Partogram, 198-199
Parturient, 75
Parturition, 121
Passenger, 54-64, 194
Passive phase of labor, second stage,
    267
Patient-controlled epidural analgesia,
    681
Pelvis
  adolescence, 8
  assessment, 98, 99*f*
  axis, 39, 39*f*
  bones, 4-5, 6*f*
    coccyx, 5
    ilium, 4
    innominate, 4-5
    ischium, 4
    pubis, 4-5
    sacrum, 5
  Caldwell-Moloy classification, 47,
    47*f*, 48*f*, 49*t*-52*t*
  cavity, 38, 39*f*
  contraction, 436-437
  diameters, 40-41
  false, 38, 39*f*
  fetal relationship, 66-75
  floor, 10-13, 10*f*
    functions, 10
    muscles, 11-12
    during parturition, 13

Pelvis (*Cont.*):
  inclination, 38-39, 39*f*
  inlet, 38, 41-43
  joints, 6-8, 6*f*
    sacrococcygeal, 7
    sacroiliac, 6
    symphysis pubis, 7-8
  ligaments, 7
  measurements, 46-47
  mobility, 8
  muscles, 11-12
    iliococcygeus, 12
    ischiococcygeus, 12
    levator ani, 11-12
    pubococcygeus, 11-12
    pubococcygeus proper, 12
    puborectalis, 12
    pubovaginalis, 11-12
  outlet, 38, 45-46, 45*f*
    anterior triangle, 46
    diameter, 46
    posterior triangle, 46
  during parturition, 13
  planes, 39-40, 40*f*
    greatest dimensions, 43
    least dimensions, 43-44, 44*f*
  thrombophlebitis
    clinical manifestation, 722
    diagnosis, 722
    treatment, 722-723, 723*t*
  true, 38, 39*f*
Pendulous maternal abdomen, 212
Perinatal asphyxia, 729-733
  APGAR score, 731-732, 731*t*
  consequences, 733
  diagnostic criteria, 730-731
  epidemiology, 730
  management, 732-733
    neuroprotection, 733
    preventive, 732
    supportive, 732-733
  risk factors for, 731
Perinatal mortality, 666*f*, 744-745
  neonatal death, 745
  stillbirth, 744-745
Perineal body, 19-20

Perineal muscles
  deep transverse, 18
  superficial transverse, 18
Perineal pouch
  deep, 18
  superficial, 17
Perineotomy, 390-399
Perineum, 16-20, 16*f*
  anal triangle in, 19
  lacerations, 399-403
    classification, 400-403
    fetal factors, 399-400
    first-degree tear, 400
    maternal causes, 399
    first-degree tear, 400
    second-degree tear, 400, 401*f*
    third-degree tear, 400, 402, 403*f*
  perineal body in, 19-20
  repair, 400-402
    complete tear, 402
    partial tear, 402
  urogenital triangle in, 16-18
Peripheral nerves, injury, 737-739
Pfannenstiel (transverse) incision, 467
Phantom application, 311, 321*f*
Phases of labor
  active, 200-201, 200*t*
  latent, 199-200, 200*t*
Pinard maneuver, 508-509
Piper forceps, 289*f*, 290, 320*f*, 500*f*, 501
Pitocin, 185
Pitressin, 185
Pituitary insufficiency, 384-385
Pituitrin, 185
Placenta
  abnormalities, 212, 354-355
    amnion nodosum, 354-355
    circumvallate, 354
    infarcts, 355
    placenta accreta, 360-365
    succenturiate lobe, 354
    twin placenta, 355
    weight, 355
  abruptio, 591-593
    concealed, 592, 592*f*

mixed, 592
revealed, 592, 592*f*
accreta. *See* Placenta accreta
birth of, 114-116, 115*f*
  control of hemorrhage, 116
  expulsion, 114, 116, 356
    Duncan method, 114, 116
    Schultze method, 116
  separation, 114, 115*f*, 356
bleeding, 373
delivery, 355-359
  active management, 355
  delayed separation, 358-359
  examination, 358
  manual removal, 359, 360*f*
  oxytocin, 355-356
  physiological management, 356-
    357
double setup examination, 598
increta, 362, 362*f*
location, 354
in monozygous twin, 543-544
  conjoined twins—monochorionic
    monoamniotic, 544
  dichorionic diamniotic, 541*f*,
    543
  monochorionic diamniotic, 542*f*,
    543
  monochorionic monoamniotic,
    542*f*, 543
normal, 354, 361*f*
organization, 354
percreta, 362, 362*f*
previa, 588-591
  associated findings, 590-591
  classification, 588-589
  clinical manifestations, 590
  diagnosis, 591
  etiology, 588
  ultrasound, 588-589, 589*f*, 590*f*
retained, postpartum hemorrhage,
    370-371
retention in utero, 359, 363
size and shape, 354
Placenta accreta
  definition, 360
  diagnosis

MRI, 365
  prenatal, 365
  ultrasonography, 365
etiology, 363
incidence, 362
management
  conservative approach,
    364-365
  hysterectomy, 364
pathology, 360-361
Placental insufficiency, 439
  IUGR and, 637-638
Placenta previa accreta, 364
Planes of pelvis, 39-40, 40*f*
  greatest dimensions, 43
  least dimensions, 43-44, 44*f*
Platypelloid pelvis, 47, 47*f*, 48*f*,
    49*t*-52*t*
Pneumonia, 618-619
Podalic version, 527
Polyhydramnios, 174
  in TRAP, 545
Position, fetal, 66, 67*t*, 70-72, 96
  diagnosis, 97*f*
  malpresentation
    persistent, management,
      231-232
    right, 220-230
  occiput anterior, 106*f*, 109*f*,
      111*f*-112*f*, 295*f*
    direct forceps, delivery, 299-303
    forceps, delivery, 303, 306*f*
    left, 102-114, 102*f*, 116-117. *See
      also* Left occiput anterior
    right, 117. *See also* Right occiput
      anterior
  occiput posterior, 295*f*
    direct, delivery, 304, 307-310,
      307*f*-308*f*
      orientation and application,
        307
    extraction of head, 309*f*
    indications for intervention, 232
    malpresentation, 219-232
  occiput transverse, 214-220, 295*f*
    left. *See* Left occiput transverse
    right, 219

Postdural puncture headache, 685-686
Posterior asynclitism, 81-83, 83*f*
Postmortem cesarean section, 440
Postpartum hemorrhage (PPH), 368-387
  clinical picture, 368
  dangers, 368
  etiology, 369-371
    atony of uterus, 369-370
    blood dyscrasias, 371
    obstetric shock, 386-387
      direct conditions, 386-387
      nonobstetric conditions, 387
      related conditions, 387
    placenta, retained, 370-371
    trauma and lacerations, 370
  investigation, 371
  late, 385-386
    non-uterine bleeding, 385-386
    uterine bleeding, 385-386
      clinical picture, 386
      etiology, 385
      mechanism, 385-386
      treatment, 386
  pituitary insufficiency, 384-385
  post-vaginal delivery, 363
  studies of maternal deaths, 368-369
  treatment, 371-384
    aortic compression, 381
    atony of uterus, 374-384
    blood transfusion, 373
    carbetocin, 375
    embolization of pelvic arteries, 381-382
    ergotamine, 375-376
    hysterectomy, 383-384
    internal iliac artery ligation, 382-383, 383*f*
    lacerations, 374, 384
    oxytocin, 375
    placental bleeding, 373
    prophylaxis, 371-372
    prostaglandin, intramyometrial, 376-378, 377*f*
    uterine artery ligation, 382

    uterine compression, 374-375, 374*f*
      sutures, 380-381, 380*f*-381*f*
    uterine exploration, 374
    uterine massage, 374
    uterine packing, 378-380, 378*f*
Postterm pregnancy
  cesarean section, 665
  complications, 664-666
    fetal and neonatal risks, 665*t*
    MAS, 666
    maternal risks, 665, 665*t*
  definition, 664
  fetal indications, 175, 664-670
  management
    algorithm, 669*f*
    identifying complications at term, 668
    labor induction *versus* expectant management, 668
    surveillance, 668-670
  prevalence, 664
  prevention
    accurate pregnancy dating, 667
    membrane sweeping, 667-668
  risk factors, 664
Postural supine hypotension, second stage labor, 274
PPH. *See* Postpartum hemorrhage
Preeclampsia, 174, 625
  manifestations, 608*t*
  as maternal complications during labor, 607-609
    laboratory investigation, 608-609
    pathophysiology, 608
  noncardiogenic pulmonary edema, 615
Pregestational diabetes, 602-604
  diabetic ketoacidosis during, 603
  important comorbidities for, 602
  intrapartum management of diabetes, 603-604
    glycemic control during labor and delivery, 603-604, 605*f*-606*f*
    timing and mode of delivery, 603
  neonatal considerations, 604

ominous signs, 603
physiologic changes in pregnancy, 602
postpartum, 604
Pregnancy
  HIV screening, 654-655
  multiple. *See* Twins
  postterm. *See* Postterm pregnancy
  post uterine rupture repair, 422
  uterine contractions, 126-127
Pregnancy dating, 667
Pre-induction cervical ripening, 178-182
Prelabor, 126-127
  spontaneous rupture of membranes, 174
Presentation, fetal, 66, 96, 177
  breech, 68-69, 69*f*, 472-512
  brow, 68, 233-240
  cephalic. *See* Cephalic presentation
  compound, 524-527
  face, 243-261
  malpresentation, 212-214
  median vertex presentation, 240-242
  twins, 556, 557*f*
Presenting part, 66
Preterm labor, 570-585
  classification, 572
  clinical features, 575-578
    differential diagnosis, 576
    examination, 575-576
    history, 575
    investigations, 576-578
      bedside fibronectin, 576
      cervical length, 576, 577*f*
      repeat vaginal examination, 578
  definition, 120
  etiology, 572-574
    abnormal uterine cavity, 573
    cervical weakness, 574
    idiopathic, 574
    infection, 572
    overdistension, 573
    surgical procedures and intercurrent illness, 573
    vascular, 573

incompetent cervix, 574
management, 580-585
  analgesia, 584
  antibiotics, 582
  augmentation, 584
  with cesarean section, 585
  communication and support, 580
  emergency cervical cerclage, 583
  fetal assessment, 582-583
  induction, 584
  magnesium sulphate, 581-582
  maternal steroids, 580-581
  mode of delivery, 584
  modification of activity, 583
  neuroprotection, 581-582
  tocolytics, 581
  in utero transfer, 583
in monochorionic twin, 545
pre-labor rupture of membranes
  clinical features, 578-580
    amniocentesis, 579-580
    differential diagnosis, 578
    examination, 578
    fern testing, 579
    fetal well-being, 580
    follow-up monitoring, 580
    genital tract swabs, 579
    highly specific swab tests, 579
    history, 578
    investigations, 579-580
    maternal well-being, 580
    nitrazine testing, 579
    ultrasound, 579
prevalence, 570-572, 570*f*, 571*f*
risk factors, 574-575
  modifiable, 575
  nonmodifiable, major, 574
  nonmodifiable, minor, 574-575
tocolysis
  beta-agonist, 581
  glyceryl trinitrate, 581
  nifedipine, 581
  nonsteroidal anti-inflammatory drugs, 581
  oxytocin antagonist, 581
  prostaglandins, 581

Primigravida, 74
Primipara, 75
Progesterone, in labor onset, 121
Prolapse
　cord, 527
　hand and arm, 524-526
　leg and foot, 524-526
　reposition, 526
　umbilical cord, 533-535, 534*f*
　　classification, 533
　　management, 535
　　occult, 533
　　risk factors, 533, 535
　　signs, 535
　uterus, 28
Prolonged labor, 199-203
　active phase, 200-201, 200*t*
　　multipara, 200, 200*t*
　　primary dysfunctional labor, 201
　　primigravidas, 200*t*
　　secondary arrest of dilatation,
　　　201
　descent of the presenting part, 201
　exhaustion, 369
　graphic analysis, 198-199, 198*f*
　latent phase, 199-200, 200*t*
　second stage, 202-203
Prominence, cephalic, 72-74, 73*f*
Propagation of contraction wave, 125
Prophylactic antibiotics, 466
Prophylaxis, postpartum hemorrhage,
　371-372
Prostaglandin
　cervical priming, 181-182
　induction labor, 181-182
　intramyometrial, postpartum
　　hemorrhage, 376-378,
　　377*f*
　in labor onset, 121
Psyche, 196
Psychological response, 167-168
Psychoprophylaxis, 672-673
Pubic symphysis, 7-8
Pubis, 4-5
Pubococcygeus muscle, 11-12
Pubococcygeus proper muscle, 12
Puborectalis muscle, 12

Pubovaginalis muscle, 11-12
Pudendal nerve block
　transperineal approach, 690
　transvaginal approach, 690-691
Puerperium, 708-723
　breastfeeding, 711-713
　deep venous thrombosis and
　　pulmonary embolism,
　　718-722
　　clinical manifestation, 719
　　pathogenesis, 718
　　risk factors, 720*t*-721*t*
　　thromboprophylaxis, 719-722,
　　　721*t*, 722
　endometritis, 713-716
　　clinical manifestation, 715
　　imaging, 715
　　laboratory studies, 715
　　pathogenesis, 714-715
　　risk factors, 714
　　treatment, 716
　normal changes, 708-711
　　breasts, 710-711
　　cardiovascular system, 711
　　cervix, 709
　　endometrium, regeneration, 709
　　fallopian tubes, 710
　　gastrointestinal tract, 711
　　lochia, 708-709
　　ovaries, 710
　　shivering, 708
　　urinary tract, 711
　　uterine involution, 708
　　vagina, 709-710
　thrombophlebitis
　　clinical manifestation, 722
　　diagnosis, 722
　　treatment, 722-723, 723*t*
　urinary tract
　　cystitis, 717
　　pyelonephritis, 718
　wound infection, 716-717
　　cesarean section incision,
　　　716-717
　　episiotomy, 717
Pulmonary edema, 613-616
　cardiogenic, 613-614

arrhythmia, 614
  ischemia and infarction, 614
  peripartum cardiomyopathy, 614
  valvular, 614
diagnosis, 613
medical management, 616
noncardiogenic, 614-615
  acute respiratory distress
      syndrome, 615
  amniotic fluid embolism, 615
  preeclampsia, 615
  tocolysis, 615
Pulmonary embolism, 616-618, 718-
      722
  clinical manifestation, 719
  diagnosis, 617-618
    history and physical examination,
        617
    imaging, 617-618
  pathogenesis, 718
  risk factors, 720t-721t
  thromboprophylaxis, 719-722, 721t
  treatment, 618
    heparin, 618
    thrombolytic therapy, 618
Pyelonephritis, 718

R
Radiography, 705-706
  lateral view, standing, 705-706
  in multiple pregnancy, 705
  pelvimetry and, 705
RDS. *See* Respiratory distress
      syndrome
Rectovaginal fistula, 409
Rectum, examination during labor,
      98-100
Respiratory distress syndrome (RDS),
      740-742
  clinical and laboratory findings, 741
  prevention, 742
  treatment of, 741-742
    positive-pressure ventilation,
        741-742
    surfactant therapy, 742
Restitution, 217
  brow presentation, 237

face presentation, 249, 255, 259
  LOA, 108, 109f, 112f
Retained placenta, 370-371
Retraction, myometrium
  ring constriction, 123
  ring retraction
    pathologic, 122, 124f
    physiologic, 122, 124f
Rhesus incompatibility, 439
Right occiput anterior (ROA), 117
Right occiput transverse
      malpresentation, 219
Ripe cervix, 130-131, 177
  evaluation, 178-179
  pre-induction, 178-182
Ritgen maneuver, 277-278
Ritodrine, tocolysis, 581
Rotation
  of fetus, in failed occipitoposterior
      assisted delivery, 310
  of uterus
    external, 108-109, 110f, 112f
      brow presentation, 237
      face presentation, 249, 255,
          259
    internal, 105-107, 106f, 111f,
        217
      breech, 479, 482
      brow presentation, 236
      face presentation, 248-249,
          255, 257, 260
    long arc, 223
Round ligament contraction, 126
Rupture of uterus, 364, 416-422,
      460
  classification
    cesarean scar dehiscence,
        418-419
    post-cesarean rupture, 418
    spontaneous rupture, 417
    traumatic, 417-418
  clinical picture, 419-420
  with delayed diagnosis, 420
  diagnosis, 420
  fetal mortality, 421-422
  incidence, 416
  management, 422

Rupture of uterus (*Cont.*):
  maternal mortality, 421
  pregnancy post repair, 422
  silent or quiet, 419
  site and time, 417
  treatment, 420-421
  types, 416-417
  usual variety, 419
  violent rupture, 419-420

S
Sacrococcygeal joint, 7
Sacroiliac joint, 6
Sacrum anterior, breech
  diagnosis, 476-478
  labor, mechanism, 477*f*, 478-483,
        479*f*, 480*f*-481*f*
Sacrum posterior, breech
  labor, mechanism, 484-485
Sagittal suture, 56
Scanzoni maneuver, 312, 313*f*-318*f*
Schultze method, placental expulsion,
  116
Second maneuver, 91*f*, 92
Secundagravida, 74
Segment, lower uterine, 25-26
Seizures, in pregnancy, 630-633
  causes, 631*t*
  diagnosis and investigations, 632
  eclampsia, 631-632
  epilepsy, 630-631
  management of, 632-633
    diazepam, 632
    IV benzodiazepines, 632
    lorazepam, 632
    magnesium sulphate, 632
  postpartum considerations, 633
  route of delivery, 633
Septate uterus, 26*f*-27*f*, 31
Septic pelvic thrombophlebitis,
  722-723
  clinical manifestation, 722
  diagnosis, 722
  treatment, 722-723, 723*t*
SFH (symphyseal-fundal height), 637
SGA (small for gestational age), 636
Shivering, puerperium, 708

Short arc rotation
  face presentation, 259-260, 259*f*
  malpresentation, 224-225,
        226*f*-227*f*, 228, 230*f*
Shoulder dystocia, 334-348, 335*f*
  clinical presentation, 334-336
  definition, 334
  diagnosis, 340
  differential diagnosis, 336
  incidence, 334
  management, 340-347
    fetal clavicle fracture, 346
    McRoberts maneuver, 341-342
    posterior arm and shoulder
        delivery, 342, 344*f*
    risk, 347
    rolling over to "all fours"
        position, 346-347
    suprapubic pressure, 341-342
    symphysiotomy, 347
    Woods' corkscrew maneuver,
        342, 344-345, 345*f*-346*f*
    Zavanelli maneuver, 347
  mechanism, 334
  risk factors, 336-338
    fetal macrosomia, 337
    history, 337
    maternal diabetes mellitus, 337
    maternal obesity, 337
  sequelae, 338-340
    birth asphyxia, 338-339
    brachial plexus injury,
        338-339
    bruises, 339
    fractures, 339
    maternal morbidity, 339-340
Shoulders, mechanism of labor,
  110-111, 113*f*
Simpson forceps, 286, 288*f*, 289
Sinciput, 57
Singleton birth *versus* higher order
  multiples, 564*t*
Skull, fetus, 55-56, 55*f*
  bosses, parietal, 57
  bregma, 57
  caput succedaneum, 60-62, 61*f*
  cephalohematoma, 61*f*, 62-63

diameters, 58-59, 58*f*
  biparietal, 58
  bitemporal, 58
  occipitofrontal, 57, 59
  submentobregmatic, 59
  suboccipitobregmatic, 59
  verticomental, 59
fontanelle, 56-57
  anterior, 57
  posterior, 57
fracture, 734
glabella, 57
molding, 56, 59-60, 60*f*
nasion, 57
occiput, 57
sinciput, 57
sutures, 56
vertex, 57
Small for gestational age (SGA), 636
Smead-Jones closure, 468, 468*f*
Sphincter
  ani, 19
  membranous urethra, 18
Spinal cord, injury, 737
Spinelli procedure, 426
Splenic rupture, 740
Spontaneous birth, head, 275-276
Stages of labor
  first, 90-100, 129-140, 133*t*,
      200*t*
    abnormal cephalic presentation,
        212-261
    amniotomy, 135-136
    breech, 493
    causes of pain, 673
    cervix
      dilatation, 130-131
      effacement, 130-131
    fetal health surveillance, 143-171
    Freidman curve, 132*f*
    management, 136-140
    passage of meconium, 136
    phase
      active, 132-133, 133*t*,
          200-201, 200*t*
      fetal descent, 133
      latent, 132, 133*t*, 199-200, 200*t*

fourth, 130, 133*t*, 140
second, 130, 133*t*, 140, 202-203,
    266-281
  breech, 494-495
  causes of pain, 673
  definition, 266
  duration, 266*t*
  dystocia, 270-271
  with epidural analgesia, 267
  etiology, 202-203
  fetal malpositioning, 271
  fetal monitoring, 268
  management, 268-274
    dystocia, 270-271
    Ottawa Hospital protocol,
        269, 270*t*
    positioning, 272-274
    postural supine hypotension,
        274
    pushing, 271-272
  phases
    active, 267, 269
    passive, 267
  principles of care, 269
  transition, 266
  without epidural analgesia, 266-
      267
  third, 130, 133*t*, 140, 390-399
Station, 78, 80-81, 80*f*, 177
Sternomastoid muscle, injury,
    739-740
Subarachnoid hemorrhage, 734
Subdural hemorrhage, 734-735
Subgaleal hematoma, 63-64
Subgaleal hemorrhage, 736
Succenturiate lobe, 354
Superficial perineal pouch, 17
Superficial transverse perineal muscle,
    18
Supine hypotensive syndrome, 674,
    678
Suprapubic pressure, 341-342
Sutures of skull, fetus, 56
  coronal, 56
  frontal, 56
  lambdoidal, 56
  sagittal, 56

Swab test, ruptured membranes, 579
Symphyseal-fundal height (SFH), 637
Symphysiotomy, 347
Symphysis pubis
    separation, 428-429
        clinical picture, 429
        diagnosis, 429
        incidence and etiology, 428-429
        pathology, 429
Synclitism, 81-85
    engagement in, 81, 82*f*
    in the pelvis, 85*f*

T
Tachysystole, 206-207
Tarnier forceps, 286, 290
Third maneuver, 91*f*, 92
Thorn maneuver, 260, 261*f*
Thrombocytopenia, in pregnancy,
        622-628
    differential diagnosis, 623*t*
    investigations, 622
    laboratory investigations to
        differentiate causes, 624*t*
    management, general guidelines,
        622
    ominous signs, 622
    specific etiologies, 623-628
        disseminated intravascular
            coagulation, 627-628
        gestational, 623-625
        HELLP syndrome, 625
        hemolytic uremic syndrome,
            626-627
        immune thrombocytopenia, 626
        preeclampsia, 625
        thrombotic thrombocytopenic
            purpura, 626-627
Thrombophlebitis, pelvic
    clinical manifestation, 722
    diagnosis, 722
    treatment, 722-723, 723*t*
Thromboprophylaxis, 466
    postpartum, 719-722
Thrombotic thrombocytopenic
        purpura (TTP), 626-627
Tocodynamometer, external, 123

Tocolysis
    indomethacin, 581
    magnesium sulphate, 581
    nifedipine, 581
    noncardiogenic pulmonary edema,
        615
    ritodrine, 581
Tonus of uterus, 123
Torsion of pregnant uterus, 34-35
Total hysterectomy, in uterine rupture,
        420
Traction by forceps, 303, 304*f*
Transabdominal ultrasound, 699
Transition, in second stage of labor,
        266
Transverse (pfannenstiel) incision,
        cesarean section, 467
Transverse lie, 69-70, 515-521,
        516*f*
    definition, 516
    diagnosis, 517-518
        abdominal examination,
            517-518
        fetal heart, 518
        ultrasonography, 518
        vaginal examination, 518
    etiology, 517
    general considerations, 516
    incidence, 517
    management, 520-521
        before labor, 520
        early labor, 521
        in good labor, 521
        neglected transverse lie, 521
    neglected, 521
    prognosis, 520
TRAP (twin reversed arterial perfusion
        sequence), 545
Trauma, postpartum hemorrhage,
        370
Trial of labor
    breech, 492-493
    brow, 239
    face, 260
    HIV management, 656
    previous cesarean section, 458-461
        considerations, 461

contraindications, 458-459
management guidelines, 459-460
prerequisites, 458
safety and results, 460-461
signs of uterine rupture, 460
Triangle
anal
anococcygeal body, 19
sphincter ani externus, 19
pelvic outlet
anterior, 46
posterior, 46
Triple descending gradient, uterine
contraction, 125-126
True labor, 128-129
True pelvis, 38, 39*f*
Trunk, fetal, mechanism of labor, 113
TTP (thrombotic thrombocytopenic
purpura), 626-627
Tucker-McLane forceps, 287, 289*f*,
290
Twin reversed arterial perfusion
sequence (TRAP), 545
Twins
conjoined
classification, 546-547
diagnosis, 547-549
fetal echocardiography, 548
MRI, 548
ultrasonography, 547-548
X-ray, 548-549
etiology, 546
incidence, 546
management, 549
method of delivery, 549-550
monoamniotic, 550-551
multifetal reduction, 551
selective intrauterine growth
restriction, 550
structural or chromosomal
anomaly, 552-553
in utero death of co-twin, 551-552
dizygous, 540
incidence, 538-539
monozygous, 540, 543
conjoined twins-monochorionic
monoamniotic, 544

dichorionic diamniotic, 543
monochorionic
diamniotic, 543
monoamniotic, 543
placentation in, 543-544
physiology, 539-543
presentation, 556, 557*f*
risks, 564*t*
ultrasonography, delivery of, 702
vanishing twin phenomenon, 539
zygosity, 544
Twin transfusion syndrome,
544-545
Two-forceps maneuver, 319*f*

U
UAE (uterine artery embolization),
364-365
Ultrasonography, 365
breech, 478, 488, 700
conjoined twin, 547-548
estimated fetal weight, 636
in fetal transverse lie, 518
head descent, fetus, 704
in intrapartum imaging, 696-705
advanced imaging, 699-703
breech presentations, 700
cord presentation, 702-703,
702*f*
head position, 699-700, 701*f*
preoperative mapping, 703
third stage complications,
703
twin delivery management,
702
amniotic fluid volume,
697, 699
basic imaging, 697-699
cervical dilatation and head
descent, 704
fetal number, 699
fetal presentation, 697, 698*f*
fetal viability, 697
invasive procedures
abnormal fetal fluid drainage,
703
amnioreduction, 703

Ultrasonography, in intrapartum
imaging (*Cont.*):
non-obstetric imaging
bladder residual volume,
703-704
catheter insertion, 704
nuchal cord identification, 704
placental localization, 699
safety, 696
intrauterine growth restriction, 637
mortality, fetal, 453
preterm pre-labor rupture of
membranes, 579
Umbilical artery, 530-531
Umbilical cord, 530-531
abnormalities, 530-532
clamping, 281
cyst, 531
delayed cord, 357
Doppler, 535-536
entanglements, 532
knots
false, 533
true, 532-533
length, 530
normal, 530
presentation, 533
ultrasonography in, 702-703
prolapse, 439, 533-535, 534*f*
classification, 533
management, 535
occult, 533
risk factors, 533, 535
signs, 535
single artery, 530-531
vasa previa, 531-532
velamentous insertion, 531
vessel aneurysm, 531-532
Unicornuate uterus, 31-32, 32*f*
Ureaplasma urealyticum, 649
Urethra
compressor, 18
sphincter of the membranous, 18
Urinary tract
damage at cesarean section,
450-451
infection, 717-718

cystitis, 717
pyelonephritis, 718
postpartum
infection, 717-718
normal, 711
Urogenital diaphragm, 17-18
bulbocavernosus muscle, 18
ischiocavernosus muscles, 18
superficial perineal pouch, 17
superficial transverse perineal
muscles, 18
Urogenital triangle, 16-18
deep perineal pouch, 18
deep transverse perineal muscles, 18
sphincter of the membranous
urethra, 18
urogenital diaphragm, 17-18
Uterine dysfunction, 436
Uteroplacental insufficiency, 144
Uterus, 22-23
abnormalities, 28-29
bicornuate, 212
complications, 28-29
prolapse, 28
treatment, 29
activity recording, 151-152
anatomy, 22
anomaly, 29-35
arcuate, 26*f*, 31
bicornuate, 32, 33*f*
complications, 30, 31
diagnosis, 30
didelphys, 33-34, 34*f*
double, 33-34, 34*f*
labor and delivery, 30-31
septate, 26*f*-27*f*, 31
torsion, 34-35
unicornuate, 31-32, 32*f*
atony, 369-370, 374-384
bleeding, 385-386
clinical picture, 386
etiology, 385
mechanism, 385-386
treatment, 386
body, 23
cervix, 23, 23*f*
complications, 28-29

compression, 374-375, 374*f*
  sutures, 380-381,
    380*f*-381*f*
contractions
  normal, 122-127. *See also*
    Contractions of uterus
  strength, 129*t*
corpus, 23
divisions, 23, 23*f*, 24*f*
dysfunction, 369
exploration, 359, 374
fundus, 23
grandmultiparity, 369
inversion, 364, 422-428
  acute, 423-426
  causes, 423
  chronic, 424, 426-427
  classification, 423-424
  clinical picture, 424-425
  diagnosis, 425
  etiology, 422-423
  pathology, 424
  predisposing factors, 423
  prognosis, 428
  prophylaxis, 425
  subacute, 424, 426
  treatment
    acute, 425-426, 427*f*
    chronic, 426, 428
    subacute, 426
involution, puerperium, 708
isthmus, 23, 24*f*, 25-26
location, 22
lower segment, 25-26
massage, postpartum hemorrhage,
    374
myomas, 370
overdistention, 369
prolapse, 28
rupture. *See* Rupture of uterus
shape, 22
size, 22

V

Vacuum extractor, 324-330, 328*f*
  application, 327-329
  complications, 329

contraindications, 325
indications, 325
morbidity and mortality, 326
prerequisites, 326-327
Vagina, 23*f*, 27-28
  damage at cesarean section, 451
  examination
    abnormal cephalic presentation,
      214-215, 222, 234,
      241, 245, 252, 257,
      476, 501
    intrapartum diagnosis, 595
    during labor, 95-98, 204
      complicated, 518
      membranes, 96
      palpation of cervix, 95-96
      position of fetus, 96
      presentation of fetus, 96
  hematomas, 409-411
    diagnosis, 410-411
    treatment, 411
  laceration
    deep, 404
    lower anterior wall, 404
    superficial small, 404
    upper, 405-406
      predisposing factors, 405
      repair technique, 406, 407*f*
  previous repair, 441
  puerperium, 709-710
Vaginal birth after cesarean (VBAC),
    458
Vaginismus, 12
Valsalva maneuver, 268
Vasa previa, 531-532, 593-595
  clinical picture, 595
  intrapartum diagnosis, 595
  ultrasound, 594*f*
VBAC (vaginal birth after cesarean),
    458
Velamentous cord insertion, 531
Venous thrombosis, 718-722
  clinical manifestation, 719
  pathogenesis, 718
  risk factors, 720*t*-721*t*
  thromboprophylaxis, 719-722, 721*t*
    contraindications, 719, 722

Version
  external cephalic, 488-490
    contraindications, 489
    prerequisites, 489
    procedure, 489-490
    risk, 490
    timing, 488-489
  internal podalic, 527
Vertex, 57
Vertical incision, cesarean section,
    468
Vesicovaginal fistula, 406-409
  management, 408-409
  occurrence, 406, 408
Vulva
  hematomas, 409-411
    diagnosis, 410-411
    treatment, 411
  lacerations, 404
    deep, 404
    location, 404

  repair, 404
  superficial small, 404

W
Wandering method, 311
Water intoxication, oxytocin, 189-190
Wigand-Martin maneuver, breech,
    499, 500*f*, 501
Woods' corkscrew maneuver, 342,
    344-345, 345*f*-346*f*
Wound infection, postpartum,
    716-717
  cesarean section incision, 716-717
  episiotomy, 717
Wrigley's forceps, 287, 289

X
Xylocaine, 688

Z
Zhang's study, 199